Clinical Nursing Skills

Core and Adva

EDITED BY

Ruth Endacott,
Phil Jevon,
and Simon Cooper

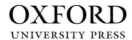

OXFORD

UNIVERSITY PRESS

OXFORD
UNIVERSITY PRESS

Great Clarendon Street, Oxford

Oxford University Press is a department of the University of Oxford.
It furthers the University's objective of excellence in research, scholarship,
and education by publishing worldwide in

Oxford New York

Auckland Cape Town Dar es Salaam Hong Kong Karachi
Kuala Lumpur Madrid Melbourne Mexico City Nairobi
New Delhi Shanghai Taipei Toronto

With offices in

Argentina Austria Brazil Chile Czech Republic France Greece
Guatemala Hungary Italy Japan Poland Portugal Singapore
South Korea Switzerland Thailand Turkey Ukraine Vietnam

Oxford is a registered trade mark of Oxford University Press
in the UK and in certain other countries

Published in the United States
by Oxford University Press Inc., New York
British Library Cataloguing in Publication Data

Data available

Library of Congress Cataloging in Publication Data

Data available

Typeset by Graphicraft Limited, Hong Kong
Printed in Italy
on acid-free paper by
L.E.G.O. SpA—Lavis TN

ISBN 978-0-19-923783-8

1 3 5 7 9 10 8 6 4 2

Preface

We hope you enjoy reading this book and that it really helps you to learn, develop, and maintain your clinical skills. International nursing practice is continuously changing and developing, so a sound evidence base and safe practice are essential. Based on these principles, this book has been written to help you develop the skills you learnt in the first year of your training and includes skills that you will begin to use in your second year of training and beyond. We include all the 'core' clinical skills that a newly qualified nurse requires, some of which may be quite 'advanced' (for example, venepuncture, ECG monitoring, and endotracheal intubation). Wherever possible we have highlighted the key evidence for the practice of each skill and encourage you to reflect on your performance and maintain and develop your ability to identify patients whose condition is deteriorating. However, it is also important to remember that no skill should be performed in isolation and a holistic overview of your patients' care is paramount.

The book has been edited by Professor Ruth Endacott, Professor of Clinical Nursing at the University of Plymouth and La Trobe University, Melbourne; Phil Jevon, Clinical Skills Lead at Manor Hospital, Walsall, and Honorary Lecturer at the University of Birmingham; and Dr Simon Cooper, Associate Professor at Monash University,

Australia. Ruth is an experienced critical care nurse, educator, and researcher; Phil has been a resuscitation officer for many years and has published widely in the field of acute care. Simon is a former intensive care nurse and resuscitation officer who has worked for an Ambulance Service and the University of Plymouth prior to moving to Australia, and he has published in the field of acute and emergency care.

It has been a great pleasure for us to draw this book together, and our sincere thanks go out to the publishing team and to the numerous professional and hardworking contributors to this book, details of whom can be found at the end of each section. We have ensured that clinicians and academics have contributed to each section to produce the best evidence and tips for best practice. All information is correct at the point of publication; however, we are aware that the field is continually developing, guidelines are updated, and practice changes, so we offer you regular updates and further information at ⓦ **www.oxfordtextbooks.co.uk/orc/endacott**.

Ruth Endacott
Phil Jevon
Simon Cooper

Acknowledgements

OUP and the authors are very grateful to the many nurses, lecturers, students, and other health care professionals who provided feedback on the draft chapters of this book. In order to maintain their anonymity they are not listed here, but their thoughtful advice has been invaluable and is highly appreciated.

Alison Hughes would like to thank the medical photography department at Walsall Manor Hospital for their assistance with Section 4.6.

Diane Kerslake would like to thank Helen Parfitt for sharing her experience as an IV trainer and Michelle Jennings for another nurse perspective on Section 5.2.

John Murray would like to thank Jane Swain for her advice on the content of Section 11.1.

Brief contents

Detailed contents

Note 🅐 indicates an advanced skill. For more details please see 'How to use this book'.

List of procedures

Note ⚫ indicates an advanced skill. For more details please see 'How to use this book'.

About the editors

Ruth Endacott is Professor of Clinical Nursing and Associate Dean (Research and Enterprise) at the University of Plymouth, and holds a professorship at La Trobe University, Australia. She has extensive experience in critical care practice, education, and research. Research grants and publications in the past 5 years focus on improving recognition of deterioration in acutely ill patients. Ruth is chair of the nursing and allied health professional section of the European Society of Intensive Care Medicine and a trustee of the British Lung Foundation.

Phil Jevon is resuscitation officer and clinical skills lead at Manor Hospital, Walsall, and an honorary clinical lecturer at Birmingham University. He is editor of the *British Journal of Resuscitation* and author of many books and articles.

Simon Cooper is Associate Professor at Monash University, Australia. He was formerly Principal Lecturer for the Masters in Advanced Practice at the University of Plymouth, UK, with a special interest in acute care and out of hospital emergency care; a field in which he has published widely. Simon previously worked as an intensive care nurse, a Resuscitation Officer, and Head of Education for an ambulance service.

Contributors

Matthew Aldridge is a Senior Lecturer in Adult Nursing at Birmingham City University (formerly UCE Birmingham). He is a Registered Nurse with 10 years of emergency nursing experience and has a particular interest in teaching and facilitating clinical skills.

Peter Allum is a Lecturer of Paramedicine at the University of Plymouth. He has had an extensive career within Westcountry Ambulance Service Trust UK, having held various teaching posts within the Clinical Educational Department and also as an Emergency Planning Officer.

Rachel Archer (RnDipHe/ENP) is a Staff Nurse and Emergency Nurse Practitioner in the Accident and Emergency department at Walsall Manor Hospital with 15 years experience within the NHS. She began her career as a Health Care Assistant and, after 8 years experience, gained sponsorship to undertake her nurse training. Upon qualifying she gained a post in Accident and Emergency nursing.

Jane Banks is a Senior Lecturer in Adult Nursing at the University of Wolverhampton. She is a Registered Nurse with clinical experience in the National Health Service, independent sector, and the Armed Forces. She has a primary health care background and teaches a range of adult nursing topics. She has specific interests in community nursing and clinical nursing skills.

Maria Bennallick is a lecturer in undergraduate programmes at the University of Plymouth, with responsibility for infection control.

Sharon Clovis is a Prostate Nurse Specialist at Guy's and St Thomas'. She graduated from Guy's and Lewisham School of Nursing in December 2001 and completed a Masters degree involving nurse prescribing in urological disease in July 2007.

Nick Conway qualified in Plymouth as an RN in 1990, working clinically within Medicine and Cardiology. Having held various nursing posts and gained his BA Education (Hons), he embarked on his teaching career in 2002. He is now project lead for the 'Productive Ward' in Plymouth, delivering at regional and national level.

Lisa Cooper (RGN, BN(Hons), MSc ANP, ALS(I), TNCC) is an Advanced Nurse Practitioner who has specialised in Emergency Care and has worked in Accident and Emergency at Walsall Manor Hospital for the past 18 years. She is also an ALS/BLS instructor and honorary lecturer at Wolverhampton University.

Dr Anu Dhillon has been a consultant anaesthetist at New Cross Hospital, Wolverhampton, for the past 10 years. He teaches anaesthetic practitioners and undergraduate medical students from Birmingham University. He specializes in Obstetrics and Ophthalmic anaesthesia.

Sarah Dodds is currently senior matron for respiratory medicine at the Royal Devon and Exeter Hospital Foundation NHS Trust. She has extensive experience in respiratory care and an interest in arterial blood gas sampling and analysis. She is an RGN with a BSc (Hons) Nursing Studies and is in the final year of her MSc in Respiratory Care.

Dan Higgins is a Senior Charge Nurse in Critical Care at the University Hospitals Birmingham NHS Foundation Trust.

Alison Hughes (RGN, MSc, BSc Hons, DPSN) is a Senior Research Facilitator at Birmingham University and was previously an Advanced Nurse Practitioner in Vascular Surgery at Walsall Manor Hospital for 9 years. She also has extensive experience in critical care and major trauma nursing.

Catherine Hughes (BSc Hons, RGN, PGCE) is a lecturer in the School of Nursing and Community Studies, University of Plymouth. Her clinical background is in vascular surgery, intensive care, and critical care outreach.

Andy Jackson (BA, RGN) is a matron in the Intensive Care Unit at the Royal Devon and Exeter Foundation Hospital NHS Trust. He has extensive experience in respiratory care, including setting up a respiratory high dependency area on the respiratory ward. He is currently a member of the ALERT faculty and leads the Care of the Critically Ill Adult course at the Trust. He is currently undertaking an MSc in Advanced Healthcare Practice.

Diane Kerslake is a lecturer at the University of Plymouth. She teaches a range of Common Foundation and Adult Nursing topics, and specializes in bioscience and acute care.

Debbie King is Infection Control Specialist at the Solihull Care Trust.

Caroline Lawson has a BSc (Hons) in Nursing Studies and has worked in a variety of different clinical settings, including working in Bangladesh for a year for VSO and Impact Foundation. In 2001 she obtained a Masters in Health Education and Health Promotion. She currently works as consultant nurse for stroke in Yeovil District Hospital NHS Trust, and is also a committee member for the RCN Forum for the Older Person.

Lisa Lewy is Interprofessional Learning Lead for the Peninsula Health Collaboration. She currently lectures on Interprofessional Education, Psychology, and Communication Skills in Health. She is also an executive member of SEEC. Previously, Lisa was Head of The Learning Development Unit at London Guildhall University. She was Chair of the Skills and Professional Development Network for the South of England for 5 years.

Andrew Lockwood is a senior physiotherapist working in critical care at the Royal Devon and Exeter Hospital, Devon.

Joe Maguire is an Elderly Care Pharmacist and Stroke Unit Pharmacist. He has worked in various hospitals in the south west of England and also in New Zealand for nearly 10 years. He joined the Royal Devon and Exeter Hospital

Foundation Trust in 2002 and specializes in elderly care and stroke.

Tracey McKenzie is the Senior Tissue Viability Clinical Nurse Specialist at the Royal Devon and Exeter Foundation NHS Trust. She has been nursing for 27 years in both private and public health care settings and has worked within her chosen speciality for the last 8 years.

Richard McShea is Principal Physiotherapist for Respiratory Services at Walsall Manor Hospital.

Tina Moore is a senior lecturer at Middlesex University. She is Programme Leader for the Acute and High Dependency modules.

John Murray (MSc, BSc, RMN, RGN) is a Lecturer in Adult Nursing at Glasgow Caledonian University. He was previously a movement and handling advisor for 8 years in a large acute NHS Trust. He specializes in adult nursing, critical care, movement and handling, integrated care pathways, and drug administration.

Mark Neal (MSc, RGN) qualified in 1985 and has worked in England and Australia with a background in intensive care nursing, hyperbaric medicine, and wound care (MSc in wound healing and tissue repair). He is based in Plymouth and is currently enjoying a flexible lifestyle as an agency intensive care nurse.

Yi-Yang Ng is an honorary clinical lecturer at the Medical School, University of Birmingham, and a Clinical Teaching Fellow of Manor Hospital, Walsall. His interests include medical education and general surgery.

Richard Ormonde (RODP, PG DIP, Affiliate Member of the Royal College of Anaesthetists) has worked in a variety of roles in his career of over twenty years, including as a Resuscitation Officer and Physician Assistant (Anaesthesia). He is currenty Practice Development Lead for Operating Theatres at the Heart of England NHS Foundation Trust.

Jacqueline Padmore is a lecturer at the University of Plymouth. Previously she was a Clinical Nurse Specialist in Tissue Viability at North Devon District Hospital. She has been module leader for the post-registration leg ulcer and tissue viability management modules at the University of Plymouth since 2002.

Clare Parkinson is a Clinical Nurse Specialist in Dermatology at the Royal Devon and Exeter Hospital with

24 years of nursing experience. She has been working in Outpatients' Dermatology for 10 years, has published articles related to skin care, and was previously on the National Executive Committee for the British Dermatological Nursing Group (BDNG).

Carol Pollard (BSc, RN Parts 12 and 15) has worked in general and neurosurgical Critical Care for 14 years. She was previously Practice Development Sister at the Neurological Critical Care Unit, and is now Lead Nurse for the Vascular Access Team, Derriford Hospital, Plymouth, UK.

Kate Roland was the Surgery Pharmacist at the Royal Devon and Exeter NHS Foundation Trust at the time of writing. She is now Domiciliary Pharmacist for Devon PCT based in Exeter.

Sharon Russell is the Education Lead for Clinical Academic Partnerships and Renal Education Manager at Plymouth Hospitals Trust. She has extensive renal experience, having worked in renal for over 25 years.

Helen Ryan qualified as a nurse in 1981 and joined the Princess Mary's Royal Air Force Nursing Service in 1984. In 1992 Helen was awarded the Associate Royal Red Cross (ARRC) for services to nursing in the Royal Air Force. In 1993 she took up the post of Senior Sister for Intensive Care at Yeovil District Hospital. Helen has been Nurse Consultant for Critical Care since 2001 and completed an MSc in Health Studies in 2005.

Vicki Shawyer is Senior Vascular Access Nurse Specialist at Royal Devon and Exeter NHS Foundation Trust. Vicki has worked in various areas including emergency medicine, diabetes, and surgery, and specialized in thoracic, upper gastrointestinal, breast, and endocrinology. She was a matron in surgery and is now developing a new Vascular Access team in Exeter.

Tim Simmonds (BSC Hons, PGDip, CPSN (ENB 100), OND) is a Clinical Nurse Specialist in Pain Management in Walsall Hospitals NHS Trust. He has extensive experience in critical care nursing. Following the award of a travel scholarship he has visited Western Australia to study pain management practices and has particular interest in the care of bariatric patients.

Pam Y Smith is a Registered Nurse and a senior lecturer at the University of Wolverhampton. She teaches a range of topics in both Common Foundation and Adult Branch pre-registration programmes and has a particular interest

in clinical skills. Her background is in acute medicine (gastroenterology).

Jane Swain is a nurse lecturer and site coordinator for clinical skills teaching at the University of Plymouth.

Elaine Swan (BN Hons, RGN, RM) is an Advanced Nurse Practitioner in colorectal/stoma care at Walsall Hospitals NHS Trust with over 20 years experience. She was instrumental in setting up these services in Walsall and has had a number of publications in this area of practice. She was previously the nurse representative to the National Council for the Association of Coloproctology of Great Britain and Ireland.

Gareth Walters (MB, ChB, MRCP(UK), AHEA, LCGI) is an honorary clinical lecturer at the University of Birmingham, and Specialist Registrar in Respiratory Medicine in the West Midlands. He regularly teaches clinical examination skills to a multiprofessional audience.

Catherine Waters is an Advanced Nurse Practitioner in General Practice and a module leader and clinical facilitator on the MSc Advanced Healthcare Practice Pathway at the University of Plymouth. She is module leader for second year clinical skills and currently has an honorary contract with a local surgery.

Louise Watson is a Clinical Specialist Physiotherapist in Respiratory Care at the Royal Devon and Exeter Hospital, Devon.

Graham R Williamson (BA, MA, PhD, PGDipEd, RGN) is a Lecturer in Adult Nursing at the University of Plymouth. He has a clinical background in acute medicine and respiratory care. He has published extensively on topics related to nurse education. He is a core member of the University of Plymouth Centre of Excellence in Professional Placement Learning (CEPPL).

Louise Winfield (RN, BSc, MSc, PGDipEd) is a lecturer at Plymouth University with a special interest in advanced nursing. She is programme lead for the university's Advanced Healthcare Practice course, which encompasses a clinical skills element.

Amanda Wirgman (RGN) qualified in 1981 and is a senior resuscitation officer working in Derriford Hospital, Plymouth, with a background in intensive care nursing and theatre recovery. She is currently undertaking an MSc in resuscitation practice.

How to use this book

Clinical Nursing Skills: Core and Advanced explains and demonstrates the clinical skills required of all adult and general nursing students through the use of specific features and learning tools. This brief tour shows you how to get the most out of this textbook package.

Background knowledge

The essential principles, evidence, and important considerations for each skill are introduced and discussed before the procedure is presented so students understand why, when, and if to undertake a clinical skill.

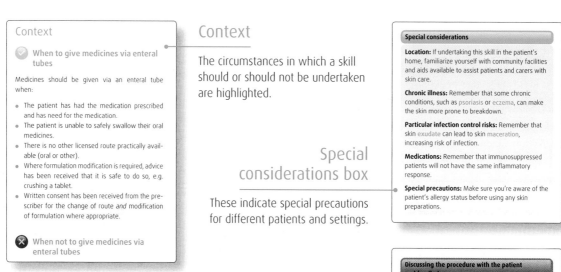

Context

Context
✔ **When to give medicines via enteral tubes**
Medicines should be given via an enteral tube when:
• The patient has had the medication prescribed and has need for the medication.
• The patient is unable to safely swallow their oral medicines.
• There is no other licensed route practically available (oral or other).
• Where formulation modification is required, advice has been received that it is safe to do so, e.g. crushing a tablet.
• Written consent has been received from the prescriber for the change of route *and* modification of formulation where appropriate.
✖ **When not to give medicines via enteral tubes**

Context

The circumstances in which a skill should or should not be undertaken are highlighted.

Special considerations box

These indicate special precautions for different patients and settings.

Special considerations
Location: If undertaking this skill in the patient's home, familiarize yourself with community facilities and aids available to assist patients and carers with skin care.
Chronic illness: Remember that some chronic conditions, such as psoriasis or eczema, can make the skin more prone to breakdown.
Particular infection control risks: Remember that skin exudate can lead to skin maceration, increasing risk of infection.
Medications: Remember that immunosuppressed patients will not have the same inflammatory response.
Special precautions: Make sure you're aware of the patient's allergy status before using any skin preparations.

Discussing the procedure with the patient box

Prior to undertaking a procedure nurses need to explain to patients what is involved in order for the patient to give consent. These boxes outline key issues to discuss.

Discussing the procedure with the patient and family/carers
■ Explain what self-administration involves and why it is done.
■ Make sure the patient understands that they don't have to self-administer – it is their choice.
■ Assure the patient that they can stop self-administration at any point during their stay, should they wish to.
■ Assure the patient that nursing or pharmacy staff will be happy to answer any questions they have about their medication.
■ Explain to the patient that their medication must be stored securely in a locked box or cupboard.

Step-by-step guidance

Step-by-step guide to undertaking nebulization

Step	Rationale
1 Introduce yourself, confirm the patient's identity, explain the procedure, and obtain consent.	To identify the patient correctly and gain informed consent.
2 Check the prescription of the drug to be given and the patient identification.	To ensure correct medication is given as prescribed.
3 Place mouthpiece in patient's mouth (see Figure 5.6) or place mask over patient's face, and turn on nebulizer. Leave on for 10 minutes. Masks, if used, must be tight-fitting and the patient should be encouraged to breathe through an open mouth.	Optimum time for nebulization of bronchodilators is 10 minutes; if it takes longer then the machine should be serviced. To avoid aerosol and droplets spreading to the eyes.
If nebulizing via a tracheostomy or non-invasive	Use T-piece to incorporate nebulizer into the circuit.

Each procedure is broken down into clear steps with accompanying rationale so students can see what to do and why. These have been carefully laid out to help learning.

When this icon appears in the Procedure Box a video of the skill is available on our Online Resource Centre (see overleaf for details).

Advanced guidance

Step-by-step guide to recording CVP using a manometer

Note: this is a complex, advanced procedure. Follow local guidance for the authority to perform this procedure, and seek guidance and assistance as required.

Step	Rationale
1 Introduce yourself, confirm the patient's identity, explain the procedure, and obtain consent.	To identify the patient correctly and gain informed consent.
2 Help the patient into a supine position, lying in either a flat or semi-recumbent position (Woodrow 2006).	Venous return may be reduced when in the upright position, and increased when lying flat.
3 Locate a point midaxilla in line with the fourth intercostal space, which is taken to be in line with the right atrium. Using the spirit level for accuracy, adjust the manometer	This approximates the level of the right atrium (the phlebostatic axis). If the alternative zero point is used, this should be recorded so that subsequent readings can be compared accurately.

When you see this icon and the procedure table is in gold, this is an **advanced skill**. Readers must check local Trust policy before undertaking the skill and must ensure they receive additional supervision and training to complete the skill safely.

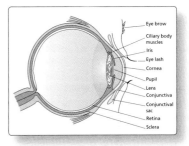

Patient deterioration box

Recognizing patient deterioration

The following may be signs of patient deterioration that you or the patient may detect during eye-care:

- Pain in, around, or behind the eye.
- Deteriorating vision.
- The patient complains of light hurting their eyes (photophobia).
- Unequal pupils.

These indicate to the reader the potential 'warning signs' that a clinical skill could indicate.

Scenarios

Q Patient scenarios

Consider what you should do in the following situations, then turn to the end of this skill to check your answers.

1 Patient A has a NG tube and it is coming up to the time that their Simvastatin dose is due. The prescription has 'ORAL' written as the route and no further information regarding enteral tube administration. What should you do before administering it?

Patient scenarios at the end of each skill prompt the reader to relate the theory to a clinical situation. Answers are provided overleaf.

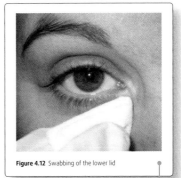

Figure 4.12 Swabbing of the lower lid

Visual demonstration

Colour drawings help to relate the underlying anatomy to the clinical skill whilst colour photographs demonstrate to students how to undertake a skill.

Support for further learning and assignments

At the end of each skill there are specific sections to aid reflection and further learning as well as reminders of key points. Each skill ends with references and a list of key further reading material.

How to use the Online Resource Center

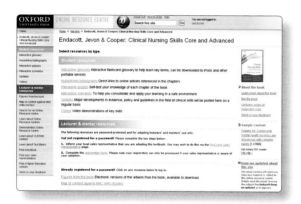

This textbook is accompanied by an Online Resource Centre (ORC) that provides students, lecturers, and mentors with interactive resources to develop clinical nursing skills. You can access the ORC from any computer with internet access and so you will find it helpful to save the web address in to your 'favourites' at the earliest opportunity:
www.oxfordtextbooks.co.uk/orc/endacott/

Videos

A selection of key clinical skills videos are available to watch on the ORC. Where you see the video icon in the chapter text, watch the accompanying video at your earliest convenienice to consolidate the procedures in the book. Please note that in some instances the videos show alternative approaches to the step by step procedures in the text. However, the videos follow the overall principles presented in the text and are accurate and evidence based.

 To access the videos, visit the home page for the ORC and click on the 'videos' link.

Updates

Major developments in evidence, policy, and guidelines in the field of clinical skills will be posted to the Online Resource Centre on a regular basis. Sign up to be alerted to the updates by clicking on the link 'Keep me updated about this site' on the home page of the ORC **www.oxfordtextbooks.co.uk/orc/endacott/**

Chapter specific resources

Each chapter is supported by the following resources to help readers apply and develop their skills.

Interactive scenarios
Give students the opportunity to try out their skills in a safe environment prior to placements.

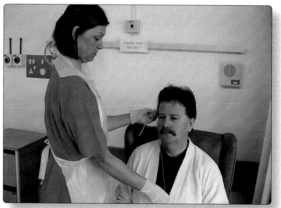

Quizzes
Reinforce students' knowledge and understanding.

Hyperlinked bibliography
Direct links to online articles referenced in the chapter (institutional subscriptions are required for access to full papers).

Interactive glossary
Technical terms from each skill are presented in an interactive 'flashcard' format to help students learn terms and concepts.

For lecturers

- Figures from the book to download and use in teaching
- Map of content against NMC skills clusters

Introduction

1

SIMON COOPER

We broadly define clinical skills as the range of skills that may be practised in the adult and general nursing environment and have therefore included core skills such as communication, essential skills such as infection control, pain management, and drug administration, and the specific skills related to each anatomical system, for example monitoring oxygen saturation, recording a blood pressure, care of the unconscious, bladder lavage, bowel care, and moving and handling patients.

This book is designed to provide nursing students with a comprehensive description of adult and general nursing clinical skills, for use in both primary care and hospital settings. Each section includes practical instruction with a balanced account of the background theory and evidence. Most of the skills you learnt in the first year of your training are repeated, but to the level expected of more senior students. We include all of the skills required of student nurses according to professional bodies (namely the Nursing and Midwifery Council in the UK), as well as additional skills that will help you develop your own repertoire and to assist Registered Nurses. We also include skills that may be used upon registration as a newly qualified nurse, so this book is still there for you at the start of your career.

We have described skills in a way that will help novice practitioners to reach a high standard of understanding and competency, but remember that some prior experience and knowledge are required, as we assume that students have completed the first year of a standard nursing programme. We have not included skills that are only pertinent to child, mental health, or learning disability nursing.

While you may be tempted to use the book to focus on specific skills, it is important to ensure that you are competent in the **essential skills** in Chapters 2, 3, and 4. These are placed at the beginning of the book as they provide the background for many of the specific skills. For example, the specific assessments identified in Section 6.1 (*Visual assessment of the cardiac patient*) and Section 7.1 (*Visual respiratory assessment*) assume that a comprehensive patient assessment was undertaken when the patient was admitted (Section 3.1). Similarly, we encourage you to read each skill section in the sequence listed and **not** to read the procedure section in isolation. Remember that as a novice practitioner, you should never perform a skill without having practised in an educational setting and with the support of a mentor or senior clinician.

We believe that clinical skills are not just isolated tasks to be learnt robotically, and that the current health care climate requires newly Registered Nurses to demonstrate sound **decision-making skills** before, during, and after implementation of skills. For this reason most skill sections list the prior knowledge requirements, a description of how the intervention works, when not to use it, alternative procedures, potential problems, and next stages.

Each section also includes **contemporary evidence** (at the point of publication) to support the use and practice of each skill. However, we are aware that local employers and universities may have their own policies on who can practise specific skills and the specific procedures that should be followed. Please therefore, where applicable, always refer to your local guidelines prior to practice. We are also aware that clinical practice varies and that evidence is lacking for some procedures. In these situations, writing teams have endeavoured to make decisions in light of patient safety and 'normal' best practice. If in doubt about a procedure, readers should refer to senior staff and their employer's policies and guidelines. In addition, an icon in the list of contents indicates that for some 'advanced' skills, the reader should check their local employer's policies before undertaking the skill ⚠ . Remember that additional practise and supervision will be required in order to complete these skills correctly and safely.

A theme throughout this book and emphasized in each chapter highlights the need to **identify deteriorating patients**. It is rare, however, for a patient to be identified as deteriorating from one parameter, e.g. their pulse. You should be aware of the global nature of assessment skills and the importance of monitoring changes in patient parameters, i.e. a pulse that is increasing and a blood pressure that is decreasing.

Additional guidance can be obtained from the National Patient Safety Agency 'Foresight' training programme (National Patient Safety Agency 2008) and from courses and publications such as ALERT (Smith 2000). However, new guidelines, protocols, and practice procedures are published regularly. To reflect this, readers have access to a dedicated online resource, **http://www.oxfordtextbooks.co.uk/ orc/endacott**, where the writing team will **regularly upload any changes in guidelines and policy** (e.g. Resuscitation Council guidelines). We would encourage you to register at the website to receive automated e-mail prompts when updates are available.

How to use this book and develop a skill

You'll have seen in the colourful opening pages just how the features in this book have been designed to help you (see page 16 onwards) – here we wish to explain in a little more detail how you can use the book for learning both at university and during placement.

Where possible we have used a standardized format; however, in some sections (e.g. *Communication skills*) it has been necessary to deviate slightly from this outline. In general, each section includes a definition and summary of the skill, and for some skills there is a video demonstration that should be watched in full prior to performing the skill. A section follows that highlights the key issues that you should remember and what prior knowledge you

require. These include references to basic bioscience (physiology, pharmacology, microbiology, etc.) and are supported by an online question bank to enable you to test your underpinning knowledge in each area.

The essential background to the skill is clearly described, including, for example: how the skill relates to anatomy and physiology; patient safety issues; hygiene and infection control; and applicable medical conditions. We then list the key contextual issues, including when to use and when not to use the skill, and alternative procedures, e.g. 'Have you tried x, y, and z before considering catheterizing the patient?' Indications for assistance are listed, i.e. the additional expertise or resources that are needed to complete the skill successfully, and we include indicators of potential problems (such as adverse reactions) during the skill. How readings can be interpreted (especially normal ranges and specific problems) is described, and any specific observations that may be relevant.

Most skills have a section entitled 'special considerations'. Here we highlight special precautions (say with the elderly, in pregnancy, or in acute illness) or the additional steps to take when the skill is undertaken, for example, outside of the hospital setting.

The procedure or intervention is then described, including the equipment that needs organizing beforehand, effective communication issues, the procedure itself, and things that need doing on completion, e.g. the key observations. We follow this with the key issues to be aware of in order to identify patients who are deteriorating.

The final subsections include guided questions for reflection and evaluation, what you should do next, some patient scenarios, and reminders; these are all designed to highlight and emphasize good and safe practice.

Key notes

For ease of reading, the term 'hospital' is used throughout the text. However, we recognize that students will be working in a range of settings, for example a residential home or the patient's own home, when they observe or undertake these skills. We also understand that where we advise that patient consent should be obtained, this may not be possible (or required) in an emergency. In addition, where reference is made to documenting aspects of care in the patient's health record, this includes completing documentation relevant to the integrated care pathway. Finally, we are also aware that the term 'patient' can be contentious and is not strictly accurate in every skill situation; however, for ease of reading we have used this term throughout the text.

Universal precautions and health and safety issues are emphasized throughout the book, but there are some generic issues that we are not able to make explicit under every skill, for example the risk of latex allergy from gloves.

Additional website resources

Again, you'll have seen at the start of the book colourful pages explaining how to use the accompanying online resource centre (page 16 onward). We urge you now to save the URL into your Favourites page on your home computer, and when at university to use as your login URL: **http://www.oxfordtextbooks.co.uk/orc/endacott**.

It would be a good idea to sign up for the UPDATES at the same time. On the Home page, simply choose 'Register here for email updates'.

We wish you all the best of luck in your future nursing career and hope that this book is a useful contemporary resource that supports your learning for many years to come.

References

National Patient Safety Agency (2008). Foresight training programme [online], **http://www.npsa.nhs.uk/patientsafety/improvingpatientsafety/humanfactors/foresight/** accessed 07/07/08.

Smith G (2000). *Acute Life Threatening Events Recognition and Management (ALERT): a multi-professional course in care of the acutely ill patient*. University of Portsmouth.

2 Communication skills

SIMON COOPER AND LISA LEWY

Definition

Communication is the two-way process of giving and receiving information, both verbally and non-verbally. It is a key and essential aspect of nursing care. Communication is a core dimension in the *NHS Knowledge and Skills Framework* (Department of Health 2004) and within the Nursing and Midwifery Council (NMC) *Code of Standards* (Nursing and Midwifery Council 2008). Both refer to the requirements for communication with a range of people (colleagues, external agencies, and patients) on a variety of simple and complex matters. The Quality Assurance Agency (2006: 6) also lists communication as a key subject benchmark, stating that health and social care staff should be able to:

- 'Make active, effective and purposeful contact with individuals and organizations, utilizing appropriate means such as verbal, paper-based and electronic communication.
- Build and sustain relationships with individuals, groups and organizations.
- Work with others to effect positive change and deliver professional and service accountability.'

Nurses must be able to assess, identify, and prioritize patients' needs, facilitate the expression of feelings, and build a relationship for effective care (Dougherty and Lister 2008).

It is important to remember that:

- Communication requirements vary dependent on the situation. The nurse must be prepared to adapt to the needs of the situation. Examples include breaking bad news, cultural differences in communication, communicating with children or the elderly, or the specific requirements of those with physical or learning disabilities.
- Communication competence varies depending on an individual's character and background. It is central to the patient's experience and therefore essential that all nurses throughout their career reflect on and (where appropriate) develop their communication skills as an integral part of professional development.

Prior knowledge

Prior to reading the following sections, consider your communication experiences to date, how these have influenced your development, and the skills you will need to develop in your nursing career. For example:

- How do children communicate?
- Do nurses need to adapt their communication skills for the working environment?
- What influences the development of communication styles?
- What forms of communication are there?
- Who are nurses required to communicate with?
- What are the communication barriers?

Background

Effective communication in the health care setting improves recovery rates and reduces pain and complications rates (Wilkinson *et al.* 2003). However, poor communication is cited in many NHS complaints (Bayer 2003). Catherine McCabe (2004) found that patients felt that nurses' communication skills needed to be improved, as they concentrated more on clinical tasks than talking to patients. She emphasizes the importance of 'patient-centred communication' and its central role in delivering quality patient care.

Models of communication

A number of communication models have been proposed, with descriptions of the processes and templates for best practice. Ellis *et al.* (2003: 5) describe the basic components of communication (shown in **Figure 2.1**) as being context specific, i.e. they should change depending on the situation. The sender (patient, nurse, doctor) aims to convey a message to a receiver who may or may not interpret it as intended. The message may have been misread due to contradictory body language, misheard or not heard at all, or generally 'lost in translation'.

Effective communicators rely on feedback from the receiver (two-way communication) requiring understanding or additional messages from the sender. Good communicators tend therefore to send messages in a consistent and clear way, their non-verbal and verbal language conveying the same message. For example, 'How are you feeling today Mrs Jones?' is said with empathy and concern, while waiting patiently at the bed for a reply, and then responding appropriately.

Ley (1988) developed a useful evidence-based model for improving patient communication and for improving medication compliance rates. Compliance rates can be quite low, for example Haynes *et al.* (2005) suggest that those prescribed self-administered medication

may take less than half their prescribed medication. Ley found that where understanding and memory were enhanced, patients were more satisfied with their care and more likely to comply with treatment.

Understanding and memory can be improved by avoiding jargon, simplifying language, and highlighting key issues at the start of the consultation, at the end, and where they are important, a process known as primacy, recency, and importance. Written explanations in the form of patient information or mail and e-mail reminders are also important, as well as telephone texting (texting4health 2008). Finally, satisfaction can also be improved by reducing waiting times, maintaining a friendly attitude, and allowing patients to tell their story in their own words and to express their worries and expectations.

A key model and set of skills for managing a patient consultation have been produced in the form of the Calgary–Cambridge Guides (Silverman *et al.* 2005). This model has been well researched and evaluated. The general principles can be used for nurse assessments with patients. Stages of consultation/assessment are listed as:

- 'Initiating the session' – where a rapport is built and the reasons for the meeting established.
- 'Gathering information' – for an exploration of the patient's problems, using skills such as listening to the patient's own story and identifying concerns and expectations.
- 'Building a relationship' – through appropriate verbal and non-verbal behaviour.
- 'Explanation and planning' – through the provision of information and shared decision-making.
- 'Closing the session' – with reference to further action and planning for unexpected outcomes (safety netting).

In the following sections we break down the stages of communication into three phases: the set, dialogue, and closure (Mackway-Jones and Walker 1998).

- 'Set' is the preparation phase – reading the patient's notes, introductions, ensuring that the patient and/or family are comfortable, etc.
- 'Dialogue' is the active communication stage, involving, for example, listening skills, verbal and non-verbal skills, and open and closed questioning.
- 'Closure' is the summary phase, with checks on understanding and safety netting.

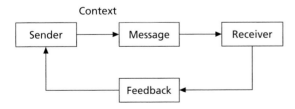

Figure 2.1 The components of communication. In a nursing context; the nurse may act as the 'sender', e.g. explaining to the patient what a procedure will involve, or as the 'receiver', e.g. listening to a patient's description of their pain symptoms.

Set

Where possible the nurse should become familiar with the patient's history prior to any meeting and should be updated on their condition as long as they remain in the nurse's care. An applicable amount of time should be allocated to each meeting to ensure that it is not rushed. However, where unavoidable interruptions occur, the patient should be reassured of the nurse's return. Special consideration should be given to assessing communication needs, which are categorized by Hilton (2004) as:

- Physical aspects such as hearing, talking, and writing skills.
- Psychological issues such as anxiety, intelligence, and anger.
- Sociocultural aspects in relation to dialect, first language, and cultural and religious issues.
- Environmental constraints such as temperature, noise, safety, and physical barriers to communication such as beds and desks.

In establishing an initial relationship, the nurse should greet the patient (and family if applicable), introduce themselves, and explain their role. Where required, informed consent should be gained for treatment (Dougherty and Lister 2008). Appropriate dress should be worn and the nurse should use a friendly and professional approach, aiming to make patients feel welcomed and supported (Pendleton *et al.* 2003). Particular attention should be paid to the environment, ensuring that the patient is comfortable, warm, and safe, and that privacy and confidentiality are maintained, especially in busy wards where curtains are the only dividers.

The reason for the meeting should be identified and the consultation developed through open questions, e.g. 'What is the problem today?' or 'How can I help you?' and, where appropriate, through closed questions such as 'How old are you?' and 'Where does it hurt?' (Hilton 2004, Silverman *et al.* 2005). The nurse should encourage the patient to discuss their problems/issues openly while listening closely, maintaining an awareness of their emotional state, and 'showing empathy, concern and optimism' (Kruijver *et al.* 2001).

Dialogue

Once the ice is broken and the initial introductions are completed there are a number of communication elements that the nurse should be aware of. The ability to develop rapport is important; treatment goals are more likely to be achieved when the patient is comfortable and relaxed, and where the nurse is non-judgemental, values opinions, and acknowledges individuals' views.

This 'accepting response' is described by Silverman *et al.* (2005) as a process of acknowledgement. It is achieved through the reiteration and clarification of patients' concerns (using comments such as 'So, you're concerned that the tablets have given you an ulcer') and by acknowledging their rights ('I can see that you may want to get a second opinion on that') or by giving them the 'space' to say more, through appropriate pauses and non-verbal behaviour.

This 'acceptance' does not imply agreement but places a value on patients' beliefs. For example, it would be inappropriate to dismiss patients' concerns with a comment such as 'There is nothing to worry about,' and more appropriate to acknowledge their concerns by stating 'I can understand why you are worried; we will make sure we check it out and let you know as soon as possible.'

A second and essential element is the ability to listen actively and demonstrate or clarify that we have 'heard' our patients correctly. In diabetes research, patients claimed that their knowledge about their condition and its management was not heard by health care professionals (Pooley *et al.* 2001). Hawkins and Lindsay (2006) highlight the significance of listening to patients' stories to enhance health professionals' understanding and to improve patients' 'physical and psychological healing'.

Gask and Usherwood (2002) describe a number of communication and active listening skills that should be used during a consultation. These include:

- Open and closed questions. Questions that encourage patients to expand on their answer but give 'yes' or 'no' responses where applicable.
- Checking. Repeat back patient responses to ensure joint understanding.
- Demonstrating empathy. For example, 'I am so sorry, this is clearly a concern to you.'
- Facilitation. Encouraging patient responses by non-verbal responses, e.g. nodding, or by verbal responses, e.g. 'Yes – and then what?'
- Offering support. Questions such as 'How can I support you with this condition?'

- Legitimizing feelings. Expressing your concern and understanding about the problem.
- Negotiating priorities. Decide, with the patient, the key priorities for their care.
- Summarizing. Clarify and summarize your agreement with the patient prior to closing the consultation.

A key element of communication is the nonverbal component (Ellis *et al.* 2003, Dougherty and Lister 2008), which includes your own and the patient's non-verbal behaviour. When working with patients, think about how they respond to you, bearing in mind cultural differences. Consider the following:

- Their body language and personal distance – do they move their chair away from you, or are they reluctant to sit down?
- Level of eye contact (Ruusuvuori 2001). Do they avoid your gaze? Do they constantly look around? What is their facial expression/gaze like?
- What are their voice, tone, inflection, and volume like?
- Do they have an open or closed posture – for example do they look relaxed and casual or do they have tightly folded arms and face away from you? Do they avoid your touch?
- Are they well dressed and groomed or do they look dishevelled and unclean?
- How are they moving? Are they slow and lethargic or is their gait awkward or shuffling?

As a nurse, consider how you may need to adapt your behaviour for specific situations. For example, nurses in elderly care have been found to display more non-verbal behaviours, such as touch, smiling, and patient-directed gaze, than community nurses (Caris-Verhallen *et al.* 1999).

Barriers to effective communication skills

Environmental factors can have major influences on the way we communicate. In hospitals and nursing homes, nurses who care for the elderly have been found to use communication as a means of maintaining power over vulnerable patients (Brown and Draper 2003). Chant *et al.* (2002) found that nursing work and high stress levels can act as 'barriers to empathy and communication skills implementation', while Yam and Rossiter (2000) refer to the hierarchical nature of health care and how this may have negative impacts on communication and patient

care. Environmental influences and interruptions, e.g. phones, children, and door bells, may also hinder effective communication.

Throughout all phases, but particularly during the dialogue, consider how communication can be hindered. Think about privacy issues and the patient's level of anxiety, for example are they tachycardic, hypertensive, or perspiring (Grandis *et al.* 2003)? Are there physical restrictions to communication, for example a tracheostomy, or perhaps the patient has had a laryngectomy? Request a translator if the patient or family are non-English speakers (many health providers maintain a list of foreign language speakers for this purpose).

Avoid the use of medical jargon and think about your speech rhythm, pace, emphasis, intonation, pitch, and tone. These are known as paralinguistic features ('features of the spoken message that are not contained in the message alone,' Ellis *et al.* 2003) and care must be taken to ensure that the patient does not misinterpret your meaning. For example, depending on the word emphasis, 'I will see you in the ward at 10 o'clock' may be considered a command to be in the ward at 10 o'clock, or alternatively a friendly and reassuring promise of your return.

It is important to remember that there may be a number of patient-related communication barriers, which Park and Song (2004) list as:

- Tiredness.
- Pre-health conditions (physical disability, poor hearing or sight, impaired levels of understanding).
- Life stresses related and unrelated to the illness.
- A short attention span.
- Low education levels.
- Differing social norms.
- Lack of trust.
- Accent issues.
- The withholding of information.
- Generation gaps.

In summary, Silverman *et al.* (2005) describe the key elements of the 'dialogue' as building a relationship and exploring of the patient's problems, including encouraging them to tell their own story, using open and closed questions, listening, picking up on verbal and non-verbal clues, and clarifying and checking on the story. Explanations should be clear and provided in small 'chunks', with appropriate use of repetition and checks on patient understanding, aiming for a shared decision by the end of the consultation.

Closure

Appropriate summing up, emphasis, checks on understanding, and future plans are the final essential elements of any patient communication episode. It is important that this phase is relatively short and sharp to ensure that the key elements of the communication remain salient.

Silverman *et al.* (2005) have again produced a very useful template for closing a consultation, suggesting that the 'next steps' should be discussed and safety issues should be raised, covering what to do if the plan is not working and how to seek help (safety nets). Sessions should be summarized with final checks on agreement, plans, and questions.

Where applicable, documentation should be completed, ideally in a multidisciplinary format (Dougherty and Lister 2008) to ensure that all health professionals are kept up to date. Finally, again where applicable, close attention should be given to handover procedures; for example, in the Accident and Emergency setting, Jenkin *et al.* (2007) found that listening skills, repetition, and a phased approach to handover are important. A British Medical Association (2004) report also concludes that multidisciplinary handovers are an important element of good communication and that effective handovers are vital for patient safety – safe handovers = safe patients.

As Information Communication Technology (ICT) develops, the traditional models of communication will need to be reviewed. Health care providers are rapidly investigating how ICT can be utilized in improving health care. Wahlberg *et al.* (2003) discuss the development of 'telephone nurses' and the prospect of e-mail and virtual nurses. This study highlights the importance of supporting nurses who are delivering health care without direct visual contact and the impact this has on telephone nurses' ability to make informed decisions.

These ICT developments bring with them different communication cultures and a requirement for training and development. For example, nurses will need to adapt their approach on the phone to draw out information and to focus on the problem, while being reassuring and confident. In fact, Wahlberg *et al.* (2003) found that 'nurses seemed to lack confidence in their competence'

when delivering telephone-based health care, which may be due to the lack of visual contact and communication feedback issues.

Context

In the communication setting there are a number of special considerations that the nurse should be aware of. Below an outline of these is all that is possible, as in all of the following situations there will be individual and context-specific requirements.

Learning disabilities

Key considerations for patients with learning disabilities are their mode of communication and level of understanding (Grandis *et al.* 2003). Their mode of communication includes their likes and dislikes, ways of expressing discomfort and pain, sign language, and level of self-help. The level of understanding and comprehension will influence how the nurse structures information for the patient, and the degree of professional support required.

It may, for example, be necessary to refer the patient for speech therapy or request guidance from a learning disability nurse. As Grandis *et al.* (2003: 213) suggest, 'the responsibility here lies with the nurse to find a suitable and appropriate means of communication in order to establish a mutual frame of reference.'

Workplace violence

Communication is a two-way process, and patients and colleagues have an equal responsibility to communicate with you in an appropriate manner. However, violence in the workplace is increasingly common (Department of Health 2001, International Labour Organization *et al.* 2005), especially in the A & E setting.

Hilton (2004: 168) lists four 'A's for managing aggression, with the objective of awareness and avoidance wherever possible:

- *Awareness* of the likelihood of aggression. For example, patients who have taken drink or drugs, or those who portray unusual or threatening body language.
- *Alertness* to situations and changing moods.
- *Avoidance* if at all possible; being aware of the patient history or the presenting case.

- *Appropriate* and prompt responses. For example, carrying of personal attack alarms and ensuring that there is an escape route and police support.

Braithwaite (2001) also discusses ways of managing aggression, including body language, assertiveness, and diffusion techniques, which Bibby (1995) describes as the calming, reaching, and controlling stages. These stages consist of: 'calming' by talking and listening in an unthreatening posture; 'reaching' the aggressor by encouraging them to explain their grievances; and 'controlling' by working together, setting joint, realistic agreements, and admitting mistakes where applicable.

Breaking bad news

Breaking bad news is one of the most difficult and emotional experiences in the nurse's role and is often poorly managed by health professionals (Dias *et al.* 2003). Faulkner and Maguire (1994) suggest that health professionals tend to 'block' the emotional flow by, for example, ignoring cues, selective attention, inappropriate encouragement, giving premature and false reassurance, and switching topics.

The Resuscitation Council (UK) (2006) provides comprehensive guidance suggesting that wherever possible, bad news should be delivered face to face in a private, quiet, and homely setting without fear of interruption. Key issues for consideration are:

- Where possible, take time to prepare yourself before going into the meeting and, if available, take a colleague with you.
- Allocate a suitable amount of time, so that the exchange is not rushed.
- Check that you are talking to the correct relatives and exchange introductions.
- Maintain eye contact and be direct, honest, and sensitive throughout.
- Give accurate and clear explanations, avoiding the use of terminology, e.g. 'Her heart has stopped', instead of 'She has had a cardiac arrest.' Say '. . . he has died', instead of euphemisms such as '. . . he has gone to a better place.'
- Be prepared for questions and a wide variety of emotions and use touch if it feels right.
- Avoid platitudes such as 'I know what it feels like.'

- Explain and discuss with the family what will happen next and identify any culturally specific requirements, for example the management of the body after death.

Cultural considerations

Nurses deliver health care to a wide range of patients/clients from a wide range of cultural backgrounds. Nurses need to be aware of and respect cultural differences and recognize potential weaknesses in traditional communication methods. Rhodes and Nocon (2003) outline the differences in communication in ethnic minority communities and report that there are gaps in communication when interpreters are used. For example, the interpreter may not speak the dialect, may miss critical information, may lack rapport, or may not pass on information using caring and applicable language. For interpreters to be effective, they need to be integrated within the health care service and gain an understanding of the concerns of patients/clients. However, such integration may prove difficult in rural areas with small ethnic minority communities. It is therefore important to be aware of the services available in each area, for example refugee centres or relevant ethnic community groups.

The elderly

Communicating with the elderly may take time and patience. As with all patients, but especially with the elderly, you should check their previous health care records to determine if their condition will affect their ability to understand and respond to you, for example if they have had a stroke, or have diabetes or dementia. It is then important to establish if the elderly person can hear, see, and understand you.

At all times, avoid behaviour that may be interpreted as patronizing, for example speaking to the individual as if they were a child or carrying out procedures without explanation or permission. Brown and Draper (2003) demonstrated that it is common within elderly health care for nurses to use 'accommodation speech', defined as being simplified, projected in a high pitched tone, and involving increased use of questions, imperatives, and repetition. La Tourette and Meeks (2001) emphasized the need to listen to the elderly and found that nurses were rated more highly when they used non-patronizing speech.

Finally, there is some evidence that technology may help the elderly. For example, Savenstedt *et al.* (2005) found that video conferencing had a positive effect on elderly patients suffering from dementia.

Interdisciplinary/interprofessional working and teamwork

Key to team building and communication within health care is communication between the professions (Molyneux 2001), a process known as interprofessional working. Interprofessional working is described by the Centre for the Advancement of Interprofessional Education (CAIPE 2002) as 'occasions when two or more professions learn with, from and about each other to improve collaboration and the quality of care'.

Of course an interprofessional approach should be adopted even where the individual is not a formal member of a 'team'. The need to communicate well with your colleagues, as well as your patient, is critical to the continued development of and improvement in patient care (Ginsbury and Tregunno 2005). For example poor communication between midwives and medical staff can lead to an increase in mortality rates (Revill 2004). Good communication practices between professionals, on the other hand, improve discharge planning (Pethybridge 2004), and in multidisciplinary teams where trained supervisors are allocated to each team, there are improvements in cohesion, joint decision-making, and communication (Hyrkas and Appelqvist-Schmidlechner 2003). Training also makes a difference to communication skills; for example, leadership training improves workplace performance (Cooper 2003).

It is important to remember that the communication skills used with colleagues may differ from the skills used with patients. However, there are core competencies for interprofessional working that are relevant to any communication episodes (CAIPE 2002):

- Equity – all contributions are valued.
- Respect differences.
- Confidentiality.
- Avoid or explain jargon.
- Check understanding.
- Identify mutual goals and where there are differences.

- Discuss the challenges of collaborative working.
- Identify a strategy to deal with disagreements.

Procedure

Box 2.1 lists the key requirements for effective communication. Note that the stages and emphasis may change depending on the situation.

Reflection and evaluation

Reflect on each communication episode you've been involved in and think about the following issues.

- Did you make the patient feel welcome and supported?
- Were you aware of the patient's emotional state?
- Did you encourage the patient to 'open up' and raise any problems and issues?
- Did you recognize and value cultural diversity?
- Did you consider treatment options and agree a plan?
- Did you identify a multiprofessional patient care pathway, where applicable?
- Did you develop a rapport by:
  - Being non-judgemental?
  - Acknowledging that the patient is an individual and has a right to their view?
  - Valuing the patient?

Further learning opportunities

Communication is improved with practice so develop your skills in role play scenario situations with your colleagues. Where communication is likely to be challenging, for example breaking bad news, observe an experienced colleague first and ask for their support on later occasions to develop your competence and confidence.

Reminders

As you practise talking to patients/staff and build your communication skills, remember the following points:

- Communication is critical to the patient experience.
- Adopt a patient-centred communication approach.
- Be culturally aware in your approach and acknowledge that in 'translation' your empathetic

Box 2.1 The key elements of each phase of communication

Set (preparation and lead in)

Preparation

Consider the context of the forthcoming communication by:

- Reading the patient's notes and records.
- Communicating with the multidisciplinary team.

Will it involve patients who have:

- Learning disabilities?
- Understanding or memory problems?
- Specific language requirements?
- Cultural differences?

Or patients who are:

- Elderly or infirm?
- Angry or violent?

Anticipate and rapidly assess communication issues:

- Hearing.
- Verbal communication.
- Anxiety levels.

Lead in

Prepare the environment:

- Personal dress/uniform.
- Temperature.
- Seating.
- Privacy.
- Comfort.

Initiate the session:

- Greet – introductions and preferred names.
- Consent to treatment (where applicable).
- Identify the key issues.
- Jointly plan the agenda.

Dialogue (active communication)

Build a rapport by:

- Being non-judgemental.
- Valuing opinions.

- Acknowledging views.
- Accepting and acknowledging concerns.
- Active listening (maintaining an open posture, eye contact, attention, and waiting and pausing).
- Using open and closed questions.
- Being sensitive and supportive.

Consider your own and the patient's verbal and non-verbal behaviour:

- Personal space.
- Eye contact.
- Posture (open or closed?).
- Movement.
- Dress and grooming.
- Voice, tone, inflection, and volume.

Maintain a structured approach by:

- Considering the sequence of the discussion.
- Exploring problems and issues through the patient's story, using listening skills and open and closed questions.
- Restricting the use of medical terminology.
- Supplying applicable information.
- Repeating information.
- Explanation and feedback.
- Reinforcing information with written and illustrative feedback (e.g. using an anatomical model or showing an X-ray).
- Emphasizing and highlighting key issues at the start and end of the conversation.

Closure (summary)

Close the session by:

- Summarizing the discussion.
- Ensuring that there is shared understanding.
- Safety netting (how to seek additional help and what to do if outcomes are unexpected).
- Confirming final agreed plans.

---

approach may be lost. It is important therefore to use your non-verbal communication skills to demonstrate concern and openness.

- Actively listen to your patients, 'hearing' what they say and 'seeing' how they feel.
- Ensure excellent communication skills are adopted with your colleagues.
- Make sure you value communication exchanges and seek support where there are difficulties.

 Patient scenarios

Consider what you should do in the following situations, then turn to the end of this skill to check your answers.

1. Patient care advice

Miss Kosovich has recently been diagnosed as diabetic. You are responsible for advising her on her diet. However, Miss Kosovich is very outgoing, loves drinking and smoking, and is extremely depressed that her lifestyle may change. You notice from her records that she has been given health promotion advice but that she appears to be ignoring it. She has collapsed four times during the past month after not taking her insulin and drinking alcohol in excess. How are you going to deal with Miss Kosovich?

2. Patient referral

Mr Dorrington has missed three appointments but managed to turn up today. However, he appears disorientated and his behaviour concerns you. He keeps jumping up and down saying that people are following him. You are a nurse who is advising him on his back pain. What should you do?

3. Communication with colleagues

You are a nurse attending a meeting to discuss one of the patients on the rehabilitation ward where you work. The senior registrar is at the meeting, together with the physiotherapist. The senior registrar and the physiotherapist are discussing the patient's health care and use terms you are not familiar with. You are the lead nurse for this patient's care. How would you approach this situation to ensure maximization of patient care?

4. Patient assessment

Miranda, a frequent attendee, arrives in Alison's (a nurse practitioner) office concerned about numbness in her left hand. Alison ascertains that she has had the symptoms for a week. After a full examination she refers Miranda to her GP for further investigations. She is concerned that Miranda may have the early signs of multiple sclerosis.

Miranda does not keep the GP appointment but returns to Alison's office a few months later complaining of fatigue and feeling more emotional than usual, crying over the smallest issues. Alison focuses on these issues and suggests a number of stress management techniques.

A few days later, while at work, Miranda suddenly finds the numbness in her hand has returned but now also includes her face, and she is unable to focus due to blurred vision. She immediately arranges an appointment with her GP. Her GP is concerned that Alison has not mentioned Miranda and her previous visits. He

immediately refers her for further investigations to a colleague who specializes in conditions that affect the nervous system.

Website

 http://www.oxfordtextbooks.co.uk/orc/ endacott

You may find it helpful to work through our short online quiz and additional scenarios intended to help you to develop and apply the skills in this chapter.

References

Bayer A (2003). Telling older patients and their families what they want to know. *Reviews in Clinical Gerontology*, **13**(4), 269–72.

Bibby P (1995). *Personal safety for health care workers*. Ashgate, Aldershot.

Braithwaite R (2001). *Managing aggression*. Routledge, London.

British Medical Association (2004). *Safe handover: safe patients. Guidance on clinical handover for clinicians and managers*. British Medical Association, London.

Brown A and Draper P (2003). Accommodative speech and terms of endearment: elements of a language mode often experienced by older adults. *Journal of Advanced Nursing*, **41**(1), 15–21.

Caris-Verhallen WMCN, Kerkstra A, and Bensing JM (1999). Non-verbal behaviour in nurse–elderly patient communication. *Journal of Advanced Nursing*, **29**(4), 808–18.

Centre for the Advancement of Interprofessional Education (2002). [online] **http://www. caipe.org.uk/** accessed 27/02/07.

Chant S, Jenkinson T, Randle J, and Russell G (2002). Communication skills: some problems in nursing education and practice. *Journal of Clinical Nursing*, **11**(1), 12–21.

Cooper SJR (2003). Does LEO roar: an evaluation of the Leading Empowered Organisations leadership development programme. *Nursing Standard*, 14 Feb, 33–9.

Department of Health (2001). *National Task Force on Violence Against Social Care Staff – Report and National Action Plan* [online] **http://www. dh.gov.uk/en/Publicationsandstatistics/ Publications/PublicationsPolicyAndGuidance/ DH_4010625** accessed 18/08/08.

Department of Health (2004). *The NHS Knowledge and Skills Framework (NHS KSF) and the development review process. Appendix 2: core dimension 1: communication*. Department of Health Publications, London.

Dias L, Chabner BA, Lynch TJ, and Penson RT (2003). Breaking bad news: a patient's perspective. *The Oncologist*, **8**, 587–96.

Dougherty L and Lister S (2008). *The Royal Marsden Hospital manual of clinical nursing procedures*, 7th edition. Blackwell Publishing, Oxford.

Ellis RB, Gates B, and Kenworthy N (2003). *Interpersonal communication in nursing. Theory and practice*, 2nd edition. Churchill Livingstone, London.

Faulkner A and Maguire P (1994). *Talking to cancer patients and their relatives*. Oxford University Press, Oxford.

Gask L and Usherwood T (2002). ABC of psychological medicine. *BMJ*, **324**(7353), 1567–9.

Ginsbury L and Tregunno D (2005). New approaches to interprofessional education and collaborative practice: lessons from the organisational change literature. *Journal of Interprofessional Care*, **1**, 177–87.

Grandis S, Long G, Glasper A, and Jackson P (2003). *Foundation studies in nursing. Using enquiry-based learning*. Palgrave Macmillan, Basingstoke.

Hawkins J and Lindsay L (2006). We listen but do we hear? The importance of patient stories. *British Journal of Community Nursing*, **11**(9), 6–14.

Haynes RB, Ackloo E, Sahota N, McDonald HP, Yao X. *Interventions for enhancing medication adherence*. Cochrane Database of Systematic Reviews 2008, Issue 2. Art No.: CD000011.DOI:10.1002/14651858.CD000011.pub3

Hilton PA (2004). *Fundamental nursing skills*. Whurr Publishers, London.

Hyrkas K and Appelqvist-Schmidlechner K (2003). Team supervision in multi-professional teams: team members' descriptions of the effects as highlighted by group interviews. *Journal of Clinical Nursing*, **12**(2), 188–97.

International Labour Organization, International Council of Nurses, World Health Organization, and Public Services International (2005). *Framework guidelines for addressing workplace violence in the health sector. The training manual*. International Labour Office, Geneva.

Jenkin A, Cooper S, and Abelson-Mitchell N (2007). Patient handover: time for a change? *Journal of Accident and Emergency Nursing*, **15**, 141–7.

Kruijver IPM, Kerkstra A, Bensing JM, and Van der Weil HBM (2001). Communication skills of nurses during Interactions with simulated cancer patients. *Journal of Advanced Nursing*, **34**(6), 772–9.

La Tourette R and Meeks S (2000). Perceptions of patronizing speech by older women in nursing homes and in the community. *Journal of Language and Social Psychology*, **19**(4), 463–73.

Ley P (1988). *Communicating with patients. Improving communication, satisfaction and compliance*. Croom Helm, London.

Mackway-Jones K and Walker M (1998). *Pocket guide to teaching for medical instructors*. BMJ Books, London.

McCabe C (2004). Nurse–patient communication: an exploration of patients' experiences. *Journal of Clinical Nursing*, **13**, 41–9.

Molyneux J (2001). Interprofessional team working: what makes teams work well? *Journal of Interprofessional Care*, **15**(1), 29–35.

Nursing and Midwifery Council (2008). *The Code: standards of conduct, performance and ethics for nurses and midwives*. Nursing and Midwifery Council, London.

Park EK and Song M (2004). Communication barriers perceived by older patients and nurses. *International Journal of Nursing Studies*, **42**, 159–66.

Pendleton D, Schofield T, Tate P, and Havelock P (2003). *The new consultation*. Oxford University Press, Oxford.

Pethybridge J (2004). How team working influences discharge planning from hospital: a study of four multi-disciplinary teams in an acute hospital in England. *Journal of Interprofessional Care*, **18**(1), 29–41.

Pooley C, Gerrard C, Hollis S, Morton S, and Astbury J (2001). Oh it's a wonderful practice . . . you can talk to them: a qualitative study of patients' and health professionals' views on the management of type 2 diabetes. *Health and Social Care in the Community*, **9**(5), 318–26.

Quality Assurance Agency (2006). *Statement of common purpose for subject benchmark statements for the health and social care professions* [online] **http://www.qaa.ac.uk/academicinfrastructure/benchmark/health/StatementofCommonPurpose06.pdf** accessed 18/08/08.

Resuscitation Council (UK) (2006). *Advanced life support*, 5th edition. Resuscitation Council (UK), London.

Revill J (2004). *When the baby is forgotten,* March 7 [online] **http://www.guardian.co.uk/medicine/story/0,,1164082,00.html** accessed 18/08/08.

Rhodes P and Nocon A (2003). A problem of communication? Diabetes care among Bangladeshi people in Bradford. *Health and Social Care in the Community*, **11**(1), 45–54.

Ruusuvuori J (2001). Looking means listening: co-ordinating displays of engagement in doctor–patient interaction. *Social Science and Medicine*, **52**, 1093–108.

Savenstedt S, Zingmark K, Hyden LC, and Brulin C (2005). Establishing joint attention in remote talks with the elderly about health: a study of nurses' conversations with elderly persons in teleconsultations. *Scandinavian Journal of Caring Sciences*, **19**, 317–24.

Silverman J, Kurtz S, and Draper J (2005). *Skills for communicating with patients*. Radcliffe Publishing, Oxford.

Texting4health (2004). [online] **http://www. texting4health.org** accessed 18/08/08.

Wahlberg AC, Cedersand E, and Wredling R (2003). Telephone nurses' experiences of problems with telephone advice in Sweden. *Journal of Clinical Nursing*, **12**(1), 37–45.

Wilkinson SM, Leliopoulou C, Gambles M, and Roberts A (2003). Can intensive three-day programmes improve nurses' communication skills in cancer care. *Psycho-oncology*, **12**(8), 747–59.

Yam B and Rossiter JR (2000). Caring In nursing: perceptions of Hong Kong nurses. *Journal Of Clinical Nursing*, **9**(2), 293–302.

Useful further reading and websites

 Check **http://www.oxfordtextbooks.co.uk/ orc/endacott** for updated research and guidelines.

http://www.healthline.com – general communication information.

http://www.skillscascade.com – good resources website.

http://www.bmj.com – free articles on medical communication.

http://www.cisco.com/uk/humannetwork – virtual networking.

http://www.cardiff.ac.uk/encap/hcrc/helcomassoc. html – health communications research centre.

Guly HR (1996). *History taking, examination and record keeping in emergency medicine*. Oxford University Press, Oxford.

 Answers to patient scenarios

1   Miss Kosovich has concerns regarding her diagnosis, and fears that being diabetic means her life will dramatically change. You need to adopt a communication approach that recognizes Miss Kosovich's dilemma and values her views, even if they conflict with your own. You both need to discuss relevant role models and management of diabetes within her lifestyle. She needs to know that life can still be exciting and that her character does not need to change, but that her view on diabetes may need to be integrated into her social activities so she can enjoy her life long term.

2   As a general nurse, mental health issues are outside your professional expertise, but you may have colleagues within your multiprofessional team who have the necessary experience. If you don't, you can make an appropriate referral, but you need to identify the most effective way to proceed. Referral and support is the key in the long term. If it is possible to continue the current appointment then adopt a reassuring communication method, acknowledge his anxiety, but focus on his back pain. If this fails, the most appropriate step would be to stop the appointment and arrange another date. In the interim contact other health care professionals for advice.

3   It is important that you do not feel devalued or undermined as this may lead to defensive behaviour, which will limit communication. Ask your colleagues to explain terms that you are not familiar with and describe your experience of the patient in full.

4   Emphasis on the importance of keeping referral appointments is essential and it is good practice to check that appointments have been kept. Communicating with other health care professionals is also essential.

3 The patient pathway

Skills

3.1 **Principles of good record keeping**

Definition

A health record is defined as 'any electronic or paper information recorded about a person for the purpose of managing their health care' (Data Protection Act 1998) and includes 'medical records, patient records and notes, case notes and obstetric records' (National Health Service Litigation Authority (NHSLA) 2005).

Health records provide evidence of health professionals' involvement with patients (Griffith 2004) and demonstrate the delivery of 'safe and effective care based on current evidence, best practice and, where applicable, validated research' (Nursing and Midwifery Council (NMC) 2007a). This section includes: completing an entry in a health care record; use of diaries for clinical information; using computer-based records; standardizing patient wristbands; and writing an incident report.

It is important to remember that:

- The purpose of health records is to provide a current picture of the patient's problems, management, and response to treatment.
- Health records hold the key to identifying changes in the patient's condition, from physiological parameters to progress with rehabilitation. To fulfil this purpose, records must be complete, accurate, and timely.
- An ultimate outcome of poor record keeping is poor quality care and inappropriate patient management.

- The best health care record is the product of communication between members of the health care team and the patient/client (NMC 2007a).
- Information about patients must be treated as confidential and used only for the purposes for which it was given. NMC guidance about confidentiality applies to verbal and written (paper and computer-based) patient information.

Prior knowledge

Before completing an entry in a health care record, make sure you are familiar with:

1 NMC (2008) *The Code: standards of conduct, performance and ethics for nurses and midwives*.
2 NMC (2007c) *Standards for medicines management*.
3 NMC advice sheets on: confidentiality, delegation, and accountability (see the Further reading section at the end of this skill).
4 NMC (2005b) *An NMC guide for students of nursing and midwifery*.
5 Your employer's policy for record keeping.

Background

In order to understand why good record keeping is central to delivering good quality patient care, it's helpful to examine circumstances in which records have been found to be inadequate. The NMC (2005a) identified that 39% of charges brought before the professional conduct committee concerned clinical practice, with 6% related to poor record keeping. In addition, much of the research concerning poor management of patients who deteriorate emphasizes incomplete recording of vital signs (e.g. National Confidential Enquiry into Patient Outcome and Death 2005, Endacott *et al*. 2007). Factors that contribute to effective record keeping are summarized in **Box 3.1**.

The content of health records should meet the following requirements:

1 Be recorded, wherever possible, with the involvement of the patient/client or their carer.
2 Be recorded in terms that the patient/client can understand.
3 Be consecutive.
4 Identify risk and/or problems that have arisen and the action taken to rectify them.

Box 3.1 Effective record keeping

Patient/client records should:

- Be factual, consistent, and accurate, recorded so that the meaning is clear.
- Be recorded as soon as possible after an event has occurred, providing current information on the care and condition of the patient/client.
- Be recorded clearly and in such a manner that the text cannot be erased or deleted without a record of the change.
- Be recorded in such a manner that any justifiable alterations or additions are dated, timed, and signed or clearly attributed to a named person in an identifiable role, and so that the original entry can still be read clearly.
- Be accurately dated, timed, and signed, with the signature printed alongside the first entry where this is a written record, and attributed to a named person in an identifiable role for electronic records.
- Not include abbreviations, jargon, meaningless phrases, irrelevant speculation, or offensive or subjective statements.
- Be readable when photocopied or scanned.

NMC (2007a)

5 Provide clear evidence of the care planned, the decisions made, the care delivered, and the information shared.
NMC (2007a)

These requirements and the factors identified by the NMC in Box 3.1 should be applied to both paper and electronic health records.

When discussing health records with the patient, it is important to explain what is being recorded and why, and to identify goals that are important to the patient.

Completing an entry in a health care record

When completing a health care record, the principles in **Table 3.1** must be followed.

Retention of records

The period for which heath records are required to be kept will depend on local and government health department policies. Such policies and protocols usually state

Table 3.1 Principles of record keeping

Principle	Rationale
Write legibly	In order to meet the stated purpose of managing [patient's] health care (Data Protection Act 1998), records need to be read accurately by others.
Include date and time	The sequence of events is important when reviewing patient progress and, more importantly, patient deterioration, as well as providing evidence of chronology in legal cases.
Sign all entries and print name	The person providing care has accountability for that care. (See also guidance on delegated accountability and record keeping in Box 3.5.)
Use only approved, unambiguous abbreviations	Abbreviations may be clear to one group of professionals but ambiguous to others. Abbreviations can also become outdated; records may be reviewed many years after they are written, either for legal reasons or, more usually, in an attempt to understand more about treatment the patient received in the past.
Do not alter entries or disguise additions made at a later stage	It is essential that any changes to records are legible and dated.
Do not use offensive, personal, or humorous language	Such language is easily misinterpreted, even if intended as a reflection of the patient's situation.
Check everything you've written/typed before adding your signature	Some programmes used for electronic health records do not include spellcheckers; it is easy to miss errors.
Ensure reports (e.g. investigations) are seen, evaluated, and initialled before being filed in the patient's records (follow your local Trust policy)	Overdiligent filing of reports can result in abnormal results being overlooked.
Do not destroy patient records	Incomplete records can result in unsafe patient care. Trusts have local policies for storing of health records, for example some Trusts keep fluid balance charts while others do not.

Adapted from Norwell's *Ten Commandments of record keeping* (1997).

that records should be kept for a minimum period of 8 years and, in the case of a child, at least to the date of the child's 21st birthday (NMC 2007a). The recording of patient information in diaries is a controversial area; advice from the NMC is provided in **Box 3.2**.

Terminology used in patient records

Consistency in terminology is crucial; Zeleznik *et al.* (2003) found that language used by doctors and nurses to describe skin ulcers in patient records varied considerably.

They found a total of 66 different terms (including 38 non-medical, non-specific, or ambiguous terms) used to describe skin ulcers; the most frequently omitted component was the size of the ulcer.

Ambiguity in terminology was also highlighted in a legal case where different interpretations of a term used in ophthalmology led a surgeon to conclude that a patient had deteriorated. The surgeon consequently undertook surgery that resulted in severe complications and was held to be negligent (*Scheck v. Dart High Court*, 22/10/04, cited in NHSLA 2006). Particular care should be taken to

Box 3.2 Advice from the NMC (2007a) regarding use of diaries for clinical information

Diaries containing clinical information are considered part of a patient or client's clinical record and should be kept for the minimum period of eight years or to a child's 21st birthday in the case of children's records.

The NMC recommends that clinical information should not be recorded in diaries. Where it is, then the information must be transcribed into the patient or client's records within 48 hours. Registrants should, however, be aware of local policies, as many state that diaries should only be used as a tool enabling registrants to log appointments. Providing the diary contains no clinical information or that this has been transcribed into the patient/client's own records, they should be retained for one year from the date of their completion.

Box 3.3 NHS Code of Practice for Confidentiality: specific guidance for electronic record keeping

Staff must:

- Always log out of any computer system or application when work on it is finished.
- Not leave a terminal unattended and logged in.
- Not share logins with other people. If other staff need to access records, then appropriate access should be organized for them – this must not be by using others' access identities.
- Not reveal passwords to others.
- Change passwords at regular intervals to prevent anyone else using them.
- Avoid using short passwords, or using names or words that are known to be associated with them (e.g. children's or pets' names or birthdays).
- Always clear the screen of a previous patient's information before seeing another.
- Use a password-protected screensaver to prevent casual viewing of patient information by others.

(**http://www.connectingforhealth.nhs.uk/resources/resources/
nhs_code_of_practice.pdf**)

avoid communication-related errors when using terms that sound or look similar, for example prefixes such as anti and ante, ab(duction) and ad(duction) (Lyons 2008).

Using computer-based records

Major drawbacks with paper-based health records include difficulty in retrieving vital information about the patient and different document designs, even within the same organization (Taylor 2003). Computerbased records (or electronic health records, EHRs) may be one solution to these problems; however, they are themselves not without difficulties. Researchers in the USA found that patient attitudes to EHRs (including web messaging and online access to their EHR) were more positive than those of clinicians (Hassol *et al.* 2004). A review of 26 studies by Delpierre *et al.* (2004) found that user and patient satisfaction were improved with the use of computer-based records, although the impact of EHRs on patient outcomes was inconclusive.

In a survey of 225 primary care nurses and doctors, Linder *et al.* (2006) found a number of barriers to using the EHR during a patient visit, the most common reported as: loss of eye contact with patients (62%); falling behind (52%); computers too slow (49%); inability to type quickly enough (32%); feeling that using the computer in front of the patient is rude (31%); and preferring to write long prose notes (28%). However, the electronic health care record is a cornerstone of future developments in

patient documentation (see NHS *Connecting for Health*, **http://www.connectingforhealth.nhs.uk**) and hence it is important that these barriers are overcome. The NHS *Code of Practice for Confidentiality* guidance on electronic data storage provides helpful guidance (see **Box 3.3**).

In order to maintain patient confidentiality, care records should only be accessed by those involved in the patient's care. Under the NHS Care Record Scheme, an **audit trail** will be kept of all staff who access an individual patient record (BMA/NHS Connecting for Health 2008) and patients will be able to request a copy of their audit trail.

The move to electronic records opens up a number of different ways of sharing patient information, for example:

1 Access to records by clinicians in different settings. This is particularly useful when patients may access more than one health care provider, for example a number of different walk-in centres in the same area (Colucci 2007).
2 Electronic transfer of vital signs data. In an attempt to improve recognition and timely management of

patients with abnormal vital signs, some hospitals are using PDAs to record vital signs, linked to a central monitoring system (Smith *et al.* 2006).

Further initiatives such as drugs trolleys accessed/ secured by thumbprint are currently being piloted by some hospitals.

Standardizing wristbands

Complete, legible, and up-to-date health records are crucial to provide safe and timely patient care. Safe care is also dependent on correct patient identification; the National Patient Safety Agency (NPSA) reported 2900 instances of incorrect patient identification due to inadequate documentation on patient wristbands in England and Wales in 2006. As a result, new guidelines were issued in 2007 (**http://www.npsa.nhs.uk/display? contentId=6076**); the requirements from July 2008 are listed in **Box 3.4**.

Writing incident reports

If you are asked to write a report about a clinical incident, it is important to remember the following:

- Identify what happened, to whom, and how.
- Identify where the incident happened.

Box 3.4 NPSA requirements for wristband use

- Wristbands will have to meet NPSA requirements.
- Wristbands must only include the patient's last name, first name, date of birth, and NHS number (or a temporary identification number).
- Organizations must develop clear and consistent processes specifying who can produce, apply, and check wristbands.
- Wristbands must be white with black text.
- Patients with known risks such as allergies, or patients who do not wish to receive blood products, should be given a red wristband with text in black.
- Wristbands should be generated and printed from the hospital patient information system, at the bedside wherever possible.
- In Wales the first line of the patient's address must be included.

(NPSA 2007, **http://www.npsa.nhs.uk/display?contentId=6076**)

- Report facts only – do not be tempted to provide an opinion about why the incident might have happened.
- Include, in a factual manner, any unusual circumstances (e.g. unexpected staff sickness/ absence) or unusual workload issues (e.g. an emergency with another patient).

One of the goals of clinical governance, in the light of the Bristol Inquiry (Kennedy 2001), is that a more 'open' culture should be evident when clinical incidents occur, for example:

- Focusing not on who went wrong but on what went wrong.
- Talking through the incident rather than instigating an investigation.
- Treating the incident as a training point rather than a disciplinary matter.
- Learning lessons and changing systems as appropriate.

The processes used by most NHS Trusts follow the root cause analysis method (see **http://www.npsa.nhs.uk/ health/reporting/reportanincident**).

Reviewing health records

Health records should be regularly audited as part of NHS Trust risk management processes. Records may, however, also be reviewed some time after they were written to ascertain whether safe and appropriate care was provided. This type of review may be part of a legal case or a professional misconduct hearing. **Tables 3.2** and **3.3** identify lessons to be learnt about health care records from both types of case.

Other aspects of documentation

Delegation

As a Registered Nurse or midwife, you are responsible for any activity you have decided to delegate to others. The NMC Code (2008) states:

You must establish that anyone you delegate to is able to carry out your instructions. You must confirm that the outcome of any delegated task meets required standards. You must make sure that everyone you are responsible for is supervised and supported.

Table 3.2 Lessons to be learnt from legal cases

Detail	Key lessons
Saunders v. Leeds Western HA [1993] Healthy 4-year-old child suffered cardiac arrest and brain damage during an arthroplasty operation. Operating department team claimed that the child's heart had simply stopped abruptly. There was no evidence in the records of a sequence of events leading to the heart stopping. The Health Authority was found to be negligent.	Records need to be sufficiently detailed to demonstrate an appropriate standard of care.
McLennan v. Newcastle HA [1992] A patient claimed she had not been told of the relatively high risk associated with her operation. The surgeon had written in the notes that the risks were explained and understood by the patient. The court found in favour of the Health Authority.	It is essential to record details of conversations with patients at the time they occur (a contemporaneous record). If the procedure for which the patient is giving consent is particularly rare or complex, a written patient information sheet is also helpful.
Prendergast v. Sam Dee [1989] An illegible prescription from a GP resulted in the patient being given the wrong drug by a pharmacist. The patient suffered harm as a result. The pharmacist was held to be 75% liable for the harm and the GP 25% liable due to his poor handwriting.	Illegible writing can result in harm to patients and liability for those responsible.

Table 3.3 Cases reviewed by the Nursing and Midwifery Council Fitness to Practise Committee (reported in NMC Annual Report 2004–05)

Proven charges	Implications
An adult nurse (RN) working as an emergency nurse practitioner based in a hospital: ■ failed to triage patients properly ■ failed to complete triage documentation ■ falsely represented that she had completed triage documentation ■ failed to deal properly with a complaint relating to a patient in the triage process. Similar issues had been raised in the past concerning the quality of the nurse's triage and record keeping.	Appropriate treatment was delayed with potentially serious consequences; this was compounded by false recording. The nurse's actions clearly demonstrated unsafe practice and had been repeated on previous occasions. **NMC decision:** **Removed from the register**
An adult nurse (RN) was employed as a staff nurse at a nursing home and admitted the following charges: ■ failed to update the notes of a diabetic patient whose condition was poor ■ failed to give drugs at the correct time ■ signed for a medication when there was doubt whether it was given ■ signed for medication when it had not been given ■ on 14 occasions failed to record the pulse of a patient on digoxin.	The nurse failed in her obligations to keep proper and accurate records. The nurse's actions demonstrated a lack of understanding regarding the administration of medicines and the essential requirements of good record keeping. **NMC decision:** **Removed from the register**

Box 3.5 NMC advice regarding documentation of delegation

- The registrant has a responsibility to ensure that any aspect of care delegated has been documented appropriately.
- Documentation should clearly outline any decision-making processes and must be patient/client specific.
- The most appropriate place to record this information should be decided based on the working environment, i.e. patient held records/ care plans.
- At each delegation, the names of those being delegated to must be clearly stated.

NMC (2007b)

Delegation to others must also be documented appropriately (NMC 2007b); see **Box 3.5**.

Documentation of care, including any discussions with the patient or relatives about care management, is the responsibility of the person who has undertaken the care. This will include those to whom care has been delegated, e.g. unregistered staff and students. The Registered Nurse/midwife who has delegated the activity may be required to countersign the record, according to local Trust policy. All entries in patient records made by students must be countersigned by a Registered Nurse or midwife (NMC 2005b). Don't forget that documenting care should only be delegated to others if the Registered Nurse/midwife has evidence of their competence in this skill.

Reflection and evaluation

When you have completed an entry in the patient's records, think about the following questions:

1 Is my entry clear, unambiguous, legible, dated, timed, and signed? Review the entries made by others; do these also meet these requirements?

2 Have I used available opportunities to discuss the health record entry with the patient? Is the patient aware of the goals that have been set and the actions planned?

3 Would I be able to provide safe care for the patient based on the information in the health record?

Further learning outcomes

Look at the records written by experienced colleagues. How do their entries differ from yours?

As electronic health records become more commonplace, look at the steps taken in your workplace (or placement venues) to protect patient confidentiality.

Reminders

Don't forget to:

- Check all entries you make in health records to ensure they meet the requirements of Table 3.1.
- Ensure that you maintain the confidentiality of patient information held in health records.

 Patient scenarios

Consider what you should do in the following situations, then turn to the end of this skill to check your answers.

1 Mr Jones has chronic obstructive pulmonary disease and asked to see his health records. He is alarmed that the GP has written that he might need to be considered for 'LTOT', and the practice nurse has reported that on attending the practice respiratory clinic, he is increasingly 'SOB'. He assumes that the nurse is calling him a 'son of a bitch' and the GP is making some detrimental reference to his occasional drinking habit. How can this situation be avoided?

2 You are a student working on a medical ward. A doctor from the Emergency Department requests to see the notes of his sister-in-law, who has been admitted for investigations. What action should you take?

Website

 http://www.oxfordtextbooks.co.uk/orc/ endacott

You may find it helpful to work through our short online quiz and additional scenarios intended to help you to develop and apply the skills in this chapter.

References

British Medical Association/NHS Connecting for Health (2008). *Joint Guidance on Protecting*

Electronic Patient Information [online]
**http://www.connectingforhealth.nhs.uk/
systemsandservices/nhscrs/publications/
staff/jointguidance.pdf** accessed 12/08/08.

Colucci M (2007). Moving to a paperless walk-in centre. *British Journal of Healthcare Computing and Information Management*, **24**(4), 14–16.

The Data Protection Act (1998). [online]
http://www.hmso.gov.uk accessed 12/08/08.

Delpierre C, Cuzin L, Fillaux J, Alvarez M, Massip P, and Lang T (2004). A systematic review of computer-based patient record systems and quality of care: more randomized trials or a broader approach? *International Journal for Quality in Health Care*, **16**(5), 407–16.

Endacott R, Kidd T, Chaboyer W, and Edington J (2007). Recognition and communication of patient deterioration in a regional hospital: a multi-methods study. *Australian Critical Care* **20**(3), 100–5.

Griffith R (2004). Putting the record straight: the importance of documentation. *British Journal of Community Nursing*, **9**(3), 122–5.

Hassol A, Walker JM, Kidder D, *et al.* (2004). Patient experiences and attitudes about access to a patient electronic health care record and linked web messaging. *Journal of American Informatics Association*, **11**(6), 505–13.

Kennedy I (2001). *The report of the public inquiry into children's heart surgery at the Bristol Royal Infirmary 1984–1995: Learning from Bristol*. The Stationary Office, London.

Linder JA, Schnipper JL, Tsurikova R, Meinikas AJ, Volk LA, and Middleton B (2006). Barriers to electronic health record use during patient visits. *AMIA Annual Symposium Proceedings*, 499–503.

Lyons M (2008). Do classical origins of medical terms endanger patients? *The Lancet*, **371**, 1321–2.

National Confidential Enquiry into Patient Outcome and Death (NCEPOD) (2005). *An acute problem*? NCEPOD, London. [online] **http://www.ncepod.org.uk** accessed 20/08/07.

National Health Service Litigation Authority (2005). *CNST general clinical risk management standards*. NHSLA, London.

National Health Service Litigation Authority (2006). Clinical cases. *NHSLA Journal*, **5**, 8–9.

Norwell N (1997). The ten commandments of record keeping. *Journal of the MDU*, **13**(1), 8–9.

Nursing and Midwifery Council (2005a). *Fitness to practise annual report 2004–2005*. NMC, London.

Nursing and Midwifery Council (2005b). *An NMC Guide for Students of Nursing and Midwifery* [online]
**http://www.nmc-uk.org/aFrameDisplay.aspx?
DocumentID=1896** accessed 20/08/08.

Nursing and Midwifery Council (2007a). *Advice sheet on record keeping*. NMC, London.

Nursing and Midwifery Council (2007b). *Advice sheet on delegation*. NMC, London.

Nursing and Midwifery Council (2007c). *Standards for medicines management* [online] **http://www.nmc-uk.org/aFrameDisplay.aspx?DocumentID=4092** accessed 20/08/08.

Nursing and Midwifery Council (2008). *The Code: standards of conduct, performance and ethics for nurses and midwives*. NMC, London.

Smith GB, Prytherch DR, Schmidt P, *et al.* (2006). Hospital-wide physiological surveillance – a new approach to the early identification and management of the sick patient. *Resuscitation*, **71**, 19–28.

Taylor H (2003). An exploration of the factors that affect nurses' record keeping. *British Journal of Nursing*, 12, 751–8.

Zeleznik J, Agard-Henriques B, Schnebel B, and Smith DL (2003). Terminology used by different health care providers to document skin ulcers: the blind men and the elephant. *Journal of Wound, Ostomy and Continence Nursing*, **30**(6), 324–33.

Useful further reading and websites

Department of Health (2004). *The NHS Knowledge and Skills Framework (NHS KSF) and the development review process*. DH, London. [online]
http://www.dh.gov.uk.

Nursing and Midwifery Council (NMC) advice sheets:
Confidentiality (**http://www.nmc-uk.org/
aFrameDisplay.aspx?DocumentID=1560**)
Delegation (**http://www.nmc-uk.org/
aFrameDisplay.aspx?DocumentID=3076**)
Accountability (**http://www.nmc-uk.org/
aFrameDisplay.aspx?DocumentID=1551**)

Royal College of Nursing (2006). *Competencies: an integrated career and competency framework for information sharing in nursing practice*. RCN, London. [online] **http://www.rcn.org.uk/publications/
pdf/information_sharing_in_nursing_practice.pdf**

Electronic health record websites for England, Scotland, Wales, and Northern Ireland:
Connecting for Health (England) –
http://www.connectingforhealth.nhs.uk

The e-health programme (Scotland) –
   http://www.ehealth.scot.nhs.uk
Informing health care (Wales) –
   http://www.wales.nhs.uk
HPSS ICT programme (Northern Ireland) –
   http://www.dhsspsni.gov.uk
See **http://www.hmso.gov.uk** for details of Acts
   relating to information and health care.

 Answers to patient scenarios

1 All records should be written with the assumption
   that they will be read by the patient and/or relatives.
   All abbreviations should be fully explained with the
   full version (e.g. LTOT – long-term oxygen therapy)
   written in the narrative. When a patient requests
   their notes, the records should be scanned to identify abbreviations that are acceptable across health
   professions but ambiguous to the patient. If time
   allows, a health professional should be available to
   answer any queries the patient may have.

2 The ED doctor has no right to view the records of
   his sister-in-law. The only circumstance in which the
   doctor would be allowed to view the notes is with
   the express permission of the patient. Local Trust
   policy may require this to be given in writing. It is the
   responsibility of Registered Nurses and midwives to
   protect confidential information (NMC 2008). The
   management of this scenario is beyond the expected
   competence of a student, so you should refer the
   doctor to a Registered Nurse.

3.2 **Completing an effective patient admission assessment**

Definition

Patient assessment on admission can be defined as the
act of evaluation of a patient's condition and welfare, in
order to plan and implement appropriate care on admission to a health care setting.

It is important to remember that:

● An effective admission assessment is essential to
   ensure that the patient's needs are identified and

met as fully as possible, and that the patient is fully
and appropriately prepared for discharge.

● Good record keeping within the patient assessment
   will also allow for effective continuity of care and
   promotes communication and sharing of information
   between members of the interprofessional health
   care team (NMC 2007).

● Nursing records are subject to audit as part of the
   clinical governance cycle. Therefore, any patient
   assessment you undertake may be subject to review.
   The level of detail you include may assist in the
   development of health care when the quality review
   cycle takes place.

● As part of the *Access to Health Records Act* (1990),
   any nursing assessment made after 1 November
   1991 may also be viewed by the patients you have
   cared for, at any time.

● *Any* patient record can be used as evidence to
   investigate potential discrepancies either at the local
   level or in a court of law. Keep in mind that the detail
   you record today may reliably assist you in
   remembering the care you delivered to your patients
   in many years to come.

Prior knowledge

Before undertaking a patient admission assessment,
make sure you are familiar with:

1 Section 3.1 of this book, *Principles of good record
   keeping.*
2 The NMC guidelines for records and record keeping
   (NMC 2007).
3 *Going lean in the NHS* (NHS Institute for Innovation
   and Improvement 2007).
4 Local policies and guidelines relating to record keeping.

Background

There is currently no single model or template for a
quality admission assessment; however, in England the
NHS is seeking to standardize and improve communication
and record keeping by implementing a new integrated
information technology system. 'NHS Connecting for
Health' is providing the delivery of these systems and
services, enabling information to be shared between NHS
organizations across England. Similar projects are taking
place across Scotland, Wales, and Ireland.

Assessment models

Across health care settings, different modes of assessment may be used dependent on anticipated patient needs. An acute NHS medical inpatient unit will initially want to focus on managing the patient's presenting condition and the assessment will reflect this. However, a Stroke Rehabilitation Unit may need to address the development needs of the patient in order for them to maintain their own care; the format of the assessment will reflect this.

Most assessment tools are based on a cyclical process that enables appropriate assessment, planning, implementation, and evaluation of care; in nursing this has been referred to as the nursing process, first described in the 1960s (Orlando 1961). The frameworks developed to tailor the assessment to patient needs are usually referred to as nursing models and became popular in nursing practice in the 1980s. These models tend to be tailored according to the eventual goal for the patient – for example the self-care model first described by Orem (1971) or the adaptation model described by Roy (1976). In the twenty-first century these have been described as outdated and remote theories, full of 'pretentious jargon' (Salvage 2006).

One of the most widely used nursing models in the UK was developed in 1980 by three nursing leaders who were significantly disenchanted with the existing 'biomedical' approach to nursing care (Salvage 2006). The Roper, Logan, and Tierney (RLT) model of nursing (Roper *et al*. 1983) started out as a nursing education tool but was rapidly adopted as a framework for planning patient care. The model uses 12 activities of living as the basis for assessing the patient and planning/evaluating care (see **Figure 3.1**).

In 2000 the authors wrote their final account of *The Roper-Logan-Tierney model of nursing* (Roper *et al*. 2000) but suggested that others may choose to develop it as the face of nursing develops and progresses. Re-evaluation of the processes used to plan care is vital and, as a student or newly Registered Nurse, your fresh eyes may note areas of weakness where improvements could be made.

Whichever mode of assessment your department uses, the principles remain the same. The aim is to achieve the best possible account of the patient's needs on admission and, through effective record keeping, to provide optimum care throughout the hospital stay and the best possible outcome on discharge. Best practice promoted by the NMC (2007) requires assessment of the patient's

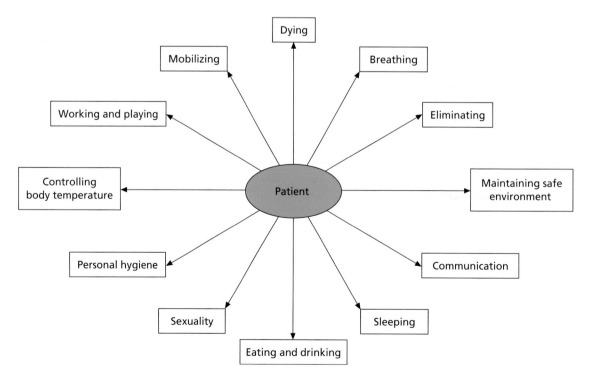

Figure 3.1 The Roper, Logan, and Tierney activities of living model.

immediate needs within 4 hours of the patient's arrival, followed by full documentation within 24 hours.

There may be variations in the detailed requirements for admission assessment in public and private hospitals, nursing homes, and community settings. However, the principles of admission assessment remain the same throughout different care settings. For the purpose of this chapter, the example of a patient arriving for care within the NHS acute sector via an 'Admissions Unit' is used.

Clinical observations

If the patient is acutely ill, your admission assessment is likely to include the following clinical measurements:

- Blood pressure
- Temperature
- Respirations
- Pulse
- Oxygen saturation
- Neurological status

The purpose of this chapter is to prepare you to undertake a baseline admission assessment. More details of specific physiological assessments are provided in the following sections: 6.1 *Visual assessment of the cardiac patient*; 6.2 *Measuring and recording the pulse*; 6.3 *Measuring and recording blood pressure*; 7.1 *Visual respiratory assessment*; and 10.1 *Nutritional assessment*.

The quality of the written patient assessment is dependent on the care taken by the person making the record. It therefore has the potential to fall foul of human error. Remember that all documentation you complete is a 'window' of your practice, so give thought to the detail you include in your assessment. Some examples of legal cases and cases of misconduct reported to the NMC that related to patient documentation are provided in Section 3.1. The mandatory standard for nursing documentation is also made explicit in the guidelines from the NMC (2007) shown in Box 3.1 on page 16.

Context

 When to undertake an admission assessment

All patients should be assessed when they first enter a different health care setting. For example, a patient transferred from hospital to a nursing home will require an assessment to identify needs specific to that setting. The detail of the assessment will be tailored according to circumstances, for example a patient admitted to the resuscitation area of an Emergency Department will require rapid assessment and prioritizing of their life-threatening condition.

Do not undertake this task until you have observed others undertaking it and feel suitably prepared for your first time. You are not letting anybody down by taking your time and learning the skill. Better to take your time and ensure accuracy than to rush and miss a vital part of the admission assessment.

Alternative interventions

Use all sources of information available to you; this may include family members and paramedic/ambulance staff. This should not be considered 'alternative' but should be a normal dimension of admission assessment. However, most of the admission assessment detail depends on communication with the patient. Where this is not possible, for example if the patient is unconscious, as much detail as possible should be gleaned from family and other professionals.

Procedure

Preparation

Prepare yourself

Ensure you have all relevant information about the patient to hand. As far as possible, plan your workload in order to undertake the admission assessment with the minimum of interruptions.

Prepare the patient

Undoubtedly, wherever you work, your area will be busy and high expectations will have been placed upon you. When the patient arrives on the ward, take the opportunity to take a step back and put yourself in their position. Consider how the patient is possibly feeling at that moment:

- Unwell
- Unclean
- In discomfort

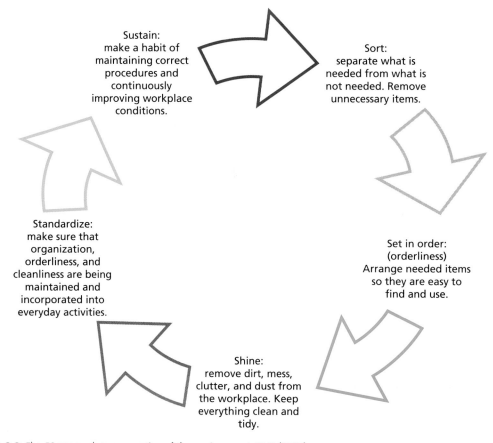

Figure 3.2 The 5S approach to preparation of the environment. NHS (2007).

- Vulnerable
- Anxious

With this in mind, consider your response. A welcoming smile and an indication that you are prepared for them could put the patient at ease. If the patient's arrival is unexpected or there are going to be any delays in facilitating their admission, then try not to look blank or too busy to be concerned. Take sufficient time to reassure the patient and assist them into a bed space as expediently as possible, ensuring that you provide appropriate care and consideration for relatives as required.

Prepare the equipment/environment

Prior to the patient's arrival on the ward, think about the materials and information you will need and prepare your area.

Be aware that some of the equipment used to record clinical observations is electronic and will require charging.

Therefore, before you use any equipment, check that it is sufficiently charged and in full working order. After use, check that it is clean, in good working order, and returned to its designated area for charging. If your clinical area is likely to receive these admissions, hopefully it will have adopted the NHS '5S' approach (NHS Institute for Innovation and Improvement 2007) to the preparation of its environment (see **Figure 3.2**). You will then find that an allocated area will have been designated for this purpose.

With equipment available and ready for use, your patient should experience minimal delay in the assessment process and you as a nurse will endure less frustration in delivering your practice.

Documentation Once again, if the '5S' principle is used, this would allow for the unit to have admission packs ready prepared and easily to hand. This achieves two possible benefits when the patient arrives into your care:

firstly, it ensures maximum nursing time is available for direct patient care and, secondly, it demonstrates a professional approach to the patient.

Ensure that the documentation is relevant to the patient you are admitting. It may include items from the following list:

- Admission pack
- Medical notes
- X-ray/Blood/Culture/Investigation request forms
- Manual handling score chart
- Dietary assessment tool
- Observation record sheets
- Physio/OT/Social services referral forms

- Pressure area record sheet (e.g. Waterlow Scoring Tool)

It may be advantageous throughout the admission process for your area to consider the development of a checklist approach. This would ensure that you had everything to hand and also ready to operate at the right time.

Bed space Prior to the patient's arrival (preferably at the start of your shift), assess your patient bed space and ensure that it is clean, tidy, and fit for purpose, e.g. oxygen port and mask. Finally check that the patient name board has been completed, together with locally required additional information, e.g. admitting physician.

Step-by-step guide to undertaking an admission assessment

Step		Rationale
1	Introduce yourself, confirm the patient's identity, explain the procedure, and obtain consent.	To identify the patient correctly and gain informed consent.
2	For each of the activities of living, consider how your patient normally coped at home prior to the onset of the admission and also how they are at the time of assessment.	This will provide a baseline and allow early planning for discharge.
3	Assess each of the activities of living using the questions in the following sections.	To ensure a systematic approach is followed. The patient may have a set of symptoms (e.g. respiratory difficulties) that take priority, but may also have problems with other activities of living.
4	Confirm contact details regarding next of kin; check that they are aware of the patient's admission.	To ensure that next of kin can be contacted quickly should an emergency arise.
5	When the assessment is complete, ensure the patient is as comfortable as possible and aware of the next stages in their care.	To alleviate patient anxiety as far as possible.

Assessment framework

1. Breathing

As you speak with the patient, consider how the patient is breathing on arrival. There are a variety of signs to look

for and each of these may indicate a particular illness. Points to consider include:

- Is it laboured?
- Is it shallow?

- Is the patient mouth breathing?
- Is the patient using diaphragmatic breathing?
- If oxygen is required, is the patient distressed? Would a mouthpiece be more effective than a mask?
- Does the patient have chronic obstructive pulmonary disease (COPD)? If so, remember that patients with advanced COPD may be dependent on low oxygen saturation to maintain their respiratory drive, and high levels of oxygen should only be used under written medical advice.
- Would the patient prefer to be sitting up? How many pillows are required?

Ask questions that establish answers to the above or use your observation skills to decide for yourself. Careful documentation and reporting of findings could prevent serious patient deterioration (Smith 2003) or potential fatality.

2. Elimination

Think about what you are asking. This is not just about ascertaining bowel movements. When at home, how does your patient manage with the passing of urine and faeces? Consider:

- How often does the patient pass urine?
- What volume?
- Does the patient experience nocturnal micturition?
- Does the patient require diuretics?
- How often does the patient open their bowels?
- How formed are bowel motions?
- Does the patient suffer from an irritable bowel?
- Does the patient take iron medication?
- Does the patient require laxatives/aperients?
- Does the patient require assistance?
- Are any aids required to ease elimination?

These questions are not exhaustive but will allow you to delve deeper into the patient's normal elimination habits and provide assistance when normal habits change. Remember that reduced mobility and changes to fluid intake and diet will have effects on your patient. Daily assessment will demonstrate changes early and therefore aid you in preventing complications. This will also include the need to undertake urinalysis on a regular basis, dependent on the needs of the patient. This will assist in indicating issues such as infection or potential diabetes.

3. Maintaining a safe environment

Throughout your patient's stay, they will have to negotiate a period of their life through illness. This may be a short- or long-term event but your care will hopefully allow this period to be as comfortable as possible. On admission, consider the needs of the patient during their hospital stay and what their needs may be on discharge.

Assess the patient for any factors that may make them unsafe in a different environment. For example, if the patient suffers from any loss of sight, how can you best promote their care? Can you place them near the nurses' station and within easy reach of the toilet with uninterrupted passage? The patient's safety is particularly dependent on their ability to communicate their needs; specific assessment questions for this are detailed in the next section.

4. Communication

The ability of the patient to communicate is dependent on a number of interrelated factors (e.g. intact speech, sight, and hearing). It is important to assess these when you first meet the patient to ensure they are as involved in planning their care as possible. The following questions are helpful:

- How does your patient appear on arrival to the ward?
- Is the patient alert and orientated?
- Is the patient relaxed and communicating well or anxious and only able to provide closed answers?
- Does the patient have any speech or hearing difficulty?

Don't judge the patient as being 'awkward' if their answers are clipped. There may be predisposing factors that are leading to this, such as respiratory illness causing breathlessness. All sorts of external factors could potentially influence your patient's response and you as a professional need to identify these. For a patient who is giving restricted responses but their partner is speaking for them, ensure you take time to assess their communication when their partner has left.

In order to review and improve your own communication skills, please refer to Chapter 2 for further information.

5. Sleeping

At home, what is the patient's usual routine? Do we meet this when we are providing care? Reflect on your own night-time routines: how do you settle to sleep at night?

Do you have a milky drink at 8.30 p.m. with lights out at 11.30 p.m.? Do you fall asleep and then have someone wake you at 12.30 a.m. to give you your night sedation?

As nurses we cannot totally break with ward routine and our routine will be different from the patient's usual experience. Therefore, what can we do to ensure they obtain a good night's sleep? Firstly, your admission assessment should obtain usual habits and ascertain if any night sedation is required. Are they awoken by the need for nocturnal micturition? Once this information has been collated, we can be aware of and prepared for any difficulties the patient may experience. We can also establish if there has been a change in the patient's normal habits.

6. Eating and drinking

So often, meaningless phrases are used, e.g. 'Patient maintains a normal diet'. What is normal? Each of us has different needs and there is much to be questioned here.

- How many meals does the patient have per day?
- Are these cooked independently or provided by a service such as 'meals on wheels'?
- Does the patient have any special dietary needs, e.g. gluten free, vegetarian?
- How many litres of fluid does the patient drink a day and in what capacity? (The patient is likely to answer this question in terms of numbers of cups of tea, etc., with no knowledge of fluid volume.)

7. Personal hygiene

Each patient admitted to hospital will have their own standards of personal hygiene, and as health care professionals we should endeavour to meet these. Patient hygiene may not appear particularly 'high tech' but the provision of this to a high standard can improve the patient experience considerably. Further detail regarding assessment of the patient's skin care requirements and usual practices can be found in Section 4.2.

Throughout the assessment process, we need to ascertain what the patient's normal standard is so this can be met. Points to consider include:

- How often does the patient wish to be washed?
- Does the patient prefer to bath or shower?
- Has the patient brought provisions to hospital to maintain hygiene needs?

- How often does the patient wash their hair? Will this be achievable in hospital?
- Does the patient wish to use soap on their face?
- Does the patient like the use of flannels? If so, how many? (Some people use four flannels for different parts of the body.)
- How much assistance is usually required to meet hygiene needs?
- On return home, is it likely they will need assistance/ equipment provided in order to maintain hygiene?

8. Controlling body temperature

This is not necessarily an area of concern for many patients, but for some patients, temperature control can be problematic. There are a variety of methods that can be used to assist patients to warm up or cool down; however, it is important also to consider how your actions may influence other patients. For those patients who feel the cold, it would be considerate to move them away from draughty doorways.

9. Working and playing

Patients who have been admitted may experience considerable anxiety in relation to their condition. Preparing for returning home and to work can add to this stress and therefore we need to consider how this will impact on their progress.

Consider the 52-year-old gentleman working as a sales representative who is trying to achieve targets and needs to be on the road, meeting customers. How is the news that he has had a myocardial infarction going to impact on his life? How likely is it that he will heed your advice to take it easy? Consider his need for counselling and support to facilitate this.

For most patients, admission to hospital removes them from their social life. It is useful to ask about their usual social habits when the patient is admitted, as these can provide useful goals for rehabilitation.

10. Mobilizing

On admission, health professionals tend to restrict the movement of patients to reduce any worsening of their presenting condition. Therefore, we may subconsciously view them in a different light to how they 'normally' mobilize.

The 74-year-old lady presenting with a fractured scaphoid, following a trip at home, may be admitted and nursed in a bed. Unable to bear weight on the affected wrist, she may require assistance to move up the bed. Yet at home, the same lady may be fully able to drive long distances and maintain a household independently.

It is vital we are aware of patients' 'normal' ability in relation to mobility, so that we may be able to return them as closely as possible to this position.

11. Sexuality

In this present era of the NHS, mixed wards are a necessity for most NHS Trusts. However, in keeping with government policy (Department of Health 2007), mixed bays are kept to a minimum. Yet patients do hold this as important to their own values. Therefore, as health care professionals, where possible we need to promote and uphold patients' needs in relation to sexuality.

This equally applies to patients who may be preparing for gender reassignment, etc., and these views need to be considered. Considering a person's view of their sexuality pre-admission is vital in ensuring the same standard is provided throughout the hospital stay and in preparation for discharge.

Throughout the patient's stay, it is also of high importance that we as practitioners consider the needs of patients in the same way that we may consider our own. Being in hospital does not stop the need for an individual to feel at their best where possible, and the use of make-up or relevant prosthetics may enhance the patient experience.

12. Dying

While death is part of everyone's life, it will always remain a difficult area to be faced by our patients and colleagues. Alterations to our normal way of life through illness will often present a question of our own mortality, and dealing with this can be difficult.

As health professionals, we need to be prepared and trained for this, in order to identify fear and be able to act upon it. It will be a difficult question to ask on admission and it is unlikely that it will be appropriate to ask in a direct manner. However, the topic can be approached indirectly by asking about religious needs and ascertaining if the patient would wish to see any representative of the hospital or local spiritual community.

This may lead to further statements or questions that we need to pick up on and question, leading to provision of relevant service advice or support.

Following the admission assessment

1 Ensure the patient has a call bell and (if appropriate) a drink within reach.
2 Ensure that documentation is complete; alert colleagues if you have uncovered any patient needs that require immediate attention.
3 Refer the patient to other professionals (e.g. physiotherapist or occupational therapist) as appropriate and according to local policy.

The information offered within this chapter is not exhaustive. It is intended to provoke thought and encourage you to reflect on your own practice. The hospital admission will undoubtedly be time-consuming and cause pressure on your working time. However, the detail you obtain at this important stage of the patient's illness will inform the wider health care community as to the needs of your patient, as illustrated in **Figure 3.3**.

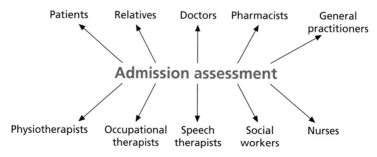

Figure 3.3 People who may access the admission assessment.

Reflection and evaluation

When you have completed an admission assessment, consider the following questions:

1 Did you find it easy to ask the patient about their normal daily activities?
2 Did any of the patient's answers surprise you?
3 Did the documentation help or hinder you in your conduct of the assessment?
4 What aspects of the documentation might you change?
5 In what circumstances might the admission assessment be less straightforward?

Further learning opportunities

1 Observe an experienced nurse undertaking an admission assessment. Take particular note of any steps taken to put the patient at ease.
2 Review admission assessments for other patients, particularly the language used to document the clinical assessment.
3 Consider liaison with family/next of kin to confirm patient perspective is shared. This holistic approach may alleviate discharge difficulties where family and patient have different views on the patient's needs.

Reminders

Don't forget that:
● The admission assessment can determine how quickly the patient's needs are addressed.
● The admission assessment should not be viewed in isolation but as the first stage of a cyclical process of assessment, planning, implementing, and evaluating care.
● Preparation is key – ensure you have the bed space ready for the patient's arrival, with documentation to hand.
● First impressions are important – make the patient feel welcome and in competent hands!

Patient scenarios

Consider what you should do in the following situations, then turn to the end of this skill to check your answers.

1 A patient is admitted to your surgical ward from a nursing home. His family live some distance away and he has to have surgery in the next 4 hours. What steps can you take during the admission assessment to reduce his anxiety?
2 You are asked to prepare a bed space for a patient waiting in the Emergency Department. The patient has chronic obstructive pulmonary disease and is thought to have an acute infection. How would you prepare the bed area?

Website

 http://www.oxfordtextbooks.co.uk/orc/ endacott

You may find it helpful to work through our short online quiz and additional scenarios intended to help you to develop and apply the skills in this chapter.

References

Access to Health Records Act (1990). HMSO, London.

Department of Health (2007). *Privacy and dignity – A report by the Chief Nursing Officer into mixed sex accommodation in hospitals* [online] **http:// www.dh.gov.uk/en/Publicationsandstatistics/ Publications/PublicationsPolicyAndGuidance/ DH_074543** accessed 20/08/08.

NHS Institute for Innovation and Improvement (2007). *Going lean in the NHS: how lean thinking will enable the NHS to get more out of the same resources.* University of Warwick.

Nursing and Midwifery Council (2007). *Advice sheet on record keeping.* NMC, London.

Orem DE (1971). *Nursing: concepts of practice.* McGraw-Hill, New York.

Orlando J (1961). *The dynamic nurse/patient relationship: function, process and principles.* GP Putnams and Sons, New York.

Roper N, Logan W, and Tierney A (1983). Nursing process, a nursing model. *Nursing Mirror*, May 25, 17–19.

Roper N, Logan W, and Tierney A (2000). *The Roper-Logan-Tierney model of nursing based on activities of living (Monograph).* Churchill Livingstone, Edinburgh.

Roy C (1976). *Introduction to nursing: an adaptational model.* Prentice Hall, Englewood Cliffs, NJ.

Salvage J (2006). Model thinking. *Nursing Standard*, **20**(17), 24–5.

Smith GB (2003). *ALERT™ Acute Life-threatening Events Recognition and Treatment: a multiprofessional course in the care of the acutely ill patient*. University of Portsmouth.

 Answers to patient scenarios

1 Introduce yourself and the patients in the immediate bed area. Ensure you take next of kin contact details from the nursing home staff or the ambulance crew and ascertain what they have been told. If the patient is able to understand, have this conversation in his presence. Orientate the patient to the ward layout and ensure he is as comfortable as possible before starting the assessment. If the nursing home has provided patient information, check the accuracy of the information with the patient and transfer relevant details onto the admission documentation.

2 Check that all relevant documentation is at the bed space. This should include: an admission pack, manual handling assessment, pressure area record sheet, observation record sheet. Ensure the bed space is clean and tidy. Attach a clean oxygen mask to the oxygen port. Check whether an intravenous infusion has been inserted in the ED; if so, put a drip stand in the bed space. Complete the patient name board.

3.3 **Planning the effective patient discharge**

Definition

Patient discharge planning can be defined as the act of facilitating the movement of a patient from one area of health care to another based on accurate assessment of their needs and subsequent implementation of an effective plan.

It is important to remember that:

- Good record keeping throughout the patient discharge will also allow for effective continuity of care and promotes communication and sharing of information between members of the interprofessional health care team (NMC 2007).
- Nursing records are subject to audit as part of the clinical governance cycle. Therefore, any discharge planning that you undertake may be subject to review. The level of detail you include may assist in the development of health care when the quality review cycle takes place.
- Planning for patient discharge should begin as soon as possible after admission; it is therefore important to engage other members of the multidisciplinary team as soon as a patient need becomes apparent.

Prior knowledge

Before getting involved in planning patient discharge, make sure you are familiar with:

- Guidelines for records and record keeping (NMC 2007).
- Local policies and guidelines relating to record keeping.
- The range of services available in the local community.
- Section 3.1 of this book, *Principles of good record keeping*.
- *Achieving timely 'simple' discharge from hospital: a toolkit for the multidisciplinary team* (Department of Health 2004).
- *Discharge from hospital: pathway, process and practice* (Department of Health 2003).
- Principles of informed consent.
- The Community Care Act *(synopsis)*.

Background

As with patient admission, there is currently no single model or template for a quality discharge plan; however, in England the NHS is seeking to standardize and improve communication and record keeping by implementing a new integrated IT system. 'NHS Connecting for Health' is providing the delivery of these systems and services, enabling information to be shared between NHS organizations across England. Similar projects are taking place across Scotland, Wales, and Ireland. This is a particularly important development when patients are discharged from a health care setting.

The patient's discharge process commences on their admission to your area. When you are questioning your patient and their carers about their present status, you need to be preparing for what will be required on discharge and putting this in place at the earliest opportunity. Patients are encouraged to expect this level of planning (see *Your guide to the NHS*, NHSE 2001) with assurance that any requirements at home will be provided as promptly as possible.

If structural changes to the home are needed, consider the amount of notice needed to facilitate this. By planning effectively, this will potentially allow the patient to maintain an optimum level of independence. For some patients, this means returning home.

If the patient has received input from social services, the service provider will need to be made aware of the patient's admission in order to suspend any support provided at home. Ensure that patient documentation prompts the person responsible for discharge planning to reinstate these resources quickly and effectively.

An effective discharge planning process enables the following to occur:

- Effective communication between health care professionals and with social services.
- The patient is able to move in a timely and safe manner to an area relevant to their needs.
- The patient is able to achieve a level of independence with support of family and social care facilities, where appropriate.

Improving discharge processes has distinct benefits for patients, the service, and health professionals (see Boxes 3.6–3.8).

Box 3.6 Benefits for patients

- Identifying expected date of discharge can help patients to plan for when they go home.
- Patients' own responsibility for elements such as transport and arrangements at home can be clarified, discussed, and agreed in advance.
- Patients' experiences can be improved when they have more information about their care and they feel included in the decisions.
- Patients have more realistic expectations of the care they will receive.
- Patients only stay in hospital for the optimum amount of time for their recovery and are less likely to pick up a health care-associated infection (HCAI). (Department of Health 2004).

Box 3.7 Benefits for the service

- Health and social care can work as a whole system, supported by a managed care approach, resulting in improved quality, better match between demand and capacity, and better use of resources such as staffed hospital beds.
- Improved discharge processes contribute to improving patient flow and the effectiveness and efficiency of the system: right patient, right place, right time.
- Increased bed days will be available for the organization, reducing queues and cancellations.
- More effective communication between hospital and community will mean more streamlined services for all.
- Consistency in approach to single assessment and services based on need – joint assessment processes mean an integrated approach and less time wasted on duplicating the assessment process by different teams (Department of Health 2004).

Box 3.8 Benefits for health professionals

- Improved discharge processes make professionals' working lives easier and clearer, seeing their role as part of the whole system with each part impacting on the effectiveness of every other part.
- The development of proactive processes and a more managed care approach to their work, potentially leading to greater job satisfaction.
- Professionals have an increased sense of responsibility, recognition, and support for the work they contribute.
- Clinical team members will be directly contributing to improving the patient's experience of health care (Department of Health 2004).

Carer involvement in the discharge process

It is essential that informal carers are engaged as early as possible and their anxieties/needs addressed throughout the hospital stay. Two decades ago, the UK Department of Health (DH) acknowledged that the majority of care is provided by informal carers and that they require sufficient help to fulfil this role (DH 1989). A more recent report identified that one in six over 65s were providing some form of informal care (Wanless 2006).

Taking on the role of carer can be viewed as a duty or obligation, and health care professionals need to assess the support that carers themselves may require. Engaging the carers from admission will allow you to identify where increased input or support is required.

Patient involvement in the discharge process

In the UK, the Department of Health promotes a partnership approach to patient discharge, with the patient taking an active role in discharge planning. A sample discharge proforma is suggested in **Figure 3.4**.

Detailed discharge planning

The 12 activities of living (Roper *et al.* 1983, 2000), used as a template for admission assessment, provide a useful framework for detailed discharge planning. For full details on these, please refer to the admission assessment skill (Section 3.2). It is essential that these questions are addressed well in advance of the time of discharge.

Consider these suggestions as prompts – they are not intended to be exhaustive:

- **Breathing** – Is any respiratory support needed? For example, oxygen at home, COPD specialist nurse?
- **Elimination** – Has the patient returned to normal bowel habit on day of discharge? Is further advice or support needed? Do they have access to a toilet on either level of home? Has a risk assessment been completed?
- **Maintaining a safe environment** – Have relevant agencies been involved in ensuring safe place of residence on discharge?
- **Communication** – Are family and external agencies aware of pending discharge? Has relevant patient and family education been provided?
- **Sleeping** – Has relevant medication been dispensed with patient, including night sedation? Has this been explained to patient and/or carers?
- **Eating and drinking** – Is patient able to maintain their own dietary needs? If not, has Meals on Wheels been contacted or have dieticians provided sufficient gastrointestinal feeds for patient prior to review by GP?

- **Personal hygiene** – Has district nurse team been contacted in order to assist patient at home on discharge? Are resources required to facilitate this? Is there provision/availability of bath chair and shower for patient at home? Can this be provided?
- **Controlling body temperature** – Has the home been prepared so patient will be warm and comfortable on arrival? Does the patient have access to hot fluids and sufficient layering of clothing at home to maintain a comfortable body temperature?
- **Working and playing** – Is patient able to return to work? If so, do they require sickness authorization for work?
- **Mobilizing** – Has the physiotherapy team been required during the hospital stay? Are they aware of discharge plan? Is transport home appropriate and has the ambulance service been contacted if required?
- **Sexuality** – Does the planned discharge environment allow for the patient to be cared for in single sex accommodation, if they wish?
- **Dying** – If relevant, has an appropriate care environment been provided to allow the patient to die with dignity or to allow them to discuss this as a concern? Has the palliative care team been contacted?

Discharging patients who have a long-term condition

Patients are increasingly discharged from health settings with a chronic condition. In general these patients fall into one of two categories: firstly, those who were living with the disease prior to their current admission and, secondly, those for whom this admission has resulted in a diagnosis of a condition that requires considerable adaptation to their previous lifestyle.

For patients with a new diagnosis, one of the goals of discharge planning is to equip them with the knowledge and skills needed to take on self-care. For some patients this will mean ensuring they have information about how to access support services. Age becomes a factor when considering communication strategies proposed for increasing self-care; sources of information are increasingly Internet-based but in 2006 less than 30% of older people (over 65) had access to the Internet and only 9% had Internet access via broadband (according to an Ofcom Consumer Panel).

Patient section **Please complete these questions and the nurse will collect the form from you.**	
Your name:	
Date:	
Is this the first time you have attended the Department?	□ Yes □ No
Do you understand your diagnosis?	□ Yes □ No
Has a clinic appointment been made for you?	□ Yes □ No □ Not sure
Have further investigations been arranged for you?	□ Yes □ No □ Not sure
Have you been prescribed any medications?	□ Yes □ No
Do you understand your medications?	□ Yes □ No □ Not sure
Do you require a sick certificate?	□ Yes □ No □ Not sure
Thank you for completing this, please hand to the nurse looking after you.	
Nurses to complete	
Clinically stable and medically fit for discharge (in notes)	□
Venflon removed	□
Discharge discussed with patient	□
GP discharge letter given to patient	□
Drugs to take home supplied and explained	□
Patient's own drugs returned	□
Dressings and equipment supplied	□
Information provided about self-care and who to contact if symptoms return	□
District nurses contacted	□
Follow-up call indicated	□ Yes □ No
Notified patient about follow-up call	□ (time)..
Clothes for discharge and keys on ward area	□
Clerical staff	
Transport arranged	□ (time)............... (how) ....
Appointments and relevant documentation	□ (with)..
Other follow-up arranged	□...
Discharging signature	(time).............................

Figure 3.4 Discharge planning proforma for completion by patient, nurse, and ward clerk. Amended from Department of Health (2004).

Accountability and responsibility

Overall legal responsibility for a patient's care remains with the named consultant during admission, hospital stay, and discharge. However, the consultant can delegate responsibility to an appropriately qualified health professional. When a task is delegated, the consultant/lead clinician assumes responsibility for delegating appropriately. The person to whom the responsibility is delegated takes on commitment and responsibility for carrying out the task in a responsible, accountable, reasonable, and logical manner in keeping with their own professional code of conduct (DH 2004).

The person to whom responsibility is delegated should be aware that they are accountable for all their actions. There should be clear lines of communication between the consultant/lead clinician and the health professional discharging the patient so that they are accessible for advice when necessary.

It is recommended that the parameters of clinical/medical stability for each individual patient are agreed with the consultant or lead clinician and recorded on a locally developed form or documented in the patient's health care record.

Reflection and evaluation

When you have completed a patient discharge, consider the following questions:

1 Did you find it easy to liaise and organize the discharge with your patient?
2 Did any events surprise you?
3 Did the documentation gained on admission help or hinder you in your conduct of the discharge?
4 What aspects of the documentation might you change?
5 In what circumstances might the discharge be less straightforward?

Further learning opportunities

1 Observe an experienced nurse planning a patient's discharge. Take particular note of any steps taken to put the patient at ease.
2 Review discharge plans for other patients, taking note of the range of professionals involved in ensuring a safe and timely discharge.

Reminders

Don't forget to:

● Initiate planning for discharge as soon as possible after admission.
● Provide appropriate support and education to enable the family to be involved as much as possible.
● Ensure communication with the multidisciplinary team is maintained.

 Patient scenarios

Consider what you should do in the following situations, then turn to the end of this skill to check your answers.

1 Mr Kershaw is adamant that he should return to his own home following major abdominal surgery. What factors should you consider when planning his discharge?
2 Mrs Jitesh is being discharged tomorrow to a residential home following surgery for breast cancer. Her wound has not yet healed and requires regular dressings. What do you need to include in your discharge planning for this patient?

Website

 http://www.oxfordtextbooks.co.uk/orc/endacott

You may find it helpful to work through our short online quiz and additional scenarios intended to help you to develop and apply the skills in this chapter.

References

Department of Health (1989). *Caring for people*. DH, London.

Department of Health (2003). *Discharge from hospital: pathway, process and practice*. DH, London.

Department of Health (2004). *Achieving timely 'simple' discharge from hospital: a toolkit for the multidisciplinary team*. DH, London.

NHS Executive (2001). *Your guide to the NHS*. HMSO, London.

Nursing and Midwifery Council (2007). *Advice sheet on record keeping*. NMC, London.

Roper N, Logan W, and Tierney A (1983). Nursing process, a nursing model. *Nursing Mirror*, May 25, 17–19.

Roper N, Logan W, and Tierney A (2000). *The Roper-Logan-Tierney model of nursing based on activities of living (Monograph)*. Churchill Livingstone, Edinburgh.

Wanless D (2006). *Securing good care for older people; taking a long term view*. London, King's Fund.

 Answers to patient scenarios

1 It is important to establish the patient's wishes as early as possible during the hospital admission; this provides as much time as possible for planning. The feasibility of Mr Kershaw's return home will depend largely on his level of independence prior to hospital admission. If he was receiving health or social services support prior to admission, these may need to be reviewed and extended. A number of other health care professionals, for example physiotherapist and occupational therapist, are likely to be involved in assessing Mr Kershaw's fitness for discharge home. This may include assessment of his home. Specific advice will be provided depending on the type of surgery, but may include avoiding stairs unless absolutely necessary; this will be difficult if he lives alone with the bathroom upstairs and kitchen downstairs. In addition, dietician advice may be required if he has to adapt his diet following surgery. If wound dressings are required, liaison with the community nursing service at an early stage is essential.

2 Ensure that community nursing services are alerted to the requirement for dressing changes and that the residential home are aware of Mrs Jitesh's needs. By their nature, residential homes do not provide nursing care; ensure Mrs Jitesh is sufficiently prepared for discharge to recognize any symptoms that may require review of the wound site. Follow your local policy for supply of wound dressings on discharge.

3.4 **Last offices**

Definition

Last offices are the last moments of care that we provide as health care professionals for patients who have recently died. It is a time in which full dignity should be provided and all religious and cultural beliefs fully met,

ensuring that the health and safety of staff, other patients, and the deceased patient's relatives is protected.

It is important to remember that:

- The deceased is your patient and you are responsible for them and their relatives/friends until they leave your care.
- As health professionals, we need to be considerate of the patient's religious and cultural needs. Local demographics will highlight changes in ethnicity; as care providers we need to be prepared to meet a wide range of needs relevant to the patient population.
- *Any* patient record can be used in evidence to investigate potential discrepancies either at local level or in a court of law. Keep in mind that the detail you record today may reliably assist you in remembering the care you delivered to your patients in many years to come. Documentation is particularly important if the patient has specific religious or cultural requirements that will affect last offices.

Prior knowledge

Before undertaking last offices, make sure you are familiar with:

1 Guidelines for records and record keeping (NMC 2007).
2 Local policies and guidelines relating to record keeping.
3 Local policies and guidelines relating to the provision of last offices.
4 Local guidelines and support on spiritual care.
5 Patient/family wishes.
6 Local infection control policies.

Background

Nursing care does not cease when a patient dies (Quested and Rudge 2003) and preparation for last offices often starts through discussion with the patient and family to ascertain their wishes.

The death of a patient can be one of the most traumatic events in your nursing career; Neuberger (2003) emphasizes the enormous demands placed on the nurse to make a difference for the dying and the bereaved when death is imminent. However, care of the dying patient can provide one of the most fulfilling periods of nursing care when carried out in a planned and organized way.

The final moment cannot be truly determined until the last breath is taken; therefore, any prior consideration to a potential death can alleviate distress for all involved. The actions included in last offices, for example washing the body, can also mark a point of closure in the relationship between the nurse and the patient (Cooke 2000).

Nurses working in specialist environments will become aware of particular conditions that are likely to result in death and can mentally prepare for this eventuality. For those nurses working in a respiratory role, for example caring for patients with cystic fibrosis, this can result in a close therapeutic relationship. However, the patient's eventual death, sometimes at a young age, can be distressing. Therefore, any planning for this likely outcome can help assure relatives and nurses that the patient's wishes are addressed.

The circumstances leading up to a patient's death vary widely, from a sudden, unexpected, traumatic death to a prolonged death surrounded by technology in an intensive care unit or a peaceful anticipated death in which symptoms are controlled.

The relationship between the nurse undertaking last offices and the deceased patient may also vary widely and you may experience a range of reactions to the death, some of which may seem out of proportion to your relationship with the patient and family. The support of colleagues is important at these times (Wilkin and Slevin 2004) and supervised reflective practice can be a useful strategy (O'Connell 2008). It is important to remember that the bereavement and counselling services offered by health services can play a useful role in supporting staff.

Verifying and certifying death

Death should be verified by a health care professional, most commonly a doctor, by checking for an apical heartbeat; some employers provide training for senior nursing staff to undertake this under agreed criteria (e.g. the expected death of a palliative care patient). An unexpected death must be verified by a doctor. Verification of death, including time and the name of the practitioner verifying death, must be recorded in the medical and nursing records.

The death must also be certified, a separate process that may occur after the body has been moved to the mortuary or funeral home; in hospital, this commonly occurs while the body is still on the ward. A death certificate must be provided by a registered medical practitioner who managed the patient during their last illness.

Rigor mortis occurs 2–6 hours after death, with full intensity within 48 hours, then disappears within another 48 hours (Robbins 1995). There are no specific requirements regarding when last offices must be completed; however, it is generally accepted practice for last offices to be undertaken as soon as possible after death, taking account of family wishes, potential infection control risks, and, in a hospital or institutional setting, the needs of other patients. It is easier to prepare the body before full rigor mortis is established.

Religious requirements

Neuberger (1999) makes it clear that it is impossible to provide last offices without knowing the patient's religious background. Therefore, it is vital that the admitting nurse establishes a full history of the patient on admission and establishes the wishes of the patient in relation to meeting religious and dying needs (Roper *et al.* 2000) – for further detail, see Section 3.2.

Having obtained this information, the nurse should take the time to understand what relevant procedures will be needed in the event of the death of the patient. This may involve some research on a particular culture or faith; health services will have prepared for this through their 'Spiritual Department' or designated representative. There should be supportive literature or a direct contact to provide advice on what will be required.

The following guidelines are provided in order to support your study (see also the Further reading section). However, these are not exhaustive, and subtle changes may exist between individuals who practise the same faith. Therefore, if in doubt, seek advice from family or an appropriate faith leader. If the patient expresses any deviation from the accepted 'norms' for their faith, ensure this is documented.

Baha'ism

- Normal last offices procedure is appropriate, but relatives may wish to pay their own respects prior to this.

- Patients of this faith must not be cremated, embalmed, or transported more than 60 minutes away from the place of death.
- A special ring may be placed on the patient's finger and under no circumstances must this be removed.
- Post-mortems or donation of bodies to medical science is perfectly acceptable should patients wish it.

Buddhism

- Nurses should be aware that there are a variety of versions of this faith so specialist advice should be sought.
- Normal last offices procedure is appropriate, but a religious representative may wish to be present.
- If prayers are required, the body should not be moved for at least 1 hour.

Christianity

- Normal last offices procedure is normally appropriate. However, there are many denominations so specialist advice should be sought.

Hinduism

- Certain readings may be required throughout the last offices so contact of local temple may assist.
- Family, in particular eldest son, may wish to be involved with the procedure and at times this may involve a large number of people. Preparation for this may be advisable. Patient should be dressed in their own clothes.
- If no relatives are present then staff of the same sex should carry out procedure wearing gloves and apron. No washing of body should be undertaken. Nurses should straighten the body, close the eyes, and support the jaw before wrapping in a sheet. No removal of jewellery should be undertaken.
- Bodies should be cremated as soon as possible and generally post-mortems are considered inappropriate.

Islam

- It is desirable in the event of death that the patient's head is facing Mecca. If this is not possible then the patient should be turned on their right side so that their face faces Mecca.
- Owing to the faith objecting to the body being touched by a non-Muslim or person of the opposite sex, the nurse should ensure they wear gloves and apron at all times. The eyes should be closed, the jaw supported, and the body straightened. The head should be turned to the right shoulder and the body covered in a white sheet.
- Toenails and fingernails should not be cut or the patient's body washed.
- Patient's body is normally taken home or to a mosque to be washed by another Muslim of the same sex. Cremation is forbidden and burial normally takes place within 24 hours.

Jehovah's Witness

- Relatives may wish to be present during last offices, either to pray or to read from the Bible. The family will inform staff should there be any special requirements, which may vary according to the patient's country of origin. Normal routine is appropriate.
- Jehovah's Witnesses usually refuse post-mortem unless absolutely necessary. Organ donation may be acceptable.

Judaism

- The family will contact their own Rabbi if they have one. If not, the hospital chaplaincy will advise. Prayers are recited by those present.
- Traditionally the body is left for about 8 minutes before being moved while a feather is placed across the lips and nose to detect any signs of breath.
- Usually close relatives will straighten the body, but nursing staff are permitted to perform any procedure for preserving dignity and honour. The body should be handled as little as possible but nurses may, while wearing gloves:
  - Close the eyes.
  - Tie up the jaw.
  - Put the arms parallel and close to the sides of the body, leaving the hands open. Straighten the patient's legs.
  - Remove tubes unless contraindicated.

● Watchers stay with the body until burial (normally completed within 24 hours of death). In the period before burial a separate non-denominational room is appreciated, where the body can be placed with its feet towards the door.

● It is not possible for funerals to take place on the Sabbath (between sunset on Friday and sunset on Saturday). If death occurs during the Sabbath, the body will remain with the watchers until the end of the Sabbath. Advice should be sought from the relatives. In some areas, the Registrar's office will arrange to open on Sundays and Bank Holidays to allow for the registration of death where speedy burial is required for religious reasons. The Jewish Burial Society will know whether this service is offered in the local area.

● Post-mortems are permitted only if required by law. Organ donation is sometimes permitted.

● Cremation is unlikely but some non-Orthodox Jews are now accepting this in preference to burial.

Sikhism

● Family members (especially the eldest son) and friends will be present if they are able.

● Usually the family takes responsibility for the last offices, but nursing staff may be asked to close the patient's eyes, support the jaw, straighten the body, and wrap it in a plain white sheet.

● The family will wash and dress the deceased person's body. Note the 5 Ks in **Box 3.10**.

● Post-mortems are only permitted if required by law. Sikhs are always cremated.

● Organ donation is permitted but some Sikhs refuse this as they do not wish the body to be mutilated.

Box 3.10 The 5 Ks in Sikhism

Do not remove the '5 *Ks*', which are personal objects sacred to Sikhs:

■ *Kesh*: do not cut hair or beard or remove turban.
■ *Kanga*: do not remove the semi-circular comb, which fixes the uncut hair.
■ *Kara*: do not remove bracelet worn on the wrist.
■ *Kaccha*: do not remove the special shorts worn as underwear.
■ *Kirpan*: do not remove the sword: usually a miniature sword is worn.

Zoroastrianism

● Customary last offices are often acceptable to Zoroastrian patients.

● The family may wish to be present during, or participate in, the preparation of the body.

● Orthodox Parsees require a priest to be present, if possible.

● After washing, the body is dressed in the *Sadra* (white cotton or muslin shirt symbolizing purity) and *Kusti* (girdle woven of 72 strands of lambs' wool symbolizing the 72 chapters of the *Yasna* (Liturgy)).

● Relatives may cover the patient's head with a white cap or scarf.

● It is important that the funeral takes place as soon as possible after death.

● Burial and cremation are acceptable. Post-mortems are forbidden unless required by law.

● Organ donation is forbidden by religious law.

Further advice is provided in *A guide to cultural and spiritual awareness* published by Nursing Standard (2005).

Special considerations

Legal requirements

There are a number of circumstances in which the procedure for last offices has to be adjusted (see **Table 3.4**).

Death of an infected patient

Infection Control Services (2006) state four key points that must be attended to when an infected patient dies:

1 Place the patient in a waterproof body bag.

2 An infected body should be handled using the same precautions that were in place when the patient was alive.

3 According to local policy, complete a risk/hazard form to accompany the patient to the mortuary.

4 No religious procedure that carries the risk of spread of infection should be carried out on an infected body.

Check your local policy to clarify what categories of infected patient would be handled in this way.

Personal interpretations of death

A patient's death will affect each member of staff differently, depending on the relationship that they have developed with the patient, together with their own cultural and religious beliefs. Be aware that the way in which you present yourself to those around you will affect their expression of grief. If you are a student assisting with last offices for the first time, look at how your colleagues handle the situation.

Nurses may add their own personal touch to the formal last offices procedure. Examples of how this may occur could include the following, observed in colleagues who displayed sensitivity and a caring approach, despite the pressure of a busy ward. Some of these may appear quirky but highlight practices that you may witness:

- After the moment of death, place the body in a relaxed position and cover with sheet.

- Where possible, leave the body in privacy for a few minutes' rest, before undertaking the last offices procedure.

- When the patient has been wrapped and labelled, place a flower on top of the sheet and tape into place before requesting porters to transport the deceased patient to the mortuary.

Although these are not required practices, they demonstrate an intrinsic disposition to care rather than perform a task. However, regardless of the personal style of individual nurses, it is important to ensure that any special considerations, either for religious or legal reasons, are adhered to.

Table 3.4 Legal requirements associated with circumstances of death

Circumstance	Requirement
Death occurring within 24 hours of an operation.	All tubes, drains, catheters, and cannulae must be left in position. Post-mortem examination will be required to establish the cause of death. Any tubes, drains, etc. may have been a major contributing factor to the death (e.g. sepsis arising from infected central venous catheter).
Unexpected death or unknown cause of death.	As above. Post-mortem examination of the body will be required to establish the cause of death.
Patient brought into hospital who is already deceased.	As above, unless patient seen by a medical practitioner within 14 days before death. In this instance the attending medical officer may complete the death certificate if they are clear as to the cause of death.
Patient who dies after insertion of radioactive material.	Wards caring for patients with radioactive implants should have procedures in place for last offices. These are likely to include: 1 Informing the medical physics department. 2 Removal of radioactive sources after death is confirmed but *before* last offices are undertaken. 3 Use of a Geiger counter to check that all sources have been removed. The time and date of removal of the sources should be recorded.
Patient and/or relative wishes to donate organs/tissues for transplantation.	Contact local transplant coordinator as soon as decision is made to donate organs/tissue and before last offices is attempted. Obtain verbal and written consent from next of kin, as per local policy. Prepare body as per transplant coordinator's instructions (Travis 2002).

Procedure

Preparation

Prepare yourself

If this is the first time you have performed last offices, ask a more experienced nurse to assist. Check the patient's records for any specific wishes to be followed after death. If the patient's religious or cultural beliefs require certain procedures that you are unfamiliar with, seek advice from an appropriate faith leader.

Prepare the family

Ensure family are informed as soon as possible after death is confirmed. Provide verbal and written information regarding sources of support. If possible, provide a private room for family. Ascertain whether relatives wish to view the body; this should happen before last offices are completed. If relatives or next of kin are not contactable by telephone or via the GP, the police will attempt to locate them.

Family members may wish to undertake or assist with last offices; for some people, this provides a degree of comfort (Wong and Chan 2007, Marie Curie 2008). This option should be available whether the patient dies in hospital, in a residential setting, or at home.

Prepare the equipment/environment

Ensure you have equipment for washing the patient, shaving, combing hair, mouth care, and covering wounds or cannula sites. In addition, gather the documentation you need, according to local policy. This will include identification labels, notification of death cards, and the hospital property record book. Ascertain whether the patient is to be dressed in a shroud or their own clothes. Check the bed for any 'sharps' that may have been left on the bed during the urgency of resuscitation and dispose of them appropriately.

Step-by-step guide to last offices

Step		Rationale
1	Put on gloves and apron.	To reduce risk of cross-infection.
2	Lay the patient on their back with the assistance of two nurses (according to your employer's manual handling policy).	
3	Remove all but one pillow. Support the jaw by placing a pillow or rolled-up towel on the chest underneath the jaw.	To maintain the patient's dignity and to assist with future management of the body.
4	Straighten the limbs. Remove any mechanical aids such as pressure-relieving pads, patient-controlled analgesia pumps, etc., subject to the advice in Table 3.4.	
5	Document actions in patient records.	
6	Close the patient's eyes by applying light pressure to the eyelids for 30 seconds.	To maintain the patient's dignity and for aesthetic reasons. Closure of eyes will also provide tissue protection in case of corneal donation (Green and Green 1992).

7	Drain the bladder by pressing on the lower abdomen.	To prevent leakage that may pose a health hazard to staff.
8	Depending on local policy, pack orifices with gauze if fluid secretion continues or is anticipated. If excessive leaking of bodily fluids occurs, consider suctioning.	To prevent leakage that may pose a health hazard to staff. In some settings, this will be undertaken by mortuary staff – check your local policy.
9	Exuding wounds should be covered with a clean absorbent dressing and secured with an occlusive dressing. **If a post-mortem is required**, existing dressings should be left *in situ* and covered.	To prevent leakage that may pose a health hazard to staff.
10	Remove drainage tubes, etc. unless otherwise stated and document actions and any tubes remaining, e.g. CVP lines. Cover open drainage sites and seal any tubes with a spigot or cannula. **If a post-mortem is required** drainage tubes, etc. should be left *in situ*.	To prevent leakage that may pose a health hazard to staff.
11	Wash the patient, unless requested not to do so for religious/cultural reasons. If necessary, shave a male patient.	For hygienic and aesthetic reasons.
12	Clean the patient's mouth using a foam stick to remove any debris and secretions. Clean dentures and replace them in the mouth if possible. If this is not possible, place dentures in a clean, labelled denture pot and send to the mortuary with the body.	For hygienic and aesthetic reasons.
13	Remove all jewellery (in the presence of another nurse) unless requested by the patient's family to do otherwise. Jewellery remaining on the patient should be documented on the 'notification of death' form. Record the jewellery and other valuables in the patient's property book and store the items according to local policy.	To address legal requirements, local policy, and relatives' wishes.
14	Dress the patient in night clothes, other personal clothing, or a shroud, depending on hospital policy or relatives' wishes.	To meet the wishes of the deceased patient and the family.
15	Label one wrist and one ankle with an identification label. In the hospital setting, include the name of the ward on which the patient died, according to local policy. Complete any documents such as notification of death cards. Tape appropriate documentation securely to clothing or shroud.	To ensure correct and easy identification of the body in the mortuary.

continued overleaf

16	Wrap the body in a mortuary sheet, ensuring that the face and feet are covered and that all limbs are held securely in position.	To avoid possible damage to the body during transfer and to prevent distress to colleagues, e.g. portering staff.
17	Secure the sheet with tape.	To avoid health and safety hazards associated with using pins.
18	Place the body in a sheet and then a body bag if leakage of body fluids is a problem or is anticipated, or if the patient has an infectious disease.	To prevent leakage that may pose a health hazard to staff.
19	Tape the second notification of death card to the outside of the sheet (or body bag).	For ease of identification of the body in the mortuary.
20	Screen off the area where removal of the body will occur.	To avoid causing unnecessary distress to other patients, relatives, and staff.
21	Remove gloves and apron. Dispose of equipment according to local policy and wash hands.	To minimize risk of cross-infection.
22	Record all details and actions in the patient records. Include time of death, names of those present, and names of those informed.	To ensure optimal communication.
23	Transfer property and patient records to the appropriate administrative department.	To facilitate timely production of death certificate and the collection of property by the next of kin.

Following the procedure

1 Ensure the patient is moved to the chapel of rest/ mortuary as soon as possible. Decomposition of the body may pose a health and safety hazard for those handling the body (Cooke 2000).

2 Other patients are often aware that a death is expected or has occurred. Be prepared to answer their questions honestly. It is also important to offer support and reassurance and to allay any misconceptions and fears.

3 If the patient is to be moved straight from the ward to the undertakers, contact the senior nurse for the hospital. There are a number of additional legal procedures to be followed including obtaining a Certificate for Burial or Cremation from the local registry office and obtaining written authority from the next of kin for removal of the body. Your employer should have policies (and a named person) in place to manage this situation.

4 If the relatives want to view the body after it has been removed from the ward, contact the mortuary staff.

The hospital chaplaincy or bereavement support officer may accompany relatives to the mortuary viewing room, according to local policy.

Reflection and evaluation

When you have completed last offices, consider the following questions:

1 Did you find it easy asking what a patient's wishes were in relation to religious and dying needs?

2 Did any events surprise you?

3 Did the documentation gained on admission help or hinder you in your conduct of last offices?

4 In what circumstances might last offices be less straightforward?

Further learning opportunities

1 Observe an experienced nurse breaking the news of a patient's death to next of kin. Take particular note

of how the experienced nurse responds to difficult questions.

2 Observe an experienced nurse break the news of a patient's death to fellow patients.

Reminders

Don't forget:

- That you are responsible for the deceased person and their family until they leave your care.
- That you too may need help and support after participating in last offices.

Patient scenarios

Consider what you should do in the following situations, then turn to the end of this skill to check your answers.

1 A patient dies unexpectedly 6 hours after surgery. What do you need to consider when preparing to undertake last offices?

2 Why is the admission assessment important when preparing to undertake last offices?

Website

 http://www.oxfordtextbooks.co.uk/orc/ endacott

You may find it helpful to work through our short online quiz and additional scenarios intended to help you to develop and apply the skills in this chapter.

References

Cooke H (2000). *A practical guide to holistic care at the end of life*. Butterworth-Heinemann, Oxford.

Green J and Green M (1992). *Dealing with death: practices and procedures*. Chapman and Hall, London.

Infection Control Services (2006). *Last offices on infected patients* [online] **http://www. infectioncontrolservices.co.uk/documents/policies/ Last%20Offices%20on%20Infected%20Patients% 20Policy%202006.pdf** accessed 20/08/08.

Marie Curie Cancer Care (2008). *Bereavement: helping you to deal with the death of someone close to you* [online] **http://www.mariecurie.org.uk/**

NR/rdonlyres/CB08CE6E-C711-4227-910A- A694704BBD54/0/Bereavementbooklet.pdf accessed 20/08/08.

Neuberger J (1999). *Caring for dying people of different faiths*. Lisa Sainsbury Foundation, London.

Neuberger J (2003). Commentary: a good death is possible in the NHS. *British Medical Journal*, 326, 34.

Nursing and Midwifery Council (2007). *Advice sheet on record keeping*. NMC, London.

Nursing Standard (2005). *A guide to cultural and spiritual awareness* [online] **http://www. crusebereavementcare.org.uk/BPPResearch/ CulturalAware.pdf** accessed 13/08/08.

O'Connell E (2008). Therapeutic relationships in critical care nursing: a reflection on practice. *Nursing in Critical Care*, 13, 138–143.

Quested B and Rudge T (2003). Nursing care of dead bodies: a discursive analysis of last offices. *Journal of Advanced Nursing*, 41, 553–60.

Robbins J, ed. (1995). *Caring for the dying patient and the family*, 3rd edition. Chapman and Hall, London.

Roper N, Logan W, and Tierney A (2000). *The Roper-Logan-Tierney model of nursing based on activities of living (Monograph)*. Churchill Livingstone, Edinburgh.

Travis S (2002). *Procedure for the care of patients who die in hospital*. Royal Marsden NHS Trust, London.

Wilkin K and Slevin E (2004). The meaning of caring to nurses: an investigation into the nature of caring work in an intensive care unit. *Journal of Clinical Nursing*, 13, 50–59.

Wong MS and Chan SWC (2007). The experiences of Chinese family members of terminally ill patients – a qualitative study. *Journal of Clinical Nursing*, 16, 2359–64.

Useful further reading and websites

Further advice regarding religious practices can be found at the following websites:

Baha'ism – **http://www.bahai.org.uk**
Buddhism – **http://www.nbo.org.uk**
Christianity – **http://www.ccj.org.uk**
Hinduism – **http://www.hinducounciluk.org**
Islam – **http://www.mcb.org.uk**
Jehovah's Witness – **http://www.watchtower.org/**
Judaism – **http://www.bod.org.uk**
Sikhism – **http://www.sikhs.org**
Zoroastrianism – **http://www.avesta.org**

Answers to patient scenarios

1 Ensure the relatives are told immediately. It is possible that they haven't visited the patient since before surgery so they may wish to view the body. This should take place before last offices. The patient will undergo a post-mortem to ascertain cause of death, so all drains, cannulae, catheters, and tubes must be left in place. The religion of the patient may mean that post-mortem is unacceptable; the medical staff should be alerted to this as soon as possible in order for appropriate discussions to take place with the family.

2 Essential information is gathered during the admission assessment, including next of kin contact details, the patient's religious preferences, and the storage (or return to relatives) of any valuables that the patient may have brought into hospital. Admission assessment also provides an opportunity to talk with patients and relatives about the possibility of dying.

Essential skills

Skills

4.1 **Infection prevention and control**

Definition

Health care-associated infections (HCAIs) are infections acquired as a result of a person's health care treatment (Department of Health (DH) 2006). Infection prevention and control can be defined as a series of strategies and practices that aim to reduce the risk of infection to staff, patients, and others where care is delivered. This can be achieved by practising the following skills, which help prevent the transmission of organisms:

- Hand washing.
- Putting on sterile and non-sterile gloves.
- Use of disposable aprons.
- Use and disposal of sharps.
- Waste disposal.
- Dealing with spillages.
- Providing source isolation.
- Aseptic technique.

It is important to remember that:

- Many HCAIs are preventable.
- Each health care worker has a duty to provide safe care to the patients under their care.
- Following best practice in infection prevention will contribute to the delivery of safe care.

Prior knowledge

Before undertaking the skills associated with infection prevention and control, make sure you are familiar with:

1 Principles of microbiology – for example how bacteria multiply; how infection is spread; how microorganisms enter the body; differences in structure and mode of action between viruses, bacteria, and fungi.
2 The inflammatory response.
3 Your employer's infection control policies.
4 Steps taken to reduce MRSA in your place of employment.

Background

The estimated cost per year of HCAIs is approximately £1 billion; around 9% of patients in hospitals in England at any one time have an HCAI (National Audit Office (NAO) 2000). In 20 000 patients per year in England, an HCAI is a contributory factor towards their deaths, while 5000 patients have their deaths attributable directly to an HCAI. It has been estimated that 15–30% of these infections are preventable (Plowman *et al.* 1999). Good infection prevention and control reduces morbidity and mortality, thereby reducing costs to the health care community (Wilson 2006).

Chain of infection

For infection to spread from person to person, certain factors need to be in place. These are termed 'the chain of infection' and are represented in **Figure** 4.1.

Infectious agent

Microorganisms such as bacteria and viruses are the causative agents of most HCAIs. These can be either endogenous organisms (part of the body's normal flora) or exogenous (originating from outside the body) (Bannister *et al.* 2000).

Source of infection

The reservoir of infection is where microorganisms such as bacteria and viruses can survive and may be a patient or member of staff with an infection, a piece of equipment, food or water, the environment, or an animal (McCulloch 2000).

Portal of exit

Organisms have to be able to leave the reservoir to enable them to spread. The route by which they leave the reservoir, or source, varies according to the organism and their mode of transmission.

Modes of transmission

There are three main methods used by microorganisms to travel away from the source or reservoir of infection:

- Direct contact – this can be with body surfaces or fluids of an infected individual.
- Indirect contact – people, animals, or inanimate objects can be vehicles on which organisms can be transferred. Food, water, and equipment may also provide means by which organisms are able to spread.
- Air – organisms need to be carried through the air on particles such as water, respiratory droplets, or dust. (Wilson 2006)

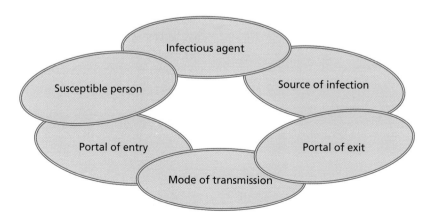

Figure 4.1 The chain of infection. These factors need to be in place for infection to spread from person to person.

Portal of entry

The chain of infection is complete when a microorganism enters the susceptible individual, enabling the development of an infection. The portals of entry are the skin, ingestion, inhalation, mucous membranes, invasive procedures, and sexual contact.

Susceptible person

Some groups of individuals are more at risk than others of acquiring an infection. These groups include:

- The very young
- The very old
- Surgical patients
- Individuals with underlying conditions such as diabetes
- Immunosuppressed individuals
- Those undergoing invasive procedures
- The malnourished
  (McCulloch 2000)

Breaking the chain of infection

As with any chain, it becomes useless if any one of the links is broken. Infection prevention and control policies, procedures, and practices are designed to break various links of the chain of infection. These include source isolation, use of personal protective clothing, and hand decontamination.

Standard principles for preventing HCAIs

Standard precautions should be applied at all times by all health care practitioners when caring for all patients. They comprise:

1 Environmental hygiene.
2 Decontamination of equipment.
3 Hand hygiene.
4 Use of personal protective equipment.
5 Use and disposal of sharps.
6 Disposal of waste.
  (DH 2007, Pratt *et al.* 2007).

1. Environmental hygiene

Good hygiene in clinical environments is recognized as an important factor in preventing and controlling HCAIs. Investigations of outbreaks of infection suggest that there is an association between poor environmental hygiene

and the transmission of organisms that may cause HCAIs (Pratt *et al.* 2007). All health care staff have a responsibility to follow local policies relating to the decontamination of the environment as well as the decontamination of equipment that is used by more than one patient.

2. Decontamination of equipment

It is imperative that equipment and medical devices that are to be used as part of care delivery have been decontaminated appropriately and are safe to be used. Manufacturers' recommendations should always be followed when decontaminating equipment of any sort.

Single-use devices

Single-use products are labelled with the words 'single use' or similar and marked with the symbol: ②

A single-use device, for example a needle or a urinary catheter, should be used once only and then discarded. Therefore, any piece of equipment designated as single-use should not be decontaminated and re-used but should be disposed of as clinical waste after use.

Single patient use

An item that has been designated as 'single patient use' may be used on more than one occasion but must only be used by one patient, e.g. nebulizers, nasal cannulae. The piece of equipment should be decontaminated after each use and then disposed of when no longer required by that patient or at the duration recommended by the manufacturer (NHS Estates 2004).

It is important that equipment that should be sterile is checked before use on a patient. Equipment should be checked for any breaks in the wrapping. If the wrapping has become wet, the equipment should not be used as this would allow organism transmission through the wrapping and present a risk of microbial contamination.

There are three levels of decontamination:

- **Cleaning**, which is the physical removal of organic matter and organisms using detergent and water, is required for items to be used on intact skin. It is also a prerequisite for items that are going to be disinfected or sterilized.
- **Disinfection** is a process by which harmful organisms are removed but spores are not usually

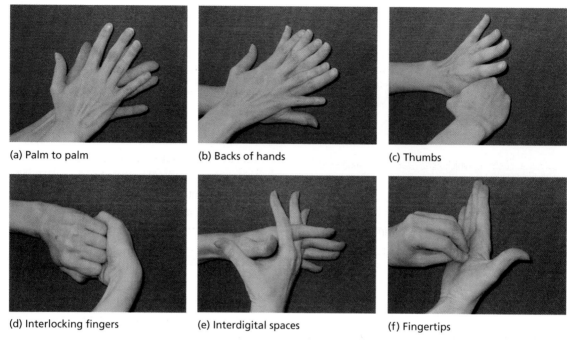

(a) Palm to palm   (b) Backs of hands   (c) Thumbs

(d) Interlocking fingers   (e) Interdigital spaces   (f) Fingertips

Figure 4.2 The six-step hand wash technique (with kind permission of Kate Burke).

destroyed. This process is necessary for equipment that has been used on the mucous membranes or that is likely to be contaminated with organisms that are easily transferable.

- **Sterilization** destroys all microorganisms and spores and is required for high-risk equipment that penetrates the skin and/or mucous membranes or enters a sterile cavity of the body.

3. Hand hygiene

Although there is no conclusive evidence that the presence of a pathogenic organism in the environment is necessarily the cause of HCAIs, the evidence does support the need for hand hygiene before patient contact to remove any prior contamination of the hands from the environment. As the hands are covered in microorganisms, they are a potential route of infection spread and must therefore be decontaminated appropriately. Some of the organisms are part of the resident flora and others can be classified as transient. Transient microorganisms can be picked up during care activities and may be transported to another person, increasing the risk of an infection.

Decontamination of the hands is a key aspect of infection prevention and control. It is important that the hands are decontaminated using the correct technique (Ayliffe *et al.* 1978) at the appropriate times and using the most suitable decontamination agents. Ayliffe *et al.* specified six steps that must be carried out during hand washing, as shown in **Figure 4.2**.

Hands must be decontaminated before and after each episode of patient contact (Pratt *et al.* 2007).

It is important to look after your hands when working in health care. Moisturizing hands and maintaining skin integrity is necessary outside of working hours. Nails should be kept short and smooth. Any rough edges around the nails and nail beds can provide an environment for microbial growth.

Hands *must* be decontaminated before and after contact with a patient or their environment, after any contact that may result in hands becoming contaminated, before handling food and medicines, and at the beginning and end of duty (even when going for breaks!). **Figure 4.3** shows how to choose which hand decontamination product to use.

Soap and water should be used when removing organic matter from the hands and when decontaminating

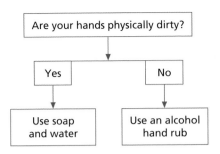

Figure 4.3 Choosing which hand decontamination product to use.

hands while caring for patients with diarrhoea which may be related to *Clostridium difficile* (Pratt *et al.* 2007). *Clostridium difficile* spores are not killed by alcohol-based skin disinfectants.

It is preferable to use a hand washbasin with elbow-operated or non-touch mixer taps when undertaking hand washing. Liquid soap or antimicrobial skin disinfectant should also be available in appropriate containers, and disposable paper hand towels should be used for drying hands. These should be disposed of in a foot-operated waste bin. However, in the community it is often difficult to achieve this. Portable preparations of liquid soap are available for community staff. If elbow-operated taps are not available then the used paper towel should be used to turn off the taps.

Alcohol-based hand rubs can be used as an alternative agent to soap and water where hands are physically clean (i.e. not contaminated with organic matter or soil). In addition, most manufacturers recommend that hands are washed with soap and water after every five applications of alcohol hand gel.

Alcohol-based hand rub or gel or **antimicrobial hand wash** should be used prior to performing an invasive procedure.

It is essential to remember that alcohol hand disinfection products must only be used on physically clean hands.

Step-by-step guide to hand washing with soap and water

▶ Step	Rationale
1 Set the taps to run water at a temperature and speed that is comfortable, and wet hands.	Washing hands is likely to be more effective if the water is at a comfortable temperature.
2 Apply enough liquid soap or skin disinfectant to create a lather.	There should be sufficient soap applied to allow lathering of all surfaces of the hands.
3 Rub the soap into all areas of the hands and wrists.	Any surfaces that are not covered may leave contamination on the hands.
4 Rinse the lather off the hands, ensuring it is all removed.	Organisms will be rinsed away with the lather.
5 Turn off the taps using elbows or a non-touch technique.	Avoid recontamination of the hands by touching taps.
6 Dry the hands thoroughly using disposable paper towels, starting with the fingertips and working down the rest of the hands and wrists.	Thorough drying of the hands reduces the risk of sore skin and produces a less favourable environment for microbial growth.
7 Dispose of the paper towels in a foot-operated waste bin using a non-touch technique.	Avoid recontamination of the hands by touching the lid of the waste bin.

Step-by-step guide to hand decontamination with alcohol

Step		Rationale
1	Apply alcohol rub/gel in sufficient quantity to cover both hands and wrists.	There should be sufficient product applied to allow coverage of all surfaces of the hands.
2	Rub the hands together briskly for approximately 10–15 seconds, ensuring that all areas of the hands and wrists are covered with gel.	Any surfaces that are not covered may leave contamination on the hands.
3	Keep rubbing hands until they feel dry and not sticky.	Rubbing the hands will help the effectiveness of the product.

4. Use of personal protective equipment

Personal protective equipment (PPE) such as non-sterile gloves, disposable aprons, and eye and mouth protection helps protect staff from infection spread and reduces the opportunity for microorganism transmission (Infection Control Nurses Association 1999). The type of PPE required relates to the level of risk associated with the activity about to be undertaken:

- When there is no risk of contact with blood and/or body fluids, no protective clothing is required.
- When contact with blood and/or body fluids is expected but there is a **low risk of splashing**, non-sterile gloves and a disposable apron should be worn.
- When contact with blood and/or body fluids is expected and there is also a **high risk of splashing**, non-sterile gloves, a disposable apron, and facial protection for eyes, nose, and mouth are required.
- When caring for patients in source isolation, PPE should be worn. Details of specific equipment required will be dependent on the organism being isolated. Local policies should be followed (Wilson 2006).

Figure 4.4 provides an overview of which type of gloves to use in different situations. Non-sterile latex, vinyl, or nitrile gloves should be used as single-use items. They should be put on immediately before carrying out a clinical procedure and be removed immediately after completion of the procedure (Pratt *et al.* 2007). Gloves must comply with the standard set by the British Standards Institution (2000).

If staff or patients have natural rubber latex allergies, alternatives to latex gloves should be available for their use.

Use of masks and eye protection

Eye protection and masks should be available for use in clinical settings where there is a risk of splashing of blood and/or body fluids onto the face. Surgical and obstetric procedures are those most commonly requiring this type of PPE (Wilson 2006).

All PPE should be stored appropriately to prevent the risk of contamination prior to use. Community staff should be aware of how PPE is stored in patients' homes to reduce contamination prior to use.

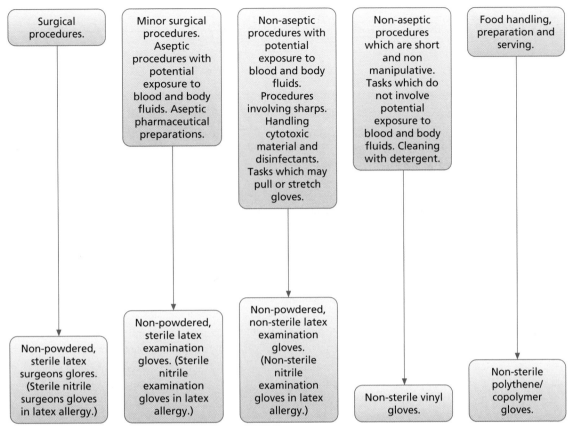

Figure 4.4 Choosing which type of gloves to use.

Step-by-step guide to putting on non-sterile gloves

Step		Rationale
1	Hands should be decontaminated before putting on gloves.	The warm, moist environment inside the gloves encourages microbial growth.
2	Well-fitting gloves should be chosen.	This will ease the donning process and improve dexterity while wearing the gloves.
3	After use, gloves should be removed without contaminating the wrists or hands.	Organisms and organic matter should not be transferred onto the hands during the disposal process.
4	Gloves should be disposed of in a clinical waste bin.	Used gloves are classified as clinical waste.
5	Hands should be thoroughly decontaminated.	Any contamination of the hands that may have occurred during the activity must be removed to avoid transmitting infection.

Step-by-step guide to using disposable aprons

Step		Rationale
1	Decontaminate hands.	Hands should be decontaminated before and after every clinical procedure.
2	Place the apron over the head, avoiding contact with clothing and hair.	Avoid contaminating the hands while putting on the apron.
3	Tie loosely around the waist.	The apron needs to be securely tied.
4	After use, the apron should be removed by snapping the neckband, folding down the top part of the apron, snapping the ties around the waist, and then folding the apron while only making contact with the inside of the apron.	Avoid handling the parts of the apron that are likely to be contaminated.
5	Dispose of used apron into a clinical waste bin.	Used disposable aprons are classified as clinical waste.
6	Thoroughly decontaminate hands.	Hands should be decontaminated before and after every clinical procedure.

5. Use and disposal of sharps

A 'sharp' is any item that may cause a laceration or puncture the skin, e.g. needles, scalpel blades, suture removers, glass (Wilson 2006).

An 'inoculation injury' is an injury sustained following contact with a 'sharp' or splashing of blood or body fluid onto mucous membranes or non-intact skin.

The risk of a health care worker acquiring an infection from an inoculation injury is related to the level of contamination of the sharp, the severity of the injury sustained, and the presence of a pathogenic organism in the blood or body fluid. There have been a number of cases of health care workers who have acquired a blood-borne virus such as human immunodeficiency virus (HIV) or hepatitis B virus (HBV) through such injuries (Wilson 2006).

Staff working in the community should ensure that they have a dedicated community-sized sharps container and that it is closed using its temporary closure mechanism when in transit to reduce risks of spillage and injury.

Step-by-step guide to use and disposal of sharps

Step	Rationale
1 Take a sharps disposal container with you when carrying out a procedure that entails the disposal of a used sharp.	Disposal of used sharps as near as possible avoids the need for carrying an item that may cause injury.
2 Never re-sheath a used needle.	Re-sheathing of a used needle increases the risk of an inoculation injury.
3 Dispose of the used needle and syringe as a complete item into an approved container.	Manipulation of used sharp instruments increases the risk of inoculation injury.
4 Always dispose of sharps that you have used and do not pass them to anyone else to dispose of.	Handing sharp instruments to someone else for disposal increases the risk of an inoculation injury.
5 Sharps disposal containers should be sealed when two-thirds full and disposed of according to hospital policy. They should *not* be placed inside a yellow bag for disposal.	Overfilling sharps disposal containers increases the risk of waste handlers and other users sustaining an injury.

6. Disposal of waste

It is important that any waste produced in the clinical setting is segregated appropriately at the point of production. This is to ensure that the waste enters the correct waste management stream and therefore poses the minimum of risk to waste handlers (Wilson 2006). There are also considerable financial and environmental costs involved in waste disposal that are optimized when the correct procedures are followed (Hilton 2004).

Step-by-step guide to use and disposal of sharps

Step-by-step guide to waste disposal

Step		Rationale
1	Place waste in the correct colour-coded bag according to local policy.	Different bags are treated according to the type of waste they contain and the level of risk that is posed to handlers.
2	All waste bags should be labelled with details of the source of waste.	Waste should be traceable to the point of production in case of incident in the handling process.
3	Never fill a waste bag more than two-thirds full.	Overfilled bags are difficult to seal and can cause problems for waste handlers.
4	Always wear PPE when changing or handling waste bags.	This will protect the skin in case of incident.
5	Use the swan neck technique when sealing bags ready for disposal.	This safe method of sealing bags reduces risk of spillage.
6	If a bag splits or spills, put on PPE and re-bag in the appropriate colour bag.	Minimal handling of bag contents will reduce the risk of injury.

Spillages

All spillages of blood and/or body fluids should be dealt with promptly by an appropriate member of staff. The procedure for dealing with such a spillage will vary between organizations but the key principles set out here will apply.

Staff working in the community should be aware that using hypochlorite on patients' own soft furnishings is not recommended. Refer to local policies for advice.

Step-by-step guide to dealing with a spillage

Step		Rationale
1	Put on a disposable apron and disposable, non-sterile gloves.	Protective clothing reduces the risk of contamination of clothing and hands.
2	Facial protection against aerosolization may be required for large spills.	Some organisms that may be present in the spillage may pose a risk of infection by the inhalation route.
3	Absorb liquid using disposable paper towels and dispose of these in a yellow clinical waste bag, or use chlorine-based granules to absorb liquid.	This will reduce the area of contamination.

4	Clear with disposable paper towels and dispose of these in a clinical waste bag.	Contaminated waste should be treated as clinical waste and disposed of accordingly.
5	Clean and dry the area using general purpose detergent, following local cleaning procedures.	Any organic matter will need to be removed to render the area safe.
6	Disinfect using 1% sodium hypochlorite solution (1000 ppm).	This will inactivate any virus particles that may be present.
7	Remove protective clothing and dispose of in a clinical waste bag.	Used protective clothing is classified as clinical waste and should be disposed of accordingly.
8	Wash and dry hands thoroughly.	Hands should be decontaminated before and after every clinical procedure.

Source isolation precautions

The purpose of source isolation is to minimize the risk of transmission of pathogenic organisms from the source patient to others at risk (Wilson 2006). Successful source isolation is achieved by ensuring that procedures are followed that are appropriate to the route of transmission of the organism being isolated.

Step-by-step guide to providing source isolation

Step		Rationale
1	Patients requiring isolation should be nursed in a single room with the door shut.	Transmission by the airborne route can be significantly reduced by nursing patients in single rooms.
2	PPE should be put on before entering the isolation room.	Gloves and aprons should be worn when dealing with infective material, e.g. respiratory secretions, diarrhoea, vomit. Masks should be worn when caring for patients with certain respiratory infections. Local policies should be followed.
3	Following care delivery the PPE should be removed and disposed of into a yellow clinical waste bag inside the isolation room.	Disposing of waste in the room reduces the risk of organisms being spread outside the isolation area.
4	Hands should be decontaminated inside the isolation room.	This is to remove any contamination of the hands acquired during the care of the patient.
5	Hands should be decontaminated using alcohol rub/gel on leaving the room.	This is to ensure any subsequent contamination of the hands is removed on leaving the room.

Aseptic technique

Many invasive procedures that are carried out in clinical practice require an aseptic technique to be used to minimize the risk of introducing pathogens into a vulnerable part of the body (Hilton 2004). The aim of the technique is to reduce contamination during the process of the invasive procedure. Clinical teams are required to demonstrate high standards of aseptic technique (DH 2003). Staff working in patients' own homes should follow the principles of asepsis, ensuring that they work wherever possible from a clean surface covered with a sterile field.

Use of sterile gloves

Sterile gloves may be required to protect the patient during clinical procedures including performing dressings, catheter insertion, and the handling of intravenous lines. Pairs of sterile gloves that may be used when carrying out an aseptic procedure are packaged with the cuffs folded down. This enables the gloves to be put on the hands without contamination. The first glove to be put on should only be handled by the cuff and the second glove should only be touched by the other gloved hand.

Step-by-step guide to putting on a pair of sterile gloves

Step		Rationale
1	Open the non-sterile outer packaging and place the gloves on a clean dry surface.	A clean environment will reduce the risk of contamination.
2	Decontaminate the hands.	Hands should always be decontaminated prior to applying sterile gloves.
3	Open the inner sterile wrapping, exposing the gloves with the cuffs facing downwards.	The position facilitates the safe donning of the gloves.
4	Pick up the first glove by the cuff, only making contact with the inside of the glove.	This is to avoid risk of contamination of the outside of the glove.
5	Holding the glove in one hand, slip the other hand into the glove making sure that nothing is touched by the gloved hand. Any adjustment of the glove to make it more comfortable should be done at a later stage.	This is to avoid risk of contamination of the outside of the glove.
6	Slide the fingers of the gloved hand under the folded cuff of the remaining glove and pick it up. Ensure that the outside of the second glove is only touched by the gloved hand.	This is to avoid risk of contamination of the outside of the glove.
7	Put the glove onto the other hand by pulling steadily through the cuff, taking care not to contaminate this glove with the ungloved hand.	A slow, steady movement is more likely to result in the glove being put on successfully.
8	Adjust the fingers of both gloves until they fit comfortably.	A comfortable fit allows any procedures to be carried out more effectively.

Step-by-step guide to undertaking an aseptic technique in an acute setting

Step		Rationale
1	Decontaminate hands and put on a disposable apron.	Use of PPE reduces the level of contamination of the clothes.
2	Ensure the trolley or other surface being used is clean. It is not always necessary to clean the surface before every use.	Local cleaning policies should always be followed.
3	Collect all equipment required for the procedure and place on the bottom shelf of the trolley, having checked for sterility and expiry date. Discard any equipment that does not meet these requirements.	All sterile equipment should be within date and have intact packaging.
4	Prepare scissors if cutting non-sterile tape by washing, drying, and decontaminating using alcohol wipes. Place scissors on the bottom shelf.	Sterile scissors are required if they are to be used on sterile equipment that is to be in contact with high risk areas of the body, to avoid contamination.
5	Take the trolley to the patient. Introduce yourself, confirm the patient's identity, explain the procedure, and obtain consent.	To identify the patient correctly and gain informed consent.
6	Open the outer packaging of the dressing pack and place on the top of the trolley without allowing the outside packaging to touch the inside wrap.	The outside wrapping is contaminated and should not come into contact with the sterile equipment inside the packaging.
7	Open the dressing pack wrapping by touching only the corners of the wrapping paper.	This will create a sterile field.
8	Pour solution for cleansing wounds and open sterile dressing etc. onto the sterile field without contamination. This should be done without making contact between the solution and the sterile field.	To avoid contamination of the sterile field.
9	Loosen the patient's dressing and decontaminate hands.	Hands should always be decontaminated prior to applying sterile gloves or handling sterile equipment.
10	Place a hand into the sterile yellow waste bag and use this to organize the contents of the dressing pack on the sterile field.*	The waste bag acts as a sterile barrier and allows handling of sterile equipment without the risk of contamination.
11	Remove the patient's soiled dressing using the hand inside the waste bag.*	Contamination will not occur if there is no direct contact with the soiled dressing.

continued overleaf

12	Turn the waste bag inside out with the used dressing inside and attach the bag to the side of the trolley nearest the patient.	Placing the bag near to the patient reduces the risk of contamination of the sterile field when disposing of soiled swabs and dressings.
13	Put on sterile gloves without contamination of the outside of the gloves (see section on how to apply sterile gloves).	Any contamination on the gloves could be transferred to the patient's wound.
14	Carry out the invasive procedure or dressing, etc. Local policies and procedures should be followed.	Following local policies and procedures ensures a safe and effective process.
15	Dispose of any sharps in a sharps bin.	See section on sharps disposal.
16	Remove gloves and place in the waste bag. Wrap all used disposable equipment in the sterile field and place in the waste bag.	See section on waste disposal.
17	Seal the waste bag and place in a clinical waste bin.	See section on waste disposal.
18	Decontaminate hands.	All clinical procedures should be followed with hand decontamination to reduce the risk of cross-infection.

*If there isn't a sterilized waste bag included in the pack, omit stage 10 and remove any old dressings (stage 11) using clean gloves before donning the sterile gloves.

Reflection and evaluation

1 Reflect on your hand washing technique. Do you wash or decontaminate your hands on every occasion that the skill is required?

2 Think about the last time you saw a patient being isolated because of infection. Did you understand the details of the clinical practices involved in their care?

3 Reflect on the type of gloves you need to wear when carrying out a range of clinical procedures. Are you sure you are wearing sterile gloves when required?

4 Do you always dispose of waste in an appropriate container?

Further learning opportunities

- Try to use an ultraviolet light source with light-sensitive gel to assess your hand hygiene technique.
- Reflect on your own practice in relation to standard precautions. Do you comply with them at all times?
- Observe other clinicians as they go about their work. Are you able to recognize the good and the poor role models?

Reminders

Don't forget that:

- Effective hand hygiene is the single most important practice in reducing the risk of HCAI.
- You are saving patients' lives when carrying out infection prevention practices such as hand washing and isolating patients with infections.

Patient scenarios

Consider what you should do in the following situations, then turn to the end of this skill to check your answers.

1 Stanley Johnson is a 75-year-old retired bus driver. He was diagnosed with cancer of the prostate 2 years ago and has undergone surgery and chemotherapy for the treatment of this condition. He has a urinary catheter *in situ* as he has been left with post-operative incontinence. He has been readmitted to hospital for treatment of a chest infection.

A Identify the main factors that increase Mr Johnson's susceptibility to infection.

B What symptom may result as a side effect of antibiotic therapy administered for the treatment of Mr Johnson's chest infection?

C Which organism is likely to be causing those symptoms?

D How would you care for Mr Johnson to reduce the risk of infection to others on the ward?

2 Mrs Li is a 67-year-old woman who has been having problems with a painful knee for the last 3 years. She had inpatient treatment for breast cancer 5 years ago and has been told that this was successful. She has been given an appointment for a pre-admission clinic during which swabs are taken to test for the presence of MRSA.

The following week, Mrs Li is told that the MRSA screen was positive.

A What does MRSA stand for?

B Which sites are normally swabbed when carrying out an MRSA screen?

C How might Mrs Li have acquired MRSA?

D What action might be taken to reduce the risk of post-operative MRSA infection for Mrs Li?

3 You are working on a medical ward in a district general hospital when you notice that a patient in a six-bedded bay suddenly vomits. Within 2 hours, another patient in the bay complains of feeling sick and a member of staff also tells you that she has just vomited in the sluice room.

A What is the most likely cause of these symptoms?

B What actions should be taken immediately to respond to the situation?

C How long should staff be advised to stay away from work?

D What advice should be given to members of the public visiting patients on the ward?

Website

 http://www.oxfordtextbooks.co.uk/orc/ endacott

You may find it helpful to work through our short online quiz and additional scenarios intended to help you to develop and apply the skills in this chapter.

References

Ayliffe GAJ, Babb JR, and Quoraishi AH (1978). A test for hygienic hand disinfection. *Journal of Clinical Pathology*, **31**, 923.

Bannister BA, Begg NT, and Gillespie SH (2000). *Infectious disease*, 2nd edition. Blackwell Science, Oxford.

Department of Health (2003). *Winning ways: working together to reduce healthcare associated infection in England*. DH, London.

Department of Health (2006). *The Health Act 2006: code of practice for the prevention and control of health care associated infections*. DH, London.

Department of Health (2007). *Environment and sustainability health technical memorandum 07-01: safe management of healthcare waste*. DH, London.

Hilton P (2004). *Fundamental nursing skills*. Whurr, London.

Infection Control Nurses Association (1999). *Glove usage guidelines*. ICNA and Regent Medical, London.

McCulloch J (2000). *Infection control, science, management and practice*. Whurr, London.

National Audit Office (2000). *The challenge of hospital acquired infection*. The Stationery Office, London.

NHS Estates (2004). *Healthcare facilities cleaning manual*. The Stationery Office, London.

Plowman R, Graves N, Taylor L *et al.* (1999). *Socio-economic burden of hospital acquired infections*. DH, London.

Pratt RJ, Pellowe CM, Wilson JA *et al.* (2007). Epic 2: national evidence-based guidelines for preventing healthcare associated infections in NHS hospitals in England. *Journal of Hospital Infection*, **65S**, S1–S64.

Wilson J (2006). *Infection control in clinical practice*. Bailliere Tindall, London.

 Answers to patient scenarios

1 A Age, immunosuppression, invasive device *in situ*, hospital inpatient, surgery.

B Diarrhoea.

C *Clostridium difficile*.

D Nurse in isolation until 48 hours clear of symptoms, monitoring of diarrhoea, administer antibiotic therapy as prescribed.

2 A Methicillin-resistant *Staphylococcus aureus*.

B Nose, axillae, groin, wounds, urine (if patient is catheterized), sputum (if patient has a productive cough).

C During her previous hospital admission.

D Decolonization prior to admission (chlorhexidine washes, mupirocin nasal ointment), rescreening, isolation on admission, and possibly the use of prophylactic antibiotics.

3   A   Norovirus.

   B   Patients with symptoms should be nursed in isolation or in a cohorted bay. Stool or vomit specimens should be sent to the microbiology laboratory. The environment should be thoroughly cleaned. Admissions to the ward should be stopped (following appropriate management involvement). Symptomatic staff should be sent home.

   C   Until 48 hours after they have been free of symptoms.

   D   They should be told that there is an outbreak of infection on the ward and they should only enter the ward if necessary. They should be asked to decontaminate their hands on leaving the ward.

4.2 **Skin care**

Definition

Skin care (sometimes referred to as personal hygiene) is undertaken when an individual is unable to meet their own hygiene needs. Hygiene is one of the *Essence of care* benchmarks (DH 2001) and is usually performed or supervised by a Registered Nurse.

It is important to remember that:

- The purpose of skin care is to allow the skin to function normally and promote comfort.
- Skin care is an intimate aspect of nursing care and due respect should be given to cultural and religious differences.
- Skin care provides opportunities for physical assessment, assessment of mental health and well-being, health education, and encouraging patient mobility.
- 'Skin disease affects between one quarter and one third of the population at any one time. It accounts for up to one fifth of all GP consultations' (DH 2003: 2).

Prior knowledge

Before undertaking skin care, make sure you are familiar with:

1   Anatomy and physiology of the skin.
2   Communication skills (see Chapter 2).
3   Cultural or religious-specific skin care practice.
4   Maintaining a healthy skin.
5   Pathophysiology of common skin diseases.
6   Mechanisms of skin repair.
7   Recognizing skin abnormalities.
8   Impact of medication on skin integrity.
9   Principles of maintaining patient safety (see Section 11.1).
10 Principles of wound assessment and management (see Section 4.5).
11 Relevant *Essence of care* benchmarks (Hygiene and Privacy and Dignity, DH 2001).
12 Prevention of cross-infection (see Section 4.1).

You may also find it useful to familiarize yourself with eye care (Section 4.3) and mouth care (Section 4.4); these are commonly provided at the same time as skin care.

Background

Skin functions

In an adult the skin weighs 6 lbs (15% of body weight), covers an area of 2 square metres, and provides a buffer between the body and the environment. **Figure 4.5** shows a cross-section of healthy skin and the structures that enable it to perform the following functions:

- Protection
- Secretion
- Excretion
- Temperature regulation
- Sensation
- Vitamin D production

In order to understand why skin care is fundamental to patient care (DH 2001), it is helpful to review these functions and their implications for skin care.

Protection

The epidermis provides protection from microorganisms. **Skin abrasions** allow the entry of bacteria, making the patient susceptible to infection, so patient documentation should include any skin injuries. It is not clear whether the sharing of an electric razor contributes to cross-infection;

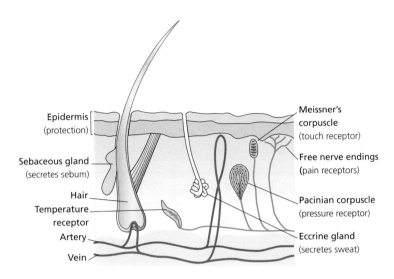

Figure 4.5 A cross-section of healthy skin.

however, male patients are generally encouraged to use their own electric razor or a disposable safety razor.

The epidermis also protects from radiation. The extent of sun protection provided by the skin depends to a certain extent on skin type (see Table 4.1 for common skin types); individuals with types I and II, people who are immunocompromised, or those with a large number of moles are considered high risk for developing skin cancer (Buchanan 2006a, 2006b). Skin care provides an ideal opportunity to educate all patients, especially those with type I or type II skin, regarding the potential additional risk of skin cancer.

Secretion

Sebum is secreted through sebaceous glands into the hair follicles; it lubricates the hair and skin and removes bacteria from hair follicles. Excess bathing (and removal of sebum) can result in drying of the skin; this is worsened if the water is too hot (Baillie and Arrowsmith 2001). In severe cases, dry skin can become cracked, compromising the protective function of the skin. Conversely, skin that is constantly moist is prone to softening, pressure ulcer formation, and breakdown. It is important to keep bed linen and clothing dry, particularly in areas prone to pressure ulceration.

Excretion

Sweat is excreted through **eccrine glands** distributed throughout the skin; this process assists with temperature

Table 4.1 Common skin types

Skin type	Defining features
I	Always burns, never tans. Tends to have freckles, red or fair hair, blue or green eyes.
II	Always burns, sometimes tans. Tends to have light hair, blue or brown eyes.
III	Sometimes burns, always tans. Tends to have brown hair and eyes.
IV	Rarely burns, always tans. Tends to have dark brown eyes and hair.
V	Naturally black-brown skin. Often has dark brown eyes and hair.
VI	Naturally black-brown skin. Usually has black-brown eyes and hair.

(After Fitzpatrick 1988)

control through evaporation. Sweat is also excreted via **apocrine glands** in the axillary and genital areas; if not removed regularly, body odour will occur as a result of bacterial decomposition.

Temperature regulation

The body conserves heat through shivering and promotes heat loss through the skin via conduction, convection, evaporation, and radiation. If the patient is unable to adjust clothing or bed linen to maintain a comfortable body temperature, you may need to do this for them.

Sensation

The skin contains nerve endings sensitive to heat, cold, touch, pain, and pressure. Any damage to skin or nerves may mean the patient is at risk of greater skin damage. Be aware that there is a potential time lag between pressure damage and its effects; for example, a patient who has been on the operating table for 4 hours or longer may not display signs of tissue damage until up to 3 days after surgery (Schoonhoven *et al*. 2002). Remember that patients with diabetes can have altered skin sensation of the hands and feet and are therefore prone to injury.

Vitamin D production

Vitamin D is manufactured by skin cells when they are exposed to sunlight. There is controversy about the impact of sunscreen use on vitamin D production (Marks *et al*. 1995, Farrerons *et al*. 1998). For up-to-date advice, visit the SunSmart website (see Further reading section).

Skin care provides an ideal opportunity for a comprehensive assessment of the patient (see also Section 6.1, *Visual assessment of the cardiac patient* and Section 7.1, *Visual respiratory assessment*). However, this also requires confident use of communication skills (see Chapter 2).

Factors influencing personal skin care

The way in which patients care for their skin is reflective of a number of factors including: socio-economic, cultural, ethnic, and religious aspects; personal preferences; psychological aspects; and physical limitations.

Socio-economic factors

Access to facilities (e.g. outside toilet/shared washing facilities in hostel-style accommodation) can lead to difficulties in maintaining personal hygiene and applying skin preparations. Some skin preparations require the patient to use a bath – this is not available in all types of accommodation, so ensure that shower products are prescribed if necessary.

Sufferers of skin diseases can be prescribed a range of products, at considerable cost to themselves.

Cultural, ethnic, and religious aspects of skin care

Many differences between cultures and religions relate to privacy and intimate aspects of care, for example the requirement for 'no touch' washing or washing when clothed. Make sure you're familiar with guidance in your local Trust; Hollins (2006) also provides a comprehensive overview of different practices.

Personal preferences

It is important to develop a plan for skin care with the patient/carer, for example some people prefer not to use soap on their face. Not all patients are used to having a full wash every day; this should be respected as far as possible when the patient comes under the care of health professionals.

Psychological aspects of skin care

It is important to take client preferences into account when providing skin care; the patient may wish to remain covered because they are embarrassed about some aspect of their condition, e.g. odour from a wound, stoma, or incontinence. It is important to remember that skin that is in contact with body fluids has a higher risk of breakdown, particularly from the corrosive effects of gastric or pancreatic drainage.

Many aspects of skin care practised by individuals are a form of personal expression, from selection of cleansing agents, perfumes, and body lotions to application of make-up. When a patient requires assistance with personal hygiene, they can interpret this as a decline in their independence and well-being (Evans 2004).

The stigma associated with skin diseases should also not be underestimated; ways in which this can affect patients are described by the British Skin Foundation (2006).

Physical limitations

Physical problems such as pain, vertigo, and restricted range of movement or dexterity not only will affect the self-care ability of the individual but should also be borne in mind when providing skin care *for* the patient. Some types of surgery may lead to temporary physical limitations (e.g. orthopaedic surgery, pacemaker insertion). Skin care should be incorporated into an overall rehabilitation plan for the individual and, ideally, undertaken when symptoms such as pain or vertigo are minimal.

It is also important to remember that providing skin care can be tiring for the patient (Verderber and Gallagher 1994). In addition, older people on bed rest are at risk of large skeletal muscle loss, particularly from the lower extremities (Kortebein *et al.* 2007), affecting their ability to participate in self-care activities such as personal hygiene.

Age-related skin care

Seventy per cent of people over 60 have skin problems and, while the majority of these are entirely treatable, many older people are either too ashamed to seek help, or do not get the right help when they ask (All Party Parliamentary Group on Skin 2000). Common skin conditions seen in elderly patients include seborrhoeic keratoses and sun damage.

The normal process of ageing influences the condition of body tissues and structures; for example, skin thins and becomes more fragile, and older men have less (protective) hair-bearing skin on the scalp. These aspects are comprehensively addressed by Smoker (1999). The condition of the skin will also be affected by the older person's ability to maintain normal nutrition, hydration, and mobility. **Figure 4.6** illustrates pressure dermatitis from sitting in the same position for prolonged periods.

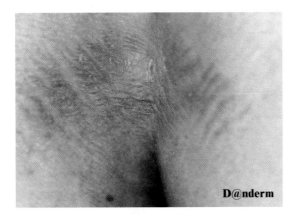

Figure 4.6 Pressure dermatitis. With permission of Danderm.

Context

When to perform skin care

As discussed earlier, skin care is particularly important when one of the functions of the skin is compromised. It also provides an ideal opportunity for patient assessment and rehabilitation, and for reinforcing normal hygiene practices, for example when the patient has a wound. See Section 4.6 (*Pre- and post-operative assessment and management*) for additional aspects of skin assessment for patients having surgery.

When not to perform skin care

There are a number of situations in which skin care has to be modified; consult the patient's health care records for specific instructions, for example:

- Specific post-operative wound care instructions.
- Radiotherapy skin care instructions.
- Patients' preferences, for example when care is palliative (see the Liverpool Care Pathway for further advice, Ellershaw and Murphy 2005).

Alternative interventions

An alternative method of washing patients in bed is towel bathing (Hancock *et al.* 2000); it has also been used with older patients who have dementia (Rader *et al.* 2006). In a comparison between soft towel bathing and the traditional 'blanket bath', Hancock *et al.* (2000) found that patient and nurse satisfaction were higher with towel bathing.

Potential problems

Potential problems that might arise with providing skin care are outlined in the previous sections on *Physical limitations* and *Age-related skin care* and in the following section, *Indications for assistance*.

Indications for assistance

If skin care requires patient handling, undertake a risk assessment for the nurse and the patient. Ensure appropriate use of slings, hoists, and low friction slides. Follow specialist advice from the physiotherapist or occupational therapist regarding patient movement (e.g. after cerebral events or orthopaedic surgery). If the patient has traction in place, seek advice. Be aware that the patient may have a poor hand grip due to soap, water, or emollients and that the bath or shower can be slippery and present a hazard. For further advice see Section 11.1, *Moving and handling of patients*.

Specific observations and monitoring

Be alert for and report any skin reactions to medication. Evaluate the effectiveness of any skin treatments (e.g. is the skin still dry? Has the itch settled? Has skin condition changed? Is there any allergic response?). Be alert for signs of infection. Skin care offers an ideal opportunity to assess the patient for pressure area development. A variety of tools is available for this purpose, for example the Waterlow scale and the Norton scale; for an overview of different systems see Russell (2002).

Special considerations

Location: if undertaking this skill in the patient's home, familiarize yourself with community facilities and aids available to assist patients and carers with skin care.

Chronic illness: remember that some chronic conditions, such as psoriasis or eczema, can make the skin more prone to breakdown.

Particular infection control risks: remember that skin exudate can lead to skin maceration, increasing risk of infection.

Medications: remember that immunosuppressed patients will not have the same inflammatory response.

Special precautions: make sure you're aware of the patient's allergy status before using any skin preparations.

Special considerations related to skin diseases

There are many specific aspects of skin care to be aware of for patients with common skin problems.

Acne skin

Use a mild, unperfumed product specific to the patient's skin type. Combination skin will need an emollient. The eye and lip area have reduced sebaceous glands; oil-removing or drying products may necessitate extra emollient care. Inflamed skin should not be exfoliated.

Dry/itchy skin

Use cool baths and pat skin dry (do not rub). Emollient emulsion can be added to bath water, or showering products are available. Apply topical emollient after bathing. Always apply emollients in the direction of hair follicles to avoid irritation or folliculitis. Wash only once per day. Use a soap substitute for skin cleansing, e.g. aqueous cream. Apply aqueous cream to dry skin and then wash off. Consider fire hazards associated with paraffin-based ointments (**http://www.npsa.nhs.uk/health/alerts**). For further information, see **http://www.eczema.org/emollient.pdf** and Dawkes (1997). See also the British National Formulary, **http://www.bnf.org**, for properties and ranges of emollients available.

Foot care

Wash daily; dry between toes. Thick skin can be routinely removed with a single patient use pumice/file-type product. Emollients containing urea can help hydrate dry, cracked skin. Avoid talcum powder as it can cake and abrade the skin (**http://www.bnf.org**).

Genital skin

Avoid perfumed products and talcum powder. Use an aqueous cream or cream skin wash. Avoid over-washing; no more than twice per day. Scented sanitary products and toilet tissue can cause irritation.

Hair

Mild shampoo can be used daily if necessary. Rinse thoroughly. A scaling, itchy scalp may need a coal tar-based product or a product containing salicylates. Rinsing with water is important. Thicker scalp scale may need a prescribed product. A greasy emollient applied and left in place under a towel wrap for several hours can help; this is potentially messy but soothing. For patients on total bed rest, a hair washing tray should be available, suitable for use when the patient is in the supine position.

Nail care

Fingernails that are kept short reduce the risk of trauma to itchy skin. Shorter nails facilitate good hand hygiene. For safety, file nails or use nail clippers. Emollients applied to the cuticle will moisturize the nail.

Psoriasis/eczema

For mild to moderate psoriasis or eczema, emollients (and/or prescribed topical treatments) should be used. For further advice see **http://www.eczema.org** and **http://www.psoriasis-association.org.uk**. A further useful resource is provided by Charman and Lawton (2006).

Sunscreen application

The British National Formulary (**http://www.bnf.org**) is a resource for the latest sunscreen products and modes of action; see also Buchanan (2006a, 2006b) and Turner (1999).

Managing skin rashes

Skin rashes could result from a variety of causes, e.g. childhood infections, drug reactions, allergy, and serious illnesses (e.g. meningitis) or blistering disorders.

Dermatitis Dermatitis describes an eczematous-type inflammation and itching of the skin and could be due to contact dermatitis. Two types of contact dermatitis skin response can occur: type I and type IV. A type IV or delayed reaction involves T cells and tends to be a true allergy to minute quantities of a substance. An eczematous rash typically appears up to 96 hours after exposure to the allergen. Type IV allergy is investigated in part by the patient's history and in part by applying patch tests to the skin for 72 hours.

A type I response is an immediate or IgE-mediated response, where an immediate wheal (i.e. oedema and erythema) is seen within a few hours. A generalized whole body response could result in anaphylaxis, which can be life-threatening. Massive histamine release from mast cells accounts for the signs and symptoms (for further details see Section 6.15). Type I allergy is tested by blood RAST tests or by skin prick testing.

Irritant contact dermatitis This occurs as a direct response by the skin to damage from soap/acids and solvents and is not due to allergy. In general, eczema does not result from any contact or allergen-driven cause. However, some individuals are 'atopic' – they may have

Box 4.1 General skin care tips for rashes

1 Keep out of the sun.
2 Keep cool.
3 Avoid soap.
4 Avoid perfume.
5 Use emollients and emollient soap substitutes to wash.
6 Wear cotton clothing.
7 Keep fingernails short if the skin is itchy.
8 Bathe in cool water that has emollient added (max. 10 minutes).
9 Pat skin dry – do not rub.

hayfever/eczema/asthma tendencies. While no direct cause can be found for these individuals' eczema, there is some evidence that allergens and irritants (chemical and physical) may play a part in periodic worsening of this condition. For further information see Charman and Lawton (2006), **http://www.anaphylaxis.org.uk**, and **http://www.allergyuk.org**.

General tips for managing skin rashes are provided in **Box 4.1**.

Procedure

Preparation

Before starting this skill:

Prepare yourself

Review the patient's records to identify any special precautions, for example with movement, and any risk factors for skin impairment. Ensure you understand how any specific skin preparations are to be applied. Wash your hands and wear an apron for personal protection (see Section 4.1, *Infection prevention and control*, for advice on how to select the appropriate level of PPE). If your assessment of the risk of infection means you should wear gloves, follow the glove use instructions in Section 4.1. Ensure you allow sufficient time to encourage the patient to participate as much as possible.

Prepare the patient

The procedure should be fully explained to the patient (see the box below). Assess the patient's ability to assist in their own skin care. Assess the patient's range of movement and ability to tolerate movement. Encourage the patient to do as much as possible in order to encourage independence, minimize loss of muscle tone, and prevent joint stiffness. Ensure the patient has had adequate pain relief and is comfortable; this may include offering a bedpan, commode, or urinal.

Prepare the equipment/environment

Get the patient to a basin or bathroom if at all possible. If the patient is seated upright they are more likely to be involved. Access to running water and privacy are also important. If the patient has to be washed in bed, put a privacy sign on the curtains. Pin curtains closed if necessary.

Ensure the room temperature and water temperature are comfortable and the bowl and all equipment are clean. Use a clean disposable cloth for washing. Use toiletries preferred by the patient. Clear the area around the bed as much as possible to provide a safe environment.

Discussing the procedure with the patient and family

- Explain what is to happen.

- Invite the patient to take part and discuss their preference for involvement.

- Encourage family involvement, if appropriate. This is particularly important if the patient will have long-term skin care needs, for example vascular insufficiency, diabetes mellitus, or eczema/psoriasis.

- Identify any personal or cultural preferences that the patient may have in relation to skin care.

Step-by-step guide to assisted washing

Step		Rationale
1	Introduce yourself, confirm the patient's identity, explain the procedure, and obtain consent.	To identify the patient correctly and gain informed consent.
2	Remove the top bed covers and cover the patient with a bath towel. Assist the patient to undress under the towel.	To maintain patient dignity and to gain access to all skin surfaces.
3	Cover the patient with a series of towels, or a bath sheet, and expose one limb at a time.	To ensure the patient is kept warm and maintain patient dignity.
4	Ensure body fluids (from wound drainage or other soiling) are removed from the skin surface; use disposable gloves according to local infection control policy.	To prevent skin damage. To prevent risk of cross-infection. Gloves should be worn for all procedures where there is potential for contact with body fluids.
5	Wash, or assist the patient to wash, the face and neck.	To minimize cross-infection. To encourage patient participation.
6	Wash the arms and chest, encouraging the patient to participate as they are able. If the patient is able to sit forward, wash their back. Apply deodorant according to patient preference. Keep IV, wound, and drain sites dry.	To promote cleanliness and maintain skin integrity. To minimize infection risk.
7	Replace pyjama top.	To maintain patient privacy and dignity.

8	Wash the patient's legs one at a time. If the patient is able to raise their knees, place the foot in a bowl of water on the bed while washing the lower leg. Examine skin condition between the patient's toes.	To promote patient comfort. To provide a more 'normal' washing environment.
9	Change the water and washing cloth. Ask consent to wash the patient's genital area. Enable the patient to wash this area themselves if they prefer. Wear disposable gloves. (See Section 9.1 for detailed description of catheter care.)	To minimize infection risk. To respect patient wishes and to maintain dignity and privacy. Gloves should be worn for all procedures where there is potential for contact with body fluids.
10	Roll the patient onto one side to wash the sacral area, using a clean, disposable cloth. Assess pressure areas. Ensure a second nurse/support worker assists with this part of the procedure.	To minimize infection risk. To prevent, identify, and manage pressure ulcers in a timely manner. To ensure nurse and patient safety and to maintain patient confidence. To comply with moving and handling guidance, as per Section 11.1.
11	Change the bottom sheet if the patient is unable to get out of bed. Remake top bedclothes.	To promote patient comfort.
12	Provide hair care and shave.	To promote patient comfort and dignity.
13	Document care given, noting any risks for skin impairment or any changes since the last skin assessment. Use appropriate terminology to describe skin condition (see Table 4.2).	To provide a baseline measurement, aid communication, and promote continuity of care. Accurate terminology improves interprofessional communication.

Following the procedure

Warn the patient that their skin may be slippery due to emollients (if used). Place the patient's call bell within reach. Ensure the patient is comfortable and safely positioned. Review the goals of skin care management and the education plan for the patient and make any adjustments necessary to the care plan. Ensure any abnormalities are reported to the clinical team.

After use, clean any equipment used to remove surface colonies of microorganisms. Store the equipment in accordance with local policy (see Section 4.1 for guidance on the type of decontamination necessary). Ensure single-use items are disposed of appropriately.

Reflection and evaluation

When you have undertaken skin care for a patient, think about the following questions:

1 Was the patient's skin in good condition?
2 Were you able to answer the patient's questions and use opportunities for patient education?

Table 4.2 Terminology used to describe skin conditions

Distribution	
Generalized	The majority of skin surface is affected by the lesions.
Localized	A few lesions (fewer than 20) are grouped together within a small area and cover only a part of one particular body area (face, neck, trunk, arm, etc.).
Linear	Lesions forming a line.
Discrete	Individual lesions.
Confluent	Lesions merging or running together, often seen in a rash.
Shape	
Guttate	Similar in shape to raindrops.
Discoid	Small discs.
Annular	Ring-shaped.
Colour	
Erythema	Redness of the skin due to congestion of the capillaries.
Hypopigmentation	Reduced pigmentation.
Hyperpigmentation	Increased pigmentation.
Non-palpable	
Macule	Discoloured spot on the skin that is not raised above the surface.
Palpable	
Papule	Elevated bump less than 5 mm.
Nodule	Elevated bump greater than 5 mm.
Tumour	Large solid lesion.
Plaque	Slightly raised, large surface area, defined edge.
Wheal	Solid elevation, sloping borders, smooth surface.
Vesicle	Small fluid-containing lesion up to 5 mm.
Bulla	Fluid-containing lesion greater than 5 mm.
Pustule	Elevated lesion containing pus.
Skin surface	
Crust	Dried serum, blood, or pus on the surface of the lesion.
Scale	Flakes of dry skin.
Lichenification	Thickening of epidermis.
Excoriation	Loss of outer layers.
Fissure	Split or crack.
Ulcer	Local loss of epidermis.
Allergy types **(type I and IV refer to the different immune response pathways)**	
Type I	Immediate hypersensitivity to allergen, e.g. anaphylactoid reaction.
Type IV	Delayed sensitivity.

3 Did your visual assessment of the patient alert you to any potential problems with skin integrity?

4 Was the patient able to participate as much as you expected?

5 Did the patient need any referral to other health care professionals (e.g. dermatology specialist or diabetes nurse)?

Further learning opportunities

- Take any opportunities to work with experienced colleagues providing skin care for patients. Observe how they encourage patients to be involved in meeting their own hygiene needs.
- Talk to patients about how they manage their hygiene needs at home.
- Discuss the particular skin care needs of people with diabetes with the diabetes nurse specialist.

Patient scenarios

Consider what you should do in the following situations, then turn to the end of this skill to check your answers.

1 A patient admitted with chronic heart disease complains of dry, itchy skin on the lower leg. What might be some of the causes?

2 An elderly patient asks you to wash their hair while they are in the bath. How would you respond?

3 A ward has had a concern expressed by two patients who felt their privacy and dignity were not considered when they were having a blanket bath. What ideas would you have to address this concern?

Website

 http://www.oxfordtextbooks.co.uk/orc/ endacott

You may find it helpful to work through our short online quiz and additional scenarios intended to help you to develop and apply the skills in this chapter.

References

All Party Parliamentary Group on Skin (2000). [online] **http://www.library.nhs.uk/ skin/ViewResource.aspx?resID=69772** accessed 20/08/08.

Baillie L and Arrowsmith V (2001). *Meeting elimination needs: developing practical skills*. Hodder Arnold, London.

British Skin Foundation (2006). *More than skin deep* [online] **http://www.britishskinfoundation.org.uk/ Uploads/documents/BSF%20BOOKLET%233%23. pdf** accessed 12/05/08.

Buchanan P (2006a). Hands on . . . sunscreens. *Dermatological Nursing*, **5**(2), 20–3.

Buchanan P (2006b). Hands on . . . recognise and protect sun damaged skin. *Dermatological Nursing*, **5**(3), 16.

Charman C and Lawton S (2006). *Eczema: the treatments and therapies that really work*. Constable & Robinson Ltd, London.

Dawkes K (1997). How to . . . apply emollients effectively. *British Journal of Dermatology Nursing*, **1**(2), 8.

Department of Health (2001). *Essence of care*. HMSO, London.

Department of Health (2003). *Action on dermatology: good practice guide*. HMSO, London.

Ellershaw JE and Murphy D (2005). The Liverpool Care Pathway (LCP) influencing the UK national agenda on care of the dying. *International Journal of Palliative Nursing*, **11**(3), 132–4.

Evans LK (2004). The bath! Reassessing a familiar elixir in old age. *Journal of American Geriatric Society*, **52**(11), 1957–8.

Farrerons J, Barnados M, Rodriguez J, *et al.* (1998). Clinically prescribed sunscreen (sun protection factor 15) does not decrease serum vitamin D concentration sufficiently either to induce changes in parathyroid function or in metabolic markers. *British Journal of Dermatology*, **139**(3), 422–7.

Hancock I, Bowman A, and Prater D (2000). 'The day of the soft towel?' Comparison of the current bed-bathing method with the soft towel bed-bathing method. *International Journal of Nursing Practice*, **6**, 207–13.

Hollins S (2006). *Religions, culture and healthcare: a practical guide for use in healthcare environments*. Radcliffe Publishing, Abingdon.

Kortebein P, Ferrando A, Lombeida J, Wolfe R, and Evans WJ (2007). Effect of 10 days of bed rest on skeletal muscle in healthy older adults. *Journal of the American Medical Association*, **297**, 1772–4.

Marks R, Foley PA, Jolley D, *et al.* (1995). The effect of regular sunscreen use on vitamin D levels in an Australian population. Results of a randomised controlled trial. *Archives of Dermatology*, **131**(4), 415–21.

Fitzpatrick TB (1988). The validity and practicality of sun-reactive skin types I-VI. *Archives of Dermatology*, **124**, 869–71.

Rader J, Barrick A, Hoeffer B, *et al.* (2006). The bathing of older adults with dementia: easing the unnecessarily unpleasant aspects of assisted bathing. *American Journal of Nursing*, **106**(4), 40–8.

Russell L (2002). Pressure ulcer classification: the systems and the pitfalls. *British Journal of Nursing*, **11**(12), S49–S59.

Schoonhoven L, Defloor T, and Grypdonck MHF (2002). Incidence of pressure ulcers due to surgery. *Journal of Clinical Nursing*, **11**, 479–87.

Smoker A (1999). Skin care in old age. *Nursing Standard*, **13**(48), 47–53.

Turner M (1999). How to . . . apply sunscreen to children. *British Journal of Dermatology Nursing*, **3**(3), 8.

Verderber A and Gallagher KJ (1994). Effects of bathing, passive range-of-motion exercises and turning on oxygen consumption in healthy men and women. *American Journal of Critical Care*, **3**(374), 374–81.

Useful further reading and websites

Dudzinski DM and Shannon SE (2006). Competent patients' refusal of nursing care. *Nursing Ethics*, **13**, 608–21.

The Merck Manual has a comprehensive section on the management of dermatological disorders: **http://www.merck.com/mmpe/sec10.html**.

The SunSmart website is a useful resource for advice for patients and professionals: **http://info.cancerresearchuk.org/healthyliving/sunsmart/**.

Wounds UK is an excellent web resource for all aspects of skin care; you can also subscribe to a free wound care e-newsletter: **http://www.woundsuk.com**.

The national Electronic Library for Health includes a skin disorders specialist library: **http://libraries.nelh.nhs.uk/skin/**.

(A) Answers to patient scenarios

1   There are three immediate possibilities to explore: polypharmacy (with interaction of drugs causing local skin irritation); stasis eczema (due to stasis of blood supply); or contact dermatitis. If this is a long-term problem, the answer could also lie in practices identified in Scenario 2, although the inappropriate

use of bathing/shampooing agents would tend to cause a more generalized drying of the skin.

2   Shampoos are not designed to be used as bathing agents and can strip the skin of its natural oils, making it dry. As older people have drier skin due to the ageing process, it is even more important to avoid this practice. Gently explain this to the patient, and to the family if this is a regular practice followed at home. Ensure you make time to wash the patient's hair with shampoo.

3   Generously fitting curtains should be used appropriately around patients' beds, with a warning sign attached when the patient is bathing. Timing of bathing should be arranged, as far as possible, to avoid visiting times. Mixed sex wards can increase anxiety for some patients; take extra steps to provide privacy in these circumstances. Where possible encourage the patient to be wheeled to a bathroom or curtained sink area. Ensure that the patient's cultural and religious practices are respected when planning care.

4.3 Eye care

Definition

Eye care is the assistance given to patients who are unable to cleanse and care for their eyes themselves. It is necessary to keep the eyes clean for patient comfort and to prevent infection.

It is important to remember that:

● The eye is a very sensitive part of the body that can easily be damaged.
● Assisting the patient with cleansing of the eye is a gentle procedure that should be undertaken with great care.

Prior knowledge

Before undertaking eye care, make sure you are familiar with:

● Anatomy and physiology of the eye.
● Physical effects of reduced levels of consciousness.

- Aseptic technique.
- Local policies for safe disposal of clinical waste.

Background

The eye is a precious organ that is vulnerable to damage and so is protected within a cone-shaped cavity in the skull called the orbit or socket. The eye is held by six muscles that regulate movement and it is surrounded by soft fatty tissues.

Inside the eyelid and covering the eye is the protective membrane, the conjunctiva. This membrane produces lubricating mucus that keeps the eye clean and moist. This mucus and tears are produced by the lacrimal glands at the upper outer aspect of the orbit (see **Figure 4.7**). When you blink a thin layer is spread over the eye; this then flows into the lacrimal sac at the inner corner of the eye and through a passage into the nose.

The structure of the eye is demonstrated in **Figure 4.8**. The outer layer of the eye is called the cornea and sclera: the sclera is the white of the eye and the cornea is the front transparent part. These layers are strong and are said to have the feel of soft leather. The cornea contains about 70 superficial nerve endings that are responsible for the intense pain that results from even slight irritation (Vaughan and Asbury 2003).

The coloured disc behind the cornea is the iris and this protects the eye from overwhelming bright light. The inner dark circle in the iris is the pupil and the size of this

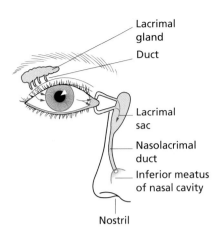

Figure 4.7 Lubrication of the eye. Tears are produced by the lacrimal gland and collect in the lacrimal sac.

determines the amount of light allowed into the eye. Directly behind the iris is the lens, and the muscles of the ciliary body make constant adjustments to the shape of the lens to focus light onto the light-sensitive cells on the inner aspect of the back of the eye, the retina. The appearance of the normal eye is summarized in **Table 4.3**.

If a patient is unable to cleanse or care for their eyes themselves, there is a serious risk of eye injury or disease (JBIEBNM 2002). Potential problems can include:

- Drying of the cornea leading to ulceration, scarring, and possibly blindness.
- Bacterial or viral infection of the conjunctiva (conjunctivitis).

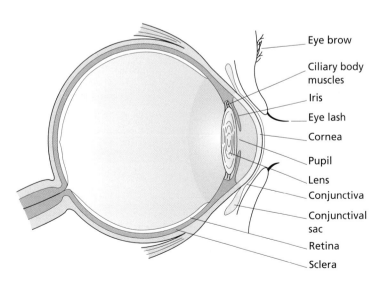

Figure 4.8 The structure of the eye.

Table 4.3 What to look for when assessing the eyes

Structure	The normal eye
Eyes	Free from signs of inflammation or infection
Conjunctiva	Clear
Sclera (white portion of the eye)	Visible
Eyelids	Fit snugly over the eyeball with lashes turned outwards
Eyebrows	Symmetrical

Tears have an essential part to play in keeping the eyes clean and free of infection. The composition of tears includes proteins and substances (beta-lysin and lysozyme) with antibacterial properties. The absence of normal tear production can give rise to the same complications as described above. The blink reflex is also important, not only to protect the eye from damage but to spread the tears across the eye and prevent the cornea from drying. The blink reflex may be absent in patients for several reasons, including those who have a facial palsy or who have a reduced level of consciousness, e.g. following a stroke.

The effective care and cleansing of the eye by the nurse should be seen as an essential procedure that can prevent complications from arising as well as contribute to the patient's comfort.

Context

 ### When to carry out eye care

Eye care may be necessary for a wide range of patients, from the alert and cooperative patient who for whatever reason is physically unable to reach their eyes and cleanse them, to the unconscious, immobile patient who is totally dependent for all their hygiene needs. Eye care should be carried out at least twice daily or whenever there is visible evidence of stickiness or discharge. The patient may also request eye care if their eyes feel dry and uncomfortable.

 ### When not to carry out eye care

If appropriate, the patient should be encouraged and/or assisted to perform this task for themselves to promote their independence and rehabilitation.

If there are signs of damage to the eye, the eye is painful, or there is new redness or discharge, the procedure should not be carried out until the patient has been reviewed by a Registered Nurse.

Indications for assistance

If at any time during the procedure the patient complains of discomfort or pain, stop immediately and ask the Registered Nurse for assistance.

Special considerations

- Unconscious patients have little or no blink reflex and so cannot protect their cornea – be extra careful when cleansing their eyes not to touch the cornea with the swab as this may scratch it. Specific aspects of eye care for critically ill patients are provided in Dawson (2005).

- The patient may have contact lenses *in situ*. If this is the case they should be removed prior to eye care being undertaken. If the patient is alert and orientated then they should be asked to remove their lenses themselves. If the patient is not able to or has a reduced level of consciousness then a qualified nurse should remove the lenses for them. Contact lenses should never be left *in situ* in unconscious patients as they may cause dryness and irritation to the cornea that could result in long-term damage or blindness.

- Remember that older patients may have increased sensitivity to glare, decreased acuity and accommodation, and decreased vision in the dark. These are normal aspects of the ageing process.

Procedure

Preparation

Prepare yourself

Make sure you are clear about the patient's condition and their likely level of understanding of the procedure you are about to undertake.

Prepare the patient

The procedure should be fully explained to the patient (see box below). This should be done even if the patient has a reduced level of consciousness – there is clear evidence that hearing is one of the last senses to be lost as a patient becomes comatose and therefore even if they appear unconscious there is a chance they may hear and understand what is being said around them (Pemberton 2000).

Prepare the equipment

You will require a clean trolley with a dressing pack (see Figure 4.9). This procedure is clinically clean as opposed to aseptic, so you may wear standard latex/plastic gloves rather than sterile gloves. You will need two gallipots of normal saline (one for each eye) and some lint-free gauze. The reason for separate trays is to minimize the risk of cross-contamination from one eye to the other (Smith 1998).

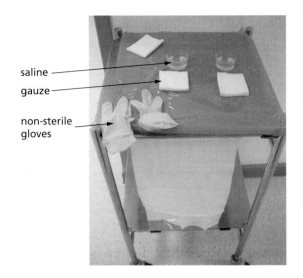

saline
gauze
non-sterile gloves

Figure 4.9 Equipment needed for eye care.

> **Discussing the procedure with the patient and family**
>
> - Explain why eye care is necessary.
>
> - Explain how you intend to carry out the procedure.
>
> - If the patient is likely to require long-term care, it may be appropriate for this skill to be taught to family members if they express a wish to assist with their relative's physical care.

Step-by-step guide to eye care

▶ Step	Rationale
1 Introduce yourself, confirm the patient's identity, explain the procedure to the patient, and obtain consent.	To identify the patient correctly and gain informed consent.
2 Place screens around the patient.	To protect their privacy and dignity.
3 Position the patient so they are sitting up with their head resting back on pillows. Ensure they are comfortable before commencing the procedure.	The patient should be relaxed with their head well supported so they do not move suddenly when you are touching close to their eyes.
4 Make sure the area is well lit but that the light is not shining in the patient's eyes.	You need to be able to see the patient clearly but it would be very uncomfortable for them if they had a light shining in their eyes.

continued overleaf

5	Wash your hands.	To prevent cross-infection.
6	Assess the condition of the patient's eyes. If there is any new redness or discharge, inform the Registered Nurse before proceeding any further.	If the patient has signs of developing an infection the Registered Nurse will want to take a swab of the eye before any cleansing takes place. The Registered Nurse will also report this finding to the doctor.

Upper eyelid

7	With the first eye to be cleansed, wipe the saline-moistened gauze from the inner aspect of the closed eye to the outer.	The eye is cleansed in this way to prevent any debris or discharge being forced into the inner aspect of the eye where it may block the lacrimal duct (see Figure 4.7).
8	Discard the gauze – for each swab across the eye a new, clean, moistened gauze is to be used.	To prevent contamination with soiled swabs.
9	Repeat the cleansing until there is no discharge or debris visible.	The eye must be thoroughly cleansed to avoid complications and maintain comfort.

Lower eyelid

10	Ask the patient to look up and gently swab the lower eyelid from the inner aspect outwards (see **Figure 4.10**).	The eye is cleansed in this way to prevent any debris or discharge being forced into the inner aspect of the eye where it may block the lacrimal duct (see Figure 4.7).
11	Repeat the cleansing until there is no discharge or debris visible.	The eye must be thoroughly cleansed to avoid complications and maintain comfort.
12	Dry the eye by swabbing once with dry gauze.	Moisture left around the eye would be uncomfortable for the patient.
13	Repeat the process with the other eye.	
14	When you have finished, ensure the patient is comfortable.	To promote comfort.
15	If the patient is unconscious then a pad moistened with saline may be left resting gently on the closed eye.	To protect the eye from drying or damage.
16	Clear the trolley and dispose of the clinical waste according to local policy.	See the guide to safe disposal of waste in Section 4.1.
17	Wash your hands.	All clinical procedures should be followed with hand decontamination to reduce the risk of cross-infection.
18	With the Registered Nurse responsible for the care of the patient, document the procedure in the patient's records, noting the condition of their eyes.	So that when the next person carries out this procedure they can refer back to your records to check if there has been any change in their condition.

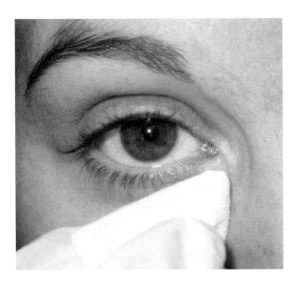

Figure 4.10 Swabbing of the lower lid.

Following the procedure

Go back to the patient and check they have all important items within easy reach (e.g. call bell and drink). If the patient has spectacles, offer to clean them if they are unable to do so for themselves.

Recognizing patient deterioration

The following may be signs of patient deterioration that you or the patient may detect during eye care:

- Pain in, around, or behind the eye.
- Deteriorating vision.
- The patient complains of light hurting their eyes (photophobia).
- Unequal pupils.

Reflection and evaluation

When you have undertaken eye care with a patient, think about the following questions:

1 Check with the patient that you have made them feel more comfortable as a result of your care. Ask the patient if you could have performed this task differently to have improved how they felt.

2 Don't forget that all patients are individuals and what suits one may not suit another. However, by gathering as much information as you can from patients you will be sure to improve your performance and techniques.

Further learning opportunities

As with most clinical skills, the technique of eye care will improve with practice, but these actions will help:

- Ask an experienced colleague to observe you and give feedback on how you carried out the procedure.
- Make a point of accompanying Registered Nurses when they are carrying out this task and when they are carrying out more advanced procedures such as administering eye medication.
- See if you can attend an Ophthalmic Clinic and observe eye examinations.
- If there are ophthalmic specialist nurses where you work, spend some time with them so you can gain extra knowledge of eye conditions and treatment.

Reminders

- The effective care and cleansing of the eye by the nurse should be seen as an essential procedure that can prevent complications from arising as well as contribute to the patient's comfort.
- If at any time during the procedure the patient complains of discomfort or pain, stop immediately and ask the Registered Nurse for assistance.
- Unconscious patients have little or no blink reflex and so cannot protect their cornea.

Ⓠ Patient scenarios

Consider what you should do in the following situations, then turn to the end of this skill to check your answers.

1 Patient A has asked for help to cleanse his eye, which has become red and has a discharge – what should you do?

2 When you are cleansing the eye of patient B, she says the swabbing is painful – should you tell the Registered Nurse immediately or when you have finished the procedure?

3 Patient C asks you to give him the swab so he can cleanse his own eye.

Website

 http://www.oxfordtextbooks.co.uk/orc/
endacott

You may find it helpful to work through our short online quiz and additional scenarios intended to help you to develop and apply the skills in this chapter.

References

Dawson D (2005). Development of a new eye care guideline for critically ill patients. *Intensive and Critical Care Nursing*, **21**, 119–22.

JBIEBNM (2002). Eye care for intensive care patients. *Best Practice*, **6**(1). Blackwell Publishing, Australia.

Pemberton L (2000). The unconscious patient. In M Alexander, J Fawcett, and P Runciman, eds. *Nursing practice, hospital and home. The adult*, 2nd edition, pp. 851–71. Churchill Livingstone, London.

Smith I (1998). Practical procedures for nurses, No. 17.1. Eye Care 1: external examination. *Nursing Times*, **94**(37), 2.

Vaughan D and Asbury T (2003). *General ophthalmology*. Lange Medical Books/McGraw-Hill, London.

Useful further reading and websites

http://www.patient.co.uk
http://www.eye-care.org.uk
http://www.eyehelp.co.uk
http://www.nurseseyesite.nhs.uk

 Answers to patient scenarios

1 Inform the Registered Nurse first so they can assess the patient's eye and take a specimen of the discharge if appropriate.

2 Stop the procedure immediately and ask the Registered Nurse for assistance.

3 If the patient feels he would like to carry out this procedure for himself then he should be allowed to do so with support. Give the patient a clear explanation as to how the procedure should be performed and observe him carrying this out to ensure he manages to achieve adequate cleansing.

4.4 **Mouth care**

Definition

Mouth care (sometimes referred to as oral hygiene) is the care of the mouth, its lining mucosa, lips, teeth, tongue, and gums. The skills involved include: assessment of the mouth; brushing the teeth; mouth rinsing; and denture care. The aim of mouth care is to prevent soreness, infection, and bad breath (**halitosis**) and to promote comfort.

It is important to remember that:

● The mouth has several functions that affect well-being. These are: the ingestion, chewing, and swallowing of food and fluid; communication through speech; and breathing (if the nose is blocked).

● If the mouth becomes colonized by pathogenic organisms, these can spread to the lungs causing life-threatening pneumonia in intensive care patients (Scannapieco *et al.* 1992, in McNeill 2000, Ross and Crumpler 2007).

Prior knowledge

Before undertaking mouth care, make sure you are familiar with:

1 Anatomy of the mouth.
2 Physiology of swallowing.
3 Infection control measures, as the performance of mouth care involves contact with a body fluid (saliva).
4 The causes and effects of dehydration and malnutrition, as patients in need of mouth care are at risk of both.
5 Pathology of fungal infection with *Candida*, and action of Nystatin, the most commonly used antifungal agent.

Background

Figure 4.11 shows the main structures of the mouth.

Physiology of the salivary glands

There are three pairs of salivary glands, which between them produce 1–2 litres of saliva a day (see **Figure 4.12**). There are two types of saliva:

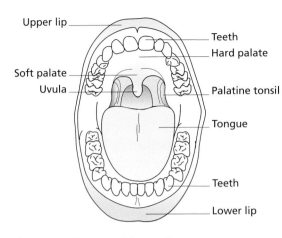

Figure 4.11 Structure of the mouth.

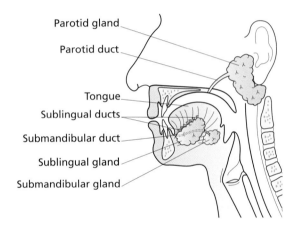

Figure 4.12 Section of the head showing salivary glands and ducts.

1 Serous saliva is 90% water and keeps the mouth wet. It contains amylase, which helps break down starch in food, and fibronectin and lysozyme, which have antibacterial actions.

2 Mucous saliva lubricates the mouth and helps chewed food to stick together into a bolus to be swallowed.

The flow of saliva is under the control of the autonomic nervous system; parasympathetic nerves stimulate the flow of saliva while sympathetic nerves suppress the flow. The presence of food in the mouth (particularly sour foods), and even the smell of food, stimulates the release of saliva through parasympathetic nerve stimulation.

The action of chewing helps promote the flow of saliva to keep the mouth moist and remove debris and bacteria, as does drinking fluids. If the flow of saliva dries up, as happens when a person becomes dehydrated or is not eating, the teeth, lips, mouth, and tongue become coated with dead cells and dried mucous saliva, and are prone to infection. These patients are therefore likely to need help to maintain a healthy mouth.

Patients at increased risk of mouth problems

Patients who are not eating or drinking or who are dehydrated, such as terminally ill patients, are particularly at risk. Also prone to mouth problems are diabetics, immunosuppressed patients, those having oxygen, radiotherapy, or chemotherapy, those with an oral endotracheal tube, and those prescribed steroids (Evans 2001). Numerous medications (notably certain hypotensive drugs, antidepressants, and diuretics) suppress production of saliva and can cause a dry mouth (Barnett 1991, cited in Holman *et al.* 2005).

After urinary tract infection, ventilator-associated pneumonia is the next most common hospital-acquired (nosocomial) infection, and is the leading cause of death due to hospital-acquired infection, with a mortality rate of up to 71% (Eggimann and Pittett 2001, Fagon 2002, Fleming *et al.* 2001, Koeman *et al.* 2001, Apostolopoulou *et al.* 2003, Berry and Davidson 2006). Bacteria from the mouth can also enter the bloodstream, causing septicaemia, or the heart, causing infective endocarditis (Kite and Pearson 1995, in McNeill 2000).

Assessing the mouth

The functions of the mouth will be impaired by a sore, infected, or dry mouth, as the patient may be reluctant to eat if their mouth is sore and unable to articulate words if it is dry. This can result in the patient becoming socially withdrawn and having a lowered self-esteem and a reduced appetite (Garcia 2004). Assessing the mouth should therefore form part of an overall patient assessment, observing for the following problems.

Fungal infection, e.g. thrush (candidiasis)
This is characterized by sore, red areas in the mouth and white patches that when wiped reveal raw areas underneath. The corners of the mouth where the lips meet may also be cracked and sore.

The fungus *Candida* is naturally present in the mouth but rarely causes infection. If the bacterial commensals in the mouth are depleted by antibiotic therapy, this may allow the *Candida* to flourish, leading to a fungal infection. Other causes are the patient being immunosuppressed, having a dry mouth, or having poor oral hygiene.

Good mouth and particularly denture care in susceptible patients will reduce the risk. Dentures can harbour the infection and reinfect the mouth if not cleaned, disinfected, and removed overnight. (Dentures should not be left in 24 hours a day for this reason.)

Nystatin oral suspension may be prescribed for this condition.

Bacterial infection

This can lead to the potentially fatal ventilator-acquired pneumonia mentioned previously. The normal flora of the mouth can consist of up to 350 different species of microorganism (Bagg *et al.* 1999). In compromised patients, increased amounts of proteases in oral secretions remove the protective coat of fibronectin. This enables pathogenic organisms such as *Pseudomonas aeruginosa* to adhere to the inside of the mouth and teeth (Gibbons 1989, cited in Berry and Davidson 2006).

Microorganisms and their toxins attach to the tooth surfaces, and, if not removed within 24–48 hours, coalesce to form dental plaque (Drgreene.com). Plaque is the commonest cause of gum disease and tooth decay. Plaque that is allowed to build up and calcify hardens into calculus (tartar), a porous deposit not removed by cleaning with a toothbrush (Drgreene.com).

Dry mouth (xerostomia)

This unpleasant condition makes speech and eating difficult, and makes the patient more susceptible to oral infections such as thrush (see earlier section). Frequent mouth care and sips of water will be needed, and some patients may find prescribed artificial saliva sprays helpful.

Ulceration of mucosa, tongue, and gums

Any trauma to the mouth, such as rough or badly fitting dentures, can cause painful ulcers. In addition to removing the cause of the trauma, regular mouth care and the prescription of pain-relieving gels or lotions will help make the patient's mouth more comfortable.

Brushing the teeth

Research shows that the toothbrush wins (nearly) every time! Research evidence over the years (from Howarth 1977, cited by Evans 2001, to Xavier 2000 and Pearson and Hutton 2002) has shown the toothbrush to be far more effective in removing debris and plaque than the alternatives such as foam sticks or gauze-covered forceps.

In spite of this, oral care packs still routinely come supplied with foam sticks and some nurses remain reluctant to use toothbrushes. This could stem from a fear of traumatizing the patient or finding it difficult to manoeuvre the toothbrush inside the mouth (Berry and Davidson 2006). However, the most effective proven tool for cleaning not only the teeth but the whole mouth remains the toothbrush (Franklin *et al.* 2000, Griffiths *et al.* 2000, cited in Berry and Davidson 2006, Pearson and Hutton 2002). It is recommended that a small-headed, soft child's toothbrush be used.

Foam sticks do have their uses but are not recommended for the routine procedure of cleaning the mouth, as they are ineffective for plaque removal (Rawlins 2001, cited in Berry and Davidson 2006, Buglass 1995). Foam sticks should only be used to clean the mouth if use of a toothbrush is contraindicated, for example if the patient has bleeding gums (Berry and Davidson 2006) or has had surgery to the mouth (Hahn and Jones 2000: 35–7).

However, foam sticks dipped in a mouthwash solution can be effective for removing toothpaste residue, and nurses' fears that a patient could bite off the end of a foam stick and choke on it have been unfounded (Berry and Davidson 2006). Foam sticks are also useful for moistening the mouth between mouth care procedures.

Rinsing the mouth

Water

Do not underestimate the benefits of using water as the solution for mouth care and mouth rinsing. Water is cheap, non-irritant, refreshing, and does not leave an unpleasant aftertaste. It has, however, no anti-plaque action.

Chlorhexidine gluconate (Corsodyl®)

This is an antiseptic with broad-spectrum antimicrobial and antifungal action. It works by binding to the mucosa and teeth, preventing bacterial build-up. It is released over up to 12 hours, giving prolonged protection (Berry and Davidson 2006). It is therefore recommended as the best antiplaque agent (Bagg *et al*. 1999).

Disadvantages are that it has an unpleasant taste (Evans 2001) and can cause tooth discoloration (Holmes 1991, cited by Evans 2001). If it is used after toothpaste, the toothpaste should first be rinsed out with water, as chlorhexidine is incompatible with some toothpaste ingredients (Netdoctor.co.uk).

It is worth remembering that there is no conclusive research evidence proving that chlorhexidine is better than water in preventing mouth infections, although several studies have been done, such as those by Dodd *et al*. (2000) and Potting *et al*. (2006).

However, for intubated patients receiving mechanical ventilation, NICE guidelines (National Institute for Health and Clinical Excellence 2007) recommend that 'Oral antiseptics (for example, 2% chlorhexidine) should be included as part of the oral hygiene regimen' in order to reduce risk of ventilator-associated pneumonia.

Benzydamine hydrochloride (Difflam®)

This a non-steroidal anti-inflammatory agent that reduces pain and inflammation in stomatitis. It should be used undiluted, rinsed out and not swallowed, and should be prescribed.

Hydrogen peroxide

Hydrogen peroxide has an antiplaque effect but must be diluted correctly, because if too strong it can irritate or even burn the mucosa (Tombes and Gallucci 1993, cited by Evans 2001, and Dougherty and Lister 2008). It leaves an unpleasant aftertaste and patients generally do not like it, so it is not recommended.

Sodium bicarbonate solution

Sodium bicarbonate makes the mucus less sticky and therefore makes the mouth easier to clean (Dodd *et al*. 2000). It does not have an aftertaste so is not unpleasant for patients. However, it must be correctly made up to 1% because if too strong a solution is used it can irritate the mucosa.

Lemon and glycerine swabs

These have appeal for the nurse in that they are ready-made and convenient, with a refreshing lemony smell. Do not be fooled by this! The lemon is acidic and has a decalcifying effect on the tooth enamel (Fitch *et al*. 1999). In addition, although salivary flow is initially stimulated (as you will notice if you try one yourself), this results in exhausting the salivary glands and quickly leads to a dry mouth (Howarth 1977, cited by Evans 2001, Miller and Kearney 2001). Lemon and glycerine swabs deserve mention here only to warn **against** their use.

Pineapple

For patients who are able to chew, unsweetened tinned pineapple helps to refresh the mouth and keep it clean. Ananase, a proteolytic enzyme in the pineapple, actively breaks down debris (Rattenbury *et al*. 1999).

Context

 ### When to use mouth care

For many immobile patients, all that is required for them to maintain comfort and a healthy mouth may be a beaker of water, a toothbrush and toothpaste (preferably fluoride), a towel, and a bowl to spit into. Once helped into a sitting position, these patients can effectively clean their own teeth and rinse their mouth out afterwards.

Unfortunately, patients frequently miss out on the opportunity to carry out this aspect of personal care if unable to walk to the bathroom (Pidsley 1989). Imagine how you would feel if you were unable to clean your teeth before settling down for the night, or first thing in the morning. An essential yet simple nursing activity is to facilitate patients to clean their teeth as frequently as they wish, at least in the mornings and evenings.

Patients who wear dentures but are unable to take themselves to the bathroom will also need to clean their teeth, and it may be appropriate for you to do this for them. You may need to assist the patient to remove their dentures (wearing gloves and an apron) and receive them into a denture pot.

Mouth care as detailed in the following sections should be carried out on all patients unable to clean their own teeth or mouth.

Assessment of the mouth

The first essential step in carrying out mouth care is to do a thorough assessment of the condition of the patient's

Table 4.4 Problems to look out for when assessing the mouth

What to look at	What to look for
Teeth	Plaque, debris, decay, how well the dentures fit
Mucous membranes and gums	Redness, coating, ulceration, bleeding
Tongue	Furring, cracks, blisters, redness
Saliva	How much and how sticky/thick
Lips	Cracks, blisters, redness, peeling

mouth. The healthy mouth has a moist, pink tongue, gums, and oral mucosa. The teeth are clean, and dentures (if any) are clean and fit well. The lips are smooth and moist and the inside of the mouth is moist with saliva (Evans 2001). Table 4.4 lists problems to look out for when assessing the mouth.

The findings should be charted in the patient's records, so that improvement or deterioration can be evaluated and the planned care modified accordingly.

Frequency

How often to carry out mouth care depends on the patient. Some may wish to clean their teeth after every meal; morning and after the last food and drink of the day should be the minimum. Dentures should be removed at night, cleaned, and then placed in a denture pot containing water or a denture-cleaning solution overnight.

Patients who are 'nil by mouth' (taking nothing orally) or dehydrated could experience discomfort and a dry mouth, and need mouth care every 2 hours (DeWalt and Haines 1969, cited by Evans 2001).

Having reviewed research evidence, Krishnasamy (1995, cited in Dougherty and Lister 2008) concluded that mouth care 4 hourly reduced the risk of infection and 2 hourly care might be needed to maintain comfort (as discussed above), but that unconscious patients, those who are mouth breathing and/or on oxygen therapy, and those with mouth infections would need 1 hourly mouth

care. Frequency therefore depends on the individual patient and should be based on the assessment findings.

Special considerations

- Mouth care should be undertaken with caution, and not by the novice, in patients with facial or mouth injuries or bleeding gums.

- Before commencing, check that the patient does not have a latex allergy, and, if they do, wear latex-free gloves, as you will be touching the patient's mouth with gloved hands.

- Care must be taken with unconscious patients because of the risk of choking on the fluid used. Unconscious patients must therefore be positioned on their side so fluid does not run to the back of the mouth before it can be removed.

Procedure

Preparation

Prepare yourself

Before you carry out mouth care for the first time, it is recommended that you practise cleaning a colleague's teeth, and get them to practise cleaning yours. It is an intimate intervention and you may both feel embarrassed, but it is useful to be able to practise on someone who is not otherwise feeling poorly and it is good to know how it feels. You may find that it is difficult to clean teeth at the back of the mouth, because you are afraid of hurting 'the patient'. You may also find that it is difficult to get rid of the toothpaste foam, so you resolve not to use so much toothpaste next time. Reflect on the experience, and decide if you have learnt any practical tips for carrying out mouth care on patients.

- Make sure you have read the nursing records and know if the patient has any special requirements (see special considerations above).
- Read the previous assessment of the patient's mouth (if there is one) so you can notice any improvement/deterioration.
- Decontaminate your hands and put on an apron. After preparing the patient, environment, and equipment, put on gloves.

Prepare the patient

Whether you are going to facilitate the patient to clean their own teeth and rinse their mouth out, or are going to carry out the teeth and mouth cleaning procedure for the patient, you must explain clearly what you require the patient to do (see box below).

Prepare the equipment/environment

Always draw bed curtains/close door to ensure privacy and dignity, as this activity is of a personal nature.

Gather together a mouth care pack containing gallipot, foam sticks, paper towel, and disposal bag (see **Figure 4.13**). In addition you will need a soft toothbrush with a small head, toothpaste (fluoride, preferably non-foaming as this is easier to remove), water (or other mouthwash solution, see earlier section) in a plastic beaker, tongue depressor, pen torch, paper tissues, gloves (non-sterile), and apron. If the patient is wearing dentures take a denture pot too.

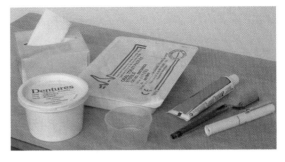

Figure 4.13 Equipment needed for mouth care.

Discussing the procedure with the patient and family

- Explain what you will need the patient to do (e.g. open their mouth or assist you to remove their dentures) and what you propose to do.

- Explain why mouth care is important.

- The explanation will need to be most thorough the first time the patient has the procedure done. This is to enable them to give their consent and cooperation.

Step-by-step guide to mouth care

Step		Rationale
1	Introduce yourself, confirm the patient's identity, explain the procedure, and obtain consent.	To identify the patient correctly and gain informed consent.
Removal of dentures		
2	If the patient is wearing dentures, these need to be removed. Most patients will be able to assist you with this, using their hands or just their tongue to push the top set forward.	You will be unable to assess or clean the mouth adequately with the dentures in place.
3	If the patient is unable to help, start by removing the top set. Hold the denture between your thumb and index finger, (with a piece of gauze if slippery), and rock up and down slightly, until the plate can be removed.	This releases the suction securing the plate to the roof of the mouth.
4	Bottom teeth can be removed by grasping between thumb and index finger, and twisting slightly to ease one side out of the mouth, then the other.	To remove the bottom set of dentures.

continued overleaf

| 5 | Dentures should be placed in the denture pot and taken to the hand washbasin for cleaning after the mouth has been cleaned (see below). | Dentures should be thoroughly cleaned and rinsed under running water to prevent reintroducing infection into the mouth (see **Figure 4.14**). |
| 6 | The denture pot should be named, and in residential settings it may be appropriate to mark the dentures too using a denture-marking pencil suitable for that purpose. | To avoid loss and ensure dentures do not get confused with other patients'/residents' dentures. |

Assessment of the mouth

| 7 | Standing in front of the patient, observe the condition of the lips, then get the patient to open their mouth. Gently hold up the upper lip to observe the condition of the teeth and gums, then repeat for lower teeth and gums. Proceed to check other structures as listed in Table 4.4. Use the tongue depressor to hold down the front third of the tongue, and use the torch to see into the back of the mouth. | Assessment will indicate how frequently mouth care should be carried out, and any other special measures that may be required, for example prescription medication. Depressing the tongue enables you to see further into the mouth. |

Brushing the teeth

8	If the patient is sitting in a chair, you should now move and position yourself beside the patient (on their right side if you are right-handed, left if you are left-handed).	You can replicate the normal position for cleaning your own teeth, with the toothbrush bristles facing you (see **Figure 4.15**).
9	If the patient is in bed, they should be on their side, and you will need to face them.	To avoid the risk of choking.
10	If possible, get into a comfortable position sitting down.	Sitting will avoid stooping and help prevent back pain.
11	Tuck a towel around the patient's neck to cover their front.	To avoid getting toothpaste on clothes.
12	Pour some of the water into the gallipot and wet the toothbrush in it. Keep water in beaker free from toothpaste.	Patient will use this water to rinse the toothpaste out of their mouth.
13	Using a pea-sized amount of toothpaste, and holding the brush at 45° to the surface of the teeth, use a circular motion to clean all top and bottom teeth from the back to the front, inside and out. Clean the biting surfaces by brushing at 90°.	Too much toothpaste will create excessive foaming and be difficult to rinse away. This ensures all surfaces of the teeth are cleaned.
14	Continue by gently brushing the gums, tongue, and roof of mouth with the toothbrush.	This will remove plaque and debris.

15	Rinse toothbrush and ask patient to rinse mouth. Give the patient a sip of mouthwash and hold a bowl under the patient's chin, to receive the mouthwash. Get the patient to do this repeatedly until all toothpaste has been removed. Wipe the patient's chin and lips with tissues.	To leave the mouth fresh and free from toothpaste and debris, and the lips and chin free from toothpaste and saliva. Toothpaste residue left in the mouth has a drying effect on the mucosa (Berry and Davidson 2006).
16	If the patient is unable to rinse their mouth out, you will need to remove the toothpaste. Use the foam sticks for this. Moisten foam sticks in water and use a twisting motion to gather toothpaste from all corners of the mouth, using a fresh foam stick for each area.	To leave the mouth fresh and free from toothpaste and debris, as above.
17	If lips look dry and cracked, apply lip salve/ petroleum jelly/lanolin sparingly.	These lip moisturizers prevent moisture loss from the lips and are soothing.

Denture care

18	Dentures, if worn, need to be taken to a hand washbasin and brushed using the patient's usual toothpaste, or even soap and water (NHS Direct 2007) making sure they are thoroughly cleaned on all surfaces and between crevices.	If dentures are not clean they can re-infect the mouth.
19	They should then be rinsed under running water and left in water or soaking in denture-cleaning solution containing sodium hypochlorite overnight.	Opening a denture pot and finding food debris from the previous day in stale water is unpleasant and unhygienic for both patient and nurse, and yet still happens.
20	Dentures should always be removed at night and stored clean and wet, and not be left in the mouth 24 hours a day.	Risk of mouth infections.

Finishing off

21	Dispose of equipment in clinical waste bin.	Contaminated with saliva, which is a body fluid.
22	Rinse toothbrush under running water and store in a pot at the bedside, so that it can dry.	Moisture encourages bacterial growth.
23	Make sure patient is comfortable before leaving bedside.	To promote comfort.
24	Wash hands with soap and water after removing gloves.	To prevent cross-infection.
25	Record result of assessment, and time of performing mouth care, in patient records.	Care plan, for example frequency of mouth care, may need modifying as a result of your assessment.

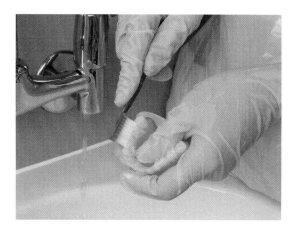

Figure 4.14 Care of dentures.

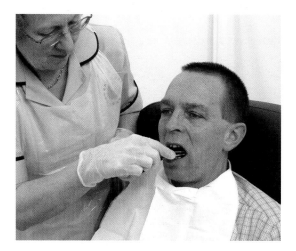

Figure 4.15 Cleaning a patient's teeth (with thanks to Jeff Knowles).

Following the procedure

Make sure the patient is as comfortable as possible and has all they need within reach (e.g. drink and call bell).

Reflection and evaluation

Having carried out a patient's mouth care, consider the following questions:

1   Do you feel you were successful in cleaning the mouth and making the patient feel more comfortable?
2   Is there anything you could have done differently?
3   Is there anything you should report to the nurse in charge?

Further learning opportunities

Even if you have already done so before, get one of your colleagues to clean your teeth for you. Take note of how comfortable it feels, how effective it was in getting your teeth clean and refreshing your mouth, and finally the psychological impact.

Now ask if you can clean your colleague's teeth and ask them for their response. Remember this experience when you next carry out mouth care for a patient.

Reminders

● Remember, toothbrush is preferable to foam stick.
● Water is as good as any other mouthwash unless the patient is particularly at risk of infection.
● Patients with a dry mouth could need mouth care as often as every 2 hours, or once hourly if they are on oxygen or unconscious.
● Do not use too much toothpaste or it will be difficult to get all the foam out of the mouth.
● Dentures should be removed at night and stored wet.
● What would *you* want if you could not clean your own teeth?

ⓠ Patient scenarios

Consider what you should do in the following situations, then turn to the end of this skill to check your answers.

1   Agnes Sheppard has just been admitted. She has dementia and is unable to care for herself. She has her own teeth. What mouth care might be appropriate for her?
2   Mrs Shaw, an 85-year-old, has returned to the ward after major gynaecological surgery. She is receiving oxygen and has regained consciousness. She is propped up in bed with several pillows, and you notice her mouth is so dry she is unable to speak to you. Her dentures are in a pot on the locker. What mouth care would be appropriate for her?
3   You are looking after a patient with an endotracheal tube in ITU. You know he needs mouth care and are aware that infections from the mouth can lead to ventilator-acquired pneumonia. How should you clean his mouth?

Website

 http://www.oxfordtextbooks.co.uk/orc/ endacott

You may find it helpful to work through our short online quiz and additional scenarios intended to help you to develop and apply the skills in this chapter.

References

Apostolopoulou E, Bakakos P, Katostaras T, and Gregorkos L (2003). Incidence and risk factors for ventilator-associated pneumonia in 4 multidisciplinary intensive care units in Athens, Greece. *Respiratory Care*, **48**(7), 552–60.

Bagg J, MacFarlane TW, Poxton IR, Miller CH, and Smith AJ (1999). *Essentials of microbiology for dental students*, 2nd edition. Oxford University Press, Oxford.

Berry A and Davidson P (2006). Beyond comfort: oral hygiene as a critical nursing activity in the intensive care unit. *Intensive and Critical Care Nursing*, **22**(6), 318–28.

Buglass E (1995). Oral hygiene. *British Journal of Adult/Elderly Care Nursing*, **4**(9), 516–9.

Dodd MJ, Dibble SL, Miaskowski C, MacPhail L, Greenspan D, and Paul SM (2000). Randomised Clinical trial of the effectiveness of 3 commonly used mouthwashes to treat chemotherapy induced mucositis. *Oral Surgery, Oral Medicine, Oral Pathology*, **90**(1), 39–47.

Dougherty L and Lister S (2008). *The Royal Marsden manual of clinical nursing procedures*, 7th edition. Blackwell Publishing, Oxford.

DrGreene.com (2007). [online] **http://drgreene.healthology.com/ dental-health/article1078.htm?pg=2** accessed 19/07/07.

Eggimann P and Pittett D (2001). Infection control in the ITU. *Chest*, **120**(6), 2059–93.

Evans G (2001). A rationale for oral care. *Nursing Standard*, **15**(43), 33–6.

Fagon J (2002). Prevention of ventilator-associated pneumonia. *Intensive Care Medicine*, **28**(7), 822–3.

Fitch JA, Munro CL, Glass CA, and Pellegrini JM (1999). Oral care in the adult intensive care unit. *American Journal of Critical Care*, **8**(5), 314–18.

Fleming C, Balaguera HU, and Craven DE (2001). Risk factors for nosocomial pneumonia. *Medical Clinics of North America*, **45**(6), 1535–63.

Franklin D, Senior N, Janes I, and Roberts G (2000). Oral health status of children in paediatric intensive care unit. *Intensive Care Medicine*, **26**, 319–24.

Garcia M (2004). Oral care of the hospitalised patient. *Cinahl Information Systems* (evidence-based care sheet), CINAHL AN: 5000001603.

Hahn MJ and Jones A (2000). *Mouth care in head and neck nursing*. Churchill Livingstone, London.

Holman C, Roberts S, and Nicol M (2005). Promoting oral hygiene. *Nursing Older People*, **16**(10), 37–8.

Koeman M, van der Van AJ, Ramsay G, Hospelman IM, and Bonten MJ (2001). Ventilator associated pneumonia: recent issues on pathogenesis, prevention and diagnosis. *Journal of Hospital Infection*, **49**(3), 155–62.

Miller M and Kearney N (2001). Oral care for patients with cancer: a review of the literature. *Cancer Nursing*, **24**(4), 241–54.

McNeill H (2000). Biting back at poor oral hygiene. *Intensive and Critical Care Nursing*, **16**, 367–72.

Netdoctor.co.uk (2007). [online] **http://www. Netdoctor.co.uk/medicines** accessed 19/07/07.

NHS Direct (2007). [online] **http:// www.nhsdirect.nhs.uk** accessed 19/07/07.

National Institute for Health and Clinical Excellence in collaboration with the National Patient Safety Agency (2007). *Patient safety consultation document: technical patient safety solutions for the prevention of ventilator-associated pneumonia*. NICE/NPSA, London.

Pearson L and Hutton J (2002). Controlled trial to compare the ability of foam sticks and toothbrushes to remove dental plaque. *Journal of Advanced Nursing*, **39**(5), 480–9.

Pidsley J (1989). *Individualised care in relation to hygiene*. University of Wales (unpublished masters dissertation).

Potting CMJ, Uitterhoeve R, Scholte OP, Reimer UW, and Van Achterberg T (2006). The effectiveness of commonly used mouthwashes for the prevention of chemotherapy-induced oral mucositis: a systematic review. *European Journal of Cancer Care*, **15**(5), 431–9.

Rattenbury N, Mooney G, and Bowen J (1999). Oral assessment and care for inpatients. *Nursing Times*, **95**(49), 52–3.

Ross A and Crumpler J (2007). The impact of an evidence-based practice education program on the role of oral care in the prevention of ventilator-associated pneumonia. *Intensive and Critical Care Nursing*, **23**(3), 132–6.

Xavier G (2000). The importance of mouth care in preventing infection. *Nursing Standard* **14**(18), 47–52.

Useful further reading and websites

Cancer Research UK website: **http://www. cancerhelp.org.uk** – mouth care for those with cancer and undergoing cancer treatment.

http://www.patient.co.uk/showdoc/27000593 gives basic advice to patients and carers on how to look after the mouth and (if applicable) dentures.

http://www.nuh.nhs.uk/qmc/PalliativeCare/ Documents/oralhygienecareplan.pdf for oral hygiene care plans for various mouth conditions.

 Answers to patient scenarios

1 Begin with an assessment of her mouth. Assist her to the washbasin morning and evening (more often if the assessment indicates), equip her with toothbrush and toothpaste, and see if she can clean her own teeth effectively. If not, sit beside her and clean her teeth with the toothbrush as described previously.

2 Offer a mouth wash of water, and sips of water to drink if allowed. Make sure her teeth have been cleaned and that there is water in the denture pot. Ask if she would like to wear her dentures.

3 You are right, effective and frequent mouth care is vitally important for this patient. You need help from the trained nurse on this one, as it is difficult to clean the mouth effectively around the endotracheal tube and the tapes holding it in place. Some staff may recommend cleaning the mouth while the tapes are being changed. This is of course very risky, as you could dislodge the tube. You should use a baby's soft-headed toothbrush, and clean extremely carefully under supervision of the trained nurse (Berry and Davidson 2006).

4.5 **Wound assessment and management**

Definition

A wound can be defined as any break in the continuity of the skin (Dealey 1999). Wound assessment is the systematic assessment of the person with a wound, their environment, and the wound itself, which leads to clear treatment objectives.

This section will consider aspects of wound healing, ranging from normal wound physiology to factors that may delay wound healing, before considering the choice of dressing for different types of wound.

It is important to remember that:

● Wounds should be assessed in a holistic manner, using a systematic approach.

● The whole of the patient should be considered, and the environment, not just the wound and the type of dressing.

Prior knowledge

Before undertaking wound assessment and management, make sure you are familiar with:

1 Anatomy, physiology, and functions of the skin.

2 Different types of wound dressing used in your area of practice.

Background

Stages of wound healing

Wound healing is a carefully orchestrated, complex series of events that depend on many factors. It can be described as the physiology by which function is restored by replacement of damaged tissue.

There are four phases of wound healing:

1 Inflammation.

2 Reconstruction.

3 Epithelialization.

4 Maturation.

These are described under various headings, depending on the publication that you read, but the principles remain the same.

Inflammation

The inflammatory stage of wound healing begins with the initial break in the skin's integrity when the epithelium is breached, and lasts 1–3 days. Bleeding occurs and the damaged ends of the blood vessels contract to stem the blood loss.

The clotting process is activated as platelets and other clotting factors are released; it is important that the body's defence mechanisms try to plug the hole as soon as possible to prevent bacteria invading the wound. A cascade is started that will enable the wound to heal.

The signs of inflammation are redness, pain, heat, and swelling, and it must be remembered that this is a normal response that should not be confused with wound infection. The capillaries become more permeable, partly because of the action of **prostaglandin**, and this enables white blood cells to enter the wound. The first to arrive are neutrophils, within 1 hour of injury, followed by monocytes which become macrophages. The purpose of all the white blood cells is to ingest bacteria. This is known as phagocytosis. Growth factors are also introduced to the wound. Growth factors stimulate cell proliferation.

During the inflammatory stage of wound healing there is an increase in **exudate**, which contains other factors necessary for wound healing. Towards the end of the inflammatory process, the function of macrophages is to control the transition between the inflammatory stage and the reconstructive stage of wound healing. Chronic wounds may remain in the inflammatory stage, with the presence of slough and necrotic tissue, and wound healing will be delayed (see **Figure 4.16**).

Reconstruction

This stage of wound healing is where **granulation** tissue forms (see **Figure 4.17**). Granulation tissue can be thought of as scaffolding on which new capillaries can

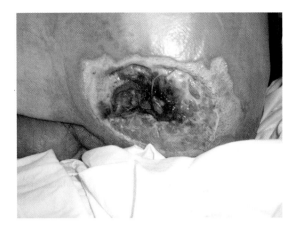

Figure 4.16 Chronic wound with slough and necrotic tissue.

grow. It fills up the wound bed and allows the wound edges to come together.

As macrophages mature, they attract **fibroblasts** to the wound. Fibroblasts are responsible for stimulating the formation of soft tissue growth, mainly collagen and elastin, and the production of blood vessels. The latter is known as angiogenesis. In normal wound healing, these begin to appear about 4 days after the initial break in the skin. These small blood vessels bleed very easily, and therefore if it is necessary to clean the wound bed, this should be done very gently to avoid damaging them. They are also the reason why the tissue is bright red.

The granulation tissue and blood vessels form on a matrix of connective tissue, known as the extracellular

(a)

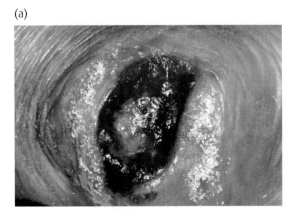

(b)

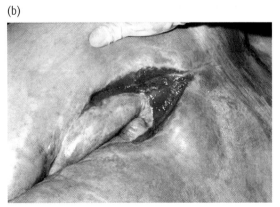

Figure 4.17 Granulating wound.

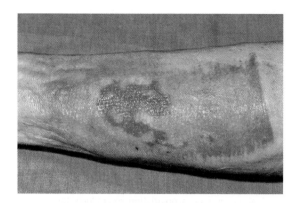

Figure 4.18 Chronic wound at epithelialization stage.

matrix. Over a period of several weeks, the granulation stage gradually gives way to the epitheliative stage. Fibroblasts are important in this process as well, because they stimulate wound contraction.

Epithelialization

Epithelialization is the term used for the skin edges contracting and the wound healing over (see **Figure 4.18**). The body will naturally try to do this as soon as possible, and in most cases of wound healing this is desirable. However, in some wounds, such as **sinuses**, early epithelialization is not ideal, until the sinus has filled up with healthy granulation tissue. If the sinus does heal over before this happens, an abscess may form under the skin, which will rupture again.

Epithelial cells, stimulated by growth factors released by macrophages, migrate from the wound edges over the surface of the granulation tissue and form a protective barrier over the wound. The wound surface needs to be moist in order for this to happen. Moist wound healing is a concept that was first developed in the 1960s. Lacerations were performed on the backs of pigs, and some were left open while others were covered in a protective film. The latter were found to heal more quickly than the dry wounds, and that is the basis of the concept of moist wound healing that we use today when selecting dressings (Winter 1962).

Maturation

This is the final stage of wound healing. The wound has 'skinned over', so it is not visible to the naked eye. The wound gains strength during this period, and the collagen is reorganized and remodelled, becoming flatter. The scar will never be as strong as unbroken skin, and is therefore vulnerable to further damage if it is knocked. The process of maturation can take up to 2 years.

Goals of wound therapy

Before any intervention begins it is essential to focus on what objectives need to be achieved to promote best practice, in both the short and long term.

Wound assessment and healing is a continuous process and it therefore follows that dressing selection will need to be considered and updated as the wound bed alters. Appropriate dressing selection should be made each time the wound is reviewed to ensure the presenting stage of wound healing is treated accordingly.

It is important to ensure that the peri-wound does not become **macerated** as this may delay the wound healing process.

Type of wound

Wounds can be either acute or chronic. An example of an acute wound is a surgical wound; an example of a chronic wound is a pressure ulcer. Acute wounds often heal uneventfully, as long as the right conditions for healing are provided. There is usually no loss of underlying tissue and the skin edges can be brought together and sutured, stapled, or glued. This is called healing by primary intention.

Chronic wounds tend to have loss of underlying tissue and this leaves a cavity that must be filled with granulation tissue before the wound edges can be brought together. This is known as healing by secondary intention. Patients who have chronic wounds often have underlying conditions that need to be addressed to help the wound to heal.

Location of the wound

This will influence the healing process. For example, a pressure ulcer on the sacrum will need to have the pressure relieved before the wound can heal, and a pre-tibial laceration may take a long time to heal because the blood supply is poor. The size, age, and extent of the wound should also be taken into consideration, as should the amount and type of exudate.

Box 4.2 Intrinsic factors affecting wound healing

- **Age:** older skin contains less collagen and is less elastic than younger skin, and it will damage more easily (Miller and Glover 1999).
- **Diabetes mellitus:** many factors can impede wound healing in the diabetic patient, and poor diabetic control can delay healing. There is an increased risk of infection (Bale *et al.* 2000).
- **Malignant disease:** patients may have a reduced nutritional status, may be treated with radiotherapy and cytotoxic drugs, or may be jaundiced. All of these factors will influence their healing status. They may also be less mobile, increasing their susceptibility to pressure ulceration.
- **Impaired blood supply:** wounds will not heal unless there is an adequate supply of oxygen and nutrients to the area.

Box 4.3 Extrinsic factors affecting wound healing

- **Nutrition:** vitamins, minerals, proteins, and carbohydrates all have an effect on wound healing (Pinchcofsky-Devin 1994). Larger wounds need more calories to heal (Williams 2002). The patient's nutritional status should be assessed using a recognized tool and, if necessary, the advice of a dietician should be sought.
- **Smoking:** carbon monoxide and nicotine have a detrimental effect on wound healing. Smoking may also act as an appetite suppressant (Dealey 1999). It also causes **vasoconstriction** and reduces the available oxygen (Siana 1992).
- **Drug therapy:** corticosteroids can suppress the healing process and can reduce inflammation (Benbow 2005). Cytotoxic drugs can impair healing by reducing cell division and can make the patient more liable to infection (Bale *et al.* 2000).
- **Infection:** all wounds contain microorganisms and these do not affect the wound healing process as long as they do not multiply and elicit a host reaction. The local signs of wound infection can include redness, heat, swelling, pain, malodour, friable tissue that bleeds easily, increased wound size, increased exudate, and formation of pus. The patient may also feel unwell or be confused. The early signs of local wound infection may be treated by topical antimicrobial agents such as silver or iodine dressings, but if the patient is unwell or confused, systemic antibiotics will be necessary. Wound swabs should be taken on the development of clinical signs, and a broad-spectrum antibiotic started immediately. When the culture confirms the type of microorganism in the wound, the antibiotic can be changed to suit the sensitivity if necessary (Kingsley 2002).
- **Psychological factors:** lack of sleep, stress, and anxiety can all affect the immune system and hence affect the wound healing process. Body image perceptions can also cause psychological problems.

Factors that may affect the wound healing process

Factors that may affect the healing process can be divided into intrinsic and extrinsic factors (see **Boxes 4.2** and **4.3**).

Rationale for three steps in wound management

Step 1 Aseptic/clean dressing technique

The aim of an aseptic technique is to prevent cross-contamination and introduction of any new pathogens to the wound being dressed. This procedure is considered best practice when dressing any type of surgical wound, including the removal of sutures, clips, and drains, or if the patient is immunocompromised. A clean technique is generally used on chronic wounds healing by secondary intention to prevent environmental and/or procedural cross-contamination. Hollingworth and Kingston (1998) clarify that when using either technique, prevention of transmission of microorganisms is the intention. To date there are no trials comparing aseptic technique with clean technique in chronic wounds (Royal College of Nursing (RCN) 2006).

Hand washing Evidence has shown that good hand hygiene is the most important factor in the prevention of spread of infection. It is therefore important that nails are kept reasonably short and clean and that hands are washed before starting a procedure. Nail varnish and artificial nails should not be worn.

Step 2 Wound cleansing

It is no longer routine practice to cleanse a wound at every dressing change, as this may be detrimental to the continued development of delicate granulation tissue.

Wound cleansing should only be done to remove:

- Superficial slough or wound exudate.
- Particulate matter, e.g. residual dressing matter.
- Visible debris, e.g. contaminated traumatic wound.
  (Towler 2000)

There has been much debate as to the use of tap water in wound cleansing. Following a systematic review conducted by Fernandez *et al.* (2003), there was no evidence of a difference in infection or healing rates as a result of using distilled, boiled, or tap water as a cleanser. There is no evidence that antiseptics confer any benefit and some evidence from studies in animals that they may be harmful (RCN 2006). Careful consideration should be given to assessing if an antiseptic is indicated, as these may have toxic effects on healing tissue and may delay healing (Morgan 1999). Products containing chlorhexidine, povidone iodine, or silver sulphadiazine may be useful in certain instances (i.e. critical colonization or wound infection) but these should only be used following a full wound assessment.

Acceptable methods of wound cleansing include:

- **Swabbing**. This should be done with gauze. Cotton wool balls should not be used because of fibre shed.
- **Irrigation**. This is generally considered preferable to swabbing as it employs a non-invasive technique. Various methods may be used to irrigate a wound such as the use of a syringe (either with or without a needle or quill), aerosol canisters, or simply pouring fluid over a wound from a sachet or capsule.
- **Bathing or showering**. This will gently cleanse the wound bed and can be useful for atraumatic dressing removal.

It should be remembered that when a wound is exposed the surface temperature falls; it may take up to 40 minutes for the wound to return to its original temperature and 3 hours for cell activity to return to normal (Miller and Dyson 1996).

Step 3 Dressing selection

This section focuses on those wounds healing by secondary intention. Before attempting to dress a wound, it is essential to consider the questions in Box 4.4.

Asking these questions will help to establish a rapport with the patient and give them a chance to discuss any

Box 4.4 Questions to address before dressing a wound

- How long has the wound been open?
- Does the patient have any known allergies?
- Does the patient have any aversions to known therapies?
- Has there been district/practice nurse involvement and, if so, what has been tried?
- Will underlying conditions affect the type of dressing utilized, i.e. is the patient diabetic, etc.?
- What does the patient understand about their wound and what troubles them most (e.g. malodour, exudate, etc.)?

concerns or questions they have. This may help to ensure concordance with any dressing regime implemented.

An ideal wound dressing: according to Morrison (1992), an ideal wound dressing should be:

- Non-adherent
- Impermeable to bacteria
- Capable of maintaining a high humidity at the wound site
- Capable of removing excess exudate
- Thermally insulating
- Non-toxic and non-allergenic
- Comfortable and conformable
- Capable of protecting the wound from further trauma
- One that doesn't require frequent changes
- Cost-effective
- Available in both hospital and in the community
- Capable of optimizing healing potential

Selection of dressings: given the amount of dressings available in both primary and secondary care settings, it is not surprising that this aspect of wound management seems to confuse many nurses. To make sense of the selection process, this part of the chapter has been broken down into sections identifying the aims to be achieved with the dressings chosen.

1. Necrotic and sloughy wounds
AIM: to remove **devitalized** or **contaminated** tissue from a wound bed until healthy tissue is exposed. Wounds that contain **necrotic** (dead) and ischaemic (low oxygen content) tissue take longer to heal and cannot be properly evaluated until debridement has taken place. It should

be remembered that necrotic tissue provides an ideal growth medium for bacteria.

Products to use:

- Alginate (e.g. Sorbsan®, Kaltostat®, Algisite®).
- Hydrocolloid (e.g. Comfeel®, Duoderm®, Granuflex®).
- Hydrofibre (e.g. Aquacel®).
- Hydrofibre and hydrocolloid mixed dressing (e.g. Versiva®).
- Hydrogel (e.g. Purilon®, Activheal®, Intrasite®).
- Hydrogel-impregnated gauze (e.g. Intrasite® conformable – note that this must be used with a film dressing to secure).
- Hydrogel sheets (e.g. Actiformcool®, Hydrosorb®).
- Honey products (e.g. Mesitran®, Medi-honey products).
- Iodine products (e.g. Iodosorb®, Iodoflex®).
- Maggot therapy.
- Topical negative pressure (e.g. VAC, Blue Sky).

2. Infected wounds

AIM: to rid the wound of infection and to prevent tissue damage and delayed healing. To address the issues of exudate control, pain management, and malodour.

Products to use:

- Alginate (if bleeding) (e.g. Kaltostat®).
- Carbon dressings (e.g. Carboflex®, Clinisorb®, Actisorb® Silver 220).
- Honey products (e.g. Mesitran®, Medi-honey products).
- Iodine products (Inadine® if not exuding, Iodosorb® or Iodoflex® if exudating).
- Silver dressings: alginates (e.g. Sorbsan® Silver, Silvercell®, Actisorb® Silver).
- Foams (e.g. Contreet Foam®, Acticoat® Moisture Control).
- Hydrocolloids (e.g. Contreet Foam®).
- Hydrofibres (e.g. Aquacel® Ag).
- Ointments (e.g. silver sulfadiazine (Flamazine®)).
- Non-adherent (e.g. Acticoat®, Urgotol® SSD).
- Topical negative pressure (e.g. VAC, Blue Sky).
- Zinc oxide products (e.g. Steripaste® – note that this must be applied either by pleating or in strips as it may constrict as it dries).

3. Cavity and granulating wounds

AIM: to provide a moist wound healing environment to aid the wound healing process. The management of the clean, granulating wound will depend on the amount of exudate. The aim is to achieve as long a wear time as possible so as not to disturb the delicate granulation tissue when removing the dressing.

Products to use:

- Alginates (e.g. Kaltostat®, Sorbsan®, Algisite®).
- Cavity fillers (e.g. Allevyn® Plus Cavity, Allevyn® Cavity fillers).
- Foam products (e.g. Allevyn®, Biatain®, Tegaderm®, Mepilex®, Activheal hydrogel foam).
- Hydrofibres (e.g. Aquacel®).
- Hydrogels (e.g. Purilon®, Activheal®, Intrasite®).
- Hydrogel-impregnated gauze (e.g. Intrasite® conformable).
- Non-adherent dressings (e.g. N-A Ultra®, Mepital®, Urgotul®, Atrauman®).
- Topical negative pressure (e.g. VAC, Blue Sky).

4. Epithelializing wounds

AIM: to protect and encourage a moist wound healing environment to assist the migration of epithelial cells across the wound margin.

Products to use:

- Film dressings (e.g. HC View®, Opsite®, Tegaderm®).
- Hydrocolloids (e.g. Comfeel®, Duoderm®, Granuflex®).
- Hydrofibre and hydrocolloid mixed dressings (e.g. Versiva®).
- Non-adherent dressings (e.g. N-A Ultra®, Mepital®, Urgotul®, Atrauman®).

5. Overgranulation

AIM: to flatten overgranulating tissue, thereby enabling epitheilialization to occur.

Products to use:

- Non-adherent dressings (e.g. N-A Ultra®, Mepital®, Urgotul®, Atrauman®).
- Foam (Lyofoam®).
- Carbon dressing (Actisorb® Silver 220).
- Iodine dressing (Inadine®).
- Steroid creams – these must be prescribed by a doctor and used for a restricted period of time (e.g. Dermovate NN®).

6. Miscellaneous dressings

AIM: to provide optimal healing for those wounds not responding to conventional therapies, or to address the problem of pain relief.

Products to use:

- Wound/exudates management bags (e.g. Option Wound Manager, Kerraboot).
- Wound balancing matrices (e.g. Prisma, Promogran).
- Ibuprofen dressings (e.g. IBU foam).
- Barrier wand/sprays (e.g. Cavilon®) (NB the barrier wand can be used on broken skin but the barrier cream cannot).

Dressings have a shelf life; this should be checked prior to applying any dressings, ensuring stock is rotated to prevent any waste.

Context

Indications for assistance

Certain wounds will be a challenge to the average practitioner who is used to dealing with relatively uncomplicated wounds. If a wound does not show signs of healing within an expected time frame, despite your best efforts, do not be afraid to ask for help. Your local employer should have care pathways for this. Examples include advice from the tissue viability nurse, or the podiatrist.

Diabetic foot ulcers should be treated with particular caution, as they can quickly become infected, leading to loss of the limb. This is an example of the necessity of a multidisciplinary approach, where other people involved are likely to be the tissue viability nurse, podiatrist, dietician, endocrinologist, possibly a surgeon, and the GP and practice/community nurse if they are being cared for at home.

Special considerations

- Whether you are nursing the patient at home or in the community will have a bearing on the way that you manage the patient's wound.
- Patients nursed at home also tend to have more autonomy than those in hospital; regardless of location, it is important that the patient understands and agrees the course of action.
- Location may also affect the types of dressing that are available.
- Identify whether there are any specific positioning requirements of the patient or the environment in which the procedure will take place.

Procedure

Preparation

Prepare yourself

Check the patient's records to ensure you have the correct dressing. Identify any problems the patient may have had previously with the wound and/or the dressing. If you are not familiar with the type of dressing required, ask for assistance from an experienced colleague. Check the patient's identity band if they are in hospital.

Prepare the patient

Before any procedure begins it is essential that full discussion with the patient and/or carer takes place. The discussion should include whether any pain relief is required prior to or during the dressing. Confirmation must be sought as to whether the patient is happy for the intervention to proceed.

Prepare the equipment/environment

Select an appropriate dressing, in light of the size and shape required, avoiding waste whenever possible. Check contraindications and recommended wear times.

Identify suitable clean area (in community setting) or use dressing trolley if available – clean the area/trolley with antimicrobial wipes (aseptic technique) or soap and water (clean technique).

Discussing the procedure with patient and family

It is very important that you discuss the wound, dressing, procedure, and likely course of events with the patient, allow them time to ask questions, and ensure that they fully understand what is going to happen. You must be honest with them and allow them to disagree if they wish. In this way, alternatives can be discussed and a concordant outcome is more likely.

Step-by-step guide to wound dressing

Note: wound dressing techniques may alter depending on local guidelines, but these generic principles are mandatory.

Step		Rationale
1	Introduce yourself, confirm the patient's identity, explain the procedure, and obtain consent.	To identify the patient correctly and gain informed consent.
2	Put on plastic apron. Cleanse hands.	To promote a clean environment.
3	Open dressing aid or dressing pack. Open packs containing sterile dressings and other items onto the sterile field without touching the sterile items.	To maintain sterility.
4	Put on non-sterile gloves and gently remove old dressing. Place dressing in appropriate plastic bag for collection/incineration. Cleanse hands.	To prevent cross-contamination during removal of contaminated dressing.
5	Put on sterile gloves. Clean wound if appropriate (see wound cleansing section). Apply new dressing (NB if packing a wound, ensure this is done with a minimal amount of force).	To prevent introduction of new pathogens during application of new dressing.
6	Dispose of all waste according to local infection control policies. Cleanse hands.	To prevent cross-contamination.

Following the procedure

1 Ensure that the patient is free from pain and is left in a comfortable position following the dressing change.
2 If appropriate, discuss the healing process of the wound with the patient, ensuring the patient is comfortable with any explanations given.
3 If appropriate, patient information leaflets may be given.
4 Discussion with the patient and carers can establish if the procedure could have been improved in any way.
5 Members of the multidisciplinary team may need to be informed of any changes that may affect rehabilitation processes.
6 All wounds should be monitored as part of the assessment process. 'Wound healing well' is a common comment on a care plan. This actually means nothing.

Considering the stages of wound healing, your documentation should include:

● Description of the wound bed and surrounding skin.
● Rationale for choice of dressing.
● An approximation of when the wound should be reviewed.

It may be that you want to photograph the wound using a digital camera. Ensure you follow your employer's guidelines for consent when photographing patients. Digital images are only as good as the person taking them, and care must be taken to try and approximate the position and lighting of the previous image if you want to make a comparison. Wounds may be traced and measured with a ruler, or measured with a commercial tool such as 'Visitrak' (Smith and Nephew). However, the size of the wound is only part of the documentation process, and you should consider the patient in a holistic manner.

Recognizing patient deterioration

Patients should not deteriorate after a dressing change but occasionally this may happen, for example if the patient is allergic to a particular dressing. It may be that the patient's whole condition worsens (not usually as the result of a dressing change), or that the wound itself deteriorates.

Should the patient's condition worsen, it is likely that the wound will show signs of breaking down. Therefore, it is extremely important that you consider the whole of the patient before you tend to the wound and take appropriate steps to rectify any problems as they arise, or to refer them to a more senior person. Should the wound deteriorate, it is important that you reassess the stages of wound healing in conjunction with the dressing selection as described above, and of course always document and pass on any changes to a more senior person.

Reflection and evaluation

Following the dressing change, think about the following questions:

1 Why is it important to review previous documentation to establish whether the healing process is proceeding satisfactorily?
2 Why should documentation be updated in a clear and precise manner?
3 Why should you ensure that there is an up-to-date description of the wound and any changes made in the choice of dressing used?
4 Why is it important to use sanctioned local wound care documentation and ensure copies are provided when a patient is discharged?

It is important to reflect on your experience in order to improve your practice. A simple model such as Driscoll's (2000) may help, for example:

What?
I was asked to dress a diabetic foot ulcer.

So what?
I prepared the patient and got consent. I set up a dressing trolley. I looked at the previous dressing type and decided to redress using the same type of dressing.

Now what?
When I looked at the wound, it appeared to be improving with evidence of granulating tissue. I asked the wound care nurse specialist to come with me at the next dressing change as I think the dressing may need to be altered. I discussed this with the patient.

Further learning opportunities

- Attend local and national study days.
- If possible, shadow a tissue viability nurse specialist.
- Subscribe to a recognized wound care journal.
- Review journal articles.
- Investigate the resources provided by the local and national tissue viability societies.

Reminders

- Assessing and managing wounds, perfecting a good dressing technique, and selecting dressings appropriately are skills that develop over time. Make sure that you allow yourself time to reflect and to practise.
- If you come across a wound or dressing that you're not familiar with, ask for assistance.
- Dressing selection is a constantly changing aspect of wound care. To ensure your patient is receiving the most appropriate care, keep up to date with the selection of products available.

Ⓠ Patient scenarios

Consider what you should do in the following situations, then turn to the end of this skill to check your answers.

1 You are caring for a patient with a wound in the reconstructive stage of wound healing. The wound bed is red, with evidence of epithelialization around the edges. How would you consider managing the cleansing of this wound?
2 You are caring for a patient who has an abdominal wound that needs to be dressed twice a day, due to the large amount of exudates. The peri-wound is becoming very excoriated.
   a What are the main aims when choosing a dressing for this wound?
   b How would you address the problem of excoriation?

3 Mrs P is a 79-year-old lady admitted to the Emergency Medical Unit following a CVE (cerebrovascular event) while on holiday abroad. She had been hospitalized abroad and on transfer to her local hospital at home was found to have a grade 4 (EPUAP) sacral pressure ulcer 15–14 cm in diameter and 6 cm deep. VAC (vacuum-assisted closure) therapy has been prescribed by the tissue viability specialist.

   a What contraindications do you need to consider before applying this therapy?

   b How often should the dressing be changed?

Website

 http://www.oxfordtextbooks.co.uk/orc/ endacott

You may find it helpful to work through our short online quiz and additional scenarios intended to help you to develop and apply the skills in this chapter.

References

Bale S, Harding DJ, and Leaper KG (2000). *An introduction to wounds.* Emap Healthcare, London.

Benbow M (2005). *Evidence based wound management.* Whurr publications, London.

Dealey C (1999). *The care of wounds: a guide for nurses,* 2nd edition. Blackwell Science, London.

Driscoll J (2000). *Practising clinical supervision: a reflective approach.* Bailliere Tindall/RCN, London: 26–8.

Fernandez R, Griffith R, and Ussia C (2003). Water for wound cleansing. *The Cochrane Library,* Issue 4. John Wiley & Sons Ltd, Chichester.

Hollingworth H and Kingston JE (1998). Using a non-sterile technique in wound care. *Professional Nurse,* **13**, 226–9.

Kingsley A (2002). Wound healing and potential therapeutic options. *Professional Nurse,* **17**(9), 539–411.

Miller M and Dyson M (1996). *Principles of wound care.* Macmillan Magazines Ltd, London.

Miller M and Glover D (1999). *Wound management: theory and practice.* Nursing Times Publications, London.

Morgan DA (1999). Wound management products in the drug tariff. *The Pharmaceutical Journal,* **263**, 820–5.

Morrison M (1992). *A colour guide to nursing management of wounds.* Macmillan, London.

Pinchcofsky-Devin (1994). Nutrition and wound healing. *Journal of Wound Care,* **3**(5), 231–4.

Royal College of Nursing (2006). *The nursing management of patients with venous leg ulcers,* 2nd edition. RCN, London.

Siana JE, Franklid S, and Gottrup F (1992). The effects of smoking on tissue function. *Journal of Wound Care,* **1**(2), 37–41.

Towler J (2000). Non-antiseptic cleansing of traumatic wounds. *Nursing Times,* **96**(23) Supplement, 14–17.

Williams L (2002). Assessing patients' nutritional needs in the wound healing process. *Journal of Wound Care,* **11**(6), 225–8.

Winter GD (1962). Formation of the scab and the rate of epithelialisation of superficial wounds in the skin of the domestic pig. *Nature,* **193**, 293–4.

Useful further reading and websites

Bryant M (2006). *Acute and chronic wounds,* 3rd edition. Mosby, London.

Dealey C (2005). *The care of wounds.* Blackwell Scientific, London.

http://www.epuap.org
http://www.dn.gov.uk
http://www.ewma.org
http://www.legulcerforum.org
http://www.nice.org.uk
http://www.rcn.org.uk
http://www.worldwidewounds.com
http://www.wounds-uk.com
http://www.tvs.org.uk

(A) Answers to patient scenarios

1 If granulation tissue is in evidence, do not disturb the wound bed. Gently clean the peri-wound to remove any excess exudates and dressing debris. Select the appropriate dressing, involving the patient in the choice, and document your decision.

2 a The main aims are to control the wound exudates and reduce the number of dressing changes; this will reduce the trauma to the peri-wound.

   b Apply a peri-wound protective barrier prior to dressing change to increase dressing wear time.

3 a VAC should not be applied to:
   - Fungating wounds.
   - Bleeding wounds.
   - Wounds with a sinus.

   b VAC dressings should be changed at least every 48 hours according to manufacturer's instructions.

4.6 **Pre- and post-operative assessment and care**

Definition

The term **pre-operative care** refers to the patient care required before surgery. This may include physical and emotional preparation of the patient and the environment to ensure that safety is maintained.

Post-operative care refers to the care that the patient will require in the immediate period following their surgery until they have recovered. The use of the nurse's observational skills is crucial during the recovery period, in order to identify potential problems, enable a safe and timely recovery, and prevent possible complications.

It is important to remember that:

- While electronic equipment is available to measure the patient's pulse, blood pressure, temperature, etc., all nurses need to be able to assess the patient's condition without relying on electronic equipment. This is particularly important when preparing the patient for and helping them recover from surgery.
- The clinical skills involved in pre- and post-operative assessment rely on the senses of the nurse. Listen to the patient – how do they feel? How does their breathing sound? Look at the patient – what is their colour like? Is their wound oozing? Touch the patient – are they sweating? Is the skin dry and sunken? A key nursing skill lies in recognizing what these assessment data mean in the context of the individual patient and acting appropriately upon that information to ensure that the patient is fit for their surgery and has an uneventful recovery.

Prior knowledge

Before attempting pre- and post-operative care, make sure you are familiar with:

1 The cardiovascular system and factors affecting heart rate, blood pressure, and cardiac output (the amount of blood that the heart pumps out with each heartbeat).
2 Pathophysiology of hypovolaemic shock: signs and symptoms and effects on the heart, circulatory system, lungs, renal system, and brain.

3 The respiratory system: factors affecting respiration and oxygen transport to the cells.
4 The renal system: production of urine and the effects of dehydration.
5 The basic requirements for clotting of the blood to take place (coagulation).
6 Normal blood values for full blood count, urea, and electrolytes, clotting screen, liver function tests, and the significance of abnormal readings for patients undergoing surgery.
7 Pharmacology: constituents of different types of intravenous fluids, e.g. crystalloids, colloids, packed cells, whole blood. Different types of analgesics, modes of action, contraindications, and side effects.
8 Microbiology: factors affecting infection in surgical patients, basic aseptic technique, hand washing technique, factors that influence cross-infection, and the importance of ward cleanliness.

Background

Undergoing surgery as an emergency or elective procedure places stress on the body. The stress response is the term used to describe the hormonal and metabolic changes that follow surgery, injury, or shock. It encompasses a wide range of endocrine, immunological, and haematological effects. In patients undergoing surgery, the magnitude of the metabolic response is proportional to the severity of the surgical trauma (Burton *et al.* 2004). Glucagon is released from the pancreas and catabolic changes occur, resulting in muscle protein loss. The overall effect is to provide additional energy sources and the regulation of sodium and water to maintain fluid volume and cardiovascular haemostasis. Other changes also occur following surgery, notably an increase in cytokine production, which is triggered locally as a tissue response to injury (Desborough 2000).

A key component of pre- and post-operative management is patient assessment. It is essential to record baseline observations to identify normal parameters for each patient pre- and post-operatively. The patient faces several risks in the immediate post-operative period: hypovolaemic shock; compromised fluid balance (see Section 6.7 for a detailed discussion of fluid balance monitoring); inadequate oxygenation; compromised safety; pain, discomfort, and nausea; and infection. Identification of these complications is dependent on comparison with baseline observations.

In order to understand the significance of recording basic observations in the surgical patient it is important to be able to perform the following manually:

- Take a radial pulse and be able to differentiate between a normal pulse and an irregular/thready pulse, as seen in the hypovolaemic patient (see Section 6.2).
- Perform a manual blood pressure measurement using a sphygmomanometer and stethoscope (see Section 6.3).
- Record a respiratory rate. Identify if a patient is using accessory muscles.
- Recognize dyspnoea and cyanosis in a patient (see Section 7.1).

These procedures require extensive practise with patients in order to gain competence and confidence. This enables the nurse to recognize significant signs and symptoms alongside the physical changes that are taking place.

Pre-operative preparation

Informed consent

Patient consent is the principle that anyone has the right to accept or decline physical interventions. There is no single statute in English law laying out the rules of patient consent. While it is not the specific duty of the nurse to gain consent for surgical procedures (such responsibility is usually undertaken by a medical colleague), the nurse is the patient's advocate (Nursing and Midwifery Council 2008) and hence has a responsibility to ensure that the patient understands the procedure being undertaken and the associated risks and complications.

Information should not be withheld from patients out of concern that it will upset them. Even when a patient specifically requests not to be told about it, health care professionals have a responsibility to ensure that they are provided with basic information about the procedure and the alternative options available.

The patient should also be given the opportunity to discuss their questions and concerns; this is a key principle underpinning informed consent. Clearly not all patients are able to make such decisions. Where a patient lacks the capacity (e.g. due to dementia, confusion,

fatigue, the effects of medication such as anaesthetic, or being unconscious) other forms of consent are feasible; however, all must be deemed to be in the patient's best interests.

Psychological preparation

Patients undergoing surgery may be very anxious and frightened for many reasons. For example: fear of a general anaesthetic; whether they will be awake during the operation; whether they will recover from the anaesthetic; whether the operation will be a success; and fear of pain. Talking to the patient may help to allay any anxieties pre-operatively (Hughes 2002, Torrance and Serginson 2000). It is therefore important that the nurse takes time to get to know the patient, using techniques such as open listening and open questioning (see Chapter 2). Encouraging the patient to voice their fears assists in forming a therapeutic relationship, and the nurse can then assess the patient's individual anxieties and plan appropriate measures to allay them.

It may be necessary to reinforce information with the patient several times to ensure they have an adequate level of understanding; patients have been shown to forget up to 60% of the information they are given due to anxiety (Bysshe 1988). Discussing with them what to expect post-operatively is important, for example whether suction/stoma care/sutures/dressings/drains/plaster cast, etc. are likely to be used and if so what care is likely to be involved. The amount and type of information should be carefully tailored to each patient's individual needs, and the nurse should take care to avoid the use of jargon and medical terminology.

Ensuring that home/social circumstances are satisfactory is also important. Simple actions such as an additional carer at home or a phone call to reassure the patient or relatives may make a big difference to the patient's levels of anxiety and help to relieve additional worries.

Food and fluid restrictions

Clear fluids are cleared rapidly from the normal stomach. A Cochrane review of randomized control trials has assessed fasting before surgery (Brady *et al.* 2003). There was no evidence of difference in volume or acidity of gastric contents when a shortened fluid fast was performed, compared to a standard fluid fast. These findings confirmed previous recommendations that clear fluids may be given to day-case patients and inpatients until 2–3 hours before surgery (Association of Anaesthetists of Great Britain and Ireland 2001, Royal College of Nursing 2005b). This would not apply to patients who are under-going emergency surgery, have gastrointestinal disease, or have had drugs such as opioids that are known to slow gastric emptying. There is insufficient evidence to address pre-operative fasting for solids, though a consensus of opinion on a fasting period of 6 hours for a light meal such as tea and toast is well established (Royal College of Nursing 2005b).

Box 4.5 Oral medications in fasting patients

- A patient's usual oral medications can and should be given pre-operatively with minimal fluid, ideally 2–3 hours before surgery.
- If the patient is fasting for an elective investigation, for example abdominal ultrasound, the patient's usual oral medications should always be given.
- It is important to avoid fatty drinks (e.g. milk) when administering oral medications prior to abdominal ultrasound, to ensure a full gall bladder.
- Seek clarification from medical staff if you are unsure whether to give oral medications prior to surgery or a procedure for which the patient is fasting.

Pre-operative marking

The National Patient Safety Agency (NPSA) and the Royal College of Surgeons of England (RCS) strongly recommend pre-operative marking to indicate clearly the intended site for elective surgical procedures (NPSA 2005).

- An indelible marker pen should be used and the mark should be an arrow that extends to (or near to) the incision site and remains visible after the application of skin preparation.
- The marking should be undertaken by the operating surgeon or a nominated deputy who will be present in the operating theatre at the time of surgery.
- The process of pre-operative marking of the intended site should involve the patient/family/significant others where possible.
- The site should, ideally, be marked on the ward or day-care area prior to patient transfer to the operating theatre.
- Marking should take place before pre-medication to ensure competent patient involvement.

- Marking should be checked against reliable documentation to confirm it is correctly located and still visible. This checking should occur at each transfer of the patient's care and end with a final verification prior to the commencement of surgery.

The NPSA *Correct site surgery verification checklist* can be downloaded from **http://www.npsa.nhs.uk**.

Assessment of past medical history prior to surgery

All patients requiring elective surgery should be assessed in a pre-operative assessment clinic, usually undertaken by trained nursing staff (Reed *et al.* 1997). Patients with a significant past medical history will also be reviewed by an anaesthetist. The anaesthetist will also discuss what type of anaesthetic is appropriate for the patient, for example:

- **General anaesthetic (GA)**, where the patient is put into a temporary state of unconsciousness by medication, including inhaled gases and intravenous drugs, and is unaware of what is happening to them.
- **Local anaesthetic (LA)**, where the area to be operated on is made 'numb', usually by injecting anaesthetic into the surrounding area.
- **Regional anaesthetic**, such as a spinal, epidural, or ring block, resulting in lack of sensation to a larger area. Both regional and local anaesthetics have the benefit of the patient being awake, thereby reducing the intra-operative risks associated with a GA.

It is important that the nurse is aware of conditions that will require additional specific pre- and post-operative care; the most common conditions are briefly outlined below.

Respiratory disease Patients with chronic respiratory diseases are at increased risk from GA and more likely to suffer with post-operative complications such as chest infections and pneumonia. It is important that patients with diseases such as asthma, chronic obstructive pulmonary disease (COPD), and emphysema are identified prior to surgery. They will require additional assessment with chest X-rays and respiratory function tests. Specific interventions such as chest physiotherapy, antibiotics, and nebulizers/inhalers may be required before and after surgery. In some cases patients may not be assessed as fit for a GA and alternative anaesthesia may be used, e.g. local anaesthetic or regional anaesthetic.

Cardiac disease Ischaemic heart disease (IHD) is caused by a narrowing or blockage in the coronary arteries that supply blood to the heart, the primary symptom being angina pain. Previous myocardial infarction (MI) may also indicate that a patient is not fit for surgery due to the increased risk of complications. A cardiologist's opinion may be sought. In elective surgery such patients may be commenced on medication (such as beta blockers) prior to surgery to reduce the workload of the heart.

Similarly, patients with an irregular heart rate and rhythm will also require more in-depth assessment. Common investigations include an electrocardiogram (ECG) to assess the rate and rhythm of the heart and an echocardiogram (echo) to assess its three-dimensional structure and function. If the patient is unable to take their usual oral medication, it is important that an alternative medication/route is considered. Medication must be given as prescribed prior to theatre.

Hypertension It is essential that the blood pressure (BP) is well controlled. NICE guidelines for hypertension (2006) describe hypertension as a persistent raised blood pressure >140/90 mmHg. Patients with high blood pressure are more likely to suffer a cerebrovascular accident (CVA) peri-/post-operatively. Patients who are known to be hypertensive pre-operatively and require elective surgery should have regular BP monitoring by their practice nurse or GP. Antihypertensive medication may need to be adjusted prior to surgery. The anaesthetist will decide which medication should/should not be given on the day of surgery. It is also important to consider that many patients will be anxious prior to surgery (Scottish Intercollegiate Guidelines Network 2004). The nurse should therefore maintain a calm and reassuring approach in order to reduce the anxiety of the patient.

Diabetes All patients requiring a GA will be required to fast before theatre for 4–6 hours. Patients with diabetes requiring regular food and oral hypoglycaemic medication or insulin to regulate blood sugar levels may develop hypoglycaemia when fasting, hence it is essential to ensure blood sugar levels are checked regularly pre- and post-operatively according to local policy. Patients with diabetes usually have an intravenous cannula inserted and may require an intravenous infusion containing glucose, e.g. dextrose/saline.

Patients who are insulin dependent will require sliding scale insulin. This involves an intravenous infusion of saline and insulin, adjusted according to the patient's blood sugar, which must be checked on an hourly basis. Patients with diabetes are at increased risk of developing infection and likely to have delayed wound healing following surgery (Bale *et al.* 2000).

Anticoagulant therapy Patients may take anticoagulant medication, which affects the clotting cascade to extend the time it takes for the blood to clot, to reduce the risk of thrombus and emboli. This may be prescribed for a variety of reasons, including irregular heart rhythm (e.g. atrial fibrillation) or a previous history of blood clotting problems such as thromboembolic events (e.g. deep vein thrombosis (DVT) or pulmonary embolism (PE)). Patients who undergo specific types of cardiovascular surgery, such as insertion of a prosthetic heart valve or peripheral bypass surgery, are also likely to be prescribed anticoagulants.

For some patients who take warfarin on a long-term basis, it may not be safe to stop taking it several days prior to surgery. In such instances the patient may require hospital admission several days prior to surgery in order to be commenced on a heparin infusion. Heparin is also an anticoagulant, and when given intravenously it has a short half-life. By stopping the heparin several hours prior to theatre, it allows the period of time that the patient is without anticoagulant to be minimized, lessening the risk of the patient having a thrombotic event. Such decisions are normally made in advance by the surgeon/anaesthetist based upon the individual patient's clinical need.

In addition, many healthy patients will also be given a modified form of heparin known as low molecular weight or fractionated heparin, which is given as a subcutaneous injection. This may be started before or after surgery, and is intended to reduce the risk of DVT (see next section).

Additional factors to be considered prior to surgery

Prevention of venous thromboembolism (VTE) (DVT and PE)

Patients undergoing surgery who are immobile for any length of time have an increased risk of a blood clot (thrombus) developing. This commonly occurs in the legs; however, a thrombus may travel through the circulatory system and lodge in a smaller vessel (an embolus). These two events can occur simultaneously in the form of a DVT in the leg followed by a PE. PE results in a lack of blood supply to the pulmonary capillaries leading to inadequate gas exchange in the alveoli, and can have fatal consequences.

A number of factors place patients at increased risk of VTE: raised body mass index (BMI); the immobility that follows some types of orthopaedic surgery; malignancy; previous DVT/PE; the elderly; females taking the contraceptive pill; and those with a family history of clotting abnormalities.

NICE guidelines for the prevention of VTE (2007) allow accurate assessment of patients at risk and propose a combination of anticoagulants (such as subcutaneous heparin) and physical methods to avoid venous stasis (e.g. antiembolic stockings and compression boots). All patients requiring surgery should be assessed for individual risk of VTE. The nurse is responsible for reassessing the patient's condition and should amend risk assessment scores accordingly.

Hygiene

Hygiene is of the utmost importance in the prevention of infection. Swabs for microbiology, culture and sensitivity, may be taken as a matter of routine in elective surgical patients. Patients identified as having MRSA prior to surgery should be treated with antimicrobial therapy according to local policy, and re-swabbed in advance of the surgery being scheduled. Many patients, particularly the elderly, immobile, and disabled, will require assistance with showering/bathing and hair removal prior to surgery in order to minimize the risks of surgical site infection post-operatively, and may need assistance with a theatre gown.

Patient comfort

Some patients may have underlying medical conditions, for example respiratory disorder or arthritis, which means it is more comfortable for them to be positioned sitting upright or to lie on a particular side supported by cushions. Try to gain the information pre-operatively so that patient comfort can be planned accordingly. Consider how effectively the patient can maintain a comfortable

body temperature. Many patients become cold when lying in bed, even though the ward environment may seem warm.

Pre-operative checklist

This is checked as the patient leaves the ward for the operating theatre. The format of pre-operative checklists varies from one health care organization to another; however, they all contain similar information including: the patient's name, date of birth, and hospital number; any known allergies; when the patient last ate and drank; whether pre-medication has been administered; and whether blood has been cross-matched (see **Box 4.6**). The patient's medical notes, investigations, and X-rays should also accompany them to theatre. The signed consent form should be filed in the medical notes and the operation site should be marked.

Immediate post-operative management

1. Observe for hypovolaemic shock

It is important to identify changes between pre- and post-operative observations that may indicate hypovolaemic shock. Patients can lose up to 30% of their circulating volume before the effects of hypovolaemia are reflected in changes in blood pressure and heart rate (Anderson 2003, Collins 2000). A falling systolic blood pressure following surgery may indicate hypovolaemic shock leading to inadequate tissue perfusion, damage to cells, and multiple organ failure (Anderson 2003).

When assessing the post-operative patient, nurses need to be alert for early signs of reduced tissue perfusion to help detect shock. These were described by Jevons and Ewens (2002) as shown in **Box 4.7**.

Whatever the cause of hypovolaemic shock, fluid/blood replacement and surgical intervention may be required in order to restore adequate tissue perfusion.

2. Observe for disrupted fluid balance

Two key factors can disrupt fluid balance following surgery:

1 Extended fasting times.
2 Fluid losses during and following surgery (which will depend on the type of surgery performed).

Box 4.6 A pre-operative checklist. Adapted from the *Oxford handbook of clinical nursing skills* (forthcoming) edited by Randle J, Bradbury M, and Coffey F, published by Oxford University Press. With special thanks to Rachel Peto.

Pre-operative checklist

Preparation

You will need the following:

Theatre gown
Identification bracelet
Hypoallergenic tape
Containers for dentures and/or hearing aid
Containers for jewellery and valuables
Equipment to record blood pressure, temperature, weight, and to undertake urinalysis
Patient's medical notes
Consent form

To do:

- Check the patient's medical notes for specific instructions.
- Ensure the patient is wearing an identification bracelet with the correct details.
- Ensure the patient has received all the information about the operation, has understood it, and has had an opportunity to ask questions. Reinforce information if necessary. Check if the patient is anxious and consider how you can alleviate this.
- Ensure the consent form has been signed and completed.
- Check and document the following:
    - Blood pressure
    - Temperature
    - Weight
    - Pulse
    - Respiration
    - Urinalysis
- Check the patient has undertaken any other pre-operative examinations and attach the following to their medical notes:
    - X-ray
    - Blood group
    - Cross-matching
- Check and document any allergies the patient has, including allergies to:
    - Medication
    - Antibiotics
    - Plaster or tape
    - Latex (NOTE: THE SURGICAL TEAM MUST BE ALERTED TO LATEX ALLERGIES)
- Undertake a risk assessment for
    - Pressure sores
    - Compression stockings
- Ensure the patient's skin has been adequately prepared (including a shower and removal of make-up, nail varnish, etc.) and check the surgical site marking.
- Check the patient has fasted. This includes:
    - Still water up to 3 hours pre-operative
    - Milk up to 6 hours pre-operative
    - A light meal up to 6 hours pre-operative (chewing gum and sweets are not allowed)
    - No alcohol 12 hours prior to procedure
- Encourage the patient to eliminate prior to the procedure.
- Assist them to get changed into their theatre gown.
- Remove any of the following that apply: prostheses, dentures, caps, crowns, loose teeth. Place in suitable containers and document.
- Leave hearing aid *in situ*.
- Remove any jewellery. Place in suitable container and document in valuables book. If applicable tape the patient's wedding ring with hypoallergenic tape.
- Administer prescribed medicines according to medical team instructions and if necessary advise the patient to remain in bed or sit afterwards; otherwise encourage circulation by moving around while they wait.
- Ensure the medical notes and investigation results accompany the patient to the operating theatre department and double-check the identification bracelet has not been removed.
- Sign the pre-operative checklist/care plan.

Box 4.7 Early signs of reduced tissue perfusion in detecting shock

- Restlessness or confusion (due to cerebral hypoperfusion or hypoxia).
- Increased respiratory rate occurs before tachycardia and hypotension.
- Tachycardia occurs when the heart attempts to compensate for low circulating blood volume.
- Low urine output (<30 ml/kg/hour) occurs as perfusion pressure to the kidney decreases. Conservation of fluid is activated by the renin–angiotensin pathway in an attempt to increase the circulating blood volume.
- Increased temperature occurs (this may also be due to the immune response).
- Cold peripheries and shivering action result in a decreased O_2 saturation signal.

It may not only be fluids that are lost but also body fluid components such as proteins, red blood cells, and electrolytes. Two further physiological mechanisms may also disrupt fluid balance:

1 Oedema may occur as a result of the inflammatory response caused by surgery (Carroll 2000, Hertz and Home 2001).
2 Renal function may be disrupted either as a result of surgery or as part of the patient's pre-existing medical condition.

The type of fluid replacement used should reflect the type of fluid that has been lost and will depend on blood loss, other drainage, and fluid losses such as nasogastric and wound drainage/oozing through dressings.

Accurate fluid balance monitoring is essential. It is the nurse's role to monitor and accurately record all fluids given to the patients, such as intravenous fluid, blood transfusions, intravenous drugs, and oral fluids. Fluid losses such as urine output, losses from wound drains, and nasogastric aspirate also need to be documented accurately on the fluid balance chart (see Section 6.7).

In order for medical staff to calculate the type and quantity of fluid replacements required, records of urine output and other fluid losses along with results of blood tests such as haematology and biochemistry results are necessary. The nurse should be aware of normal and abnormal haematology and biochemistry results and report abnormal results to medical staff in a timely manner. Additional electrolyte supplements may need to be given to maintain or restore normal electrolyte balance.

The pre-operative weight of the patient will influence the volume of fluid required. The cardiac status of the patient is also important; overadministration of fluids in patients with reduced myocardial function may result in heart failure and contribute to cardiogenic shock and death (NCEPOD 2001). Renal dysfunction may be worsened by dehydration.

3. Observe for inadequate oxygenation

Oxygen is given post-operatively for two reasons:

1 To encourage the transport of anaesthetic gases across the alveolar capillary membrane to be exhaled.
2 To meet the increased oxygen requirements resulting from the stress response/raised metabolic rate induced by surgery.

Clinical assessment of rate, rhythm, and depth of breathing needs to be made, alongside checks on the patient's colour and oxygen saturation levels.

Special consideration needs to be made for patients with chronic respiratory diseases such as COPD, as relatively low oxygen concentrations may be required to ensure an adequate respiratory drive. Arterial blood gases may be taken by medical staff in such patients, to identify whether the patient is retaining CO_2. Decisions about concentration of oxygen to be administered are made by medical staff; as a general indication O_2 should be administered at 24–28% in such patients while awaiting the blood gas analysis results.

Humidified oxygen should be provided for patients requiring long-term O_2 therapy to prevent drying out of the mucous membranes and aid expectoration of sputum. Drying of the secretions may lead to atelectasis (collapse of the alveoli) and pneumonia if the patient is unable to cough. Physiotherapy may be required to assist the patient to expectorate.

4. Initiate early warning scoring

Early warning scoring has been developed to enable more timely identification of patient deterioration. A number of versions of early warning scoring systems are available, for example the original early warning score (EWS) and the Modified EWS (MEWS) (Rees 2003).

An EWS is calculated using five simple physiological parameters:

1 Mental response rate.
2 Pulse rate.
3 Systolic blood pressure.
4 Respiratory rate.
5 Temperature.

For patients who are post-operative or unwell enough, a sixth parameter, urine output, can also be added.

The concept of early warning scoring is based on the premise that small changes in several of the above parameters will be identified earlier using EWS/MEWS than waiting for obvious changes in individual parameters, such as a marked drop in systolic blood pressure. Of all the parameters, respiratory rate is the most important for assessing the clinical state of a patient as it is the most sensitive indicator of a patient's well-being (Kenward *et al.* 2001). However, it is also the one that is least often recorded (Odell *et al.* 2007).

Patients who are acutely unwell pre-operatively and those who have undergone major surgery may be started on an EWS/MEWS chart as soon as they arrive on the ward, allowing monitoring of their clinical progress and giving early warning of any deterioration. Studies have indicated that once a patient has an early warning score of 3 or higher, urgent attention is required (Stubbe *et al.* 2003).

5. Identify psychological needs

Patients may have many psychological needs following surgery. They may be anxious about the success of the surgery, particularly if malignancy is suspected, or may have altered body image, e.g. following mastectomy or amputation. They may be dependent on the nurse for personal/hygiene care and the nurse must be sensitive to such needs and maintain patient dignity at all times. Explanations should be provided when changing dressings, emptying drain bags, etc. so the patient knows what to expect, and honesty regarding the progress of their recovery is imperative.

6. Assess risks to patient safety

It is essential to identify potential risks in the immobile patient or a patient who has received a GA or strong analgesic. Specific risks to be assessed include risk of:

- Falls
- Pressure sore development
- Unmet nutritional requirements
- VTE

Local policies and risk assessment tools will be in place for many of these aspects of patient care. These should be adhered to in order to minimize complications.

7. Assess and manage pain

Ensuring the patient's pain is kept under control is a nursing priority. For some patients, especially those requiring emergency surgery, analgesics may also be required pre-operatively. As nurses we should anticipate that all patients will experience pain following surgery. However, each person's response to pain will be different. Anxiety is known to heighten a patient's perception of pain, so pre-operative discussion with the patient regarding pain control is important.

Inadequate pain relief may cause pain on breathing and moving, which may in turn lead to postoperative complications such as chest infection, pressure sore development, constipation, and psychological distress, impeding the patient's recovery.

The use of a pain score will assist the nurse in accurately assessing the level of pain the patient is experiencing. However, Klopfenstein *et al.* (2000) reported that doctors and nurses underestimate patients' pain. Assessment of a patient's level of pain should be carried out during all contact with the patient, for example when performing observations or assisting the patient with care. It is important to reassess the patient's pain level once analgesics have been given, to ensure that pain relief is adequate. Repositioning the patient may also be beneficial. For further information regarding methods and types of analgesics, see Section 8.4 on pain management.

8. Assess and manage wounds

Initially the wound dressing should be left undisturbed for 24 hours following surgery, unless there has been excessive oozing, in which case additional padding should be applied and the medical staff informed immediately. Excessive pain from the wound should also be reported.

9. Monitor the patient during blood transfusion

Ensure patients receiving a blood transfusion are in a location where they can be closely observed. Advise the patient to notify you immediately if they begin to feel anxious or short of breath, or start shivering or flushing. Monitor the patient's pulse and temperature 15 minutes after commencement of transfusion of each unit of blood. Continue routine observations throughout the transfusion process. Adjust the flow rate so that the correct infusion rate is achieved. Document the start and finish times of each unit and record the blood unit number, component, and type. Stop the infusion immediately if you suspect a transfusion reaction. Administer as prescribed, assessing temperature every half hour during the transfusion, together with pulse and BP as described above (RCN 2005a).

Longer-term post-operative care – after 24 hours post-surgery

The following areas all need careful consideration and have been addressed in other sections of this book. Please refer to the relevant sections as identified below:

- Pain assessment and management – Section 8.4.
- Wound assessment and management – Section 4.5.
- Hygiene – Sections 4.2, 4.3, and 4.4.
- Nutrition – Sections 10.1 and 10.4.
- Elimination – Sections 10.5 and 10.6.
- Wound closure and wound drainage – Section 4.7.
- Discharge from hospital – Section 3.3.

Context

 ### When to undertake pre- and post-operative care

All patients undergoing surgical procedures need preparation and post-procedure observation. The extent of assessment, preparation, and intervention will depend on three main factors:

1. The size and significance of the surgical procedure itself, whether minor, intermediate, or major surgery.
2. The type of anaesthetic required.
3. Any previously existing disease, for example diabetes or chronic respiratory disease.

 ### When not to undertake pre- and post-operative care

Full pre-operative preparation is not possible for patients requiring emergency surgery. See the following section for essential aspects of pre-operative care for these patients.

Alternative interventions

The pre- and post-operative care described thus far relates to patients requiring elective surgery. However, some patients require urgent surgical intervention. These patients will still require initial assessment; however, the urgency of their condition may necessitate immediate surgery, so assessment needs to be expedited in these circumstances.

Patients requiring emergency surgery may have a great deal of pain and may have lost a lot of blood or have an excessive loss of bodily fluids due to vomiting or diarrhoea, resulting in dehydration and hypovolaemic shock. In these cases an accurate, speedy assessment is crucial and the patient may have to undergo a variety of invasive procedures prior to going to theatre. See **Box 4.8** for examples of emergency assessment and interventions for a patient requiring emergency surgery. Please note that not all interventions may be required for all patients; they will depend on the individual patient's assessment and circumstances. A patient identification band should be applied as soon as possible (see Section 3.1).

Special considerations

1. Past medical history

The patient's past medical history is of the utmost importance. Many elderly patients have underlying respiratory and cardiac histories that they may or may not be aware of. They will have been asked by medical staff about their past medical history but may consider their own symptoms insignificant and associate them with the ageing process, particularly if they have had their symptoms for some time and have learnt to accommodate them in everyday life. Respiratory and cardiac problems, along with hypertension, greatly increase the risk of a GA, so it is vital that patients with complicated past medical histories are identified in advance so that appropriate assessment and interventions can be initiated.

It is important to be alert for any symptoms not accounted for in the admission assessment, for example breathlessness on exertion or oedematous ankles in a patient with no identified cardiovascular or respiratory problems. Pre-assessment clinics, whether at home, at

Box 4.8 Examples of assessment and interventions for patients undergoing emergency surgery

Assessment

- Assess respiratory function: respiratory rate and depth, patient colour, and SaO$_2$.
- Assess cardiovascular status: BP, pulse, and temperature.
- Assess level of pain and administer analgesics as prescribed; assess effectiveness after 20 minutes and report to doctor if ineffective.
- Assess neurological state for responsiveness, confusion, agitation, and consciousness level.
- Assess during blood transfusion.
- Assess renal function: measure urine output and document on fluid balance chart.

Interventions

- Administer O$_2$ via face mask/nasal specs.
- Assist doctor to take blood for Hb/FBC/U+Es and group and save/cross-match.
- Assist in insertion and securing of peripheral/central venous cannulae.
- Administer intravenous fluids as prescribed and record on fluid balance chart.
- Insert nasogastric tube and measure and document drainage.
- Explanation to patient and/or family – offer explanation to patient for each of the above procedures as they are performed, reassure patient by answering questions. Ensure a calm approach to patient care is maintained.

the GP practice, or in hospital, are an ideal way of assessing the problems that patients encounter and allow safe planning for the procedure, recovery, and discharge of the patient.

2. Age

The age of the patient may also have an impact on their recovery. Wound healing is often slower in the elderly (Smoker 1999) and bed rest can result in deterioration of muscle tissue in healthy older adults (Kortebein *et al.* 2007). Elderly patients who struggle with their mobility may require assistance with simple tasks such as getting out of bed, or even changing position while in bed. Their hearing and sight are also more likely to be inadequate than in a younger adult. It is therefore important when communicating with the patient to ensure that they have their spectacles/hearing aid *in situ*.

Appetite and nutritional state may need to be assessed, and supplements offered to optimize wound healing and the recovery process.

3. Level of understanding

The patient's level of understanding and any communication problems should also be assessed. Some patients may wish to have a relative present who can later explain the information to them; however, this should not be assumed and the patient's wishes should always be respected. Cultural language barriers can be overcome with the help of interpreters.

The combination of information gained from the above will determine whether the patient is fit enough to undergo the procedure and anaesthetic as planned. Such assessments are carried out by anaesthetists; however, it is important for the nurse caring for the patient to identify and communicate any of the above problems, as well as the patient's wishes, to both the surgical team and the anaesthetist.

Interpreting readings

It is essential that nurses can assess pulse and BP recordings manually, and that they understand the significance of pulse pressure on palpation and know what a weak and thready pulse feels like. Similarly, taking a manual BP with a sphygmomanometer and stethoscope is a skill that requires practice in order to achieve competence and confidence. It is best practised on young, fit, cooperative patients before assessing severely ill patients. Ill patients may be in shock and have a labile pulse that is weak on both palpation (assessing by touch) and auscultation (listening with a stethoscope), making it difficult to assess.

What is right for this patient

Normal ranges and values are important; however, it is imperative that the nurse is aware of what the normal values are for each individual patient for direct comparison (see **Box 4.9**). Thus a baseline 'normal' pulse and BP recording along with respiratory rate and oxygen saturation are essential requirements as part of the admission assessment. It is also important that the patient's cognitive level of understanding has been assessed and any additional communication requirements are clearly identified so that pre- and post-operative interventions can be anticipated and planned for prior to surgery.

Box 4.9 Normal ranges and responses

It is essential that the nurse compares the patient's post-operative observations to those recorded pre-operatively to give a valid comparison. However, a general guide to normal values are:

- Patient is fully conscious/responds to voice or light touch.
- Respiratory rate 10–20 breaths per minute.
- Oxygen saturation >92%.
- Pulse rate 60–100 beats per minute.
- BP within 25% of pre-operative recording.
- Temperature >36°C.

Indications of potential problems and suggested actions

- An increase in pulse rate and BP may indicate pain. Check observations once pain relief is effective. Report to doctor if tachycardia and hypertension continue.
- A decrease in pulse rate may be satisfactory if patient is otherwise well. If accompanied by a decrease in BP, assess consciousness level as this change may be anaesthetic or analgesic-induced. If BP and pulse remain low when the patient wakes, report to medical staff.
- Increased respiratory rate and pulse rate followed by a fall in BP may indicate a severe hypovolaemia caused by fluid deficit. Exclude acute blood loss. Observe wound and drains for excessive losses. Assess fluid balance and check urine output. Report to medical staff immediately.

Procedure

Preparation

Prior to collecting the patient from theatre, the bed area should be prepared as shown in **Figure 4.19** to include:

- O_2 with nasal specs/face mask and suction in working order.
- Bed with clean linen/cot sides/call button to hand.
- IVI stand with fluid administration pump/syringe driver for analgesia.
- Catheter bag stand.
- Specific additional equipment, such as clip removers for a patient undergoing thyroidectomy, or spare tracheostomy tube and tracheal dilators for a patient undergoing tracheostomy.

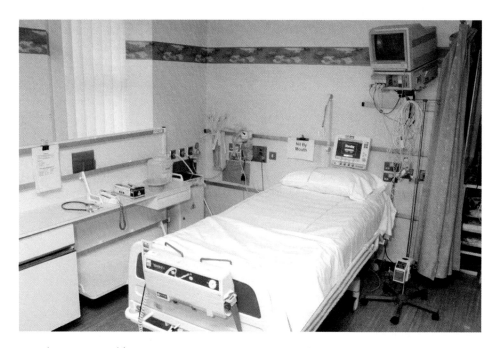

Figure 4.19 Bed space prepared for a post-operative patient.

Step-by-step guide to pre-operative care prior to theatre

Step		Rationale
1	Introduce yourself, confirm the patient's identity, explain the procedure, and obtain consent.	To identify the patient correctly and gain informed consent.
2	Undertake baseline observations of pulse, BP, respiratory rate, oxygen saturation, and temperature. Identify and report any abnormalities to medical staff.	To ensure observations are within normal limits. To provide baseline observations with which to compare post-operatively.
3	Ensure investigations have been completed and reported upon as requested, e.g. chest X-ray, ECG, echo, exercise stress test, ultrasound/CT scan, etc. Communicate any abnormal reports to medical staff.	To ensure that potential problems that could affect the proposed surgery are identified and managed prior to theatre.
4	Ensure patient consent form has been signed. Check patient's understanding of the procedure.	To ensure the patient understands the procedure being performed, including the possible risks, complications, and likely course of recovery, i.e. the patient has given *informed* consent.
5	Ensure pre-op checklist is completed.	To ensure patient is prepared for theatre safely.
6	Check patient identification details are correct on wristband and that wristband is secure.	To ensure patient is correctly identified prior to surgical procedure.
7	Ensure the patient requiring GA is nil by mouth for 4–6 hours prior to theatre (according to local policy), unless otherwise instructed.	To minimize the risk of aspiration peri-operatively.
8	Ensure hygiene needs are met, e.g. shower/theatre gown/clean bed linen. Remove nail polish. Hair removal at operation site by depilation or clippers (Tanner *et al.* 2007).	To reduce risk of infection.
9	Cover wedding ring with tape, remove any prosthesis.	To minimize risk of diathermy burns during surgery.
10	Explain to patient why each action is required, encourage patient to ask questions, offer information at a level the patient understands.	To assess and resolve patient anxiety. To ensure patient understands procedure and relevant interventions.
11	Administer pre-medication if prescribed.	To ensure patient is adequately prepared for the surgery and anaesthetic.
12	Assess pre-operative risk of DVT using recommended VTE risk assessment score. Administer antiembolic stockings/subcutaneous heparin according to risk score/local protocol.	To prevent thromboembolic events occurring post-operatively.
13	Ensure pre-operative marking is performed.	To ensure operation site is correct.

Step-by-step guide to post-operative care during the first 24 hours

Step	Rationale
1 Handover of information from the theatre/recovery nurse and review of relevant documentation of the procedure performed and any special instructions regarding nursing care.	To maintain continuity of care and promote patient safety.
2 Check patient colour, respiratory rate and depth, and oxygen saturation. Check the patient is fully conscious or responding appropriately to verbal stimuli or light touch. Observe for confusion/altered neurological state, e.g. anxiety. Administer oxygen as prescribed. Report to medical staff if patient's condition deteriorates.	To ensure patient is maintaining an airway, has an acceptable respiratory rate (10–20 breaths per minute), and adequate oxygenation is maintained (oxygen saturation >92%).
3 Initiate early warning scoring (as described earlier) if required.	To ensure any deterioration is identified at the earliest possible stage.
4 Check pulse and BP every 15 minutes for first hour. Then every 30 minutes for 2 hours, and reduce thereafter if observations are stable (increase/reduce observation rate according to patient condition). Observe skin colour for paleness, sweating, and peripheral vasoconstriction (cold extremities). Observe wound site for bleeding; report if bleeding exudes through dressing.	To observe for, recognize, and report hypovolaemic shock and haemorrhage.
5 Administer intravenous fluids as prescribed, e.g. crystalloids, colloids, blood. Undertake appropriate observations if blood transfusion in progress. Monitor urine output (report if patient has not passed urine for over 4 hours. If catheterized, report if urine output is less than 5 ml/kg of body weight per hour). Observe and record drainage, e.g. wound/nasogastric drainage. Report if excessive. Check bloods for haematology and biochemistry; report abnormal results to medical staff.	To ensure adequate fluid balance is maintained, dehydration is avoided/ corrected, and electrolyte balance restored. Renal function is maintained as pre-operatively.
6 Assess pain levels using recognized pain score (according to local protocol) when performing other observations, and record. Advise patient to let nurse know if pain develops or worsens.	To ensure patient is comfortable and pain/nausea is well controlled.

Administer analgesics and antiemetic regime as prescribed (see Section 8.4 for different modes of analgesia). Note effect and report to doctor if ineffective.

7	Assess oozing from wound through dressing each time observations are performed, and report.	To identify bleeding from wound/inadequate haemostasis/haemorrhage.
8	Change dressing as per recommendations (see NICE Guidelines due for publication October 2008). Assess wound site for heat, redness, swelling, pain, and purulent discharge. If wound exudate present, send swab for microbiology, culture and sensitivity, as per local policy. Remove sutures as instructed by medical staff. Use of appropriate dressing according to exudate level.	To optimize wound healing, identify complications such as wound infection, and treat accordingly.
9	Administer medication as prescribed (to include pre-operative medication – continue where possible, e.g. cardiorespiratory medication). Antibiotic prophylaxis/VTE prophylaxis.	To ensure treatment continues for underlying conditions. To minimize risk of infection and VTE.
10	Observe and record temperature, reporting pyrexia. Identify possible sources of infection. Send appropriate swab/specimens (e.g. wound exudate, sputum, urine) to microbiology for culture and sensitivity.	To identify possible sources of infection.
11	Use of strict hand washing technique between patient contacts. Use of gloves and other PPE when attending to patient (see Section 4.1, *Infection prevention and control*).	To minimize risk of cross-infection.
12	Assist the patient with personal hygiene as required (see Section 4.2, *Skin care*). Ensure mouth is clean and moist (see Section 4.4, *Mouth care*). Ensure good hand washing technique/appropriate use of aprons and alcohol hand gel (see Section 4.1).	To ensure the patient is clean and comfortable. To reduce infection risk.
13	Assess pressure sore risk using Waterlow score or similar. Assist patient to change position regularly, use of pressure-relieving mattress as required.	To prevent pressure sores developing.
14	Depending on type/severity of surgery and patient's general condition, assess nutritional requirements. Involvement of dietician if required.	To aid wound healing and prevent malnutrition.

Reflection and evaluation

When you have cared for a patient pre- and post-operatively, think about the following questions:

1 How did the patient feel prior to their surgery? What anxieties and concerns did they have?

2 Were you able to answer the patient's questions?

3 If so, would it be useful to provide similar information to other patients routinely or not?

4 Did you identify any problems post-operatively while carrying out post-operative observations? If so, what action did you take?

5 Did the patient suffer any complications post-operatively? If so, how could they have been prevented?

Reminders

• Ask the patient how they are feeling and listen to their response. Their pain, discomfort, etc. provide vital clues when you are performing basic observations.

• Remember to assess the patient's level of pain and comfort at all times and aim to keep them pain-free.

• Always explain to the patient what you are going to do.

• Minimize disturbances when possible if the patient is asleep.

Patient scenarios

Consider what you should do in the following situations, then turn to the end of this skill to check your answers.

1 Patient A returned from theatre an hour ago following major abdominal surgery. He looks very pale and is sweating; he is tachycardic and hypertensive with rapid, shallow breathing. What might be the problem?

2 Patient B returned from theatre 2 hours ago; he is tachycardic and hypotensive and is also pale and sweating. He is catheterized and has only passed 10 ml of urine in the last hour. What further observations would you perform and why? What action would you take next?

3 Patient C, an 85-year-old lady, had surgery last week and has a past medical history of type 2 diabetes. She complains of feeling hot and sweaty. What observations would you perform next and why?

Website

 http://www.oxfordtextbooks.co.uk/orc/endacott

You may find it helpful to work through our short online quiz and additional scenarios intended to help you to develop and apply the skills in this chapter.

References

Anderson I (2003). *Care of the critically ill surgical patient*, 2nd edition. Arnold, London.

Association of Anaesthetists of Great Britain and Ireland (2001). *Pre-operative assessment: the role of the anaesthetist* [online] **http://www.aagbi.org/publications/guidelines/docs/preoperativeaasoi.pdf** accessed 18/12/08.

Bale S, Harding DJ, and Leaper KG (2000). *An introduction to wounds*. Emap Healthcare, London.

Brady M, Kinn S, and Stuart P (2003). Pre-operative fasting for adults to prevent perioperative complications (Cochrane Review). *The Cochrane Library*, Issue 4. Wiley, Chichester.

Burton D, Nicholson G, and Hall G (2004). Endocrine and metabolic response to surgery. *Continuing Education in Anaesthesia*, **4**(5), 144–7.

Bysshe J (1988). The effect of giving information to patients before surgery. *Nursing*, **3**(30), 36–9.

Carroll H (2000). Fluid and electrolytes. In: Sheppard and Wright M, eds. *Principles and practice of high dependency nursing*, pp. 237–68. Bailliere Tindall, London.

Collins T (2000). Understanding shock. *Nursing Standard*, **14**(49), 35–9.

Desborough JP (2000). The stress response to trauma and surgery. *British Journal of Anaesthesia*, **85**(1), 109–17.

Hertz U and Home M (2001). *Acid–base balance*, 4th edition. Mosby, St Louis, MO.

Hughes E (2002). The effects of giving patients pre-operative information. *Nursing Standard*, **16**(28), 33–7.

Jevons P and Ewens B (2002). *Monitoring the critically ill patient*. Blackwell Science, Oxford.

Kenward G, Hodgetts T, and Castle N (2001). Time to put the R back in TPR. *Nursing Times*, **97**, 32–3.

Klopfenstein C, Herrmann FR, Mamie C, Van Gessel E, and Forster A (2000). Pain intensity and pain relief after surgery. *Acta Anaesthesiology Scandinavia*, **44**(1), 58.

Kortebein P, Ferrando A, Lombeida J, Wolfe R, and Evans WJ (2007). Effect of 10 days of bed rest on skeletal muscle in healthy older adults. *Journal of the American Medical Association*, **297**, 1772–4.

National Confidential Enquiry into Patient Outcome and Death (2001). *Changing the way we operate*. NCEPOD, London.

National Institute for Health and Clinical Excellence (2006). *Hypertension: management of hypertension in adults in primary care*. NICE, London.

National Institute for Health and Clinical Excellence (2007). *Clinical Guideline 46: Venous thromboembolism: reducing the risk of thromboembolism (deep vein thrombosis and pulmonary embolism) in inpatients undergoing surgery*. NICE, London.

National Patient Safety Agency (2005). *Correct site surgery verification checklist* [online] **http://www.npsa. nhs.uk/patientsafety/alerts-and-directives/ alerts/correct-site-surgery/** accessed 18/12/08.

Nursing and Midwifery Council (2008). *The Code: standards of conduct, performance and ethics for nurses and midwives*. NMC, London.

Odell M, Rechner IJ, Kapila A, *et al.* (2007). The effect of a critical care outreach service and an early warning scoring system on respiratory rate recording on the general wards. *Resuscitation*, **74**(3), 470–5.

Reed M, Wright S, and Armitage F (1997). Nurse led general surgical preoperative assessment clinic. *Journal of the Royal College of Surgeons of Edinburgh*, **42**, 310–13.

Rees JE (2003). Early warning scores. *World Anaesthesia*, **17**(10), 1–5.

Royal College of Nursing (2005a). *Right blood, right patient, right time: RCN guidance for improving transfusion practice*. RCN, London.

Royal College of Nursing (2005b). *Peri-operative fasting in adults and children: Practice guideline*. RCN, London. [online] **http://www.rcn.org.uk_data/ assets/pdf_file/0009/78678/002800.pdf** accessed 18/12/08.

Scottish Intercollegiate Guidelines Network (2004). *Postoperative management in adults: A practical guide to postoperative care for clinical staff*. SIGN, Edinburgh.

Smoker A (1999). Skin care in old age. *Nursing Standard*, **13**(48), 47–53.

Stubbe CP, Davies RG, Williams E, Rutherford P, and Gemmell L (2003). Effects of introducing the modified Early Warning Score on clinical outcomes, cardiopulmonary arrests and intensive care utilisation on acute medical admissions. *Anaesthesia*, **58**, 775–803.

Tanner J, Woodings D, and Moncaster K (2007). Preoperative hair removal to reduce surgical site infection (Cochrane Review). *The Cochrane Library*, Issue 2.

Torrance C and Serginson E (2000). *Surgical nursing*. Bailliere Tindall, London.

Useful further reading and websites

Alexander M, Fawcett J, and Runcimann P (2006). *Nursing practice hospital and home – the adult*, 3rd edition. Churchill Livingstone, London.

Richards A and Edwards S (2003). *A nurse's survival guide to the ward*. Churchill Livingstone, London.

Walker J (2002). Emotional and psychological pre-operative preparation in adults. *British Journal of Nursing*, **11**(1558), 567–75.

http://guidance.nice.org.uk/topic/surgical and **http://nhsdirect.nhs.uk/guide** (useful information regarding specific procedures)

http://www.shotuk.org (serious hazards of transfusion)

http://www.SIGN.ac.uk (outlines post-operative management in adults)

Ⓐ **Answers to patient scenarios**

1 The most likely cause of patient A's hypertension and tachycardia is pain. His breathing is likely to be shallow as normal breathing increases his pain.

2 Patient B is likely to be suffering reduced tissue perfusion as a result of hypovolaemic shock. Continue to monitor BP, pulse, and urine output. Observe for signs of restlessness or confusion. Check the wound drains and wound site for signs of haemorrhage. Alert a more senior colleague immediately. Prepare to administer IV fluids. The patient may need further surgical intervention; alert relatives to the change in his condition.

3 Immediately assess Mrs C's blood sugar to ensure she is not hypoglycaemic. Examine the wound site for redness, swelling, exudate; Mrs C will be at increased risk of wound infection due to diabetes. Record temperature and blood sugar and assess for pain. Take a wound swab for microbiology, culture and sensitivity.

4.7 **Wound closure and wound drainage**

Definition

Wound closure is defined as the bringing together of wound edges using fixation appropriate to the location and type of wound. Wound drainage refers to the steps taken when closing a wound to prevent fluid accumulating in the wound bed. The nurse's role in wound closure and drainage includes assessment of the wound, removal of sutures, observation of drainage, and removal of wound drains.

The skills covered in this section include:

- Removal of wound drains.
- Removal of sutures.
- Removal of staples.

It is important to remember that:

- The purpose of wound closure is to bring the wound edges together so that the wound can heal by primary intention.
- The purpose of wound drainage is to promote healing by preventing accumulation of fluid at the wound site.
- A wound drain is a two-way portal and can introduce infection into a wound as well as removing potentially infected material.

Prior knowledge

Before undertaking management of wound closures or wound drains, make sure you are familiar with:

1 Anatomy and physiology of the skin.
2 Mechanisms of wound healing (see Section 4.5)
3 Principles of infection control (see Section 4.1)
4 Principles of skin care (see Section 4.2)

Background

Wound closure

Surgical and traumatic wounds are closed to promote healing by primary intention. In order for this to have maximum chance of success, the wound should be clean and closed as soon as possible in most cases. However, in skin surgery the wound is sometimes left open to await histology results.

The epithelial bridge across the scar establishes rapidly and the wound appears healed within 7–10 days. Depending on the depth of the wound, it can take some time for collagen fibres to re-establish and strengthen the wound. If sutures are removed or excessive force is applied to the wound area before the wound has healed, the wound can reopen (or dehisce). The wound may be re-sutured, for example some deep abdominal wounds, or allowed to heal by secondary intention.

If the wound edges do not meet easily, for example because of traumatic tissue loss leaving a gaping irregular wound, the wound will be allowed to heal by secondary intention (see Section 4.5 for further details on mechanisms of wound healing). The wound will heal from the base upwards by laying down new tissue. Full or partial thickness skin grafts may be used to fill any defects.

Abdominal wounds contaminated with faecal material may also be left 'open' for a period of time (usually days) to minimize risk of wound infection or dehiscence; the patient is then returned to theatre for suturing (delayed primary closure, Cohn *et al.* 2001). A newer technique – the Prolene® zip – is used for these patients in some centres (Oliver and Al-Mufti 2005). Vacuum therapy is also used to help close wounds by secondary intention. Dehisced abdominal wounds may be closed in this way.

All wounds will form a scar; the best case scenario is a fine, hairline scar. However, it takes months for a scar to contract completely and remodel to its permanent form. Scarring may be excessive if sutures are left in place for a prolonged period of time. Two further problems may arise at the wound site:

1 A hypertrophic scar – this looks and feels lumpy and will usually settle in time, although this can take up to 6 months. If the outcome is cosmetically poor, the scar can be revised.
2 Formation of a keloid – an enlarged firm mass of scar tissue that extends beyond the actual site of repair and tends to be darker than the surrounding skin. A keloid results from an abnormal over-healing response to injury and has a genetic component. If the patient is prone to keloid scars, this will also be

evident in any previous wounds and minor procedures such as body piercings. Keloids can be injected with triamcinalone; the scar cannot be revised as the same overhealing response could occur, potentially in a more extreme manner.

Types of wound closure

Wounds are closed by mechanical means using sutures, staples, or adhesive. See **Figure 4.20** for three common types of suture.

When selecting a method of wound closure, the main decisions to be made relate to the closure technique (see Figure 4.20), the suture material (gauge and dissolving/non-dissolving), and the size/shape/type of needle or applicator (Leaper and Harding 2006). These decisions depend on factors such as the depth of the wound, whether it is contaminated, and the extent of likely movement of the wound edges during the healing process.

Staples Staples have the advantage of being quicker, more economical, and causing fewer infections than stitches (Leaper and Harding 2006). Disadvantages of staples include permanent scars if used inappropriately and imperfect aligning of the wound edges, which can lead to improper healing. Staples are often used on scalp lacerations and to close surgical wounds. Staples approximate and evert the wound edges well, especially on skin that might have a tendency to roll in on itself, for example neck wounds following thyroid surgery.

Adhesive Strips Wounds can be closed using adhesive strips; these are easily managed and removed by the patient, with appropriate advice (Cole 2007). A further alterative to sutures or clips is adhesive, similar to glue; this is increasingly popular for wounds in difficult areas or in children. Studies demonstrate no difference in outcomes for these methods (e.g. Mattick *et al*. 2002). A combination of these two methods (strips and adhesive) can be used in wounds that are at risk of separation after initial closure (Atkinson 2003). For facial wounds, adhesive is often used for the upper part of the face and sutures for wounds on the more mobile lower third of the face (Allonby-Neve and Okereke 2006).

The use of wound dressings for sutured wounds remains a disputed area of practice; a clear polyurethane

(a)

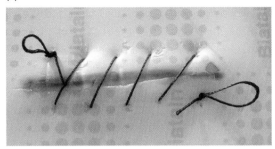

(b)

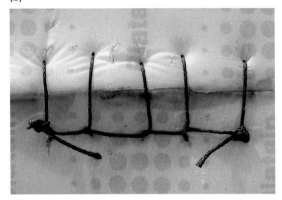

(c)

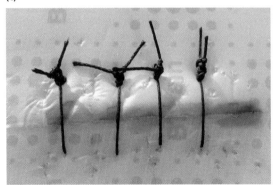

Figure 4.20 Three common types of sutures: (a) running sutures; (b) interlocking sutures; (c) interrupted sutures.

dressing allows visual inspection of the wound while an 'island' dressing, with a central gauze pad covered by a polyurethane dressing, absorbs wound exudate and reduces risk of wound leakage (Leaper and Harding 2006).

A further area of variable practice lies in whether sutured wounds should remain uncovered; guidelines published over a decade ago instruct that a wound should be kept dry and covered for 24–48 hours (Mangram *et al*. 1999). However, studies in hospital and community settings have shown no difference in infection rates whether wounds were covered or uncovered and whether the sutures are kept dry or allowed to get wet (Heal *et al.* 2006, Carragee and Vittum 1996). The use of Vaseline® and a simple island dressing is common and supports moist wound healing principles (see Section 4.5 for more information).

Wound drainage

The purpose of wound drains is to promote healing by preventing accumulation of fluid at the wound site. If allowed to accumulate, fluid collections can lead to infection or abscess formation.

Wound drains should be monitored for volume, consistency of drainage, and maintenance of suction each time post-operative observations are undertaken. Patients with diabetes have an increased risk of infection (Leaper and Harding 2006), so particular attention should be paid to monitoring wound drainage.

Your local policy for documentation of wound drainage should be followed. If wound drainage ceases suddenly, be alert for signs of haematoma formation or infection around the wound. It is important to remember that a wound drain is a two-way portal and can introduce infection into a wound as well as removing potentially infected material.

Prolonged wound drainage is a serious postoperative complication and may be influenced by a number of factors. Comparison between patients following hip arthroplasty (n=1211) and knee arthoplasty (n=1226) found that each day of prolonged wound drainage increased the risk of wound infection by 42% for patients following hip arthroplasty and 29% for patients following knee arthroplasty (Patel *et al.* 2007). Prolonged wound drainage resulted in a significantly longer hospital stay for patients in both groups (p<0.001).

Recent studies have investigated patient outcomes if no wound drain is inserted. Purushotham *et al.* (2002) found that hospital stay length was reduced, with no adverse surgical or psychological effects, in patients who did not have wound drains inserted following surgery for breast cancer. For patients undergoing elective colorectal surgery, a meta-analysis of six randomized clinical trials of patients allocated to wound drainage or no wound drainage found no significant differences across a number of outcomes, including mortality, wound breakdown (dehiscence), and wound infection (Karliczek *et al.* 2006). These studies emphasize that the evidence for use of wound drains is inconclusive for some types of surgery.

Wound drains are usually removed while the patient is still in hospital. One study evaluated outcomes for patients discharged home early after breast surgery with a wound drain *in situ*; the researchers found that patients in the early discharge group were satisfied with their care and felt early discharge was a safe option (Chapman and Purushotham 2001). However, participants also emphasized the importance of patient choice; those in the early discharge group had chosen this option.

Types of wound drain

Drains operate in two ways:

1. By passive (open) drainage: the wound drain provides a sinus tract along which drainage escapes into a dressing or drainage bag. Two examples of passive wound drainage are shown in **Figure 4.21**.
2. By active (closed) drainage: the drain is attached to a vacuum container and drainage is encouraged by a gentle negative pressure.

Wound drains are inserted either in the incision or in a stab wound lateral to the incision. A wound drain may or may not be sutured to the skin.

Context

 ### When to remove a wound drain

Wound drains are generally left *in situ* until drainage is less than 50 ml per day (Purushotham *et al.* 2002).

 ### When not to remove a wound drain

It is important not to remove drains while there is still bleeding or excess exudate from the wound.

Alternative interventions

Some types of wound drain are shortened 1 or 2 days before removal. This process brings the drain closer to the

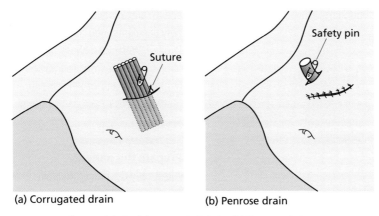

(a) Corrugated drain (b) Penrose drain

Figure 4.21 Two common types of wound drain: (a) corrugated drain; (b) Penrose drain.

Table 4.5 Types of wound exudate

	Description	Contents
Serous	Clear or slightly yellow	Plasma and extracellular fluid
Purulent	Thick, yellowish or green	Pus (dead and dying white cells)
Sanguinous	Blood-stained (bright red indicates fresh bleeding)	Whole blood, broken-down clots
Serosanguinous	Thin/watery and pink or red	Plasma and a few red blood cells

skin surface and promotes healing from the base of the wound. Follow steps 1–17 in the step-by-step guide to removing a wound drain later in this section. Then, with a gloved hand, pull the drain out of the wound as required (usually 5 cm). Place a sterile safety pin horizontally across the drain, to prevent it slipping back into the wound, and cover the drain and drain site with a sterile plastic bag.

When to remove wound closures

Wound closures (sutures/staples) should be removed when the wound surface has healed and there are no signs of infection present. If wound closures are left in place too long, excess scarring can occur. Leaper and Harding (2006) suggest that non-absorbable sutures should be removed from the scalp and face after 3–4 days, from lower limbs after 7–10 days, and from the trunk after 10–14 days.

When not to remove wound closures

If the wound is infected it may be preferable to remove some (rather than all) sutures at the infected area (or towards the bottom of a vertical wound) to allow pus to drain. Any sutures remaining at the site of infection will be a focus for infection. Seek advice from a Registered Nurse if you are asked to remove sutures from a wound that you suspect may be infected.

Potential problems

Make sure you have removed the entire drainage tube/suture material. Alert a more senior member of staff immediately if you suspect there may be drainage tube or suture material left in the wound.

Indications for assistance

If you are unsure whether the wound drain/wound closures are ready to be removed, seek advice. Ask for advice if you notice subtle signs of infection that have not been present previously.

Observations and monitoring

If the drain site has signs of infection, take a wound swab and record this in the patient records.

Common signs of infection are:

- Redness
- Increasing pain
- Swelling
- Fever
- Red streaks progressing up an arm or leg
- Discoloured exudate from the wound site or the wound drain

Special considerations

- Remember that wound healing can be impaired in the elderly; sutures and drains may need to be left in position longer than you would expect.

- If undertaking this skill in the patient's home, remember to provide explicit guidance for the patient so that they can recognize signs of infection.

- Wound healing will also be influenced by medication, for example anticoagulant therapy or anti-inflammatory medication. Anticoagulant medication may be administered as prophylaxis to prevent VTE; check the patient's prescription chart prior to removal of drains or sutures.

Procedure

Preparation

Prepare yourself

Ensure you understand what type of suture/drain you are removing. Review the patient's records to identify any special precautions, for example if the patient is receiving anticoagulants, and any risk factors for impaired wound healing. Wash your hands (see Section 4.1, *Infection prevention and control*, for advice on how to select the appropriate level of PPE). If you are unclear about what type of gloves to use, follow the glove use instructions in Section 4.1.

Prepare the patient

The procedure should be fully explained to the patient (see the box below). Ensure the patient is as comfortable as possible.

Prepare the equipment/environment

Ensure you have the appropriate stitch cutter/staple remover and forceps. Take a sharps disposal container to the bedside (see Section 4.1). Check all equipment for sterility and expiry date; all packaging should be intact. If the procedure includes cutting non-sterile tape, prepare scissors by washing, drying, and decontaminating using alcohol wipes. Sterile scissors are only required if being used on sterile equipment that is to be in contact with high-risk areas of the body.

Discussing the procedure with the patient and family

- Explain to the patient that the wound drain/wound closure is no longer needed.

- Explain what you intend to do and give the patient time to ask any questions.

- If the patient is having a drain removed, explain that this is an uncomfortable rather than painful procedure. Warn the patient to expect a slight tugging feeling as the drain is removed. Removal of wound closures is also an uncomfortable rather than painful procedure.

Step-by-step guide to removing a wound drain

Step	Rationale
1 Introduce yourself, confirm the patient's identity, explain the procedure, and obtain consent.	To identify the patient correctly and gain informed consent.
2 Decontaminate hands and put on a disposable apron.	Use of PPE reduces the level of contamination of the clothes.
3 Ensure the trolley or other surface being used is clean. Take the trolley to the patient.	Local cleaning policies should be followed.
4 Open the outer packaging of the dressing pack and place on the top of the trolley without allowing the outside packaging to touch the inside wrap.	The outside wrapping is contaminated and should not come into contact with the sterile equipment inside the packaging.
5 Open the dressing pack wrapping by touching only the corners of the wrapping paper.	This will create a sterile field.
6 Pour solution for cleansing wounds and open sterile dressing, etc. onto the sterile field without contamination. This should be done without making contact between the solution and the sterile field.	To prevent contamination of the sterile field by the wound or solution packaging.
7 Loosen the patient's dressing and decontaminate hands.	Hands should always be decontaminated prior to applying sterile gloves or handling sterile equipment.
8 Place a hand into the sterile yellow waste bag and use this to organize the contents of the dressing pack on the sterile field.*	The waste bag acts as a sterile barrier and allows handling of sterile equipment without the risk of contamination.
9 Remove the patient's soiled dressing using the hand inside the waste bag.*	Contamination will not occur if there is no direct contact with the soiled dressing.
10 Turn the waste bag inside out with the used dressing inside and attach the bag to the side of the trolley nearest the patient.	Placing the bag nearer to the patient reduces the risk of contamination of the sterile field when disposing of soiled swabs and dressings.
11 If the drain has a vacuum bottle attached, clamp the tubing and detach the bottle.	To prevent suction being applied during removal of the drain, causing pain and tissue damage.
12 Note the amount of drainage and discard the drainage bottle or bag into the clinical waste bag. According to local policy, solidify liquids with a commercially available powder to form a gel or follow the instructions for safe closure on the drainage product.	To allow accurate fluid balance recording. To ensure appropriate disposal of contaminated material.

continued overleaf

13	Adjust bed linen and patient's clothing to expose the drain site.	To allow the suture holding the drain in place to be visible.
14	Put on sterile gloves without contamination of the outside of the gloves.	See Section 4.1.
15	Clean the drain site.	To prevent contamination of the drain site.
16	Place a sterile towel under the drain tubing.	The drain will be removed onto the sterile towel.
17	Lift the suture with the forceps, cut close to the skin, and remove the suture.	To avoid pulling the contaminated stitch through the tissues.
18	Warn the patient that you're about to remove the drain. Place a sterile gauze pad over the drain site and gently remove the drain onto the sterile towel.	The patient will be ready to expect a tugging sensation.
19	Maintain pressure over the drain site until bleeding has stopped.	To stop any bleeding quickly.
20	Cover the drain site with a sterile dressing.	To reduce risk of infection.
21	Dispose of any disposable sharps in a sharps bin.	To maintain staff and patient safety.
22	Remove gloves and place in the waste bag. Wrap all used disposable equipment in the sterile field and place in the waste bag.	To prevent cross-contamination.
23	Seal the waste bag and place in a clinical waste bin.	To prevent cross-contamination.
24	Decontaminate hands.	All clinical procedures should be followed with hand decontamination to reduce the risk of cross-infection.
25	Record your actions in the nursing documentation, noting the condition of the drain site.	This provides a baseline measurement.

*If there isn't a sterilized waste bag included in the pack, omit stage 8 and remove any old dressings (stage 9) using clean gloves before donning the sterile gloves.

Step-by-step guide to removing sutures and staples

▶ Step   Rationale

	Step	Rationale
1	Introduce yourself, confirm the patient's identity, explain the procedure, and obtain consent.	To identify the patient correctly and gain informed consent.
2	Decontaminate hands and put on a disposable apron.	Use of PPE reduces the level of contamination of the clothes.
3	Ensure the trolley or other surface being used is clean. It is not always necessary to clean the surface before every use. Take the trolley to the patient.	Local cleaning policies should be followed.
4	Open the outer packaging of the dressing pack and place on the top of the trolley without allowing the outside packaging to touch the inside wrap.	The outside wrapping is contaminated and should not come into contact with the sterile equipment inside the packaging.
5	Open the dressing pack wrapping by touching only the corners of the wrapping paper.	This will create a sterile field.
6	Open the sterile dressing onto the sterile field without contamination.	This should be done without handling the dressing to reduce infection risk.
7	Loosen the patient's dressing and decontaminate hands.	Hands should always be decontaminated prior to applying sterile gloves or handling sterile equipment.
8	Place a hand into the sterile waste bag and use this to organize the contents of the dressing pack on the sterile field.*	The waste bag acts as a sterile barrier and allows handling of sterile equipment without the risk of contamination.
9	Remove the patient's soiled dressing using the hand inside the waste bag.*	Contamination will not occur if there is no direct contact with the soiled dressing.
10	Turn the waste bag inside out with the used dressing inside and attach the bag to the side of the trolley nearest the patient. Clean your hands.	Placing the bag nearer to the patient reduces the risk of contamination of the sterile field when disposing of soiled swabs and dressings.
11	Inspect the wound; seek advice if signs of inflammation or infection are present.	It may be necessary to remove a few sutures/staples to allow infection to drain. Removal of all sutures at this stage may lead to the wound breaking down (dehiscence).
12	If the wound is longer than 15 cm, remove alternate sutures/staples in the first instance.	A longer wound can take longer to heal; ensure that the wound is healed prior to removing the remaining sutures/staples.
13	**Individual sutures:** lift the suture with the forceps, cut close to the skin and remove the suture.	To avoid pulling the contaminated stitch through the tissues.

continued overleaf

14	**Continuous suture:** cut the first suture close to the skin and opposite to the knot. Remove the cut piece of suture and repeat this process for remaining sutures. Do not cut both ends of a suture.	A continuous suture must be removed in the same way as individual sutures to avoid pulling contaminated stitches through the tissues. Cutting both ends would make it difficult to remove the suture from under the skin.
15	**Staples:** use a staple remover. Ensure you have handled the remover in the treatment room or skills lab before attempting to remove the patient's staples. Insert the blade of the staple remover under the middle of the staple and squeeze hard. Discard the staple in the clinical waste bag.	The patient needs to have confidence in your ability to remove the staples. This releases the staple ends from the tissues.
16	Cover the wound site with a sterile dressing if necessary.	To reduce risk of infection where appropriate. The patient may also prefer the wound to be covered for cosmetic reasons.
17	Dispose of any disposable sharps in a sharps bin.	To maintain patient and staff safety.
18	Remove gloves and place in the waste bag. Wrap all used disposable equipment in the sterile field and place in the waste bag.	To prevent cross-contamination.
19	Seal the waste bag and place in a clinical waste bin.	To prevent cross-contamination.
20	Decontaminate hands.	All clinical procedures should be followed with hand decontamination to reduce the risk of cross-infection.
21	Record your actions in the nursing documentation, noting the condition of the wound.	This provides a baseline measurement.

*If there isn't a sterilized waste bag included in the pack, omit stage 8 and remove any old dressings (stage 9) using clean gloves before donning the sterile gloves.

Following the procedure

Ensure the patient is as comfortable as possible. Ensure the patient is able to reach their water and call bell without putting undue strain on the wound site. Allow time to discuss any concerns the patient may have about the wound, for example what will happen next to the wound. Check that the patient understands any aspect of wound care for which they have responsibility, including how to recognize signs of infection.

Reflection and evaluation

When you have removed a wound drain or wound closures, think about the following questions:

1 Did the patient have any anxieties/concerns regarding their wound?
2 Were you able to answer the patient's questions?
3 Were you able to remove the drain/wound closures without any difficulty?
4 Were you confident in your assessment of the patient's wound?

Further learning opportunities

1 Observe an experienced nurse removing sutures from a more difficult wound.

2 Ask to see any infected wounds, to improve your ability to assess for presence of infection.

3 Practise your patient education skills by explaining to a patient how to care for their wound site after discharge from hospital.

Reminders

Don't forget to:

- Give the patient the opportunity to discuss any anxieties they may have regarding the procedure.
- Check the nursing records for any factors that may delay wound healing.
- Seek assistance if you're not confident of your wound assessment.
- Document your actions and the condition of the patient's wound in the patient records.

Patient scenarios

Consider what you should do in the following situations, then turn to the end of this skill to check your answers.

1 Mrs A, a patient with diabetes, returned from theatre 3 days ago with a wound drain *in situ* following breast surgery. You are reminded that she is at increased risk of infection and to 'keep an eye on her'.

   Why is she at increased risk of infection? What signs and symptoms would alert you to the possibility of wound infection?

2 You are about to remove sutures from the wound of Mr K, who has had abdominal surgery. The patient is reluctant to let you remove the sutures as he has heard that someone's wound 'opened up' when the sutures were removed. How would you handle this situation?

3 You are asked to shorten a wound drain. You commence the procedure and the wound drain falls out when you remove the suture holding it in place. What will you do?

Website

 http://www.oxfordtextbooks.co.uk/orc/ endacott

You may find it helpful to work through our short online quiz and additional scenarios intended to help you to develop and apply the skills in this chapter.

References

Allonby-Neve CL and Okereke CD (2006). Current management of facial wounds in UK accident and emergency departments. *Annals of the Royal College of Surgeons, England*, **88**, 144–50.

Atkinson P (2003). Tissue adhesive with adhesive strips for wound closure. *Emergency Medicine Journal*, **20**, 498.

Carragee EJ and Vittum DW (1996). Wound care after posterior spinal surgery: does early bathing affect the rate of wound complications? *Spine*, **21**, 2160–2.

Chapman D and Purushotham A (2001). Acceptability of early discharge with drain in situ after breast surgery. *British Journal of Nursing*, **10**(22), 1447–50.

Cohn SM, Gianotti G, Ong AW *et al.* (2001). Prospective randomised trial of two wound management strategies for dirty abdominal wounds. *Annals of Surgery*, **233**, 409–13.

Cole E (2007). Wound closure using adhesive strips. *Nursing Standard*, **22**(9), 48–9.

Heal C, Buettner P, Raasch B *et al.* (2006). Can sutures get wet? Prospective randomised controlled trial of wound management in general practice. *BMJ*, **332**, 1053–6.

Karliczek A, Jesus EC, Matos D, Castro AA, Atallah AN, and Wiggers T (2006). Drainage or nondrainage in elective colorectal anastomosis: a systematic review and meta-analysis. *Colorectal Disease*, **8**(4), 259–65.

Leaper DJ and Harding KG (2006). ABC of wound healing: traumatic and surgical wounds. *BMJ*, **332**, 532–5.

Mangram AJ, Horan TC, Pearson ML *et al.* (1999). Guideline for the prevention of surgical site infection. *Infection Control and Hospital Epidemiology*, **20**, 250–78.

Mattick A, Clegg G, Beattie T *et al.* (2002). A randomised, controlled trial comparing a tissue adhesive (2-octylcyanoacrylate) with adhesive strips (Steristrips) for paediatric laceration repair. *Emergency Medicine*, **14**, A34.

Oliver JC and Al-Mufti R (2005). The Prolene® zip technique: prevention of wound infections in contaminated abdominal incisions. *Annals of the Royal College of Surgeons, England*, **87**, 380–9.

Patel VP, Walsh M, Sehgal B, Preston C, DeWal H, and Di Cesare PE (2007). Factors associated with prolonged wound drainage after primary total hip and knee arthroplasty. *Journal of Bone and Joint Surgery. American Volume*, **89**, 33–8.

Purushotham AD, McLatchie E, Young D *et al.* (2002). Randomized clinical trial of no wound drains and early discharge in the treatment of women with breast cancer. *British Journal of Surgery*, **89**, 286–92.

Useful further reading and websites

Bales S, Harding DJ, and Leaper KG (2000). *An introduction to wounds*. Emap Healthcare, London.

Leininger S (2002). The role of nutrition in wound healing. *Critical Care Nursing Quarterly*, **25**(1), 13–21.

http://www.worldwidewounds.com and **http://www.woundsresearch.com/** are websites providing a wealth of research, product information, and suggestions for clinical management of wounds.

Answers to patient scenarios

1   Mrs A would be at increased risk of infection as she has diabetes. You should be alert for the following signs of infection: thick yellowish or green wound drainage; sudden cessation of wound drainage; redness/pain/swelling at the wound site; pyrexia; tachycardia.

2   Informed consent is essential prior to any nursing procedure, so you cannot proceed unless the patient agrees. Explain that the sutures are no longer needed to keep the wound edges together. Ascertain the patient's level of knowledge about his surgery and how wounds heal. Explain how the wound heals and give him time to ask questions. Explain that he has subcuticular (deeper) sutures in place that are not removed; these remain strong for 3 months or longer.

If he is still unwilling for you to remove the sutures, give him the opportunity to discuss it with a more senior member of staff. In order to allay Mr K's fears, your experienced colleague may suggest removing alterative sutures, with the remainder staying in place for a further 2 days, or using adhesive strips to support the wound when sutures have been removed.

3   Assess the wound and drain site for any signs of infection or excess bleeding. Cover the drain site with a sterile dressing, using an aseptic technique. If the drain site is bleeding, call for assistance and put gentle pressure on the wound using a thick sterile pad. If there is no drainage from the drain site, make the patient comfortable and then inform a more senior member of staff. Compare your wound/drain site assessment with previous assessments documented in the patient's records and alert a senior member of staff to any change in the condition of the wound or drain site. If excess fluid remains at the wound site, the surgeon may wish to insert another drain.

5 Drug administration

Skills

5.1 Principles of drug administration

Introduction

Nurses undertake a range of roles in relation to medications, from independent prescribing (Department of Health (DH) 2006) and administering drugs, to monitoring for therapeutic effects and side effects. There are a number of issues and developments common to all routes of drug administration; these are considered in this section.

It is important to remember that:

- All preparation and administration of medication should be systematic and should promote safety, follow policies, and minimize risk of cross-infection.
- It will be necessary to explain the drug administration procedure so that the patient understands what they are receiving and gives valid consent.
- All medications should be held securely and correctly according to law. Security of medications is the responsibility of the registered practitioner in charge of the health care setting.
- Drug administration can be complex in older people, who often receive multiple drug therapies (polypharmacy).
- The patient/client is entitled to be informed of the therapeutic effect of any drug and also contraindications or likely complications (Nursing and Midwifery Council (NMC) 2007, BMA and RPSGB 2008).

Prior knowledge

Before undertaking drug administration by any route, make sure you are familiar with:

1   Pharmacokinetics – the way in which drugs are absorbed, distributed, metabolized, and eliminated (BMA and RPSGB 2008, McGavock 2005).
2   Concepts of consent, accountability, negligence, malpractice, and vicarious liability (see The NMC code (NMC 2008) and *Standards for medicines management* (NMC 2007).
3   Local policies for medicines management.
4   Principles of infection control (see Section 4.1).
5   Principles of patient education.
6   Patient Group Directions.
7   Principles of drug calculations (see Section 5.2).

Background

Basic pharmacokinetics principles

Pharmacokinetics is the study of drug transport through the body (pharma = drug, kinetics = movement), specifically the Absorption, Distribution, Metabolism, and Excretion of drugs, often written as the acronym ADME (Riviere 2003). These four phases of drug transport vary considerably for individual medications; to give just two examples:

1   Many aged patients excrete drugs slowly.
2   A drug with a narrow margin between the therapeutic (useful) dose and the toxic (harmful) dose, such as digoxin, can rapidly develop adverse effects (BMA and RPSGB 2008).

It is important to understand the four phases of drug transport as they apply to different types of medication. Where appropriate, individual examples are provided throughout this chapter.

Principles of safe drug administration

The nurse must be able to demonstrate safe, evidence-based practice, having due regard for their level of competence and the patient's safety (BMA and RPSGB 2008). The '5 Rs' memory aid (Clayton 1987) has stood the test of time as a useful checklist to ensure safe drug administration by any route:

- Right patient
- Right drug
- Right route
- Right dose
- Right time

Certain factors need to be considered with all drug administration, regardless of the route; these are summarized in **Table 5.1**. It is important to remember that the speed of action of the drug will depend on the route of administration.

Table 5.1 highlights the number of professionals involved in drug administration and the importance of good teamwork and communication in all aspects of drug administration. There is often communication between hospital and community staff regarding patient medication, for example the ward pharmacist may contact the patient's GP to clarify what the patient is usually prescribed.

In the context of drug administration, a further mnemonic serves as a reminder to consider the wider responsibilities of health care practitioners:

- **N**ever forget to check patient identity and prescription (BMA and RPSGB 2008).
- **E**ducate the patient about their medication whenever possible.
- **E**nsure hygiene, privacy, and dignity are all addressed as appropriate.
- **D**ocument what has been done.

Legislation

There are a number of legislative issues relevant to drug administration; these are summarized in **Table 5.2**. The NMC also provide guidance on professional responsibilities of Registered Nurses (NMC 2007, 2008).

Specific knowledge related to each drug

Whatever route is being used, anyone who administers a medication must have an awareness of:

- Action and indications for use of the drug.
- Side effects.
- Contraindications.
- Need for monitoring pre-/peri-/post-drug administration.

Table 5.1 Factors to be considered when administering medications

The patient	Why is the medication being prescribed? Could the medication have an effect on any concurrent illnesses or medications? What effect might size, age, and organ function have on the medication? Does the patient have preferences or particular fears, such as needle phobia?
The prescription	Are medical staff following accepted prescribing behaviour? Has national and local policy and practice been adhered to? Are the therapy choice, dose, and route appropriate? (See Section 5.6 for specific advice regarding the administration of drugs via enteral tube.) Will special monitoring be required?
The medicine supplied	Has the pharmacist reviewed the prescription? Does the local pharmacy service assist in preparing the medication? What is the usual practice for ordering and receiving medicines? Is the drug an unusual supply, e.g. requires multiple tablets or vials to meet prescribed dosage?
The nurse	Is the nurse competent to give the drug using this route? Is specialist training or experience required to give this drug? Does the nurse have the ability to accept responsibility for the administration?

(Adapted from Luker and Wolfson 1999).

- Normal therapeutic dosage and potential range.
- Storage, stability, usability (potential for contamination) and expiry date.
- Location of local drug policy.
- Who to ask for advice.

It is also important to be aware that some interactions can occur between specific foods and medications. Two examples are cranberry and warfarin, and grapefruit and carbamazepine. These interactions would be advised on the patient information leaflet for the medication, and the pharmacist will undoubtedly bring it to the attention of those administering medicines. However, it is essential that the patient/family are made aware of such interactions if the patient is to start/continue the medication at home.

Storage of medicines

All medicinal products must be stored in accordance with the patient information leaflet and any instruction on the label. The patient information label and summary of UK licensed product characteristics can be found at

http://www.emc.medicines.org.uk. This is very important for medicines requiring storage within a limited temperature range.

Controlled drugs (CDs) are subject to special legislative controls because there is a potential for abuse, causing possible harm. The government has introduced strengthened measures to make sure CDs are managed safely:

- CDs are subject to safe custody requirements and so must be stored in a locked receptacle, usually in an appropriate CD cabinet.
- The CD may be administered to a patient by any person acting in accordance with the directions of a doctor or dentist.
- A register must be kept for Schedule 2 CDs and this register must comply with the relevant regulations.
- The destruction of CDs in Schedule 2 must be appropriately authorized and the person witnessing the destruction must be authorized to do so.

The purpose of this guidance is to promote the safe, secure, and effective use of all CDs. The full document, *Safer management of controlled drugs: guidance on standard operating procedures for controlled drugs,*

Table 5.2 Legislation and guidance relevant to drug administration

Legislation	Remit
The Medicines Act 1968	Licensing system for use of medicines. Manufacture, distribution, prescription, and supply of medicines. Packaging and labelling of medicines.
The Misuse of Drugs Act 1971	Regulations governing production, supply, and possession of controlled drugs (CDs) to prevent their misuse.
Duthie Report: *Guidelines for the safe and secure handling of medicines* (DH 1988)	Regulations for the storage of all drugs. Three areas of good practice are highlighted: the '**three Rs**' of **reconciliation**, **record keeping**, and **responsibility**.
Royal Pharmaceutical Society of Great Britain (RPSGB) (2005) *The safe and secure handling of medicines: a team approach*.	An updated version of the Duthie Report.
EU Directive 92/27/EEC 1999	Drug information to be provided to patients.
Misuse of Drug Regulations (MDR) (DH 2001), Misuse of Drug Regulations 2006	The MDR delineate drugs in five schedules according to the different levels of control required. CDs are subject to highest level. These are periodically revised and amended. (See DH *Controlled drugs* website in Useful further reading.)
Health Act 2006	Primary legislation that applies to UK, although the regulations may differ in each of the devolved administrations. Part 3, Chapter 1 – concerns CDs. Safe, appropriate, and effective management and use of controlled drugs.
The Controlled Drugs (Supervision of Management and Use) Regulations 2006	These regulations set out requirements to appoint an accountable officer who would have certain duties and responsibilities to improve the management and use of CDs.

can be found at: **http://www.dh.gov.uk/en/ Publicationsandstatistics/Publications/Publications PolicyAndGuidance/DH_064824**.

Patient Group Directions (PGDs)

These are individual protocols that allow specific health care professionals who do not ordinarily have prescribing rights to supply and administer a medicine directly to a patient under the following conditions:

1 The professional is named individually on the PGD.
2 The professional has been assessed as competent.
3 The professional has signed the document.

Professionals using PGDs must be registered members of their profession and act within their code of con-

duct. Students cannot supply or administer under a PGD but would be expected to understand the principles and may be involved in the process (NMC 2007). A PGD also has legal requirements that the health care organization must adhere to. More information can be found via websites in the Useful further reading section of this skill.

Route of administration

Route of administration can be divided into two types:

1 Enteral – via the gut.
2 Parenteral – via any other route (intravenous, subcutaneous, intramuscular, or mucosal routes).

These have different modes of action (see **Table 5.3**).

Table 5.3 Mode of action for enteral and parenteral drug administration

Enteral administration	Parenteral administration
Drugs delivered via the digestive system and thus absorbed by the intestines and exposed to first-pass metabolism in the liver are termed 'enterally administered'. Enteral administration is via the mouth or rectum (see Section 5.6).	Drugs that are absorbed straight into the bloodstream, rather than through the intestines and liver, are 'parenterally administered' (Simonsen *et al.* 2006).

Crushing medication

The mechanics of crushing medicines may alter the therapeutic properties, rendering them ineffective or resulting in a very rapid rate of uptake; this practice is not covered by the product licence. Medicines should not routinely be crushed unless advised by the pharmacist (NMC 2007). For further discussion, see Section 5.6.

Covert drug administration

Covert drug administration occurs when medication is administered, disguised in food or drink, even though the patient is led to believe that they are not receiving the medication (NMC 2007). This is not good practice and the registered practitioner would be accountable for this decision. Registered practitioners should seek advice from a pharmacist or the relevant professional body (e.g. the NMC). As a student, you should not be expected to administer drugs in a covert manner.

Reporting adverse reactions

Any drug may produce unwanted or unexpected adverse reactions. The detection and recording of these are of vital importance. If you suspect that an adverse reaction may be related to a drug, you should document this in the patient's records, inform the prescriber, and initiate the Yellow Card Scheme immediately. A Yellow Card can be found in the back of the British National Formulary (BNF, BMA and RPSGB 2008) or completed online at **http://www.yellowcard.gov.uk**. This process allows the central monitoring of, and where necessary a centralized response to, drug reactions.

Potential for medication errors

There are five stages in the medication process:

1 Prescribing.
2 Dispensing.
3 Preparation.
4 Administration.
5 Monitoring.

There is potential for error at each of these stages (National Patient Safety Agency (NPSA) 2007a). Nurses have clear responsibilities for administration and monitoring of most medications, with responsibility for preparation of some medications; however, the increase in non-medical prescribing means Registered Nurses are increasingly likely to be responsible for prescribing. Since May 2006, over 9000 Registered Nurses in a range of settings have been able to independently prescribe licensed medications within their competence (NPSA 2007a).

Some examples of errors occurring during prescribing are: prescribing without taking into account the patient's clinical condition; failure to communicate essential information; and errors in transcription. In a review of reported medication incidents, omitted (or missed) medications were the second most commonly reported medication incident in hospitals (NPSA 2007a); two audits of medication charts, conducted across five NHS Trusts, found that a significant number of patients are not receiving the drugs that are prescribed for them (Endacott *et al.* 2006, 2007).

Drug administration can be complex in the elderly, who often receive multiple drug therapies (polypharmacy) (McGavock 2005). However, polypharmacy is also common in many patients with chronic conditions, as a result of higher treatment standards required by National Service Frameworks, availability of new medicines, and general advances in health care (NPSA 2007a). It is essential to monitor (and where possible prevent) adverse effects; this becomes more complicated with the more medications a patient receives.

Monitoring the effects of medication is particularly important in the community setting. In a systematic review, Howard *et al.* (2007) found that the median percentage of preventable drug-related admissions to hospital was 3.7% (range 1.4–15.4). Four main categories of drug were responsible for over 50% of these admissions: anti-platelets, diuretics, non-steroidal anti-inflammatory drugs (NSAIDs), and anticoagulants.

Patient education is an important component of monitoring the effects of medication; the patient must be informed of the therapeutic effect of any drug and also contraindications or *likely* complications (NMC 2007, BMA and RPSGB 2008). It should be recognized that the patient may not always be informed of all *potential* complications as some of these may be very rare. However, the nurse should be alert to possible unusual side effects. This applies regardless of whether the patient will only receive drugs administered by health care staff or continue with the drug and self-medicate in future. While many patients will start a drug regime in a health care setting, they need to understand how and why to continue with self-medication once at home (Kelly 2000) (see Section 5.3 for further detail on patient self-administration of medicines). Patients must also be advised how to keep medicines safe at home.

Safety in the home

Patients must be warned to keep all medicines out of reach of children. All must be dispensed in a child-resistant container unless:

- The medicine is in an original pack.
- The patient will have difficulty opening a child-resistant container.
- A specific request is made that the product shall not be in a child-resistant container.
- No suitable child-resistant container exists for a particular liquid preparation.

All patients should be advised to dispose of unwanted medicines by returning them to the supplier for destruction (BMA and RPSGB 2008).

Standardizing wristbands

Safe care is also dependent on correct patient identification; the NPSA reported 2900 instances of incorrect patient identification due to inadequate documentation on patient wristbands in England and Wales in 2006. As a result, new guidelines were issued in 2007 (**http://www.npsa.nhs.uk**); these came into effect in July 2008 and are listed in Box 3.4 (Chapter 3).

The NPSA (2007a) recommend seven key actions to improve medication safety:

1 Increase reporting and learning from medication incidents.
2 Implement NPSA safer medication practice recommendations.
3 Improve staff skills and competences.
4 Minimize dosing errors.
5 Ensure medicines are not omitted.
6 Ensure the correct medicines are given to the correct patients.
7 Document patients' medicine allergy status.

When there are difficulties in clarifying an individual's identity, such as learning disabilities, patients with dementia, or confusional state, an up-to-date photograph should be attached to the prescription chart (NMC 2007).

Indicators for potential problems

On occasion, vital signs must be recorded or blood test results obtained *prior* to administering a medication, as this will indicate whether it should be given or omitted. Below are some examples:

- The patient's pulse is recorded prior to digoxin – if below 60 bpm, seek doctor's advice.
- The patient's blood pressure is recorded prior to angiotensin-converting enzyme (ACE) inhibitors (such as captopril, enalapril, ramipril) – if systolic blood pressure below 90 mmHg, seek doctor's advice.
- The patient's capillary blood sugar is tested prior to oral antidiabetic drugs (such as glicazide, glibenclamide, metformin, rosiglitazone) or insulin – remember that hypoglycaemia can cause unconsciousness, which should always be treated as an emergency.
- A recent INR (International Normalized Ratio) level must be known prior to administration of oral anticoagulants such as warfarin. The therapeutic level must be documented on the drug chart. (The frequency of INR checks will depend upon the stability of the previous readings. This may vary from daily to every few weeks.)

For the latter two examples, the medication is commonly prescribed on a sliding scale, with the drug dose administered according to the patient's blood results. Always document the vital signs to ensure safe practice and allow monitoring of any trends in the patient's condition. Look at Chapters 6 and 7 to familiarize yourself with the recording of vital signs.

Reflection and evaluation

1 Look at the medication charts for patients in the area where you're working. For each drug, test your knowledge in the following areas:
   - Action and indications for use of the drug
   - Side effects
   - Contraindications
   - Need for monitoring pre-/peri-/post-drug administration

   Check your answers in the BNF or drug information leaflet contained in medication package.

2 Look at the wristbands for patients in your area; how many comply with the NPSA requirements stated in Box 3.4? Identify a plan of action to ensure that all wristbands comply with NPSA requirements.

   Check the patient's details verbally with them. Do not lead them by asking 'Is your name Mrs Smith?' Ask the patient to give you their full name. If you use patient addressographs (stickers), check all details such as date of birth with the patient. If you find any details are incorrect, ensure they are corrected immediately.

Further learning opportunities

Practise under supervision at different times to get an overall picture of what the patient is being prescribed, including ordering, storage, and dispensing of controlled drugs.

It is important to understand the role of each team member involved in the different stages of drug management. Arrange to work with the ward pharmacist to get a different perspective on prescription charts.

Reminders

Don't forget to:

- Check the patient's identity as per NPSA requirements.
- Check the patient's allergy status.

- Undertake any monitoring *prior* to administering the medication.
- Check the prescription chart – have all the medications been given? Check that the patient hasn't missed more than one dose of a drug.
- Check that, where medication is not given, the reason is documented.
- Clarify with the patient:
  - Are they aware what they are taking?
  - Is it their normal dose?
  - Is it the time they take it at home?
  - Is there anything missing from what they normally take?

Website

 http://www.oxfordtextbooks.co.uk/orc/ endacott

You may find it helpful to work through our short online quiz and additional scenarios intended to help you to develop and apply the skills in this chapter.

References

BMA and RPSGB (2008). *British National Formulary*, 55th edition. British Medical Association and Royal Pharmaceutical Society of Great Britain, London.

Clayton M (1987). The right way to prevent medicines errors. *Registered Nurse*, **50**, 30–1.

Department of Health (1988). *Guidelines for safe and secure handling of medicines (The Duthie Report)*. Stationery Office, London.

Department of Health (2001). *The misuse of drugs regulations*. The Stationery Office: Crown Copyright, London. [online] **http://www.opsi.gov.uk/si/ si2001/20013998.htm** accessed 19/08/08.

Department of Health (2006). *Improving patients' access to medicines – a guide to implementing nurse and pharmacist independent prescribing in England*. HMSO, London.

Endacott R, Boulanger C, Chamberlain W, Hendry J, Ryan H, and Viner J (2006). Missed medications and clinical cues in patients admitted unexpectedly to intensive care [abstract]. *Intensive Care Medicine*, **32**(Suppl), S12.

Endacott R, Warne S, Boulanger C *et al.* (2007). Missed medications in acutely ill patients [abstract]. *Intensive Care Medicine*, **33**(Suppl 2): S117.

Howard RL, Avery AJ, Slavenburg S *et al.* (2007). Which drugs cause preventable admissions to hospital? A systematic review. *British Journal of Clinical Pharmacology*, **63**(2), 136–47.

Kelly J (2000). *Adverse drug effects: a nursing concern*. Whurr Publishers, London.

Luker K and Wolfson D, eds (1999). *Medicines management for clinical nurses*. Blackwell Science, Oxford.

McGavock H (2005). *How drugs work: basic pharmacology for healthcare professionals*. Radcliffe Medical Press, Abingdon.

National Patient Safety Agency (2007a). *Safety in doses: medication safety incidents in the NHS. The fourth report from the Patient Safety Observatory*. NPSA, London. [online] **http://www.npsa.nhs.uk/ patientsafety/alerts-and-directives/ directives-guidance/safety-in-doses/** accessed 19/08/08.

National Patient Safety Agency (2007b). *Standardising wristbands improves patient safety. Safer Practice Notice*. NPSA, London. [online] **http:// www.npsa.nhs.uk/patientsafety/ alerts-and-directives/notices/wristbands/** accessed 19/08/08.

NMC (2007). *Standards for medicines management*. Nursing and Midwifery Council, London.

NMC (2008). *The Code: standards for conduct, performance and ethics*. Nursing and Midwifery Council, London.

Riviere J (2003). *Comparative pharmacokinetics: principles, techniques and applications*. Wiley-Blackwell Publishing, London.

Royal Pharmaceutical Society of Great Britain (RPSGB) (2005). *The safe and secure handling of medicines: a team approach*. [online] **http://www.rpsgb.org/ pdfs/safsechandmeds.pdf** accessed 09/04/08.

Simonsen T, Aarbakke J, Kay I, Coleman I, Sinott P, and Lysaa R (2006). *Illustrated pharmacology for nurses*. Hodder Arnold, London.

Useful further reading and websites

British National Formulary: **http://www.bnf.org**

Medicines and Healthcare Products Regulatory Agency – information and standards relating to medicines and medical equipment: **http://www.mhra.gov.uk**

Misuse of Drugs Act 1971: **http://drugs.homeoffice. gov.uk/drugs-laws/misuse-of-drugs-act/**

The Health Act 2006: **http://www.opsi.gov.uk/ acts/acts2006/pdf/ukpga_20060028_en.pdf**

The National Prescribing Centre: **http://www.npc.co.uk/**

Patient Group Directions – a practical guide and framework of competencies for all professionals using Patient Group Directions: **http://www.npc.co.uk/ publications/pgd/pgd.pdf**

NHS Patient Group Direction website: **http:// www.portal.nelm.nhs.uk/PGD/default.aspx**

A guide to good practice in the management of controlled drugs in primary care (England): **http://www.npc.co.uk/controlled_drugs/ cdpublications.htm**

Integrated Medicines Management Programme for Long Term Conditions (IMMP): **http://www.npc.co.uk/ mms/immp/immpphase2.htm**

The Department of Health set up a webpage to post all changes to regulations regarding CDs following the Shipman Inquiry: **http://www.dh.gov.uk/ controlleddrugs**

The RPSGB is the professional and regulatory body for pharmacists in England, Scotland, and Wales: **http://www.rpsgb.org.uk/**

The Clinical Knowledge Summaries service (CKS) is a resource that provides access to evidence-based clinical knowledge (this has replaced PRODIGY): **http://www.cks.library.nhs.uk/**

5.2 **Calculations**

Definition

A drug calculation is the use of simple arithmetic to ensure the right amount of medication is given. Most calculations are straightforward. Some involve several arithmetic functions or stages.

It is important to remember that:

- Medicines administration is an important professional task. When calculations are involved it is recommended that the result be checked with another registered professional practitioner to reduce the risk of error (NMC 2007).
- Students must also check the local employer policy regarding the role of the student in drug administration (see Section 5.1).

- Opinions differ as to the value of calculators (Pentin and Smith 2006, Tarnow and Werst 2000). They make arithmetic much easier, but cannot substitute for calculation problem-solving skills.
- The NMC (2007) insist that calculators must not replace arithmetic knowledge and skill. If a calculator is used, check its function first. Errors can occur if the battery is failing.

Prior knowledge

Before undertaking drug calculations, make sure you are able to:

1 Multiply, divide, add, and subtract whole numbers and decimals. There are many online or text resources to help you revise these skills.
2 Recognize the International System of Units (the standard form of the metric system, also known as the SI or Système International d'unités).

If you intend using a calculator, make sure you:

1 Understand how to make it perform basic arithmetic functions ($\times$, $\div$, $+$, $-$).
2 Know whether your calculator can perform just one arithmetic function at a time or whether it can perform several functions in the right order. See later in this section to find how to do this.

Background

The interpretation of clinical information and knowledge of some mathematical principles are key components of performing safe drug calculations (Wright 2006). Brush up on some mathematical ideas in the context of drug calculations.

Common measurements in drug calculations

The measurements you may encounter are summarized in **Table 5.4**.

Converting units of measurement

Being able to convert between the various units of a quantity or volume is vital for accurate calculation. The

Table 5.4 Common measurements used in drug calculations

Weight or mass	1 gram (g) = 1000 milligrams (mg)
	1 mg = 1000 micrograms
	Some drugs are measured in 'units' rather than milligrams or grams.
	E.g. Insulin 24 units or Heparin 5000 units.
Volumes	1 litre (l) = 1000 millilitres (ml)
Time	1 hour = 60 minutes

Note – 'micrograms' should *not* be abbreviated in prescriptions (BMA and RPSGB 2007) but it is possible that the abbreviations μg or mcg may be encountered in other contexts. Most drugs are prescribed in milligrams or micrograms. These are very small amounts, but this does not always mean a very small effect – drugs often require only small quantities to exert large effects.

use of different units causes confusion. If you want to convert something written in big units to something written in smaller units you *multiply* (think – you will need more of them!). Conversely, if you want to convert something written in small units to something written in bigger units, you *divide* (think – you will need fewer of them!).

Example 1

Oral doses of digoxin (a drug used to treat heart failure or some cardiac arrhythmias) may range from 62.5 micrograms to 1.5 mg per day (the higher doses usually being divided into two or three smaller doses). To see the range written in a single unit, convert 1.5 mg to micrograms:

- Look at the prefixes; 1 milligram = 1000 micrograms.
- To convert milligrams into micrograms you must *multiply* by 1000.
- This is the same as moving the decimal point (.) in 1.5 milligrams three places to the right.

Therefore 1.5 mg is 1500 micrograms.

Example 2

A person is prescribed 500 micrograms of betamethasone. You note that the dose range is usually 0.5–5 mg daily. You want to check whether the prescription falls into this range.

- You need to convert 500 micrograms to milligrams.
- To convert micrograms to milligrams you must *divide* by 1000.
- This is the same as moving a decimal point (which you can mentally visualize in 500.0 micrograms) three places to the left.

500 micrograms becomes .5 mg or 0.5 mg.

Decimal points and zeros

Decimal points can be hard to see; a zero before the decimal point (a leading zero) can be used to indicate the presence of the point. Zeros after the decimal point and any numbers (trailing zeros) can be confusing. They are left off to give a whole figure, e.g. 400 ml. Generally, prescriptions will be written to avoid the use of decimals.

Concentrations of a drug

The concentration (strength) of a liquid drug can be written in several ways (see **Table 5.5**).

Estimates

Estimates or rough calculations are used to predict the size of an answer. Estimating first can help you spot whether you have made a mistake in the calculation process using the actual values. Estimates are especially recommended if you do not work out drug doses often or are using a calculator. Calculations are estimated by rounding the numbers. The *estimated* calculation is then done using the rounded values. The *actual* value should be of a similar size.

The rules for rounding are:

- If the number to be rounded is 5 or more, round UP.
- If the number is less than 5, round DOWN .

E.g. 17 can be rounded UP to the nearest '10' to 20, 125 can be rounded DOWN to the nearest '100' to 100.

Context

 When to use calculations

Calculations are required when drug quantities or fluid volumes prescribed differ from the stock available, or when special delivery equipment is used.

Indications for assistance

- Even if the calculation is straightforward, consider whether the result is reasonable. Although there are exceptions, a calculation suggesting more than three or four tablets or capsules should be re-checked (Williams 1996). Few prescriptions result in half a tablet. If your calculation suggests so, consult the pharmacist and prescriber before administering the drug.
- Maximum volumes for injection vary according to type and site (Roger and King 2000, Workman 1999). Check that the route intended is appropriate for the volume calculated.

Table 5.5 How liquid drug concentrations can be written

mg/ml or micrograms/ml	The weight (milligrams or micrograms) of a drug per millilitre.
mmol/l or mmol/ml	Millimoles/litre or millimoles/millilitre.
Percentage. % (w/v)	The number of grams of drug dissolved in 100 ml of the solution.
As a ratio. 1 in . . .	Number of grams of drug in ml.
e.g. 1 in 1000	e.g. 1 in 1000 = 1 gram in 1000 ml.
1 in 10 000	1 in 10 000 = 1 gram in 10 000 ml.

- The prescriber should be consulted if the dose seems unusual, and the BNF provides further information.
- Many oral medications are coated and should not be crushed or cut. The NMC (2007) gives advice. The pharmacist can advise alternative forms of the drug and the prescriber should be consulted.

Special considerations

Time pressure, night duty, long shifts, large workloads, staffing problems, and presence of distractions can interfere with calculation performance (Allard *et al.* 2002, Armitage and Knapman 2003). Under these conditions take extra care and always check your calculations twice.

Procedure

Preparation

Plan ahead

Reduce distractions or other interference. Get a pen, paper, and calculator if you wish.

Find the information needed to solve the problem. Read the prescription, examine the available stock, and think what has to be calculated. Decide whether you have to do any unit conversions first.

Check your calculator functions

To check whether your calculator performs one arithmetic function at a time, or whether it can carry out functions in order, key in:

[5] [+] [6] [×] [7] [=]

For calculators that do the arithmetic in the right order, the display will show 47. For calculators that do one function at a time, the display will show 77.

Either type is suitable. If you have a calculator that will do only one function at a time, you must remember to key in a calculation in arithmetic function order to get the correct answer. The calculator utility of a mobile telephone is likely to be of this type.

Choose an appropriate method for calculation

There are several ways of arriving at a correct answer. Simple calculations can often be done by simple mental arithmetic but more complex ones deserve a systematic approach, each step of which can easily be checked by another to ensure accuracy.

Oral medicines

Oral medicines include tablets, capsules, or liquid preparations.

Example 3

Imagine a patient with a severe infection. Read the 'prescription' and work out the number of capsules to be given for each dose.

You have a stock bottle containing amoxicillin capsules 250 mg.

Prescription

Drug	Dose	Route	Frequency
Amoxicillin capsules	500 mg	oral	8 hourly

Plan The patient requires 500 mg each dose.
The stock is 250 mg per capsule.
Find how many '250 mg' there are in 500 mg.

Calculate (a) This is calculated by dividing 500 mg by 250 mg.

$$\text{Number of capsules needed} = \frac{500\,\text{mg}}{250\,\text{mg}}$$

As there are 'mg' on both the top and bottom of the fraction, these can be removed.

$$\text{Number of capsules needed} = \frac{500}{250} = 2 \text{ capsules.}$$

For a calculator, key in the following:

[500] [÷] [250] [=]

The display will show 2.

(b) You can probably do many straightforward calculations like these instinctively by mental arithmetic (see Figure 5.1).

Does the answer seem a reasonable number of capsules?

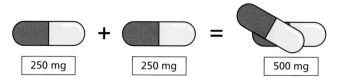

Figure 5.1 500 mg medication in 250 mg capsules.

Example 4

Imagine a patient experiencing an episode of inflamm-atory bowel disease. Read the 'prescription' and calculate the number of tablets needed per dose.

You have a stock bottle containing sulfasalazine tablets 500 mg.

Prescription

Drug	Dose	Route	Frequency
Sulfasalazine tablets	1 gram	oral	6 hourly

Plan The dose is 1 gram.

The stock is 500 mg.

Find how many '500 mg' stock tablets there are in 1 gram.

Note that the units used in the prescription and stock are different.

Convert both values to the same unit.

1 gram = 1000 mg.

Calculate (a) This can then be calculated by dividing 1000 mg by 500 mg.

$$\frac{1000 \text{ mg}}{500 \text{ mg}} = \frac{1000}{500} = 2 \text{ tablets.}$$

If the fraction seems confusing, 'simplify' or 'cancel' the fraction to make it easier to work with.

> Simplifying or cancelling a fraction in a drug calculation makes the numbers smaller and easier to work with.
>
> To simplify or cancel a fraction you must divide the top and bottom of the fraction by the same number (the common factor).

E.g. $\frac{16}{20}$ can be simplified by dividing the top and bottom by 4.

The 16 is cancelled by drawing a line through it and is replaced by 4.

The 20 is cancelled and replaced by 5.

So $\frac{16}{20}$ becomes $\frac{\cancel{16}^{4}}{\cancel{20}_{5}} = \frac{4}{5}$

Another example: $\frac{200}{40}$ can be simplified by dividing top and bottom by 10.

'Cancel' as many zeros on the top as on the bottom. Each cancelled zero is equivalent to dividing the number by 10.

$$\frac{20\cancel{0}}{4\cancel{0}} = \frac{20}{4}$$ which can further be simplified to

$$\frac{\cancel{20}^{5}}{\cancel{4}_{1}} = \frac{5}{1}$$ or just 5.

Simplify the fraction by dividing the top and bottom by 100.

$$\frac{10\cancel{00} \text{ mg}}{5\cancel{00} \text{ mg}} = \frac{10 \text{ mg}}{5 \text{ mg}} = \frac{10}{5} = 2 \text{ tablets.}$$

For a calculator, key in the following:

[1000] [÷] [500] [=]

The display will show 2.

(b) Having converted all values into the same unit, you can use mental arithmetic (see **Figure 5.2**).

Is your answer a reasonable number of tablets?

Example 5

Imagine a patient only able to swallow liquid medicines. Read the 'prescription' and calculate the volume of sus-pension you need.

You have a stock bottle containing paracetamol suspension 250 mg in 5 ml.

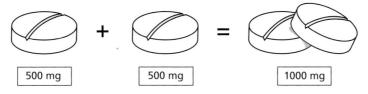

Figure 5.2 1000 mg medication in 500 mg tablets.

Prescription

Drug	Dose	Route	Frequency
Paracetamol suspension	1 gram	oral	6 hourly

Plan The dose is 1 gram of paracetamol.
The stock contains 250 mg in 5 ml.
Find what volume of stock contains 1 gram.
Note that the units used in the prescription and stock are different.
Convert both values to the same unit.
1 gram = 1000 mg.

Calculate There are several ways of answering this problem. Choose and use the method that is easiest for you.
(a) The popular 'one unit' method –
Find the volume that contains 1 mg paracetamol.
If 250 mg paracetamol is in 5 ml,

1 mg paracetamol will be in $\dfrac{5}{250}$ ml

As you want 1000 mg paracetamol, multiply $\dfrac{5}{250}$ ml by 1000.

This calculation is the same if written as $\dfrac{1000}{250} \times 5$ ml.
In words this is:

$$\frac{\text{The amount you want (dose)}}{\text{The amount you have (stock)}} \times \text{stock volume}$$

Simplify the fraction so that you only need to deal with small numbers. Divide the top and bottom by 250 – a number that both can be wholly divided by.

$$\frac{1000^4}{250_1} \times 5 \text{ ml} = \frac{4}{1} \times 5 \text{ ml} = 20 \text{ ml}.$$

For a calculator, key in the following:

[1000] [÷] [250] [×] [5] [=]

The display will show 20.
(b) The 'proportional' method –
Finding the volume:

	Stock	Need
Quantity of paracetamol (mg)	250	1000
Volume (ml)	5	?

To find the missing number (ml needed):
Find the number that you times 250 by to get 1000.
250 × (a number) = 1000
So (the number) = 1000 ÷ 250
So (the number) = 4.
Multiply 5 by 4 to get the missing volume.
Volume required = 20 ml.
(c) Using mental arithmetic –
With a little practice, this level of calculation can often be achieved by using mental arithmetic (see **Figure 5.3**). However, if a calculation does not use simple multiples like this one, it is strongly advised that you use an alternative method to ensure accuracy and avoid error.

One example where many pills may be needed is prednisolone, e.g. 50 mg = ten 5 mg tablets!

Drugs for injection

Drugs for injection (subcutaneous, intramuscular, intravenous) are calculated in the same way as for liquid oral drugs.

Example 6

Consider a patient in pain. If there is no intravenous (IV) access, or the patient is too nauseated to tolerate drugs given orally, intramuscular (IM) injections may be prescribed.

Read the 'prescription' and work out what volume of drug you will need.

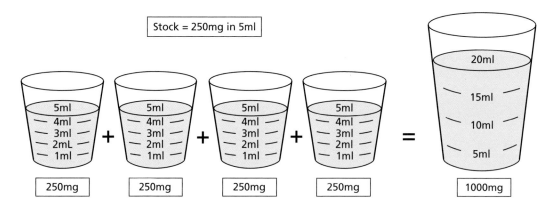

Figure 5.3 1 gram of medication using 250 mg/ml suspension.

Prescription

Drug	Dose	Route	Frequency
Tramadol	75 mg	IM	4 hourly

Plan The dose is 75 mg.

The stock contains tramadol 100 mg in 2 ml.

Find how much of the stock is needed to give 75 mg of tramadol.

Both the stock and the prescription use 'mg', so no conversions are necessary.

Calculate You can use any of the ways illustrated for oral medications to solve this problem.

(a) Using a 'one unit' method –

Find the volume that contains 1 mg tramadol.

If 100 mg of tramadol is in 2 ml,

$$1 \text{ mg of tramadol will be in } \frac{2}{100} \text{ ml}$$

As you want 75 mg tramadol, multiply $\frac{2}{100}$ ml by 75

$$75 \times \frac{2}{100} \text{ ml can also be written } \frac{75 \times 2}{100} \text{ ml}$$

Simplify the fraction. For easy stages, divide the top and bottom numbers by 25, and then again by 2.

$$\frac{^{3}\cancel{75} \times 2}{_{4}\cancel{100}} = \frac{3 \times 2}{4} = \frac{3 \times \cancel{2}^{1}}{\cancel{4}_{2}} = \frac{3}{2} = 1.5 \text{ ml}$$

Another way of using the 'one unit' method is:

$$\frac{\text{The amount you want}}{\text{The amount you have}} \times \text{stock volume}$$

$$\frac{75 \text{ mg}}{100 \text{ mg}} \times 2 \text{ ml}. \text{ This is the same calculation!}$$

If you are using a calculator, key in:

[75] [÷] [100] [×] [2] [=]

The display shows 1.5.

(b) Using the 'proportional' method –
Finding the volume:

	Stock	Need
Quantity of Tramadol (mg)	100	75
Volume (ml)	2	?

To find the missing number (ml needed):

Note that the quantity needed is less than the stock quantity.

Find the number that you times 100 by to get 75.

100 × (a number) = 75

So (the number) = 75 ÷ 100

So (the number) = 0.75

Multiply 2 ml by 0.75 to get the missing volume.

The volume required is 1.5 ml.

(c) Using mental arithmetic (see **Figure 5.4**) –

75 mg is ³⁄₄ of 100 mg.

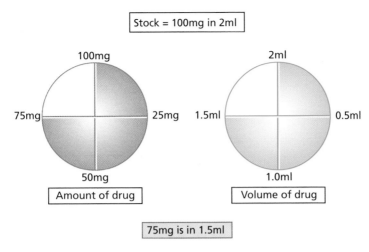

Figure 5.4 75 mg of medication using stock of 100 mg/2 ml.

If 100 mg is in 2 ml, you need to find $^3/_4$ of 2 ml.
$^1/_4$ of 2 ml is 0.5 ml, so $^3/_4$ will be 1.5 ml.

Many calculations can be resolved simply by mental arithmetic, but if the numbers are a little tricky or your calculation skills are a bit rusty, try a more structured approach, such as the methods above.

Fluids and drugs for intravenous infusion

There are several commonly used ways to deliver fluids and drugs intravenously, including:

● A simple, manual administration set and gravity.
● Pumps (volumetric or syringe).

Infusions using a simple administration set and gravity

Infusion rates are in drops per minute (dpm).

The administration set includes a dropper mechanism that delivers a defined number of drops per ml. Most manufacturers indicate how many drops constitute 1 ml on the wrapper.

Usually:

1 Standard administration sets deliver 20 drops/ml of fluid.
2 Blood administration sets deliver 15 drops/ml (fewer drops per ml as blood is thicker than clear fluids).

$$\text{Rate of infusion} = \frac{\text{Volume}}{\text{Time}}$$

Example 7

Imagine a patient has been prescribed 1 litre of 0.9% sodium chloride to be infused over 10 hours using a standard administration set. Find the infusion rate (dpm).

Plan

(i) Find how many drops make up the volume prescribed, and how many minutes make up the time prescribed.
(ii) Find the rate in drops per minute.

Calculate

(i) 1 litre is 1000 ml.
The administration set gives 20 drops per ml.
The number of drops in 1 litre = 1000 × 20 drops.
The number of minutes in 10 hours will be 10 × 60 minutes.
(ii) The rate in drops per minute is:

$$\frac{\text{Volume}}{\text{Time}} = \frac{\text{drops in 1 litre}}{\text{minutes in 10 hours}} = \frac{1000 \times 20}{10 \times 60}$$

In words this is:

$$\frac{\text{Volume prescribed (ml)} \times \text{Drops per ml}}{\text{Hours of infusion time} \times 60 \text{ (minutes per hour)}}$$

Simplify the fraction:

$$\frac{1000 \times \overset{1}{\cancel{20}}}{10 \times \underset{3}{\cancel{60}}} = \frac{1000 \times 1}{10 \times 3} = \frac{\overset{100}{\cancel{1000}} \times 1}{\underset{1}{\cancel{10}} \times 3} = \frac{100}{3}$$
$$= 33.3 \text{ drops per minute.}$$

You cannot have part of a drop so round down to 33 drops per minute.

If you are using a calculator with a memory function, key in the following:

[10] [×] [60] [=] [SM] [1000] [×] [20] [÷] [MR] [=]

The display will show 33.333333. Round to 33 drops per minute.

SM is 'store memory'; MR is 'memory recall'.

It is very important that you check the wrapper for the manufacturer's data as new equipment may differ from the standards of more familiar equipment.

Infusions using pumps

Pumps are used to deliver large fluid volumes at a prescribed rate.

Infusion rates are in ml/hour.

$$\text{Rate} = \frac{\text{Volume}}{\text{Time}} = \frac{\text{Volume (ml)}}{\text{Time (hours)}}$$

Example 8

Imagine that to maintain hydration peri-operatively, a person is prescribed 1 litre of compound sodium lactate (Hartmann's solution) intravenously over 8 hours.

Plan

(i)   Convert 1 litre to ml.
(ii) Find the flow rate in ml per hour.

Calculate

(i)   1 litre = 1000 ml.
(ii) Rate is $\frac{1000 \text{ ml}}{8 \text{ hours}}$ = 125 ml per hour.

Using a calculator, key in:

[1000] [÷] [8] [=]

The display will show 125.

Pumps used to deliver drugs

Drugs can be added to small volumes, e.g. minibags, to make up a solution of a particular concentration or for adequate dilution. Instructions are often issued by the Pharmacy as to how to do this (monographs). Alternatively, pre-prepared bags are supplied. Where a high degree of accuracy is required, smaller volumes can be given using a syringe pump.

Typically, drug doses are mg or micrograms per hour or prescribed based on the patient's weight. Doses may need to be converted to ml/hour, or volume of drug and diluent to be drawn into a syringe set at a predetermined or calculated rate.

Example 9

Dopamine is prescribed at 5 micrograms/kg body weight/min.

The pre-prepared stock is a 250 ml bag containing a total of 400 mg dopamine. The patient weighs 64 kg.

Work out the rate at which the pump should be set.

Plan

(i)   Work out the dose per minute and per hour.
(ii) Convert the dose from micrograms to mg per hour as the stock is in 'mg'.
(iii) Calculate how many ml of stock contains this amount.

Calculate

(i)   Dose per minute = 5 micrograms × 64 kg = 320 micrograms/min
      Dose per hour = 320 micrograms × 60 = 19 200 micrograms/hour
(ii) Convert this to mg/hour by dividing 19 200 by 1000 = 19.2 mg/hour.
(iii) Work out how many ml contains 19.2 mg:

If 250 ml contains 400 mg dopamine,

1 mg dopamine will be in $\frac{250}{400}$ ml

(If you are not sure which way up this fraction should be, think if 250 ml contains 400 mg dopamine, each ml will contain *more* than 1 mg dopamine. 1 mg dopamine must therefore be in *less* than 1 ml.)

19.2 mg will be in $19.2 \times \frac{250}{400}$ ml, which can also be written as $\frac{19.2 \times 250}{400}$

Simplify by dividing top and bottom by 50:

$$\frac{19.2 \times \cancel{250}^{5}}{\cancel{400}_{8}} = \frac{19.2 \times 5}{8} = \frac{96}{8} = 12 \text{ ml}$$

Using a calculator, key in:

[19.2] [×] [250] [÷] [400] [=]

The display will show 12.

To give 19.2 mg/hour, the pump must be set at 12 ml/hour.

Put another way:

$$\frac{\text{The amount you want (dose)}}{\text{The amount you have (stock)}} \times \text{stock volume}$$

In this case it is:

$$\frac{\text{Dose (mg/kg/hour)} \times \text{body weight (kg)}}{\text{Amount of stock (mg)}} \times \text{stock volume (ml)}$$

Infusions using a syringe pump

Syringe pumps are used to deliver low volumes of drugs, up to 60 ml. Most pumps accept a variety of sizes of syringe. Settings are usually in ml per hour. Graseby pumps measure millimetres per hour. For these, the size of syringe is extremely important.

A common prescription requires that the syringe is filled to give a concentration of drug of 1 mg/ml. The syringe pump rate can then be easily set.

Example 10

Insulin may be given according to a sliding scale, dependent on capillary blood glucose readings.

A 60 ml syringe is filled with 60 units of prescribed insulin, diluted to 60 ml. This gives a concentration of 1 unit/ml.

The syringe pump is set to deliver the amount of insulin needed according to the sliding scale.

If 1 unit/hour is needed, the pump is set to 1 ml/hour.

If 2 units/hour are needed, the pump is set to 2 ml/hour, and so on.

Syringe pumps can be used to give drugs at different concentrations.

Example 11

Imagine the patient in pain again. This time they are prescribed 100 mg tramadol over 5 hours. The stock of tramadol is ampoules of 50 mg per ml, which are diluted with 0.9% sodium chloride to fill a 20 ml syringe in a syringe pump already set at 2 ml per hour. Work out what volume of tramadol needs to be drawn up and how much 0.9% sodium chloride diluent is needed to fill the syringe.

Plan

(i) Work out the hourly dose.

(ii) Calculate how much drug needs to be drawn into the syringe from the stock.

(iii) Find out how much 0.9% sodium chloride needs to be added to fill the syringe.

Calculate

(i) If 100 mg tramadol is to be given over 5 hours, dose for 1 hour = $\frac{100}{5}$ mg = 20 mg/hour.

(ii) The rate of the syringe pump is already set at 2 ml per hour.

The concentration of tramadol needs to be 20 mg per 2 ml, or 10 mg per 1 ml.

If 1 ml contains 10 mg,

20 ml syringe must contain 20 × 10 mg tramadol = 200 mg.

200 mg tramadol must be drawn into the syringe.

Stock is 50 mg per ml.

To find out how much stock makes 200 mg tramadol, use:

$$\frac{\text{the amount you want}}{\text{the amount you have}} \times \text{stock volume}$$

$$\frac{200 \text{ mg}}{50 \text{ mg}} \times 1 \text{ ml} = \frac{^4\cancel{200}}{_1\cancel{50}} \times 1 \text{ ml} = 4 \text{ ml}.$$

4 ml of tramadol stock must be drawn up.

If you are using a calculator, key in:

[200] [×] [1] [÷] [50] [=]

The display will show 4.

(iii) The diluent to fill the 20 ml syringe = 20 ml − 4 ml = 16 ml.

A special caution when reconstituting from a dry powder

Some drugs are supplied as powder for reconstitution with a diluent. Some powders wholly dissolve in the diluent. For others, the reconstituted volume is greater than the volume of diluent that was added. This difference is the drug's displacement value.

Certain drugs have large displacement values that must be taken into account when the reconstituted fluid

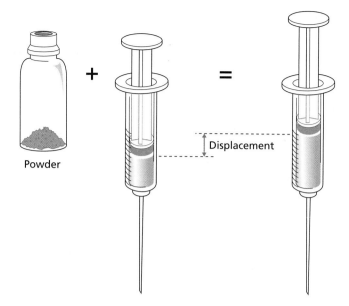

Figure 5.5 Taking account of displacement when reconstituting drugs.

is drawn up. The value can be obtained from the pharmacist, and may be included in the product information leaflet.

Example 12

The displacement value of chloramphenicol 1 gram = 0.8 ml.

To get 10 ml of final solution, only 9.2 ml diluent should be added (see **Figure 5.5**).

If only 500 mg of chloramphenicol is needed, only 5 ml needs to be withdrawn.

If, however, 10 ml of diluent has been added without acknowledging the displacement value, the final volume will be 10.8 ml.

If only 500 mg of choramphenicol is needed, 5.4 ml must be withdrawn. If only 5 ml is drawn up and used, the patient will be underdosed. This constitutes a drug error.

Reflection and evaluation

Practice, with its clinical clues, helps the maths make sense and improves performance (Hutton 1998, Wilson 2003).

Consider the following questions in your practice area:

Recognizing adverse effects

Patients may be harmed by the administration of the incorrect dose, by either underdosing (fails to have the desired benefit) or overdosing (increased incidence of undesired effects, or sometimes life-threatening acute states). As many drugs are now given intravenously, the effects of overdosage may occur very rapidly.

It is important for the nurse to have specific knowledge of the drug administered (see Section 5.1) and to watch the patient for evidence of incorrect dosage or undesired effects, e.g. anaphylaxis.

1 Have you participated in a wide range of drug and fluid calculations?
2 What or who were the main sources of help?
3 Did the use of a calculator make things easier?

Reminders

- Pen and paper are helpful. The calculation can be checked before the answer is agreed.
- Check product information leaflets and data on packaging.
- Check the requirements of each infusion pump before use.

- Drugs given via IV lines need to be flushed after administration to give the full dose. See the product information leaflet or pharmacist to check the flushing fluid compatibility.
- Your university may have a policy regarding the use of calculators in examinations.
- Mistakes should be reported immediately to line managers or employers (NMC 2007). Students should take the opportunity to reflect upon and discuss an incident with their mentor and lecturer.

Patient scenarios

Consider what you should do in the following situations, then turn to the end of this skill to check your answers.

1 Mrs Ohana is being treated for an inflammatory disorder with oral betamethasone. She takes betamethasone 2 mg once daily. Your stock tablets contain 500 micrograms. How many tablets will she need per daily dose?

2 To prevent dehydration, Miss Johnson has been prescribed 1 litre of 5% glucose to be given over 8 hours. A simple administration set and gravity is used. Calculate the drop rate (dpm) for the infusion to the nearest whole drop. The administration set delivers 20 drops per ml.

3 Isosorbide dinitrate is given undiluted via a syringe pump to control Mrs Churchill's angina. The dose is 5 mg per hour. The 50 ml syringe is filled with stock containing 500 micrograms per ml. At how many ml per hour must the pump be set?

Website

 http://www.oxfordtextbooks.co.uk/orc/ endacott

You may find it helpful to work through our short online quiz and additional scenarios intended to help you to develop and apply the skills in this chapter.

References

Allard J, Carthey J, Cope J, Pitt M, and Woodward S (2002). Medication errors: causes, prevention and reduction. *British Journal of Haematology*, **116**(2), 255–65.

Armitage G and Knapman H (2003). Adverse events in drug administration: a literature review. *Journal of Nursing Management*, **11**, 130–40.

BMA and RPSGB (2007). *British national formulary*. British Medical Association and Royal Pharmaceutical Society of Great Britain, London.

Hutton M (1998). Nursing mathematics: the importance of application. *Nursing Standard*, **13**(11), 35–8.

Nursing and Midwifery Council (2007). *Standards for medicines management*. NMC, London.

Pentin J and Smith J (2006). Drug calculations: are they safer with or without a calculator? *British Journal of Nursing*, **14**(14), 778–81.

Roger MA and King L (2000). Drawing up and administering intramuscular injections: a review of the literature. *Journal of Advanced Nursing*, **31**(3), 574–82.

Tarnow KG and Werst CL (2000). Spotlight on . . . Drug calculation examinations: do calculators make a difference? *Nurse Educator*, **25**(5), 213–15.

Williams A (1996). How to avoid mistakes in medicine administration. *Nursing Times*, **92**(14), 40–1.

Wilson A (2003). Nurse's maths: researching a practical approach. *Nursing Standard*, **17**(47), 33–6.

Workman A (1999). Safe injection techniques. *Nursing Standard*, **13**(39), 47–52.

Wright K (2006). Barriers to accurate drug calculations. *Nursing Standard*, **20**(28), 41–5.

Useful further reading and websites

BBC Schools – Bitesize: **http://www.bbc.co.uk/ schools/revision/**

Downie G, MacKenzie J, and Williams A (2006). *Calculating drug doses safely; a handbook for nurses and midwives.* Churchill Livingstone, Edinburgh.

Gatford J and Phillips N (2006). *Nursing calculations*, 7th edition. Churchill Livingstone, Edinburgh.

Lapham R and Agar H (2003). *Drug calculations for nurses: a Step by step approach*, 2nd edition. Arnold, London.

Answers to patient scenarios

1 Four tablets.
2 42 drops/min.
3 10 ml/hour.

5.3 **Patient self-administration**

Definition

Patient self-administration means that, while in hospital, patients administer their own medication under the supervision of nursing staff. Self-administration is also known as **self-medication**.

It is important to remember that:

- Self-administration is not suitable for all patients and not all patients will want to self-administer. Each patient should be assessed according to set criteria before being allowed to administer their own medication.
- Self-administration may improve concordance, increase a patient's knowledge about their medication, and allow health care staff to identify any problems the patient may have with their medication.
- The patient's own medication must be assessed as suitable before being used for self-medication.
- If the patient's condition changes, this may affect their ability to self-administer medications safely.

Prior knowledge

Before implementing patient self-administration, make sure you are familiar with:

1 Basic pharmacology of the drugs being given, e.g. how they work and what body systems they affect.
2 Understanding of what a patient's medication is being given for, the dose, and the possible side effects.

Background

Self-administration of medicines by hospital inpatients has been reported in the literature for over 50 years (Parnell 1959). Self-administration can be used to increase a patient's knowledge of their medication, to assess whether a patient is able to manage their medication before discharge, and to allow the patient to remain independent and self-caring while in hospital. Self-administration has both advantages and disadvantages (see Boxes 5.1 and 5.2).

Box 5.1 Advantages of patient self-administration of medication

- Allows patient to become familiar with their medication while in a safe environment.
- Allows identification of any problems the patient has with their medication, e.g.:
  - Side effects.
  - Problems with eyesight or memory.
  - Difficulties opening packs or bottles.
- Allows assessment of any potential support methods, e.g. reminder charts, monitored dosage systems.
- May increase patient concordance with their medication; the goal of concordance is met when the patient 'buys in' to their treatment, not just agrees to take it (compliance).
- May increase patient's understanding and knowledge of their medication.
- May reduce medication errors.
- Can improve patient comfort as they can administer their medication at the times when they need it, e.g. analgesia, sleeping tablets, Parkinson's medication.
- Allows patients to become involved in their care and make decisions about their treatment.
- Demonstrates trust of the patient and promotes independence, which can have psychological benefits.
- May save nursing time once patient is self-administering, as fewer medicines need to be given by nursing staff.

Box 5.2 Disadvantages of patient self-administration of medication

- Not suitable for all patients.
- Patients may not want to self-administer.
- Not suitable for all types of medication, e.g.:
  - Intravenous drugs.
  - New medication if unfamiliar.
  - Controlled drugs (depending on local policy).
- May be potential safety issues, e.g. over- or underdosing – accidental or intentional.
- Medication must be managed across primary and secondary care to ensure that medication remains the same on discharge.
- Can be time-consuming to set up a self-administration scheme.

Two reviews of the literature relating to patient self-administration of medication have been published (Collingsworth *et al.* 1997, Wright *et al.* 2006). Both reviews found that research into self-administration of medication was mainly descriptive and anecdotal, and that studies were not always well designed. The studies reviewed by Collingsworth *et al.* (1997) supported some benefits of self-administration, such as increased independence and empowerment and increased knowledge about aspects of their medication. They did not demonstrate that self-administration increased compliance. The studies reviewed by Wright *et al.* (2006) suggested that self-administration can contribute to increasing a patient's knowledge about their medication. They also identified that patients who have been part of a self-administration scheme feel that they have benefited from it and would be happy to take part again. Again, there was no conclusive evidence that self-administration improved compliance.

Self-administration has been advocated by various health care bodies, including the NMC, Audit Commission, Healthcare Commission, and the UK Hospital Pharmacists Group (Audit Commission 2002, Hospital Pharmacists Group 2002, NMC 2004, Commission for Healthcare Audit and Inspection 2007).

As people get older, they tend to take more medication. In the UK, 80% of people aged over 75 take at least one prescribed medicine, while 36% take four or more (DH 2001). The more medications people take, the more likely it is that they will have problems with them; as many as 50% of older patients may not take their medication as intended. Adverse reactions are implicated in 5–17% of hospital admissions (DH 2001). The *National Service Framework (NSF) for Older People* issued by the Department of Health recommends the use of self-administration schemes as a method of improving patient compliance and addressing any medication-related problems before discharge from hospital (DH 2001).

In a review of medicines management at English NHS trusts in 2005/6, the Healthcare Commission found that self-administration was 'offered on only 19.5% of wards where it was likely to be possible' (Commission for Healthcare Audit and Inspection 2007: 14). In an ideal world, all competent patients should be offered the chance to self-administer their medication. However, this can be a challenge due to the time and training needed to set up self-administration schemes. The Healthcare Commission recommends that all inpatient wards should have the resources available to support self-administration, e.g. bedside lockers for medication, policies and procedures, and trained staff (Commission for Healthcare Audit and Inspection 2007). This means that self-administration should always be an option for patients.

Self-administration requires the use of medication labelled with the patient's name, dose, and directions. This can be the patient's own drugs (PODs) brought in from home or drugs supplied by the hospital labelled as if for discharge. Most inpatient self-administration schemes run alongside a POD scheme, where a patient's own drugs are assessed before use by pharmacy staff. This assessment will check that medication is labelled correctly, with the patient's name and correct instructions, and that the label on the box or bottle matches the contents. The medication must be within its expiry date. The medication must also be suitably packaged and the physical condition of the drugs must be satisfactory. This assessment can also be carried out by nursing staff.

All medication must be stored securely in a locked cabinet or cupboard. Many hospitals have lockable bedside lockers or cabinets in which medication can be stored. Depending on local policy, patients may be given a key to this locker to enable them to self-administer. Examples of criteria used to assess a patient's suitability for self-administration are found in **Box 5.3**.

Patients will vary in their abilities and needs regarding their medication. Different levels of self-administration can be used to allow for this (see **Table 5.6**). Self-administration schemes should be flexible and patients able to move up and down the levels as appropriate during their hospital stay. For example, a patient may progress from full supervision to full self-administration as their knowledge and confidence increases. Conversely, a patient may move from full self-administration to nurse administration if they become ill, or following surgery.

Context

When to use self-administration

Self-administration in hospital may be appropriate for any patient who self-administers at home and is likely to do

Box 5.3 Criteria for patient self-administration

Assessment criteria for self-administration might include:

- Does the patient self-administer at home and will they do so on discharge?
- Have you explained self-administration to the patient, including the need for safe custody of medicines?
- Is the patient willing to self-administer?
- Can the patient open bottles/foil packets or use their inhalers or eye drops?
- Can the patient read the labels?
- Can the patient demonstrate an appropriate level of understanding of their medication?
- Have you explained:
  - Which of the medications the patient should be taking?
  - The dosage?
  - The timings?
  - The possible side effects?
- The patient cannot self-administer if *any* of the following apply:
  - The patient is confused.
  - The patient has a recent history of alcohol or drug abuse.
  - The patient may be experiencing the effects of sedation or a general anaesthetic.
  - The patient does not wish to self-medicate.

to judge a patient's abilities. Pharmacists and pharmacy technicians may also be involved, particularly if patients are having problems with their medication.

The patient must be happy to administer their own medication and must take responsibility for doing so. The patient may need to sign a form accepting responsibility for administering their own medication, depending on local policy.

Self-administration can also be of particular benefit to:

- Patients taking analgesics, as they can take them when they are needed to control pain.
- Patients who will need to take medication long term when they leave hospital. Self-administration will allow them to become familiar with their medication before going home, e.g. transplant patients on antirejection therapy or patients with inhalers for asthma.
- Patients with complicated drug regimes. Self-administration allows them to get used to managing their medication before they leave hospital and gives us the chance to provide any help that they might need.

 When not to use self-administration

Self-administration is not suitable in the following situations:

- If the patient is confused or disorientated to time and/or place.
- If the patient has a history of drug or alcohol abuse or suicidal tendencies.

so on discharge. The patient must be assessed as being able to self-administer in hospital. Assessment of patients is usually done by nursing staff as they spend the most time with patients and are therefore in the best position

Table 5.6 Levels of self-administration

0	Full nurse administration	All medicines are administered by nursing staff.
1	Full supervision	Nurses and/or other health care professionals teach the patient/carers what the purpose of the medication is and how to administer it. The nurse may still administer the medication.
2	Close supervision	Patient requests their medication from nursing staff at the appropriate times. Patient is self-administering but checking medication with nurse.
3	Full self-administration	Patient is allowed to administer their medication themselves without any supervision. The patient should be given responsibility for the key to their drug locker or cabinet.

- If the patient is undergoing a test, procedure, or operation that requires them to be sedated or have a general anaesthetic or for an *appropriate* time frame afterwards.
- Patients may not be allowed to self-administer CDs, such as morphine. This will depend on local policy.
- If any alterations are made to a patient's medication or new medication is started, these drugs are usually given by nursing staff until the patient becomes familiar with them. Once the nurse and patient are happy, a patient may begin to self-administer these items.
- Some medication may not be suitable for self-administration, e.g. IV medication, CDs.

Alternative interventions

If a patient is not suitable to self-administer or does not wish to, nursing staff will administer their medication during their stay in hospital.

Additional expertise

When supervising a patient self-administering their medicines, it is essential to understand what the medication is and why the patient is taking it. Knowledge of a drug's potential side effects is also important, to allow you to identify these and refer the patient to their doctors. If you are unsure, ask a pharmacist or other nursing staff. Use the *British National Formulary* (BNF) to look up drug information.

Self-administration is also an opportunity to identify any problems the patient might have with their medication. These could include side effects, physical problems such as poor eyesight or difficulty opening packets, or poor memory. You need to be aware of how these problems could be overcome. A pharmacist or pharmacy technician will be able to advise you of appropriate ways to help. Some solutions include use of large print labels, use of non-click-lock or easy-open lids for bottles, or devices to help with the administration of eye drops or aerosol inhalers.

Patients with poor memory may be helped by reminder charts or use of monitored dosage systems (MDS) such as 'dosette' or 'medidos' boxes or weekly blister packs. These MDS devices usually contain a week's worth of medication in separate slots for times of day and days of the week. These devices can be given to patients in hospital and on discharge but you must ensure that arrangements are made for them to be filled.

Potential problems

As mentioned earlier, patients will differ in their ability and confidence in managing their medication. This may vary during their inpatient stay. It is important to reassess your patients regularly to ensure that they are still suitable to self-administer. Potential problems may include side effects, physical problems with taking medication, or problems remembering when to take medication.

Special considerations

- Remember that patients' needs and abilities may vary greatly regardless of age. Some 'elderly' patients may be far more able to manage their own medication than younger patients.

- Remember that the patient must be able to manage their medication in their own home as well as in hospital. Be aware that differences in routine, or the amount of assistance the patient receives at home, may affect their ability to self-administer their medication.

- When giving people information about their medication, be aware that patients will differ in their level of understanding and desire for information. Also, remember that English may not be the patient's first language and that this may affect their understanding.

Procedure

Preparation

Prepare yourself

Ensure you understand the criteria for self-administration used in your hospital, what the patient's medication is, why they are on it, and what the potential side effects could be. Make sure you have completed any relevant documentation.

Prepare the patient

Make sure the patient understands what self-administration means and is happy with the procedure.

Prepare the medication

Make sure that all of the patient's medication is available and appropriate for use.

Discussing the procedure with the patient and family/carers

- Explain what self-administration involves and why it is done.
- Make sure the patient understands that they don't have to self-administer – it is their choice.
- Assure the patient that they can stop self-administration at any point during their stay, should they wish to.
- Assure the patient that nursing or pharmacy staff will be happy to answer any questions they have about their medication.
- Explain to the patient that their medication must be stored securely in a locked box or cupboard.

Step-by-step guide to patient self-administration

Step		Rationale
1	Introduce yourself, confirm the patient's identity, explain the procedure, and obtain consent.	To identify the patient correctly and gain informed consent.
2	Ensure the patient has a fully completed drug chart with all the patient's medicines recorded, including dose and frequency. Ensure that the chart is signed and dated by a doctor.	To meet legal requirements.
3	Discuss the patient's medication history with them or their carers on admission. Ensure an accurate record has been made of all medication (prescribed or otherwise), herbal medicines, dietary supplements, complementary therapies, and allergies or intolerances.	To allow assessment of patient understanding of their medication and possible problems with administration. To allow you to identify patients who currently have MDS or other devices to help them manage their medication.
4	Review the inpatient prescription chart with the pharmacist and ensure that this matches the details given by the patient and their own medication.	To ensure that the drug chart is an accurate record of what the patient takes. If frequent changes of dose or frequency are likely, it may be impractical to allow patients to self-administer.
5	Assess the patient's ability to self-administer. Use the sample criteria in Box 5.3 or your own hospital guidelines. Different levels of self-administration may be suitable for different patients or for the same patient at different times during their hospital stay (see Table 5.6).	If the patient is not suitable or does not wish to self-administer, administer the drugs as normal. Some drugs may not be suitable for self-administration, e.g. IV drugs, new medication.

| 6 | Document this assessment in the nursing notes. Depending on your hospital policy, you may need to complete a patient assessment form and get the patient to sign a form accepting responsibility for administering their own medication. | Hospital policy must be followed at all times. |

| 7 | Consider whether the patient will have any problems with self-administration and how they might be overcome, e.g. poor sight, difficulty opening packets. Discuss this with appropriate members of the multidisciplinary team. | To encourage successful and safe self-administration and ensure that a patient's medication is dispensed and labelled appropriately for their needs. If compliance aids such as 'dosette' boxes or weekly 'blister packs' are used, responsibility for filling and labelling the aid must be agreed according to local policy. It must also be ensured that the aid can be filled and monitored once the patient is discharged. |

| 8 | If the patient's own medication is being used, ensure that it is suitable for use. This assessment may be done by pharmacy or nursing staff. The medication must be labelled correctly, with the patient's name and correct instructions. The label and contents must be the same. The medication must be within its expiry date. The medication must be suitably packaged and the physical condition of the drugs must be satisfactory. | Patient's own drugs must be assessed before use for reasons of safety and efficacy, according to your local policy. |

| 9 | Monitor the patient and continue to reassess their ability to self-administer. Regularly discuss their medication and any problems that they might be having. Teach any skills needed, e.g. inhaler technique. | A patient's ability may differ during their stay so it is important that you continue to reassess them frequently. Self-administration is an opportunity for patients to learn about their medication and increase their confidence, becoming involved in their own care. You can support them by providing information and advice about their drugs. Other health care professionals, such as pharmacists, can help you with this. |

| 10 | Ensure that medication is taken as intended, and that the appropriate records are kept. | To ensure that responsibility is taken for administration of the patient's medication. To record who has taken this responsibility, nurse or patient. The method of recording will usually be the patient's drug chart but this may vary according to local policy. |

| 11 | Check when drug supplies are going to run out and ensure that a resupply is made. Organize medication for discharge ('to take out', TTOs) as far in advance as possible. | To ensure that treatment is not interrupted by lack of medication. To facilitate discharge planning by arranging medications as early as possible. |

| 12 | Evaluate whether self-administration has been effective for your patient. Record any problems encountered and any interventions you have made. | To identify any further learning needs for you or your patient. To enable modification of the care plan to account for problems or interventions. |

Following the procedure

Monitor changes in your patient's prescription

New items may not be suitable for self-administration initially. It is important to ensure that any changes are explained to the patient and that the patient's medication is altered as necessary. Any discontinued drugs should be retrieved. Document actions in the nursing care plan.

Reflection and evaluation

1   How easy was it to assess your patient's ability to self-administer? Were they happy to do so? If they weren't, why do you think this was?

2   How easy did you find it to explain to patients what their medication was for and how to take it? Do you feel more confident in your knowledge now that you have supervised patients' self-administering?

3   Do you think there are enough opportunities for patients to self-administer their medication? Are there ways in which the ward routine could be changed to make this easier?

4   What do you think are the benefits of self-administration? Are there any groups of patients for whom you think self-administration would be particularly beneficial or important?

Further learning opportunities

Practise your skills in communicating with patients. Take every opportunity to provide explanations to a range of patients about their drugs.

Talk to the ward pharmacist about some of the challenges of implementing self-administration.

Identify any areas of patient teaching where you need to improve your skills, for example teaching patients to use an inhaler.

Reminders

Don't forget to:

• Keep assessing the patient's suitability to self-medicate – this may change during their stay.

• Reassure the patient that self-administration is not compulsory and they may choose not to at any time.

• Make sure you know what the medication is for and how it should be given.

Patient scenarios

Consider what you should do in the following situations, then turn to the end of this skill to check your answers.

1   Patient A has been administering his own medication since his admission to hospital. He is about to undergo a procedure that requires him to have a general anaesthetic. Will this affect his self-administration?

2   Patient B has been administering her own medication at home. When you supervise her self-administering on the ward, you notice that she has difficulty remembering when to take her medication and often gets her tablets muddled up. What could you do to help her?

3   Patient C is admitted to your ward. He has all his own medication with him. What would you want to check before you allowed him to self-administer?

Website

 http://www.oxfordtextbooks.co.uk/orc/ endacott

You may find it helpful to work through our short online quiz and additional scenarios intended to help you to develop and apply the skills in this chapter.

References

Audit Commission (2002). *Medicines management – Review of national findings*. Audit Commission, London.

Collingsworth S, Gould D, and Wainwright S (1997). Patient self-administration of medication: a review of the literature. *International Journal of Nursing Studies*, **34**(4), 256–69.

Commission for Healthcare Audit and Inspection (2007). *The best medicine – the management of medicines in acute and specialist trusts*. Commission for Healthcare Audit and Inspection, London.

Department of Health (2001). *Medicines and older people – Implementing medicines-related aspects of the NSF for Older People*. DH, London.

Hospital Pharmacists Group (2002). One-stop dispensing, use of patients' own drugs and self-administration schemes. *Hospital Pharmacist*, **9**(3), 81–6.

Nursing and Midwifery Council (2004). *Guidelines for the administration of medicines*. NMC, London.

Parnell MA (1959). Medicines at the bedside. *American Journal of Nursing*, 59, 1417–8.

Wright J, Emerson A, Stephens M, and Lennan E (2006). Hospital inpatient self-administration of medicine programmes: a critical literature review. *Pharmacy World and Science*, **28**, 140–51.

Useful further reading and websites

Audit Commission (2001). *A spoonful of sugar – medicines management in NHS hospitals*. Audit Commission, London.

Mehta DK, ed (2007). *British National Formulary 54 – September 2007*. BMJ Publishing Group and RPS Publishing, London.

Commission for Healthcare Audit and Inspection (2002). *Self-administration of medicines by hospital inpatients*. Briefing document from Salford Royal Hospital [online] **http://www.healthcarecommission.org.uk/_db/ _documents/04002747.pdf** accessed 19/08/08.

http://www.medicines.org.uk contains online versions of manufacturers' summaries of product characteristics and patient information leaflets for most UK licensed drugs.

(A) Answers to patient scenarios

1   Patients should not be allowed to self-administer after any procedure or operation requiring them to be sedated or have a general anaesthetic. You would need to reassess the patient daily until you think he is able to self-administer. Be aware that strong analgesia can have sedative effects in some patients.

2   There are a number of things that could be done to help. First you would need to talk to the patient and find out what the problem is. Find out whether she has problems with her medication at home. Is there anything else that could be causing her confusion? You could ask a pharmacist to review the patient's medication to see whether it can be simplified, e.g. giving medications at the same time or using a formulation that can be given once a day instead of twice or three times. The patient could also be given a reminder chart or a compliance aid such as a weekly 'dosette' box or blister pack.

3   Check through the criteria for self-administration used in your hospital. An example of the criteria is given in Box 5.3. If the patient is going to use his own medication, make sure this is assessed as suitable before it is used.

5.4 Nebulized drugs

Definition

When medications are delivered in a format that allows easy uptake by the lungs, this is called 'nebulization'. Nebulization involves air or oxygen being driven through a solution of a drug. The resulting fine mist is then inhaled directly into the lungs via a facemask or a mouthpiece (Trounce and Gould 2000).

It is important to remember that:

-   If a patient has never had a nebulizer before then the nurse should fully explain the procedure and be available during nebulization.
-   A rate of gas flow of 6–8 litres per minute is required to produce an aerosol where 50% of the particles are less than five microns in diameter (Francis 2006).
-   Air should be used for patients with **type 2 respiratory failure** and oxygen for patients with **type 1 respiratory failure**.
-   All nebulizers will retain a residual volume of medication within the storage chamber when the nebulization is complete. This residual volume will vary between different devices and can be found on the product information leaflet.
-   Nebulization time should be 5–10 minutes for bronchodilators; however, some medication might take longer (Edmond 2001), e.g. pentamidine (see Table 5.7).
-   Compressors should be serviced on a regular basis according to your local policy, to ensure that they continue to work efficiently.

It is important that the immediate effect of any new inhaled drug is monitored, by performing respiratory

Table 5.7 Commonly nebulized drugs

Class of drug	Name of drug
Bronchodilators: beta₂ agonists	e.g. Salbutamol (Ventolin®), terbutaline (Bricanyl®)
Bronchodilators: antimuscarinics/anticholinergics	e.g. ipratropium bromide (Atrovent®)
Bronchodilators: combined	Salbutamol and Ipratropium (Combivent®)
Steroids	Budesonide (Pulmicort®) and fluticasone (Flixotide®)
Antibiotics	e.g. Colistin, gentamicin, tobramycin, ceftazidime, piperacillin
RhDNase	Dornase alpha (Pulmozyme®)
Saline	normal or hypertonic saline
Opioids	Diamorphine, morphine, fentanyl
Local anaesthetics	Lidocaine: palliative care – non-productive cough. Administer only under strict medical supervision.
Adrenaline	
Antiviral	Tribavirin
Mucolytics	N-Acetylcysteine (rare)
Antifungal *Pneumocystis* prophylaxis	Pentamidine isethionate – COSHH regulations apply.

function tests before and after nebulization. Occasionally there may be a change or deterioration in lung function due to irritation of the airways causing bronchospasm. If the patient feels that the nebulized treatment makes them worse it should be stopped immediately. The requirement for lung function assessment should be discussed with the prescribing doctor.

Prior knowledge

Before using nebulizers, make sure you are familiar with:

- Respiratory anatomy, including the anatomical structures of the respiratory tract from the mouth, through the trachea, into the bronchi and alveoli.
- Physiology of respiration, including a basic understanding of the role of respiration in maintaining and regulating oxygen and carbon dioxide concentrations in the body.

- **Pathophysiology** of common respiratory diseases including asthma, chronic obstructive pulmonary disease (COPD), emphysema, lung cancer.
- The nebulizer compressors used in the hospital or in the community.
- The groups of patients requiring nebulization.
- The correct drug delivery device required and observations necessary for patients receiving the first dose of the drug.
- The potential side effects of the drugs being used.

Background

Nebulizers are used to give patients concentrated doses of medications that are easily inhaled and are thus made quickly available to the lungs and the body generally. A compressor machine delivers pressurized air to **aerosolize** (turn into fine droplets with the appearance of steam) a liquid drug in a nebulizer pot. Nebulizers and inhalers both utilize the properties of aerosols to deliver their medication.

The medication particle size is important for deposition within the lungs. Aerosols are generally composed of a range of particle sizes; particles that are less than three microns in diameter will penetrate the alveoli, and those that are 3–5 microns in diameter will distribute throughout the lung (Benson and Prankered 1998).

- Jet nebulizers push jets of air (from compressors) through the liquid drug to aerosolize the medication.
- Ultrasonic 'nebulizers' generate an aerosol by vibrating the liquid drug placed within them.

Air should be used as the driving gas for patients with known **type 2 respiratory failure** (patients who have low levels of oxygen and high levels of carbon dioxide). Oxygen should be the driving gas for those with **type 1 respiratory failure** (patients with low levels of oxygen).

When the respiratory system cannot maintain the body's blood gas values within a safe range, this is known as respiratory failure.

In type 1 respiratory failure, the patient is hypoxic without retaining carbon dioxide, and can safely be given high concentrations of oxygen (35% +) while the underlying cause is identified and treated. If this does not occur rapidly, mechanical ventilation may be necessary. Where there is a longstanding chronic cause, the patient may be assessed for long-term oxygen therapy (LTOT).

In type 2 respiratory failure, the patient has hypoxia with retention of carbon dioxide. This is like a breath-hold, also called alveolar hyperventilation. Excess carbon dioxide, hypercapnia, also termed intoxication or CO_2 narcosis, is poisonous to the central nervous system. Giving these patients high levels of oxygen causes their CO_2 to increase further. This is because their hypoxia is driving their respiratory rate and if their oxygen level increases, they will breathe more slowly and less deeply.

Type 2 respiratory failure is normally caused by central nervous system disturbance or obstruction of the upper airways (secondary alveolar hypoventilation). Very occasionally it may be caused by failure of the central respiratory drive (primary alveolar hypoventilation).

Nebulizers are often given via special nebulizer masks, which, while appropriate for sick patients who may find holding mouthpieces difficult, are less suitable for others who can hold a mouthpiece correctly in their teeth and coordinate the work of inhaling at the same time.

Mouthpieces deliver the nebulized medication more effectively to the lungs without depositing it around the face and mouth.

Mouthpieces are recommended for nebulized ipratropium (Atrovent®) as prolonged pupillary dilatation occurs if ipratropium is sprayed directly into the eyes. The addition of salbutamol (Ventolin®) intensifies the risk, especially in patients with glaucoma (Kendrick *et al*. 1997). A mouthpiece should also be used for nebulized antibiotics, steroids, and rhDNase: Dornase alpha (Pulmozyme®) to reduce drug deposition on the face. Drugs commonly delivered via nebulizer are identified in Table 5.7.

Context

 When to use a nebulizer

The main indications for using a nebulized route of administration are as follows:

- To deliver a beta agonist or ipratropium to a patient in acute exacerbation of asthma or airways obstruction.
- To deliver a beta agonist or ipratropium on a regular basis to a patient with asthma or airways obstruction who has been shown to benefit from high doses of medication.
- To deliver prophylactic medication such as corticosteroids where a patient is unable to use any other types of inhalation device.
- To deliver antibiotics such as colistin to a patient with chronic respiratory infection such as in cystic fibrosis.
- To deliver prophylaxis and treatment with pentamidine for *Pneumocystis* pneumonia to a patient with AIDS.
- In palliative care, to deliver opioids and local anaesthetics for troublesome dyspnoea, pain, and distressing coughs.
- To give adrenaline in emergency situations such as croup, and possibly for anaphylaxis.

(BMA and Royal Pharmaceutical Society of Great Britain 2004).

 When not to use a nebulizer

Nebulizers should not be used when a patient is unwilling or unable to tolerate them. If they are unable to tolerate them this may be because they are too acutely unwell to make respiratory effort sufficiently to inhale the drugs by this route.

In routine care, a patient with an acute exacerbation of COPD or asthma will no longer require nebulization as their condition improves. This is a decision to be made by the medical team but will require nurses' input from observations and peak flow measurements.

Alternative interventions

A patient who is too unwell for nebulization is likely to require ventilation support as an emergency procedure, either invasively by endotracheal intubation or by non-invasive ventilation.

A patient unwilling to take medication by nebulization may tolerate inhalers or may be offered oral medication, although this is unlikely if they are acutely unwell.

Potential problems

The nurse should observe the patient to make sure that the medications are being inhaled correctly. If not, further explanation and assistance should be given, for example holding the nebulizer mask or mouthpiece for the patient and encouraging them to inhale correctly.

Indications for assistance

A patient will need assistance with setting up and administering medications via a nebulizer if they have not done so before, or if they are too unwell to manage the compressor switches and the nebulizer pots.

Special considerations

Although medications are delivered in a mist, they are still medications. As such they can have unpleasant side effects such as tremor (shakiness), dizziness, tachycardia, and dry mouth. These must be explained. Also, nurses should limit their exposure to patients' nebulizers, and where possible they should be used in open and well-ventilated spaces. It is important to wash the nebulizer pots and mouthpieces thoroughly and allow them to dry between uses, to reduce infection control risks. Similarly, compressor filters and other equipment should be regularly changed.

Concordance

Even though nebulizer therapy should make the patient feel better almost immediately, patients can still be unwilling to use them as side effects such as shakiness and dizziness can be a problem. In order to assist concordance, the risks and benefits should be explained and re-iterated by nurses, and every effort made to minimize the length of time patients spend on nebulized medications by converting to inhaled (rather than nebulized) medications whenever possible. If a patient is to have medications long-term by nebulizer, they must understand the rationale for this and be made aware of the importance of continuing with the therapy.

Procedure

Preparation

Prepare yourself
Ensure you understand how the nebulizer compressor works and the side effects of the drug being nebulized.

Prepare the patient
The procedure should be fully explained to the patient, including an explanation of the potential side effects of the drug being nebulized.

Prepare the equipment
Place the jet nebulizer compressor next to the patient; ensure that it is placed on a hard surface. Collect the correct nebulizer pot for the drug being nebulized and place the drug in the nebulizer pot. Using a peak flow meter, record the patient's peak expired flow rate.

Discussing the procedure with the patient and family

- It is essential that the patient and their relatives are prepared for the procedure if this is their first time using a nebulizer.

- The nurse should explain what drug is being given, why this route has been chosen, and any potential side effects.

- The patient should be shown the equipment to be used, such as a compressor and the mask or mouthpiece with which the drug will be inhaled. This should be fitted securely but comfortably for the patient, who should be shown how to remove it and clean it as necessary. The on/off controls for the compressor should be demonstrated so that the patient knows how to discontinue it when the treatment has finished.

- The patient should be made aware that some compressors are very noisy, and that nebulizer pots do not usually empty fully, leaving a residual amount of the drug treatment in the bottom. This is normal but the patient should beware of spilling it.

- Any other issues such as the need to take and record peak flow readings before and after treatment should also be explained.

Step-by-step guide to undertaking nebulization

Step		Rationale
1	Introduce yourself, confirm the patient's identity, explain the procedure, and obtain consent.	To identify the patient correctly and gain informed consent.
2	Check the prescription of the drug to be given and the patient identification.	To ensure correct medication is given as prescribed.
3	Place mouthpiece in patient's mouth (see **Figure 5.6**) or place mask over patient's face, and turn on nebulizer. Leave on for 10 minutes. Masks, if used, must be tight-fitting and the patient should be encouraged to breathe through an open mouth. If nebulizing via a tracheostomy or non-invasive ventilation, a T-piece should be used.	Optimum time for nebulization of bronchodilators is 10 minutes; if it takes longer then the machine should be serviced. To avoid aerosol and droplets spreading to the eyes. Use T-piece to incorporate nebulizer into the circuit.
4	On completion of each nebulization, dispose of any residue into a clinical waste bin. The nebulizer pot should be washed and dried thoroughly.	Safe disposal of medications. Manufacturers recommend that nebulizer pots are dismantled and washed in warm soapy water, rinsed, and dried thoroughly after use (Respironics 2007). Care must be taken to ensure that none of the nebulizer parts are lost.
5	Record and document the peak expired flow rate 30 minutes after nebulization.	To monitor the effect of the nebulizer and document the readings so that response to treatment can be assessed along with related trends.

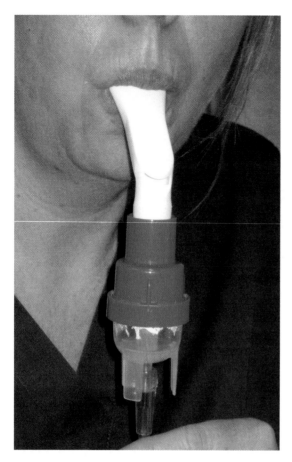

Figure 5.6 How to use a nebulizer. Courtesy of Respironics, Inc. and its subsidiaries.

Following the procedure

1   Observe the patient and ask them how they felt after receiving this nebulizer. Did it change their breathing?
2   Find out if the patient experienced any side effects such as racing heart or dizziness. If they did, make sure this is reported to the doctor.

Recognizing patient deterioration

Patient deterioration immediately upon commencing nebulization is unlikely in routine administration of nebulizers. Patient deterioration immediately after nebulization in a situation where the patient is acutely unwell is an indication that their underlying condition is worsening. For example, in an acute exacerbation of asthma, the patient's breathing rate or pattern may

change, becoming shallower and more rapid than previously. The patient may become cyanosed. In this scenario it is essential to call senior help immediately and prepare resuscitation equipment including oxygen, as the patient may suffer cardiopulmonary arrest imminently.

Reflection and evaluation

When you have administered a drug via nebulization, think about the following questions:

- Think through your role in the administration of the nebulized drug.
- Did you understand what the patient was having and why they were having it?
- Did you ensure that they understood what was happening?
- Did you explain the procedure thoroughly?

Further learning opportunities

Practise the skills listed previously and the sensitivity described in the 'Discussing the procedure with patient and family' box. It is not recommended that students practise using nebulized drugs on themselves, but it may be useful to try fitting a mask to oneself to get an idea of how they feel and how the prolonged use of one might feel for the patient. Also, make a note of how noisy the compressor is. Is there anything that can be done to make it less noisy, especially in a bay of patients?

For a demonstration of a nebulization procedure, see **http://www.yourstudioa.com/?p=238**, which shows a hand-held nebulizer being set up. This video is aimed at pre-hospital care staff such as ambulance crews and is not the same as the in-hospital procedure as a cylinder rather than a compressor is being used, but is nevertheless an interesting demonstration.

Reminders

- Nebulization allows medications to be delivered to the lungs in an easily accessible format. It involves air or oxygen being driven through a solution of a drug. The resulting fine mist is then inhaled directly into the lungs via a facemask or a mouthpiece.

- Patients may be acutely unwell when having nebulized drug therapy and require close monitoring, including assessment of respiratory rate.
- Patients having nebulizers for the first time may find this anxiety-provoking and will need explanation and reassurance.

Patient scenarios

Consider what you should do in the following situations, then turn to the end of this skill to check your answers.

1 Patient 1 has been prescribed Colistin for administration via a nebulizer. Ten minutes after the first dose of this drug, he becomes more short of breath and wheezy. What might have caused this to occur?

2 Patient 2 has been admitted to hospital and is confused and distressed, mainly due to hypoxia. He has been prescribed regular nebulizers but is refusing to use them via a mouthpiece; what is the best way to manage this situation?

3 Patient 3 is receiving non-invasive ventilation through a tracheostomy and has been prescribed regular nebulizers; what delivery device will you choose?

Website

 http://www.oxfordtextbooks.co.uk/orc/ endacott

You may find it helpful to work through our short online quiz and additional scenarios intended to help you to develop and apply the skills in this chapter.

References

Benson HA and Prankered RJ (1998). Optimisation of drug delivery – pulmonary drug delivery. *Australian Journal of Hospital Pharmacy*, **28**, 18–23.

BMA and Royal Pharmaceutical Society of Great Britain (2004). *British National Formulary*. MBA/BPSGB, London.

Edmond G (2001). *Respiratory nursing*. Churchill Livingstone, Edinburgh.

Francis C (2006). *Respiratory care: essential clinical skills for nurses*. Blackwell Publishing, Oxford.

Kendrick AH, Smith EC, and Wilson RS (1997). Selecting and using nebulizer equipment. *Thorax*, **52**(suppl 2), S92–S101.

Respironics (2007). *Patient handbook for nebulizer compressor*. Respironics, Chichester.

Trounce J and Gould D (2000). *Clinical pharmacology for nurses*, 16th edition. Churchill Livingstone, London.

Useful further reading and websites

Bourke SJ (2007). *Lecture notes on respiratory Medicine*, 7th edition. Blackwell Publishing Ltd, Oxford.

Jevon P (2007). Respiratory procedures. Part 3 – use of a nebulizer. *Nursing Times*, **103**(34), 24–5.

Porter-Jones G (2000). Nebulizers, part 1: preparation. Practical procedures for nurses, part 44.1. *Nursing Times*, **96**(36), 45–6.

Porter-Jones G (2000). Nebulizers, part 2: administration. Practical procedures for nurses, part 44.2. *Nursing Times*, **96**(37), 51–2.

Answers to patient scenarios

1 Occasionally when a patient is given a nebulized drug for the first time it can cause them to have bronchospasm, which will cause shortness of breath and a possible wheeze. If this occurs, the drug should be discontinued and an alternative sought. It is useful if spirometry and peak expired flow rate are measured prior to the first dose of the drug and 45 minutes after the dose to establish if there is any adverse effect of the drug.

2 Ideally, the patient should use a mouthpiece to improve drug deposition to the lungs and prevent droplets spreading to the eyes. On this occasion, however, it may be more appropriate to use a facemask, and then remain with the patient to help and reassure them.

3 A T-piece within the circuit is the correct device to use.

5.5 **Use of inhalers**

Definition

An inhaler is a small device that allows the delivery of small doses of medication in a form that can be easily inhaled and absorbed through a patient's lungs, using the principle of aerosolization. Aerosolization involves passing a metered volume of a solution of drug in an **inert dilutent** through a valve under pressure, which enables the delivery to the patient of a measured dose of drug in a fine spray of controlled particle size.

It is important to remember that:

- Although a very small total dose of drug is administered, the concentration achieved at the site of action is high.
- Rapid and effective control of symptoms is achieved without the side effects often associated with the oral dose of the drug.
- Ensuring a good inhaler technique is vital in the treatment of all patients. Involving them in the assessment and choice of inhaler device may help with compliance of use.

Prior knowledge

Before using an inhaler with a patient, make sure you are familiar with:

- Respiratory anatomy, including the anatomical structures of the respiratory tract from the mouth, through the trachea, into the bronchi and alveoli.
- Physiology of respiration, including a basic understanding of the role of respiration in maintaining and regulating oxygen and carbon dioxide concentrations in the body.
- Pathophysiology of common respiratory diseases including asthma, chronic obstructive pulmonary disease (COPD), emphysema, and lung cancer.
- The side effects of the commonly used inhaled drugs.

Background

Inhalers are commonly used for a variety of respiratory conditions such as asthma and COPD, and patients often use inhalers to give themselves maintenance doses of their medication. There are several types of drug delivery devices used, including:

- Pressurized metered dose inhalers, which propel the drug out of the device ready to be inhaled quickly by the patient – see **Figure 5.7(a)**.
- Breath-actuated inhalers, where a patient's brisk inhalation triggers the drug delivery, for example a Handihaler – see **Figure 5.7(b)**.

- Dry powder inhalers, which deliver a dose of medication without propellant gases, for example Accuhaler® and Turbohaler® – see **Figure 5.7(c)**.
- Spacer devices (**Figure 5.8**), which reduce the velocity of the **propellant** by allowing the patient to fire the drug into a large plastic chamber, and increase the uptake of the drug.

For patients who might be physically restricted by arthritis and find it difficult to compress a canister, a 'haleraid' can be given that fits on the inhaler and makes it easier to depress the moveable part to fire the device (Maher 2006).

Inhaler technique

Good inhaler technique is essential; even with good inhaler technique only 10–20% of the inhaled dose is likely to reach the lower respiratory tract (Benson and Prankered 1998, Brown 2004). Instructing the patient to hold their breath at the end of inspiration will ensure that a high proportion of the inhaled dose reaches the lower airways (Barnett 2007).

Choice of device will depend on several factors:

- Any coexisting problems such as arthritis, poor eyesight, cognitive impairment.
- Manual dexterity requirements and any breath coordination required.
- Availability of the drug for use in the device chosen.

Patients will generally use at least two different inhalers at a time, and where possible the same delivery device should be chosen.

Spacer devices

The use of a spacer device (see Figure 5.8) is recommended for metered dose inhalers (British Thoracic Society/Scottish Intercollegiate Guideline Network 2003, National Institute for Health and Clinical Excellence (NICE) 2004). These are plastic holding chambers that collect the aerosolized drug when the metered dose inhaler is activated. They improve medication deposition within the lungs to 40–60% and therefore the use of a spacer should be encouraged for all patients using a metered dose inhaler. They also reduce the side effects in the mouth and throat, particularly when inhaled steroids are used.

(a)

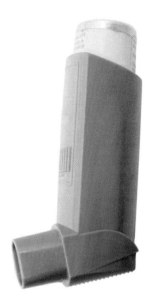

(b)

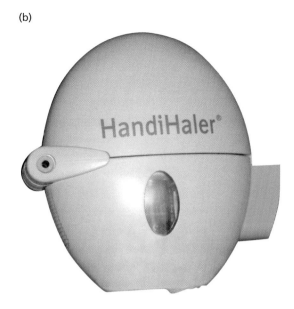

(c)

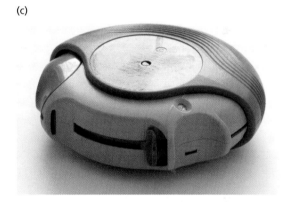

Figure 5.7 (a) An inhaler, courtesy of Ian Jeffery/istockphoto.com. (b) A Handihaler®, courtesy of Boehringer Ingelheim. (c) An Accuhaler, courtesy of Rob Bouwman/istockphoto.com.

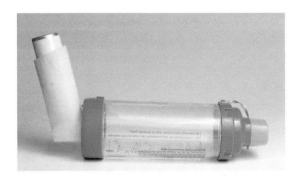

Figure 5.8 A spacer device, courtesy of Robert Byron/istockphoto.com.

Context

 ### When to use an inhaler

An inhaler would be used when metered doses of a medication are required, usually for maintenance doses and occasionally in acute situations. The patient must be able to administer these doses for themselves, or have sufficient support in the community to be able to do so.

 ### When not to use an inhaler

Although it is possible to give larger doses of some medication using inhalers and spacer devices, in acute exacerbations of asthma and COPD it is frequently necessary to give very large doses, and these are best given using nebulizing equipment (see Section 5.4).

It will not be possible for a patient who has poor technique, physical impairment, or a lack of understanding to self-administer inhalers. Poor technique will lead to the drug not being delivered in a way that makes it possible for the patient to inhale it in the correct manner and with sufficient coordination, meaning that the correct dosage will not be inhaled. It may be difficult for children to coordinate sufficiently the delivery and inhalation aspects of self-medication by inhalers.

Indications for assistance

Assistance will be required by patients with poor technique, lack of understanding, or physical impairment, and by those whose condition may be deteriorating.

Procedures

Preparation

Prepare yourself

Ensure you understand how the inhaler works and the side effects of the drug that is being inhaled. Check the patient's care records for any previous problems with inhaler use.

Prepare the patient

The procedure should be fully explained to the patient, including an explanation of the potential side effects of the drug being inhaled.

Prepare the equipment

Collect the necessary equipment and allow the patient to become familiar with it. Using a peak flow meter, record the patient's peak expired flow rate.

Discussing the procedure with the patient and family

- It is essential that the patient and their relatives are prepared for the procedure if this is their first time using an inhaler.

- The nurse should explain what drug is being given, why this route has been chosen, and any potential side effects.

- The patient should be shown the equipment to be used, such as a metered dose inhaler with a spacer, and should receive instruction concerning good inhaler technique.

- It is often possible to obtain placebo inhalers to allow health care staff to demonstrate technique and patients to practise without using the real drug.

- Any other issues such as the need to take and record peak flow readings before and after treatment should also be explained.

Step-by-step guide to using a metered dose inhaler

Patients should be advised to take their short-acting bronchodilator first, and to wait at least 5 minutes before taking their next inhaler (Barnett 2007). This is because the short-acting bronchodilator opens the airways rapidly and thus allows for better deposition of the other medications.

Step		Rationale
1	Introduce yourself, confirm the patient's identity, explain the procedure, and obtain consent.	To identify the patient correctly and gain informed consent.
2	Shake the inhaler and remove the dust cap.	To ensure drug is mixed effectively, as it is suspended in propellant.
3	Breathe out gently and fully.	To empty the lungs.
4	Place the mouthpiece between the teeth and seal the lips around it.	To prevent any loss of the drug via the mouth.
5	When breathing in fully and steadily, press the inhaler to release the dose, breathing in to full inspiration.	To optimize the drug deposition.

6	Remove the inhaler from the mouth and hold the breath for up to 10 seconds. For a second dose, wait for 60 seconds and repeat the process.	To ensure a high proportion of the inhaled dose reaches the lower airways.
7	Patients should be advised to rinse their mouth and gargle after any inhaler that contains a steroid.	To prevent the potential side effect of oral candidiasis.

If using a large volume spacer, there are two methods recommended:

1 **Holding the breath prior to expiration:** this procedure is suitable for most adults.

2 **Tidal breathing:** this procedure is useful for patients such as children or the elderly who may have difficulty coordinating inspiration and the actuation of the metered dose inhaler, as it removes the need for good coordination.

Procedure for tidal breathing through a large volume spacer

- Shake inhaler and place securely into the spacer.
- Put mouthpiece of spacer into the mouth and form a tight seal around it.
- Press the canister and inhale and exhale five times (tidal breathing).

(Francis 2006)

Procedure for holding the breath through a large volume spacer

- Shake inhaler and place in the spacer.
- Put mouthpiece of spacer into the mouth and form a tight seal around it.
- Press the canister and then take a deep breath from the mouthpiece. Hold the breath for a count of 10 prior to expiration.

(Francis 2006)

Step-by-step guide to using a Turbohaler (a dry powder device)

Step   Rationale

1	Introduce yourself, confirm the patient's identity, explain the procedure, and obtain consent.	To identify the patient correctly and gain informed consent.
2	Unscrew the dust cap. Hold the inhaler upright and twist the grip forwards and backwards until it clicks.	To load the inhaler ready for delivery.
3	Breathe out fully, put the mouthpiece between the lips, and take a deep breath in.	To prevent any loss of the drug via the mouth and aid drug deposition.
4	Remove the inhaler from the mouth and hold the breath for 10 seconds. Replace the dust cap.	To ensure a high proportion of the inhaled dose reaches the lower airways.
5	A dose counter will indicate when the inhaler is about to run out. Remind the patient that when they shake the inhaler it will seem that there is still some powder remaining; however, this is the desiccant that is used in each inhaler.	Indicates to the patient when they need to get another inhaler.

Step-by-step guide to using an Accuhaler (a dry powder device)

Step		Rationale
1	Introduce yourself, confirm the patient's identity, explain the procedure, and obtain consent.	To identify the patient correctly and gain informed consent.
2	Hold the inhaler and push the thumb grip away.	To open the inhaler case.
3	Slide the lever down.	To activate the dose.
4	Breathe out fully. Keeping the inhaler horizontal, place mouthpiece in mouth and breathe in deeply.	To prevent any loss of the drug via the mouth and aid drug deposition.
5	Remove from the mouth and hold breath for 10 seconds.	To ensure a high proportion of the inhaled dose reaches the lower airways.
6	Close the inhaler by pushing the thumb grip back.	Closes the inhaler.

Step-by-step guide to using a Handihaler

Step		Rationale
1	Introduce yourself, confirm the patient's identity, explain the procedure, and obtain consent.	To identify the patient correctly and gain informed consent.
2	Open the dust cap and mouthpiece.	To enable capsule to be placed in chamber.
3	Place the capsule in the chamber and close the mouthpiece until it clicks, leaving the dust cap open.	To ensure correct preparation of inhaler for use.
4	Holding the inhaler, push the green button once.	To pierce the capsule.
5	Breathe out fully, put the mouthpiece between the lips, and breathe in slowly.	To prevent any loss of the drug via the mouth and aid drug deposition.
6	Remove the inhaler from the mouth and hold the breath for 10 seconds.	To ensure a high proportion of the inhaled dose reaches the lower airways.
7	Replace the mouthpiece in the mouth and repeat the breath in.	To ensure that the capsule is empty.
8	Open the mouthpiece and dispose of the used capsule. Replace mouthpiece and dust cap.	To prepare inhaler for next dose.

Following the procedure

When using any inhaler device it is useful to demonstrate its use to the patient and to supplement this with written information.

Recognizing patient deterioration

Patient deterioration immediately after inhaler use is unlikely in routine administration. Patient deterioration immediately after inhaler use in a situation where the patient is acutely unwell is an indication that their underlying condition is worsening. For example, in an acute exacerbation of asthma, the patient's breathing rate or pattern may change, becoming shallower and more rapid than previously. The patient may become cyanosed. In this scenario it is essential to call senior help immediately and prepare equipment for nebulization and oxygen administration as the patient may suffer severe shortness of breath.

Reflection and evaluation

When you have used an inhaler with a patient, think about the following questions:

1 Did you feel you helped the patient in understanding and using the equipment?
2 Were there questions you could not answer?
3 Do you need to do further reading about inhalers and inhaler technique?

By using the placebo equipment, the nurse can get an idea of what the patient will need to do when taking medication in this manner.

Further learning opportunities

There are several placebo devices available for the different inhalers; obtain some of these and practise inhaler technique. Obtain some placebo training devices for use with the patient and demonstrate the technique to them, then observe their technique. If placebo devices are used for more than one patient, they should be decontaminated between each patient (NICE 2003). Use a large volume spacer and see if the patient notices a difference and if this is easier for them to coordinate.

Reminder

- The choice of inhaler device is vital in ensuring compliance and efficacy of drug delivery.

 Patient scenarios

Consider what you should do in the following situations, then turn to the end of this skill to check your answers.

1 Patient 1 is a patient with rheumatoid arthritis of the hands who is finding it difficult to depress the canister on their metered dose inhaler. What additional device would you obtain for them?
2 Patient 2 is an elderly patient who finds it difficult to coordinate their breathing with depressing the canister of a metered dose inhaler. What might you suggest to improve this and why?
3 Patient 3 has to use three different inhalers and is unclear about the sequence of taking the inhalers or how long they should wait between each inhaler. What advice would you give them?

Website

 http://www.oxfordtextbooks.co.uk/orc/endacott

You may find it helpful to work through our short online quiz and additional scenarios intended to help you to develop and apply the skills in this chapter.

References

Barnett M (2007). Managing COPD: inhaler therapy. *Journal of Community Nursing*, **21**(4), 31–5.

Benson HA and Prankered RJ (1998). Optimisation of drug delivery – pulmonary drug delivery. *Australian Journal of Hospital Pharmacy*, **28**, 18–23.

British Thoracic Society/Scottish Intercollegiate Guideline Network (2003). British guideline on the management of asthma, a national clinical guideline. *Thorax*, **58**(Suppl 1), i1–i94.

Brown R (2004). Drug delivery systems 2. Pulmonary and parenteral formulations. *Airways Journal*, **2**(1), 43–6.

Francis C (2006). *Respiratory care: essential clinical skills for nurses*. Blackwell Publishing Ltd., Oxford.

Maher A (2006). Inhalers and the elderly. *Airways Journal*, **4**(1), 50–3.

National Institute for Health and Clinical Excellence (2003). *Infection control. Prevention of healthcare-associated infection in primary and community care. Clinical Guideline 2*. NICE, London.

National Institute for Health and Clinical Excellence (2004). Chronic obstructive pulmonary disease; national clinical guideline in adults in primary and secondary care. *Thorax*, **59**(Suppl 1), 1–232.

Useful further reading and websites

Bourke SJ (2007). *Lecture notes on respiratory medicine*, 7th edition. Blackwell Publishing Ltd., Oxford.

Leyshon J (2007). Correct technique for using aerosol inhaler devices. *Nursing Standard*, **21**(52), 38–40.

About.com has a short video on inhalers at: **http://video.about.com/asthma/Inhalers.htm**

You can find a number of podcasts on the 'Builth surgery' website at: **http://www.builthsurgery.co.uk/pages/gallery/video.htm**

Patient UK has a useful factsheet on different devices at: **http://www.patient.co.uk/showdoc/23069155/**

Medicines.org.uk has a list of inhaler devices and videos about how to use them at: **http://medguides.medicines.org.uk/demonstrations.aspx**

 Answers to patient scenarios

1 A haleraid should be provided to use with the inhaler.

2 The patient should be instructed to perform tidal breathing via a large volume spacer.

3 A bronchodilator should be given first; the patient should wait 1 minute between each breath and 5 minutes between each inhaler.

5.6 **Enteral tube administration of drugs**

Introduction

The **enteral tube** can provide a useful alternative route to administer patients' medicines where conventional licensed routes (e.g. oral) are unavailable. However, there are a number of important issues to be aware of before administering medicines in this way.

It is important to remember that:

- Just because a patient has an enteral tube does not mean it should automatically be used for medicine administration.
- The actual medicine administration via enteral tubes can be straightforward but is dependent upon advice on the safest and most appropriate route and formulation. Without this advice, medicine administration via enteral tube can be dangerous.
- The risks of wrong route errors can be minimized by following best practice examples and using the correct type of syringes for enteral tube administration.

Prior knowledge

Before administering medications via an enteral tube, make sure you are familiar with:

1 Gastrointestinal anatomy, encompassing the anatomical structures of the gastrointestinal (GI) tract from the mouth, through the stomach, and into the small and large intestine. Also knowledge of the anatomical divisions of the small intestine: duodenum, jejunum, and ileum.

2 Upper respiratory tract anatomy, including anatomy of the mouth, nose, and trachea.

3 Neck anatomy, especially the division between the upper GI and respiratory tracts (see Section 10.3 for more information).

4 Physiology of digestion, including the basic functions of the GI tract (stomach and large and small intestines).

5 Basic pharmacology of any medicines you will be administering.

6 Nasogastric (and other enteral tube) feeding – see Section 10.3.

Background

Nasogastric tubes are one of many types of enteral tube (meaning: into the GI tract) and are commonly abbreviated to 'NG' [tube]. Other common types of enteral tube and their abbreviations are listed in **Table 5.8**. For more information regarding enteral tubes and feeding, see Section 10.3.

Table 5.8 Types of enteral tube

Enteral tube type	Abbreviation	Terminates in
Nasogastric	NG	Stomach
Nasojejunal	NJ	Jejunum
Percutaneous endoscopic gastrostomy	PEG	Stomach
Percutaneous endoscopic jejunostomy	PEJ	Jejunum
Radiologically inserted gastrostomy	RIG	Stomach

The administration of medicines via enteral tubes is generally **unlicensed** and can have more unpredictable effects than **licensed** routes. Therefore, where a patient has an enteral tube, alternative *licensed* routes (e.g. intravenous, rectal, topical, etc.) should always be used in preference.

There are two important legal issues involved with enteral tube administration of medicines:

1 The enteral tube as the route of medicine administration.
2 Formulation manipulations to make medicines enteral tube compatible, e.g. crushing tablets.

Enteral tubes as a route of medicine administration

Medicines are not designed for enteral tube administration and their use in this way will virtually always fall outside of their **product licence**. Therefore, any harm that the patient comes to because of receiving their medicine in this way will be the responsibility of the team looking after them, potentially including the person administering the medicine.

Nurses should be aware that the only person who is legally allowed to recommend an unlicensed use of a medicine (e.g. via an NG tube) is a medical practitioner. This may sometimes be termed an off-licence use of a medicine to avoid confusion between unlicensed and licensed products. Most commonly, these practitioners are doctors by profession, but dentists and now independent prescribers (pharmacists) may also be included in this group. This restriction is specified in the 1968 Medicines Act, and so it is crucial that a nurse gains written permission, i.e. on the prescription. This can be achieved by having the doctor specify 'NG' in the route section of the inpatient drug chart, or as a part of the directions.

If a nurse were to give a medicine via enteral tube without written consent, it could result in a finding of professional misconduct as it is against the 1968 Act. Even where a doctor has specified an unlicensed route of administration for a medicine, some responsibility remains with the person administering the medication.

Manipulation of medicine formulations

As the formulation of medicines is *not* generally designed for enteral tubes, the person administering them may need to manipulate the medicine so that it can successfully be given via enteral tube. Examples of this are: opening capsules; crushing tablets; or dispersing a tablet inside the barrel of an enteral syringe. These manipulations should be authorized in writing by the prescriber, as changes to medicines in this way nearly always constitute an unlicensed use of the medicine.

Manipulation should only be done where absolutely necessary and if it is deemed safe to do so.

Often there will be an alternative way of administering the medicine to the patient that is within the product licence. This may mean choosing an alternative route, e.g. intravenous, topical (patches), rectal (suppositories), or a more enteral tube appropriate form, e.g. liquids.

The practice of crushing tablets (or opening capsules) appears widespread (Wright 1992) and, although appearing harmless, has on occasion caused fatalities (Schier *et al.* 2003). This practice must not be done unless absolutely necessary and advice must be sought to ensure safety. Examples of the types of medicine that should *not* be considered for crushing/opening are listed in **Table 5.9**.

Medicines often appear similar but the science of formulation (putting together a medicine) is very complicated, so appearances can be deceptive. **Table 5.10** gives examples of the huge range of formulation types/subtypes that are available for oral use. Great care must therefore

Table 5.9 Types of tablet/capsule that should not be crushed/opened

Formulation	How to identify	Rationale
Modified release	Suffixes: MR, LA, SR, XL, CR, Chrono, Retard Prefixes: Slow- Other patented terms: GITS®, SPANSULE®, DURULE®, RETARD®, etc. Check on original packaging or in the BNF for form information. If in doubt check with a pharmacist.	Modified release products are designed to release the drug in a controlled and specific way. Destroying this by tablet crushing or opening capsules will change the way in which the drug is absorbed. This can result in exaggerated effects, adverse effects, or toxicity effects, and hence patient harm.
Enteric-coated	Suffixes: EC, EN, GR Check on original packaging or in e.g. the BNF for form information.	An **enteric coating** is a layer on medicines to stop them from breaking up and dissolving in the acidic environment of the stomach. They are used to stop medicines irritating the stomach, or to prevent the stomach acid destroying the active drug.
Hormonal	Look up the medicine's indication(s) in the BNF.	Crushing tablets and opening capsules will result in a small amount of medicine being released into the air. Staff inhaling this could be affected and come to harm. Extreme caution in pregnant/breastfeeding staff.
Cytotoxic	Box/bottle labels and drug charts should state a cytotoxic warning. You can also look up the medicine's indication(s) in the BNF.	Crushing tablets and opening capsules will result in a small amount of medicine being released into the air. Staff inhaling this could be affected and come to harm. Extreme caution in pregnant/breastfeeding staff.
Antibiotics	Look up the medicine's indication(s) e.g. in the BNF.	Crushing tablets and opening capsules will result in a small amount of medicine being released into the air. Staff inhaling this could be affected and come to harm. Extreme caution in pregnant/breastfeeding staff.

be taken when administering all medicines via enteral tubes. The best source of advice and knowledge relating to safety and appropriateness of formulation manipulation is the pharmacist. There are some general guidelines to follow on when not to crush tablets and these are included later in this skill.

Another factor to be aware of is that although some preparations *appear* to be enteral tube compatible, they may not be. Good examples of this are some liquid suspensions, as they obviously appear to be in an ideal form (liquid) for enteral tube administration but contain particles that may have the potential to block tubes, e.g. some brands of clarithromycin suspension. This specific issue is

more problematic with narrower bore tubes and reinforces the need to refer to the pharmacist for advice about formulation.

Types of syringe

When administering medicines via an enteral tube, a catheter-tipped bladder syringe, female reverse luer (slip or lock), or an oral syringe should always be used. Avoid the use of male luer (slip or lock) intravenous type syringes as these have been shown to increase the risk of wrong route errors, i.e. administering *oral* medicines *intravenously*. This type of error can prove fatal and is an

Table 5.10 Types of pharmaceutical formulation

Basic form	Formulation subtypes
Liquids	Suspension
	Elixir
	Solution
	Syrup
Tablets	Tablets
	Soluble tablets
	Dispersible tablets
	Enteric-coated tablets
	Modified release tablets
	Buccal tablets
	Chewable tablets
	Orodispersible tablets
Capsules	Powder-filled capsules
	Bead-filled capsules
	Capsules with enteric-coated contents
	Enteric-coated 'shell' capsules
	Modified release capsules
	Gel-filled capsules
	Liquid-filled capsules

area being closely looked at by the National Patient Safety Association (NPSA) (2007).

Where liquid medicines need to be *measured accurately*, only a graduated oral/enteral syringe should be used. Catheter-tipped syringes are inaccurate for small volumes. Familiarize yourself with any policies on approved syringe types in your local practice. Not all syringes are compatible with the ports on enteral tubes. Different types of syringe are identified in **Figure 5.9**.

Context

 ### When to give medicines via enteral tubes

Medicines should be given via an enteral tube when:

- The patient has had the medication prescribed and has need for the medication.
- The patient is unable to swallow their oral medicines safely.
- There is no other licensed route practically available (oral or other).

- Where formulation modification is required, advice has been received that it is safe to do so, e.g. crushing a tablet.
- Written consent has been received from the prescriber for the change of route *and* modification of formulation where appropriate.

 ### When not to give medicines via enteral tubes

Medicines should *not* be given via enteral tubes when:

- There is no immediate medical need for the medicine. Some medicines can be omitted short term without a problem, but this must be confirmed by the doctor.
- There has been no written confirmation from the prescriber that the medicine should be administered via the enteral tube.
- The prescriber has not confirmed in writing that it is acceptable to modify the medicine form.
- You do not know it is safe to do so (Tip: ask for advice).
- There are alternative licensed routes for the medication available. The prescriber may prefer NG to IV for cost reasons, e.g. antibiotics.
- The medicine has *not* been prepared in one uninterrupted process and the syringe is not labelled with the patient's name, date and time of preparation, drug name, and strength.

See **Figure 5.10** for further guidance.

Alternative interventions

It is always worth checking with the prescriber if you suspect the medicine could be safely omitted for a short period. Licensed non-enteral routes should be used where available and practical, e.g. IV, rectal, topical (patches), etc. This will avoid the unlicensed use of medicines and also any formulation modification with the associated risks of exaggerated, adverse, or toxic effects.

Potential problems

Enteral tubes can become blocked during or after drug administration. This can be minimized by ensuring that only compatible products are selected for administration

Syringe type	Connector	Tip detail	Enteral tube recommended?
Male luer slip	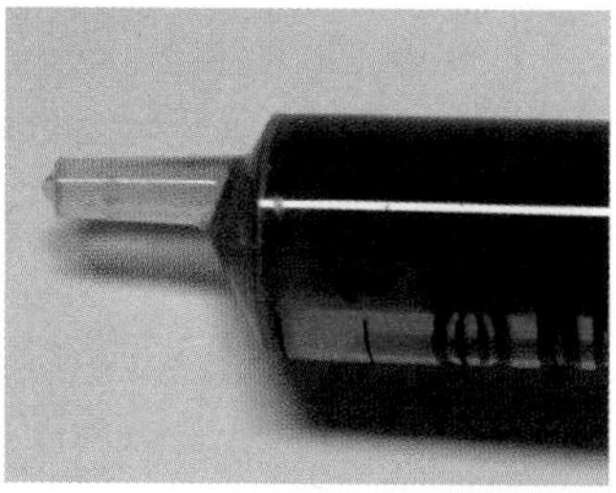	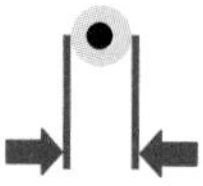 4.0 mm	✗
Male luer lock	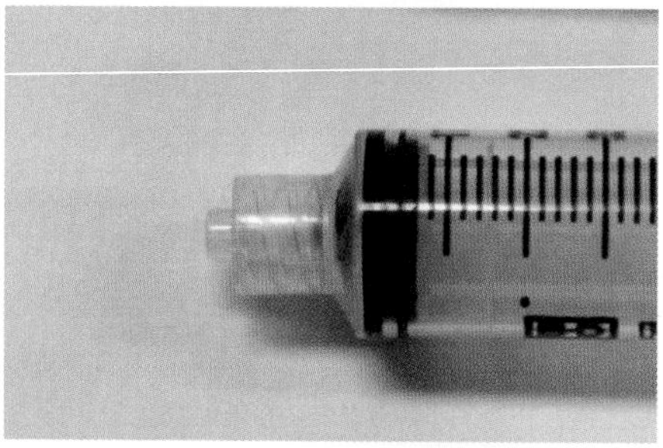	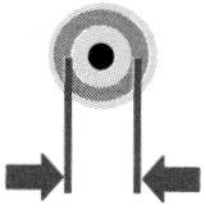 4.0 mm	✗
Female (or reverse) luer lock	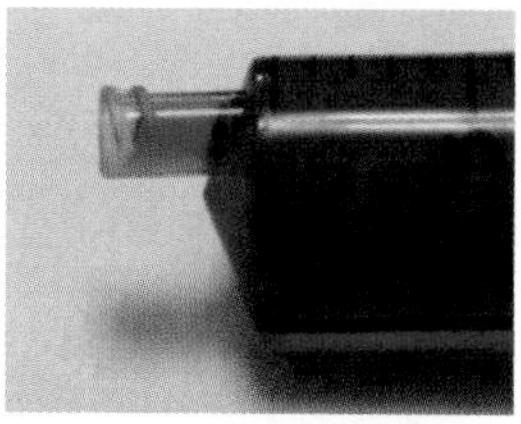	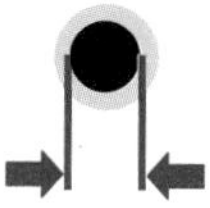 4.3 mm	✓
Oral	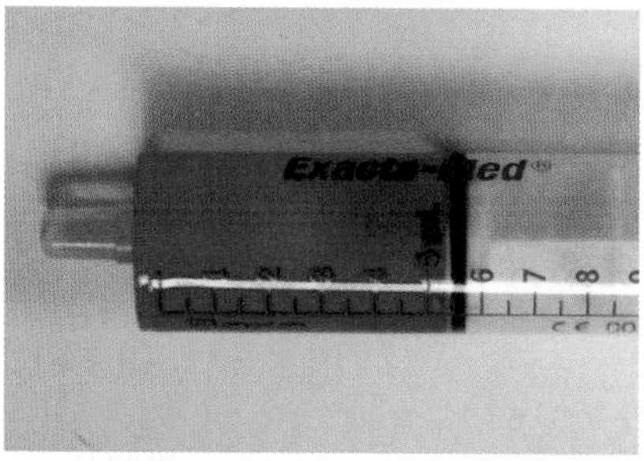	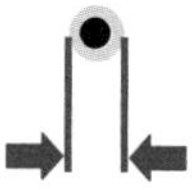 5.0 mm	✓ * *Often incompatible without an adapter
Catheter-tipped 'bladder' syringe	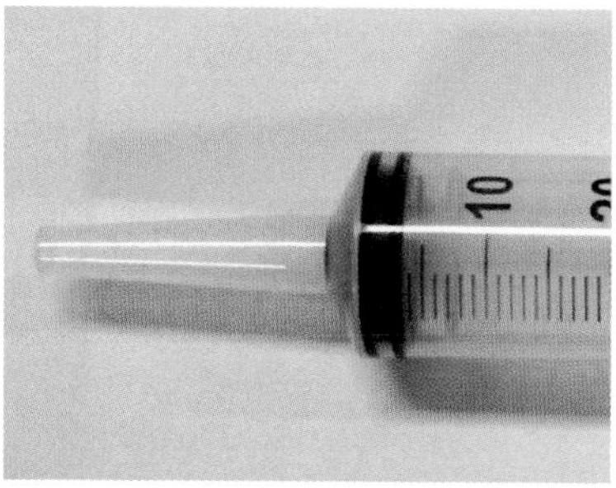	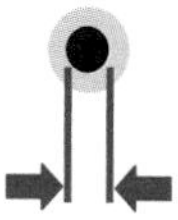 4.0 mm	✓

Figure 5.9 Suitability of different syringes for enteral medication administration.

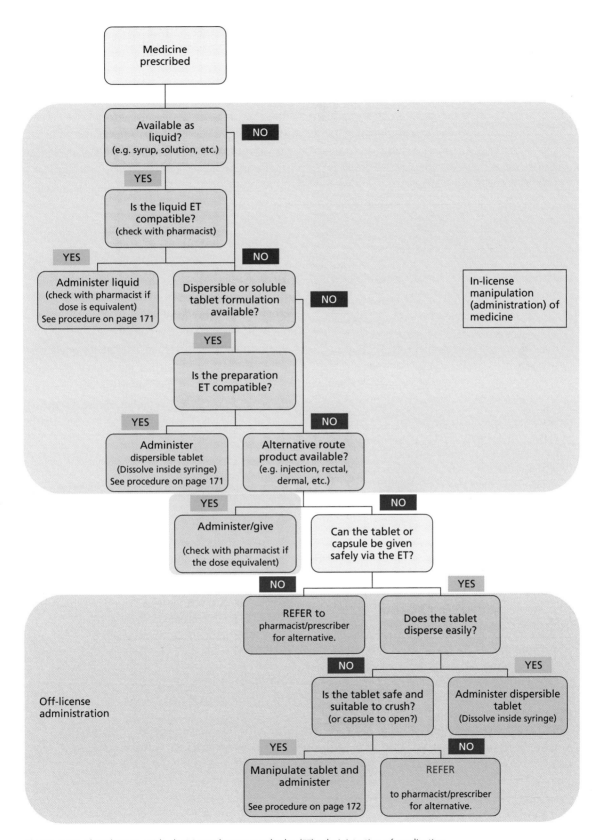

Figure 5.10 Flowchart to guide decisions about enteral tube (ET) administration of medication.

and flushing is done thoroughly before and after each drug. Advice on product selection should be sought from a pharmacist. If blockage does occur there are methods that can be used to resolve it (see Section 10.3).

Special considerations

- If the enteral tube terminates lower down the GI tract than the stomach, ensure that any flushes are done with sterile water, i.e. not tap water.

- A graduated oral or enteral syringe should be used when measuring out liquid medications. Catheter-tipped bladder syringes are not accurate when measuring small volumes.

- Where possible, avoid using intravenous syringes to measure out or administer medicines.

- The preparation and administration of medicines for enteral tube administration should be done in one uninterrupted process. If this is not achievable, the syringe must be labelled with the name and strength of the medicine, patient's name, and the date and time of preparation.

- Dissolving a tablet inside the enteral/oral syringe **may** be a useful way to protect yourself and others from hazardous (e.g. hormonal, antibiotic, or cytotoxic) medicines. Advice on hazardous medicines administration **must always** be sought.

Indications for assistance

If you are not sure if it is safe to administer a medicine or modify a medicine formulation, you must ask for advice. Always check the prescription for endorsements specifying how the medicine should be administered if off-licence.

Procedure

Preparation

Prepare yourself

Ensure you understand what the medicine is for and have a form that is suitable for administration via an enteral tube. Check the patient's records for any fluid restrictions. Check if the medicine is supposed to be given in a feed-free period (see step 1 of stepby-step guide to enteral administration). Wash your hands.

Prepare the patient

The procedure should be fully explained to the patient (see Discussion box).

Prepare the equipment

Select the medicine that is prescribed on the patient's drug chart in the form most appropriate for enteral tube administration. Gather together the equipment needed to prepare and/or measure the medicine. Clean any equipment, e.g. mortars and pestles. Ensure syringes are labelled clearly with the patient's name, the date, and the words 'oral use only'.

Discussing the procedure with the patient and family

- Explain what the enteral tube is being used for.

- Explain when the medicines are being used off-licence and seek patient consent.

- Give details of why the medicines being administered may look different from those given/taken previously, e.g. liquids to replace tablets.

Step-by-step guide to preparing and administering capsules and tablets that dissolve, disintegrate, or disperse via an enteral tube

Step	Rationale
1 Introduce yourself, confirm the patient's identity, explain the procedure, and obtain consent.	To identify the patient correctly and gain informed consent.
2 Ensure protective clothing is worn (gloves, etc.).	Some medicines are toxic, hormonal, or may cause sensitivity reactions. Wearing gloves will protect your hands if you need to handle tablets or capsules directly.
3 Remove plunger from enteral syringe and ensure syringe is capped.	This will enable you to drop the tablet into the syringe barrel.
4 Place whole tablet or total capsule contents into a capped syringe barrel.	This will seal the tablet inside the syringe, minimizing any contamination of equipment/surfaces and exposure to staff or patients. It should also ensure a complete dose is given (no residue on equipment used to crush, etc.).
5 Replace syringe plunger, and press until near to the tablet or capsule contents.	To prepare syringe for dissolving contents.
6 Uncap the syringe and draw up 10–20 ml of tap (drinkable) water into syringe barrel.	To dissolve/disperse tablet/capsule contents.
7 Upturn syringe, decap, and remove excess air by gently pressing plunger. You want a small amount of air to remain.	This will enable step 8 to happen more easily, as it will encourage the tablet to disperse and dissolve more readily.
8 Recap syringe and gently shake until tablet is dissolved or dispersed, i.e. no visible lumps.	This will ensure that minimal amounts of the tablet/capsule contents are left in the syringe barrel after administration, so the patient will receive the full dose.
9 Attach syringe to enteral tube port and administer liquid/suspension. See step-by-step guide to enteral administration.	To administer contents of syringe.
10 Remove syringe, draw up another 10–20 ml of water to rinse inside of barrel, and administer via the enteral tube (see step-by-step guide to enteral administration).	This will ensure that any drug remaining is given so that the full dose is received.
11 If syringe has been used to administer cytotoxic or hormonal medication, discard appropriately.	This will help prevent the hazardous medicine contaminating any other equipment or work surfaces, and ensure low risk of other patient/staff exposure.

Step-by-step guide to administering tablets that need to be crushed (if safe and essential to do so)

Step	Rationale
1 Ensure protective clothing is worn (gloves, etc.).	Some medicines are toxic, hormonal, or may cause adverse reactions, e.g. sensitivity. Crushing tablets will create a fine mist of the powder and exposure to this should be minimized.
2 Place tablet(s) into mortar and crush the tablet(s) into a powder with pestle. Care is needed to avoid powder leaving mortar. **[!] Only ever crush tablets of the same drug/type together.**	It is important to avoid part doses being given.
3 Add 5–10 ml of tap water and mix to a smooth paste (no lumps).	This should help minimize lumps in the preparation, and hence prevent tube blockage.
4 Add a further 5–10 ml and mix well. Withdraw liquid with a suitable syringe.	This should help minimize lumps in the preparation, and hence prevent tube blockage.
5 Rinse mortar with a further 10–15 ml and mix with pestle. Withdraw liquid into suitable syringe.	This will ensure that the patient receives the full dose.
6 Continue onto step-by-step guide to enteral administration.	

Step-by-step guide to enteral administration of the medicine

Step	Rationale
1 Check if the medicine needs to be given in a feed-free period.	Feeds are not designed to come into contact with medicines and can interact and cause tube blockages. Potable water can be used unless the enteral tube terminates below the stomach, where sterile water should be used.
2 Introduce yourself, confirm the patient's identity, explain the procedure, and obtain consent.	To identify the patient correctly and gain informed consent.
3 Stop enteral feed and flush with 30 ml of water.	The absorption of some medicines is significantly reduced by the presence of feed in the stomach, so a feed-free period will allow the stomach to empty.

4	Select the prescribed medicine in the most suitable form. Assemble and clean any equipment needed for administration, e.g. mortar, pestle, syringes, etc.	You will need different equipment depending on what medicine and form you are administering.
5	Prepare the medicine for enteral tube administration, e.g. dissolve/crush tablets, open capsules, dilute viscous liquids, shake liquid suspensions, etc. (see previous step-by-step guides).	Depending on the medicine formulation, you may need to prepare it so that it is suitable for enteral tube administration. This will ensure the patient receives the full dose and reduces risk of tube blockage.
6	Administer the medicine. Do not use excessive force.	If prepared correctly, most medicines are relatively easy to administer and do not require excessive force.
7	Flush the enteral tube. If it is the final medicine, flush with 25–30 ml of water. If another medicine is due to be administered, flush with 10–15 ml of water (then return to step 4 above).	Medicines are not designed or tested to be given together through tubes. They could interact and produce unpredictable results. Flushing between each drug minimizes the potential for interaction.
8	Leave a feed-free period where necessary.	See step 3.
9	Restart the feed.	This ensures minimal interruption in patient nutrition and hydration.
10	Document that the medicine has been given on the patient's drug chart.	So others know that the medicine has been administered.
11	Document amount of fluid used to flush the tube on the patient's fluid balance chart (where appropriate).	Some patients who require enteral feeding and drug administration will also require accurate monitoring of fluid intake and output.
12	Thoroughly clean any equipment used, e.g. mortars, pestles, etc.	Poor cleaning will result in patients receiving small quantities of the wrong medicine.

Following the procedure

After use, clean any equipment. This is especially important with equipment that is shared among patients, e.g. a mortar and pestle or tablet crusher. This will ensure small quantities of medicine are not inadvertently given to the wrong patient. It will also reduce any bacterial growth or contamination of the equipment.

Remember to report any tube blockages even if they are unblocked afterwards. Medication formulations are changed and improved continuously and so it is important to identify those that are problematic to give through tubes.

This will enable colleagues to avoid the medicine or take precautions when it is required in the future. Blockages often mean that the patient hasn't received some or all of the dose, so the prescription may need to be changed.

Reflection and evaluation

When you have administered medicines via an enteral tube, think about the following questions:

1 Was the administration straightforward or did you have any difficulties?

2 Were you able to answer the patient's/relative's/carer's questions?

3 If you had any difficulties in administration, would you do anything different next time?

4 Was your administration technique satisfactory?

Further learning opportunities

Have a colleague (e.g. nurse or pharmacist) watch you administer the medicines via enteral tube and offer advice for improving your technique.

Ask whether your ward pharmacist may be able to come and talk to you and your colleagues in a teaching session to update you about the administration of medicines generally or specific medicines used in your clinical area.

Reminders

- Always check a medicine is suitable for enteral tube administration and that the instructions to crush or open tablets are on the prescription/drug chart.
- Be methodical when administering medicine via an enteral tube and do not cut corners (e.g. crushing different medicines together for administration). Your safety and that of the patient are at risk.
- The pharmacist is the most knowledgeable professional about formulation.

 Patient scenarios

Consider what you should do in the following situations, then turn to the end of this skill to check your answers.

1 Patient A has a NG tube and it is coming up to the time that their Simvastatin dose is due. The prescription has 'ORAL' written as the route and no further information regarding enteral tube administration. What should you do before administering it?

2 Patient B has just had a NG tube inserted. The junior doctor has prescribed MST 20 mg modified release tablets, orally every 12 hours. What should you do?

3 Patient C has just arrived on the ward after having a PEG tube inserted and is currently prescribed a medicine that you know is available only as tablets and suppositories. The prescription states 'PEG' as the route. What will you do?

Website

 http://www.oxfordtextbooks.co.uk/orc/ endacott

You may find it helpful to work through our short online quiz and additional scenarios intended to help you to develop and apply the skills in this chapter.

References

National Patient Safety Agency (2007). *Safety in doses: improving the use of medicines in the NHS*. NPSA, London.

Schier JG, Howland MA, Hoffman RS, and Nelson LS (2003). Fatality from administration of labetalol and crushed extended-release nifedipine. *Annals of Pharmacotherapy*, **37**, 1420–3.

Wright D (1992). Tablet crushing is a widespread practice but it is not safe and may not be legal. *The Pharmaceutical Journal*, **269**, 132.

Useful further reading and websites

BAPEN (2003). *Tube feeding and your medicines*. British Association of Parenteral and Enteral Nutrition [online] **http://www.bapen.org.uk/pdfs/d_and_e/ de_gp_guide.pdf** accessed 20/08/08.

NHS National Patient Safety Agency (2007). *Patient Safety Alert 19: promoting safer measurement and administration of liquid medicines via oral and other enteral routes*. NPSA, London.

Ramsay SJ, Gomersall CD, and Joynt GM (2003). The dangers of trying to make ends meet: accidental intravenous administration of enteral feed. *Anaesthesia and Intensive Care*, **31**(3), 324–7.

Useful websites:

Palliativedrugs.com – administering drugs via feeding tubes: **http://www.palliativedrugs.com/ book.php?Appendix10**

http://www.nursingtimes.net/ntclinical/the_legal_ and_clinical_implications_of_crushing_tablet_ medication.html

http://www.nursingtimes.net/ntclinical/drug_ administration_via_a_nasogastric_tube.html

Note that you will need to register for instantaneous free access to the *Nursing Times* website.

 Answers to patient scenarios

1 Find the doctor and explain that they need to write on the change of route and 'crush tablet' before you

can legally and safely give the medicine. The doctor may advise omitting the statin while the patient has an enteral tube. Check whether the patient can swallow the medication; enteral tubes are sometimes used solely to provide additional nutrition and not because the patient has an unsafe swallow reflex.

2 As this medicine is modified release it should *not* be crushed (patients have come to harm from people crushing MST for administration). You should talk to the doctor and get the prescription changed, and possibly seek out the pharmacist for advice on suitable alternatives that the doctor could prescribe.

3 You should clarify with the doctor that they still wish to use the PEG route, despite a licensed route being available in the form of suppositories. If the doctor insists that the PEG is the chosen route (e.g. if the patient has diarrhoea), ensure that the drug chart/prescription is properly endorsed with 'crush tablet'. You should also check with the pharmacist that it is safe to do so if you have not previously.

5.7 Administering a subcutaneous injection

Definition

A subcutaneous injection is given beneath the epidermis into the fat and connective tissue underlying the dermis. Prescriptions are usually written as 'subcut' or 'SC'.

It is important to remember that:

- You will carry out this skill under direct supervision at all times, with the supervising registered practitioner taking full responsibility for the clinical procedure.
- As there is a poorer blood supply than in muscle, concentrations in the blood rise more slowly than if the drug is given by the intramuscular (IM) route (Simonsen *et al.* 2006, Hunter 2008).
- If the peripheral circulation is poor, absorption can be delayed.
- Effective hand hygiene and the correct disposal of waste are important for the safety of yourself and the patient.

- Gloves are required for all invasive procedures (Pratt *et al.* 2007).
- Any injection involves the use of 'sharps' and thus requires safe disposal after use.
- Subcutaneous injection is relatively more painful than IM due to the mass effect of a bolus of fluid being injected into the tight layer of connective tissue. For this reason, subcutaneous medications are usually in small volumes (<2 ml).

Prior knowledge

Before administering a subcutaneous injection, make sure you are familiar with:

1 Pharmacokinetics – the way in which the drug being administered is absorbed, distributed, metabolized, and eliminated (Riviere 2003, McGavock 2005). See Section 5.1, *Principles of drug administration*.

2 Concepts of consent, accountability, negligence, malpractice, and vicarious liability – see The NMC Code (NMC 2008) and *Standards for medicines management* (NMC 2007).

3 Principles of infection control (see Section 4.1).

4 Principles of patient education.

5 Specific knowledge related to each drug (see Section 5.1, *Principles of drug administration*).

6 The pathophysiology of lipohypertrophy in diabetic patients.

7 Common sites used for subcutaneous injection.

8 Local policies for medicines management.

Background

The subcutaneous route is used when medication requires a slow, continuous absorption rate.

The medication is injected beneath the epidermis into the fat and connective tissue underlying the dermis, where there is less blood flow and therefore a slower absorption rate (see **Figure 5.11**). The volume of medication that can be injected ranges from 0.5 to 2 ml. Subcutaneous injections can be given at a 45 degree angle if using an Orange 25G needle or at a 90 degree angle if using the shorter needles that are becoming more common with insulin or prefilled syringes (see **Figure 5.12**).

Medications commonly administered by subcutaneous injection include insulin and heparin. Regardless of the

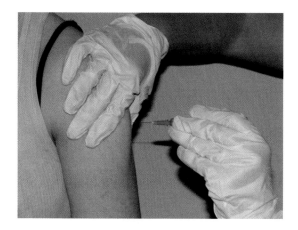

Figure 5.11 Subcutaneous injection.

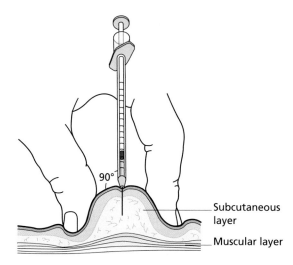

90°

Subcutaneous layer

Muscular layer

Figure 5.12 A subcutaneous injection at a 90° angle.

angle of delivery, absorption of the medication is slower through the subcutaneous route than the intramuscular route. Patients often receive subcutaneous injections on a regular basis, for example once or twice daily insulin injections, or regular anticoagulant therapy.

Three steps are taken to decrease the likelihood of irritation or tissue damage and maximize absorption of the drug:

1 Avoid using alcohol wipes to clean the skin as this can harden the skin. It is not necessary to clean the skin prior to injection (see Section 5.8). However, if the skin is visibly dirty then washing the area may be necessary (Downie *et al.* 2000).

2 Rotate the injection sites to prevent scarring and hardening of adipose (fatty) tissue, which will interfere with the absorption of medication.

3 Do not massage the site after the injection as this may cause bruising and can increase the absorption of the medication.

It is not necessary to pull back the plunger to ensure the needle is not in the vein; it is unlikely the needle will be near any blood vessels (McAskill and Goodhand 2007, Hunter 2008).

Injection sites

The following sites are commonly used (see **Figure 5.13**) as the subcutaneous tissue contains few blood vessels, so this injection route is appropriate for slow, steady absorption of a small volume of non-irritating medication:

● The outer area of the upper arm.
● The abdomen, except the area right around the navel (a 2-inch circle).
● The lateral aspect of the thighs.

The suitability of these sites will vary depending on the size of the person. The principle to be borne in mind is that the drug must be administered into the fat or connective tissue underlying the dermis, not the muscle.

A number of checks need to be made when giving any drug by injection (see **Box 5.4**).

Box 5.4 Steps for administration of any injection

■ Check prescription chart for patient details including date of birth and hospital number.
■ Check correct route.
■ Ensure prescription is clear, dated, and legible.
■ If you are not sure of any of the above, don't give the injection!
■ Check correct time.
■ Any observations to be undertaken, for example capillary blood sugar prior to insulin.
■ Check expiry date of the medication.
■ Calculate how much is needed (see Section 5.2).
■ Check prescription chart against patient ID band and clarify patient date of birth at the bedside.
■ Once given, sign prescription chart (with qualified practitioner countersigning if necessary).

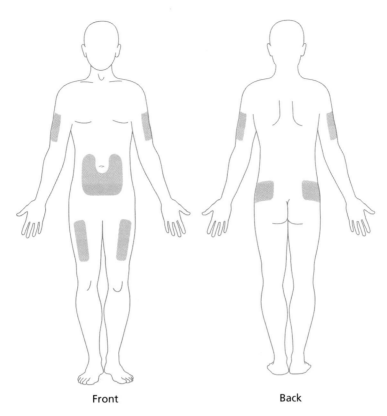

Front   Back

Figure 5.13 Suitable sites for subcutaneous injections.

Context

 ### When to give a medication via subcutaneous injection

A drug is given via the subcutaneous route when either the drug is not suitable for oral administration or the patient is unable to take the drug by mouth. The injected medication is generally absorbed more slowly, sometimes over 24 hours. Examples of medications that can be injected subcutaneously include: growth hormone, insulin, adrenaline, and heparin.

 ### When not to give a medication via the subcutaneous route

The site must be chosen carefully, avoiding any areas that are burned, inflamed, or oedematous, or sites that contain moles, birthmarks, scar tissue, or other lesions. Do not inject the area right around the navel (a 2-inch circle).

Not all medications are suitable for administration via the subcutaneous route; consult the BNF, drug information leaflet, or local pharmacy guides. If in doubt, check with the pharmacist.

Alternative interventions

Assess whether the patient can take the drug orally or if this is the only route the drug can be administered. Check the BNF or your local pharmacy guidelines.

Potential problems

Anaphylaxis is a severe, immediate hypersensitivity reaction triggered by a variety of agents. It can be life-threatening because of the rapid onset of compromise to the airway (causing stridor), breathing (causing severe wheeze), or circulation (causing shock); although in most cases a rash is the only symptom. For further details, see Section 6.15, *Anaphylaxis*.

Indications for assistance

Never give medications that you have not witnessed being drawn up.

It is essential that all students are supervised by a registered practitioner so that you can develop safe and competent practice. Any documentation or prescription must be countersigned by the registered practitioner supervising you (NMC 2007).

Procedure

Preparation

Prepare yourself

Refer to your local infection control policy with regard to hand hygiene.

Prepare the patient

The procedure should be fully explained to the patient (see Discussion box).

Prepare the equipment

Ensure you prepare the correct equipment to be used, avoiding complacent manipulation of equipment.

Discussing the procedure with the patient and family

- Involve the patient in decisions about which site to use; the patient receiving drugs via the subcutaneous route is often on long-term drug therapy.

- Identify how involved the patient and/or family wish to be in the procedure.

- Explore the patient's and family members' understanding of the drug and how to recognize any side effects. Correct any misunderstanding.

- Explain aspects of the procedure as appropriate, for example why sites are rotated and why the skin is not cleaned with an alcohol swab.

Step-by-step guide to administering a subcutaneous injection

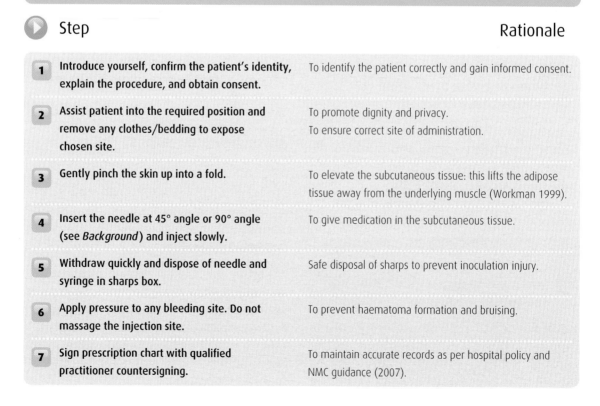

▶ Step	Rationale
1 Introduce yourself, confirm the patient's identity, explain the procedure, and obtain consent.	To identify the patient correctly and gain informed consent.
2 Assist patient into the required position and remove any clothes/bedding to expose chosen site.	To promote dignity and privacy. To ensure correct site of administration.
3 Gently pinch the skin up into a fold.	To elevate the subcutaneous tissue: this lifts the adipose tissue away from the underlying muscle (Workman 1999).
4 Insert the needle at 45° angle or 90° angle (see *Background*) and inject slowly.	To give medication in the subcutaneous tissue.
5 Withdraw quickly and dispose of needle and syringe in sharps box.	Safe disposal of sharps to prevent inoculation injury.
6 Apply pressure to any bleeding site. Do not massage the injection site.	To prevent haematoma formation and bruising.
7 Sign prescription chart with qualified practitioner countersigning.	To maintain accurate records as per hospital policy and NMC guidance (2007).

Following the procedure

- Ensure the patient is comfortable.
- Record any problems with injection site in the patient record (e.g. any pain, bruising, or swelling).
- Identify and evaluate any further learning needs if the patient or family member is learning how to administer the medication.

Reflection and evaluation

When you have administered a subcutaneous injection, think about the following questions:

1 Consider how the patient felt during the procedure; were they comfortable?
2 Will it be necessary for the patient to overcome needle phobia if they are to self-administer in future?

Further learning opportunities

- Practise under supervision; this should include the administration of heparin and insulin.
- Observe a patient self-injecting their medication. Does the patient need to be re-educated about rotating the injection sites? Is the patient following the principles of self-medication? See Section 5.3, *Patient self-administration*, for guidelines.

Reminders

Don't forget to:

- Reassure the patient.
- Ensure privacy and dignity are maintained by pulling the curtains around or closing the door.
- Gloves help prevent cross-infection and protect the practitioner when preparing the medication, as some can be absorbed through your skin. However, they do not protect you from needlestick injury. Dispose of sharp immediately after the injection.
- Document what has been done.

Patient scenarios

Consider what you should do in the following situations, then turn to the end of this skill to check your answers.

1 A patient says they always use one site for administration of insulin as it hurts less, but the site is now feeling 'lumpy'. What would you recommend?
2 A patient complains of bruising around their heparin injection sites. How will you explain this?
3 A patient is not at their bed. What do you do with the medication you have drawn up?

Website

http://www.oxfordtextbooks.co.uk/orc/endacott

You may find it helpful to work through our short online quiz and additional scenarios intended to help you to develop and apply the skills in this chapter.

References

Downie G, Mackenzie J, and Williams A (2000). Administration of medicines. In G Downie, J Mackenzie, and A Williams, eds. *Pharmacology and drugs management for nurses*, 2nd edition, pp. 495–557. Churchill Livingstone, London.

Hunter J (2008). Subcutaneous injection technique. *Nursing Standard*, **22**(21), 41–4.

McAskill H and Goodhand K (2007). Administration of medicines. In EM Jamieson, LA Whyte, and JM McCall, eds. *Clinical nursing practices*, 5th edition, pp. 13–33. Churchill Livingstone Elsevier, Edinburgh.

McGavock H (2005). *How drugs work: basic pharmacology for healthcare professionals*. Radcliffe Medical Press, Abingdon.

NMC (2007). *Standards for medicines management*. Nursing and Midwifery Council, London.

NMC (2008). *The Code: standards for conduct, performance and ethics for nurses and midwives*. Nursing and Midwifery Council, London.

Pratt RJ, Pellowe CM, Wilson JA *et al.* (2007). Epic 2: national evidence-based guidelines for preventing healthcare-associated infections in NHS hospitals in England. *Journal of Hospital Infection*, **65S**, S1–S64.

Riviere J (2003). *Comparative pharmacokinetics: principles, techniques and applications*. Wiley-Blackwell publishing, London.

Simonsen T, Aarbakke J, Kay I, Coleman I, Sinott P, and Lysaa R (2006). *Illustrated pharmacology for nurses*. Hodder Arnold, London.

Workman B (1999). Safe injection techniques. *Nursing Standard*, **13**(39), 47–52.

Useful further reading and websites

Henshaw N (2006). Aspiration not recommended in subcutaneous injection. *Nursing Standard*, **20**(30), 39.

Oven S (2007). Student experiences in the real world of nursing: starting out. *Nursing Standard*, **21**(52), 29.

Rushing J (2008). Administering an enoxaparin injection. *Nursing*, **38**(3), 19.

Patient information leaflet produced by National Institutes of Health: **http://www.cc.nih.gov/ccc/patient_education/pepubs/subq.pdf**

 Answers to patient scenarios

1 Ask the patient to show you where they inject. If it is the same place each time and is hard and lumpy, this indicates they could have lipohypertrophy. This is a swelling that occurs at the site of repeated insulin injections; these are usually painless as there are no nerve endings in the tissue. The risk is that these lumpy areas delay the absorption of insulin. Advise the patient to rotate the sites of injections around the body, not to use a swab to clean the skin, and to change the needle for each injection.

2 Heparin is an anticoagulant drug that lengthens the time blood takes to clot. As it is injected into the subcutaneous layer it may cause local bleeding under the skin (a bruise). Avoid rubbing the injection site, which can cause more trauma.

3 The risk is that the injection could be accidentally given to another patient if left out, or could be tampered with. The safest practice is to dispose of the injection into a sharps box and try to locate your patient. This will be an omission unless you document what happened and why.

5.8 **Administering an intramuscular injection**

Definition

An intramuscular injection delivers the medication directly into a muscle where it is absorbed quickly. This is frequently written as IM.

It is important to remember that:

- You will carry out this skill under direct supervision at all times, with the supervising registered practitioner taking full responsibility for the clinical procedure.
- You should be able to demonstrate safe, evidencebased practice, having due regard for the patient's safety and your level of competence.
- You should explain the procedure so the patient understands and gives their valid consent.
- You should demonstrate a sound knowledge of the drug's actions, side effects, and contraindications before administering.
- Effective hand hygiene and the correct disposal of waste are important for the safety of yourself and the patient.
- Gloves are required for all invasive procedures (Pratt *et al.* 2007).
- Drugs given IM frequently require reconstitution from a powder state, so storage, stability, and usability (potential for contamination) should all be considered.

Prior knowledge

Before administering an IM injection, make sure you are familiar with:

1 Pharmacokinetics – the way in which the drug being administered is absorbed, distributed, metabolized, and eliminated (Riviere 2003, McGavock 2005) – see Section 5.1, *Principles of drug administration*.

2 Principles of patient education.

3 Sites commonly used for IM injection.

4 Concepts of consent, accountability, negligence, malpractice, and vicarious liability – see The NMC Code (NMC 2008) and *Standards for medicines management* (NMC 2007).

5 Principles of infection control (see Section 4.1).

6 Specific knowledge related to each drug (see Section 5.1).

7 Local policies for medicines management.

8 Local policies for drug administration and storage.

Background

The intramuscular route is used to administer medication requiring a relatively quick uptake by the body (usually within 20 minutes) but where a prolonged mode of action is required (Rodger and King 2000, Hunter 2008). The medication is injected into the denser part of the muscle fascia below the subcutaneous tissues, allowing more volume to be absorbed (1–5 ml depending on the muscle bed) in tissue with fewer pain nerve endings. This means IM injections can be less painful when done correctly and can be used to inject concentrated and irritant drugs that could damage subcutaneous tissue (Greenway 2004).

There is a risk the medication will be accidentally given via the intravenous route, so aspiration (withdrawing the plunger to check that the needle is not in a vein) is an important step in the process of IM drug administration.

The needle should be long enough to penetrate the muscle and still allow a quarter of the needle to remain outside of the skin. Intramuscular injections should be given at 90 degrees to ensure the needle reaches the muscle (Workman 1999, King 2003, Zaybak *et al.* 2007). The most common needles used are 21G (green) or 23G

(blue). It is important to be aware that the older person may have decreased muscle mass, so IM medications can be absorbed more quickly than expected.

Skin cleansing prior to injection has been debated over many decades, with studies demonstrating that skin cleansing is *not* necessary (Dann 1969, Koivistov and Felig 1978, Workman 1999, Little 2000, Wynaden *et al.* 2005). However, there are some exceptions:

- If the patient is immunosuppressed, the skin *should* be cleansed with a solution containing 70% isopropyl alcohol (Downie *et al.* 2000).
- If the skin is visibly dirty, then washing the area may be necessary (Downie *et al.* 2000).

Injection sites

Current research evidence suggests there are five IM injection sites (Hunter 2008, Rodger and King 2000), as shown in **Figure 5.14**.

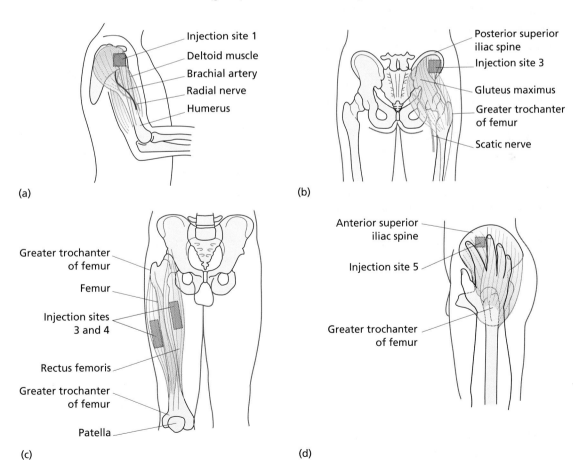

(a)

(b)

(c)

(d)

Figure 5.14 Injection sites suitable for intramuscular injection.

1 **Mid-deltoid (upper arm)**. This site is easily accessible. The area is small so the number and volume of injections is limited. The maximum volume should be 1 ml (Rodger and King 2000).

The following four sites are used for deep and Z-track injections. Assessment should take account of the age and condition of the patient; muscle mass is likely to have atrophied in the older person and will be reduced in very thin or immobile patients. Other factors to take into account when selecting the injection site include the volume of medication to be injected and the frequency of the injections.

2 **Dorsogluteal (upper outer quadrant of buttock)**. A maximum volume of 4 ml can be injected. The main concern is the high risk of hitting the sciatic nerve or the superior gluteal arteries.
3 **Rectus femoris (anterior quadriceps muscle, middle of thigh)**. Up to 5 ml can be injected.
4 **Vastus lateralis (associated with the quadriceps muscles)**. Not used much – up to 5 ml can be injected.
5 **Ventrogluteal (outer thigh)**. Most commonly used – up to 2.5 ml can be injected (Rodger and King 2000).

Z-track injection

The Z-track method of IM injection is used primarily when giving dark-coloured medication solutions, such as iron solutions, that can stain the subcutaneous tissue or skin. It is also the method of choice when giving IM medications that are very irritating to the tissue, such as haloperidol or hydroxyzine.

Z-track injection is a method of injecting medication into a large muscle. This method seals the medication deeply within the muscle and allows no exit path back into the subcutaneous tissue and skin. This is accomplished by displacing the skin and subcutaneous tissue 1–1.5 inches (2.5–3.75 cm) laterally prior to injection and releasing the tissue immediately after the injection.

This skill requires especially careful attention to technique because leakage into the subcutaneous tissue can cause discomfort to the patient and permanently stain some tissues.

A number of checks need to be made when giving any drug by injection (see Box 5.4).

Context

 ### When to give a drug via the intramuscular route

A drug is given via the IM route when the drug is not suitable for oral administration, the patient is unable to take the drug by mouth, or the medication is known to be irritant and could damage the subcutaneous tissue. Refer to the drug information leaflet.

Injecting directly into the muscle causes a delayed absorption by the body.

 ### When not to give a drug via the intramuscular route

The site must be chosen carefully, avoiding any areas that are inflamed, oedematous, or that contain moles, birthmarks, scar tissue, or other lesions. IM injections may also be contraindicated after thrombolytic treatment, during acute myocardial infarction, and in patients with impaired coagulation response, peripheral vascular disease, or shock, because these conditions impair peripheral absorption.

The IM route should not be used if the drug is not suitable for administration via this route according to the BNF, drug information leaflet, or local pharmacy guides.

Alternative interventions

Assess whether the patient can take the drug orally or if this is the only route the drug can be administered. Check the BNF or your local pharmacy guidelines.

Indications for assistance

Never give medications that you have not witnessed being drawn up.

It is essential that all students are supervised by a registered practitioner so that you can develop safe and competent practice. Any documentation or prescription must be countersigned by the registered practitioner supervising you (NMC 2007).

Indicators of adverse reactions

Anaphylaxis is a severe, immediate hypersensitivity reaction triggered by a variety of agents. It can be life-threatening because of the rapid onset of compromise to the airway (causing stridor), breathing (causing severe wheeze), or circulation (causing shock); although in most cases a rash is the only symptom. For more detail, see Section 6.15 on *Anaphylaxis*.

Procedure

Preparation

Prepare yourself
Refer to the local infection control policy with regard to hand hygiene.

Prepare the patient
The procedure should be fully explained to the patient (see Discussion box).

Prepare the equipment
Ensure you prepare the correct equipment to be used, avoiding complacent manipulation of equipment.

Discussing the procedure with the patient and family

- Involve the patient in decisions about which site to use if the patient is receiving long-term drug therapy.
- Explain aspects of the procedure as appropriate, for example why sites are rotated and why the skin is not cleaned with an alcohol swab.

Step-by-step guide to administering an intramuscular injection

▶ Step	Rationale
1 Introduce yourself, confirm the patient's identity, explain the procedure, and obtain consent.	To identify the patient correctly and gain informed consent.
2 Assist patient into required position and remove any clothes/bedding to expose chosen site.	To promote dignity and privacy. To ensure correct site of administration.
3 Place non-dominant hand on patient and stretch skin using thumb and forefinger.	To displace the underlying subcutaneous tissue (see **Figure 5.15**).
4 Insert the needle in a dart-like action at a 90° angle and pull back plunger.	To check for any blood aspiration.
5 If blood is aspirated into syringe, withdraw needle and syringe promptly and discard into sharps box. Prepare new syringe.	To prevent medication being given intravenously.
6 If no blood appears, continue to inject about 1 ml every 10 seconds.	To allow muscle fibres to expand and allow the drug to be absorbed.
7 Wait another 10 seconds before you withdraw needle.	To allow the drug to diffuse.
8 Withdraw quickly and dispose of needle and syringe in sharps box.	Safe disposal of sharps to prevent inoculation injury.
9 Apply pressure to any bleeding site.	To prevent haematoma formation.
10 Sign prescription chart with qualified practitioner countersigning.	To maintain accurate records as per hospital policy and NMC (2007).

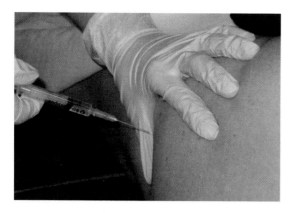

Figure 5.15 Intramuscular injection technique.

Following the procedure

- Ensure the patient is comfortable.
- Record any problems with the injection site in the patient record.

Reminders

Don't forget to:

- Reassure the patient.
- Ensure privacy and dignity is maintained by pulling the curtains around or closing the door.
- Gloves help prevent cross-infection and protect the practitioner when preparing the medication, as some can be absorbed through your skin. However, they do not protect you from needlestick injury. Dispose of sharps immediately after the injection.
- Document your actions.

Reflection and evaluation

When you have administered an intramuscular injection, think about the following questions:

1 Consider how the patient felt. Did the patient's body language reflect more discomfort than they stated?
2 How can needle phobia be managed effectively?

Further learning opportunities

- Practise giving IM injections, as these are being used less frequently in the clinical field.
- Observe and then practise Z-track injections.

 Patient scenarios

Consider what you should do in the following situations, then turn to the end of this skill to check your answers.

1 A Z-track injection is required and the patient asks why. How do you respond?
2 You are asked to administer a medication that you have not witnessed being drawn up. What do you do?

Website

 http://www.oxfordtextbooks.co.uk/orc/ endacott

You may find it helpful to work through our short online quiz and additional scenarios intended to help you to develop and apply the skills in this chapter.

References

Dann TC (1969). Routine skin preparation before injection: an unnecessary procedure. *Lancet*, **2**, 96–7.

Downie G, Mackenzie J, and Williams A (2000). Administration of medicines. In G Downie, J Mackenzie, and A Williams, eds. *Pharmacology and drugs management for nurses*, 2nd edition, pp. 495–557. Churchill Livingstone, London.

Greenway K (2004). Using the ventrogluteal site for intramuscular injection. *Nursing Standard*, **18**(25), 39–42.

Hunter J (2008). Intramuscular injection techniques. *Nursing Standard*, **22**(24), 35–40.

King L (2003). Subcutaneous injection technique. *Nursing Standard*, **17**(34), 45–52.

Koivistov V and Felig P (1978). Is skin preparation necessary before insulin injection? *Lancet* **1**, 1072–3.

Little K (2000). Skin preparation for intramuscular injections. *Nursing Times*, **96**(46), 6–8.

McGavock H (2005). *How drugs work: basic pharmacology for healthcare professionals*. Radcliffe Medical Press, Abingdon.

NMC (2007). *Standards for medicines management*. Nursing and Midwifery Council, London.

NMC (2008). *The Code: standards for conduct, performance and ethics for nurses and midwives*. Nursing and Midwifery Council, London.

Pratt RJ, Pellowe CM, Wilson JA *et al.* (2007). Epic 2: national evidence-based guidelines for preventing healthcare-associated infections in NHS hospitals in England. *Journal of Hospital Infection*, **65S**; S1–S64.

Riviere J (2003). *Comparative pharmacokinetics: principles, techniques and applications.* Wiley-Blackwell Publishing, London.

Rodger MA and King L (2000). Drawing up and administering intramuscular injection; a review of the literature. *Journal of Advanced Nursing,* **31**(3), 574–82.

Workman B (1999). Safe injection techniques. *Nursing Standard,* **13**(39), 47–52.

Wynaden D, Landsborough I, Chapman R, McGowan S, Lapsley J, and Finn M (2005). Establishing best practice guidelines for administering intramuscular injections in the adult: a systematic review of the literature. *Contemporary Nurse,* **20**(2), 267–77.

Zaybak A, Gunes U, Tamsel S, Khorshid L, and Eser I (2007). Does obesity prevent the needle from reaching muscle in intramuscular injections? *Journal of Advanced Nursing,* **58**(6), 552–6.

Useful further reading and websites

Parsons A and White J (2008). Learning from reflection on intramuscular injections. *Nursing Standard,* **22**(17), 35–40.

Small S (2004). Preventing sciatic nerve injury from intramuscular injections: literature review. *Journal of Advanced Nursing,* **47**(3), 287–96.

(A) Answers to patient scenarios

1 Explain to the patient that it is important to use this technique for drugs that might irritate the tissues.

2 You are accountable for the medications you administer to any patient. You have to be certain that what you are about to give is the medication that has been prescribed. If you have not witnessed it being drawn up, you cannot be absolutely sure what the syringe contains! Be polite but refuse to administer the medication.

5.9 Administering an intravenous injection

Definition

Intravenous (IV) medication administration refers to the process of giving medication directly into a patient's vein. Methods of administering IV medication may include giving the medication by rapid injection (bolus) into the vein using a syringe, into an injection port in an administration set, or directly into a vascular access device such as a cannula.

It is important to remember that:

- You will carry out this skill under direct supervision at all times, with the supervising registered practitioner taking full responsibility for the clinical procedure.
- It is vital in the management of IV therapy that prevention of complications or early detection is held in high regard. Many of the complications can be avoided or reduced when practitioners have underpinning knowledge.
- You should be able to demonstrate safe, evidence-based practice, having due regard for the patient's safety and your level of competence.
- You should demonstrate a sound knowledge of the drug's actions, side effects, and contraindications before administering.
- Effective hand hygiene is of particular importance, as IV-administered drugs and hence contaminants (infection) are delivered directly into the bloodstream.
- Gloves are required for all invasive procedures (Pratt *et al.* 2007).
- Correct disposal of waste is vital as the IV administration equipment will be contaminated with body fluids.
- Drugs given IV frequently require reconstitution from a powder state so storage/stability/usability (and potential for contamination) should all be considered.
- Many health services will also have specific training programmes associated with IV drug administration and the practitioner should be aware of the local policy.
- You are accountable for evaluating and monitoring the effectiveness of prescribed therapy, documenting patient response, adverse events, and interventions, and achieving effective delivery of the prescribed therapy (NMC 2007).

Prior knowledge

Before assisting with or undertaking IV drug administration, make sure you are familiar with:

- Anatomy and physiology of the circulation.
- Pharmacokinetics – the way in which the drug being administered is absorbed, distributed, metabolized, and eliminated (Riviere 2003, McGavock 2005). See Section 5.1, *Principles of drug administration*.
- Concepts of consent, accountability, negligence, malpractice, and vicarious liability – see The NMC Code (NMC 2008) and *Standards for medicines management* (NMC 2007).
- Principles of patient education.
- Use of the Visual Infusion Phlebitis (VIP) Score.
- Symptoms of anaphylaxis and related emergency management.
- Principles of infection control (see Section 4.1).
- Specific knowledge related to each drug (see Section 5.1).
- Local policies for medicines management.

Background

The primary purpose of giving IV medications is to initiate a rapid systemic response to medication. It is one of the fastest ways to deliver medication. The drug is immediately available to the body. It is easier to control the actual amount of drug delivered to the body by using the IV method and it is also easier to maintain drug levels in the blood for therapeutic response. The IV route for medication administration may be used if the medication to be delivered would be destroyed by digestive enzymes, is poorly absorbed by the tissue, or is painful or irritating when given by intramuscular (IM) or subcutaneous (SC) injection.

As the IV infusion device provides direct access to the circulatory system, the importance of scrupulous attention to asepsis cannot be overemphasized. The patient's vital signs, fluid balance, and device entry site should all be monitored regularly to identify and prevent complications. It is important to ensure prompt removal of IV access devices once they are no longer required.

The practitioner must also familiarize themselves with all the equipment used for any IV therapy within their area of practice. There are many different types of IV-giving sets, some for specific types of fluids and others for specific patient groups (e.g. children). There is also a wide range of electronic pumps and syringe drivers, designed to deliver fluids at specific rates.

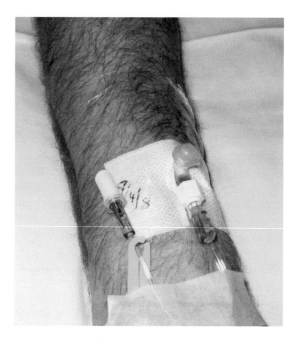

Figure 5.16 Peripheral intravenous cannula *in situ*.

A peripheral cannula consists of a short catheter (a few centimetres long) inserted through the skin into a peripheral vein (see **Figure 5.16**). A peripheral cannula cannot be left in the vein indefinitely because of the risk of insertion-site infection leading to phlebitis, cellulitis, and bacteraemias. The Department of Health (2007) advise that cannulae are replaced every 72–96 hours.

Context

 When to give drugs via the intravenous route

Intravenous administration allows a fast and accurate delivery of fluids and drugs to the patient and is used when oral or other routes are not practical or acceptable.

 When not to give drugs via the intravenous route

The intravenous cannula must not be used if any of the complications listed below are present:

- Phlebitis – see **Table 5.14**, Visual Infusion Phlebitis (VIP) Score tool.

- Infiltration – see *Potential problems* section.
- Extravasation – see *Potential problems* section.

Alternative interventions

To reduce the risk of bacteraemia, alternative and less invasive routes should be used where possible. The duration of IV antibiotic administration should be frequently reviewed by the medical team; the patient may be able to take oral antibiotics if they are apyrexial and infection markers such as CRP (C-reactive protein) are returning to normal parameters.

Potential problems

Some patients who require IV drug administration will also have an infusion running through the cannula. A number of problems can arise at the cannula site, regardless of whether an infusion is running through the cannula. Early recognition and prevention of these problems is key. **Tables 5.11–5.13** identify cause, recognition, treatment, and prevention of three common complications of IV drug or infusion administration: phlebitis, infiltration, and extravasation. Many of the actions below would be undertaken under the supervision of a Registered Nurse.

Further detail regarding the management of IV infusions is provided in Section 6.7.

Indicators of adverse reactions during IV drug administration

Anaphylaxis is a severe, immediate hypersensitivity reaction triggered by a variety of agents. It can be life-threatening because of the rapid onset of compromise to the airway (causing stridor), breathing (causing severe wheeze), or circulation (causing shock); although in most cases a rash is the only symptom.

Specific observations

All patients with an intravenous access device in place must have the IV site checked each time the cannula is accessed for infusion phlebitis.

Procedure

Preparation

Prepare yourself
Refer to the local infection control policy with regard to hand hygiene. Gloves must be worn where necessary to protect you from absorbing the medications you prepare.

Prepare the patient
The procedure should be fully explained to the patient.

Table 5.11 Causes, prevention, recognition, and management of phlebitis

Phlebitis: inflammation of the wall of a vein.

Causes: mechanical – cannula; chemical – toxicity; reactive – foreign body; bacterial – infection, poor technique.

Recognition: some or all of the following – swelling, redness, firmness to touch, heat, tenderness, exudate, fever, tracking (red lines) (see Table 5.14, *Visual Infusion Phlebitis (VIP) Score tool*).

Action	Prevention
Stop IV infusion. Remove cannula. If there is no other IV access, try to get the cannula replaced first if possible. It is not good practice to be without IV access in acutely unwell patients. Swab exit site. Consider sending tip of cannula for culture depending on local policy. Re-site the cannula. Analgesia. Document and inform doctor.	Apply infection control principles. Sterile dressing and dated. Observe site at staff handover. Secure cannula. Documentation.

Table 5.12 Causes, prevention, recognition, and management of infiltration

Infiltration: fluids that are not irritant (vesicant) are accidentally infused into surrounding tissue. Example: normal saline 0.9%.

Causes: dislodged cannula; inappropriate insertion of cannula; wrong size cannula; puncturing vein; cannula not secured properly.

Recognition: swelling, redness, boggy or firm to touch, cool to touch, slow IVI, pain, resistance to flush.

Action	Prevention
Stop IV infusion.	Apply infection control principles.
Remove cannula.	Sterile dressing and dated.
Swab exit site.	Observe cannula site at staff handover.
Re-site the cannula.	Secure cannula.
Analgesia.	Observe site during IV drug administration.
Document and inform doctor.	Documentation.

Table 5.13 Causes, prevention, recognition, and management of extravasation

Extravasation: infiltration of vesicant (irritant) medications or fluids into surrounding tissues, causing tissue damage and necrosis. Possible causes: total parenteral nutrition, phenytoin, 10% dextrose, aciclovir, vancomycin, cytotoxic drugs.

Causes: dislodged cannula; inappropriate insertion of cannula (should be flushed prior to use); wrong size cannula; puncturing vein; cannula not secured properly; severe phlebitis.

Recognition: swelling, redness, boggy to touch, wet dressing/leakage, slow IVI, pain, resistance to flush.

Action	Prevention
Stop IV infusion.	Good cannulation procedure.
Leave cannula *in situ*.	Follow specific drug information advice regarding speed of administration.
Inform medical staff.	Avoid dragging of the cannula.
Inform pharmacy: is an antidote available?	
Observe site.	
Medical staff may consult the plastic surgeons if the wound does not improve or heal.	
Analgesia.	
Documentation.	

NB for some vesicant drugs (e.g. cytotoxic drugs), breakdown of tissues can occur within 6 hours and may advance to deep structures such as tendons.

Prepare the equipment

Ensure you prepare the correct equipment to be used.

Table 5.14 Visual Infusion Phlebitis (VIP) Score tool for vascular access devices

Observations	Score	Judgement	Action
Absence of erythema and no purulent discharge	0	No signs of phlebitis	Observe cannula
Slight pain or slight erythema at IV site	1	Possible first signs	Observe cannula
Two of the following are evident: • pain at IV site • erythema • swelling	2	Early stage of phlebitis	Remove cannula Re-site cannula if still required
Increased erythema, pyrexia, pain, purulent discharge from IV site	3	Phlebitis	Remove cannula Send tip Send blood cultures Re-site cannula if still required Consider treatment

Jackson (1997).

Step-by-step guide to administering an IV injection

Step	Rationale
1 Introduce yourself, confirm the patient's identity, explain the procedure, and obtain consent.	To identify the patient correctly and gain informed consent.
2 Check the prescription to confirm you have the correct medication.	To prevent the patient from harm and a drug error.
3 Prepare correct equipment to be used, avoiding complacent manipulation of equipment.	To prevent risk of infection.
4 Prepare flush of appropriate nature (discard sharp as per Trust infection control and health and safety policies). Usually normal saline 0.9% is best to use as a flush; water is hypotonic so may cause swelling of tissue and increase risk of infiltration/extravasation.	To use pre-IV medication to check for patency of cannula, and post-IV medication to flush any remaining solution away from cannula.
5 Put appropriate needle size on each flush/drug for administration (25G orange) if using membraned connector.	Ampoules pose a risk of particulate contamination, especially glass. Vials pose a risk of fragments of rubber stopper being cut out by the needle, known as 'coring'.
6 Look at cannula site and check the VIP Score. Document.	To reduce complications associated with phlebitis and infection.

continued overleaf

7	Observe cannula site for usability. Look for signs of local infection – purulent drainage, tenderness, erythema, **warmth**, induration **of the vein (sources of bacteria – blood, skin, air).**	To reduce complications associated with phlebitis and infection.
8	Avoid breaking the closed system by use of separate needles for each bolus/flush if using a membraned connector.	To prevent risk of infection.
9	If infusion in progress, turn off via roller clamp.	To prevent drug interaction.
10	Clean IV connector with 2% chlorhexidine gluconate in 70% isopropyl alcohol, and allow to dry prior to accessing the cannula (DH 2007).	To reduce the potential for direct microbial entry into the bloodstream.
11	Administer pre-IV appropriate flush observing for signs of pain, cannula occlusion, or venous spasm.	To check patency of cannula and detect complications such as infiltration of extravasation at an early stage.
12	Inject the medication at a steady slow speed according to the pharmacy guidelines.	To prevent speed shock.
13	Administer post-IV appropriate flush.	To ensure all dose delivered and avoid interaction with any other drug that may be left in the cannula.
14	Withdraw quickly and dispose of equipment in sharps box as per local infection control and health and safety policies.	To avoid needlestick injury if using needle and syringe in membraned connector.
15	If the patient had an IV infusion running, ensure the infusion is recommenced at prescribed rate following administration of drug therapy.	To continue prescribed therapy.
16	Sign prescription chart with qualified practitioner countersigning. In the patient records, document the condition of the cannula site, according to local policy.	To maintain accurate records in line with hospital policy and NMC guidance (2007).

Following the procedure

Make sure the patient is comfortable and clothing/bedding is arranged in such a way as to avoid the cannula catching on anything. Ensure the patient has all they need within easy reach. Does the patient require any monitoring or specific observations post-medication? Look at Chapters 6 and 7 to familiarize yourself with the recording of vital signs.

Reflection and evaluation

When you have administered an intravenous injection, think about the following:

- Consider the actions to take after the administration of an incorrect drug.
- Undertake calculations associated with the appropriate drug dosage for children.

- Displacement values when a powder is diluted in a solution and the overall volume changes may be significant when dealing with doses for neonates.

Further learning opportunities

As a student, you should practise giving IV drugs in your area under direct supervision so you can build up your confidence ready for when you qualify as a registered practitioner.

Reminders

Don't forget to:

- Reassure the patient.
- Observe the cannula site each time it is accessed. Use the VIP Score tool.
- Check the need for the cannula and ask medical team if it can be removed if not required.
- Gloves help prevent cross-infection and protect the practitioner when preparing the medication, as some can be absorbed through your skin. However, they do not protect you from needlestick injury. Dispose of sharps immediately after the procedure.
- Document what has been done.

 Patient scenarios

Consider what you should do in the following situations, then turn to the end of this skill to check your answers.

1 The cannula site looks red and inflamed with a VIP Score of 2. What do you do?
2 You inject a flush into a cannula and the patient tells you it is painful. What do you do?
3 A patient has been prescribed Benzylpenicillin. Prior to administration they explain that they are allergic to Penicillin. What do you do?

Website

 http://www.oxfordtextbooks.co.uk/orc/ endacott

You may find it helpful to work through our short online quiz and additional scenarios intended to help you to develop and apply the skills in this chapter.

References

Department of Health (2007). *Saving lives. High impact intervention No 2. Peripheral intravenous cannula care bundle*. DH, London.

Jackson A (1997). A battle in vein: infusion phlebitis. *Nursing Times*, **94**(4), 68–71.

McGavock H (2005). *How drugs work: basic pharmacology for healthcare professionals*. Radcliffe Medical Press, Abingdon.

NMC (2007). *Standards for medicines management*. Nursing and Midwifery Council, London.

NMC (2008). *The Code: Standards for conduct, performance and ethics for nurses and midwives*. Nursing and Midwifery Council, London.

Pratt RJ, Pellowe CM, Wilson JA *et al.* (2007). Epic 2: national evidence-based guidelines for preventing healthcare-associated infections in NHS hospitals in England. *Journal of Hospital Infection*, **65S**, S1–S64.

Riviere J (2003). *Comparative pharmacokinetics: principles, techniques and applications*. Wiley-Blackwell Publishing, London.

Useful further reading and websites

Finlay T (2004). *Intravenous therapy: essential clinical skills for nurses*. Blackwell Publishing, Oxford.

Royal College of Nursing (2007). *Standards for infusion therapy*. RCN, London.

Shawyer V, Copp A, Dobrijevic J, and Goding L (2007). Nursing students and the administration of IV drugs. *Nursing Times*, **103**(4), 32–3.

British National Formulary: **http://www.bnf.org**

Extravasation website: **http://www. extravasation.org.uk/home.html**

The IV Team website provides up-to-date guidance for all aspects of IV drug and fluid administration: **http://www.ivteam.com/**

Up-to-date advice from the RCN IV Therapy Forum: **http://www.rcn.org.uk**

 Answers to patient scenarios

1 A VIP Score of 2 means the cannula is showing early stages of phlebitis. The cannula must be re-sited.
2 This indicates again that the early stages of phlebitis are occurring in the vein (VIP Score of 1). The cannula site may not always be red or inflamed. Monitor this

carefully as it is likely to develop to a VIP Score of 2.

3   Identify from the patient in what way they are allergic. Do *not* give the medication. They may have had an anaphylactic reaction. Inform the medical team and ensure the patient has a red wristband as per NPSA guidelines (see Section 5.1, *Principles of drug administration*). The medical team will decide whether the patient has a true allergy or whether they have experienced side effects such as nausea, vomiting, or diarrhoea (these are sometimes described by patients as an allergy but can often be tolerated once the rationale is explained to the patient and they have been reassured). If the patient has a history of anaphylaxis, ensure it is documented on the prescription chart and medical notes for future reference.

6 Cardiovascular system

Skills

6.1 Visual assessment of the cardiac patient

Definition

Visual assessment of the cardiac patient requires the nurse to use the power of observational skills to make a clinical judgement about the patient's condition. Many clues to the cardiac condition can be detected with a simple visual inspection and it should be used in conjunction with objective clinical data. Visual assessment is an ongoing assessment and it should become second nature to observe the patient continually, as well as using this skill in a structured way to aid the clinical decision-making process.

Section 6.9 refers to the recognition of cardiac pulmonary collapse and the ABCDE of assessment. Sections 6.1 and 6.9 are mutually complementary and should be read together to gain a greater understanding of cardiac assessment.

It is important to remember that:

The presentation of cardiovascular disease (CVD) is extremely variable, and appearances can often be deceptive. Therefore, it is essential that visual assessment is supported by objective data, for example pulse rate and rhythm, respiratory rate, blood pressure, etc.

Prior knowledge

Before attempting visual assessment of the cardiac patient, make sure you are familiar with:

1 The anatomy and physiology of the cardiovascular and respiratory systems.
2 Pathophysiology of common cardiovascular diseases (myocardial infarction, heart failure, atrial fibrillation, hypertension, shock, atherosclerosis, thrombosis/ embolism, anaemia).

Background

In order to understand how to assess any patient visually, it is vital to be aware of the range of normal appearances. Skin colour, tone, and texture vary from individual to individual, while body temperature, pulse rate, and respiratory rate have degrees of normal. An observant nurse will have an understanding of the diversity of normal, healthy presentations and be able to recognize subtle changes in physical appearance that denote worsening of a patient's condition.

Whitehead *et al.* (2002) state 'It is essential to notice a patient's deteriorating condition if timely intervention is to have a chance of saving that patient's life.' Signs of respiratory distress and alterations in mental state are critical warning signs indicating deterioration in a patient's condition, and indeed are the most commonly disturbed variables prior to cardiac arrest (Whitehead *et al.* 2002).

An important skill to master early is the ability to make an overall assessment of a patient's condition as soon as you see them. For example, how is their demeanour, are they happy or sad, are they tidy, are they wearing clothes appropriate to season, are they engaging verbally and non-verbally? All of these will give the health professional clues to the health status of the patient.

The recognition of deterioration by looking at the patient has an element of intuitive subconscious decision-making (Christensen and Hewitt-Taylor 2006), which is difficult to quantify and evaluate or to teach, and will develop with experience. However, you can ask yourself four key questions to aid the identification of patients at risk of deterioration:

- Has the patient's colour changed?
- Has the patient's mental condition altered; are they agitated?
- Are there any changes, even marginal ones, in their vital signs?
- Is the patient complaining of 'just not feeling right'?

Skin colour

There are a number of key observations (see *Procedure* sections) but one of the most important is skin colour. The colour of skin depends primarily on a pigment called melanin; the amount of melanin in our skin depends on a combination of inherited factors and degree of light exposure. Other pigments that contribute to skin colour include haemoglobin (oxygen-carrying pigment in red blood cells), which results in skin being redder in places where the blood vessels come closer to the surface, e.g. lips. Carotene (fat-soluble pigment found in green and yellow leafy vegetables and yellow fruits) also has an influence on the finer subtleties of the pigmentation of the skin.

However, it is important to remember that skin colour is also influenced by the blood flow through the skin, for example waste products transported in the blood and the oxygen concentration, and can be a useful marker of disease. Furthermore, when assessing the colour of the skin and mucous membranes, it is important to consider the patient's ethnic origins as there may be significant normal variations in underlying skin tone.

Pallor

Pallor (paleness) is a result of decreased blood flow through the skin, i.e. less red colouring from oxyhaemoglobin, as in conditions such as anaemia and shock. It is most easily discerned where the epidermis is thinnest, e.g. fingernails, lips, mucous membrane of mouth, and palpebral conjunctiva (around the eyelid).

Cyanosis

Cyanosis is a blue discoloration of the skin and mucous membranes caused by a lack of oxygen in the blood.

Oxygen is normally transported as oxyhaemoglobin, which is red in colour. When oxygen levels drop, high levels of deoxygenated haemoglobin are seen. This is a purplish colour, and when seen by the naked eye it gives the skin and mucous membranes the characteristic blue hue of cyanosis (Talley and O'Connor 2005).

There are two types of cyanosis:

Central cyanosis Central cyanosis is blue discoloration of mucosal surfaces such as the tongue, as well as the extremities. It is a late sign of low oxygen levels and is most likely to be caused by severely impaired gaseous exchange in the lungs. Possible causes include:

- Chronic respiratory disease such as chronic obstructive pulmonary disease (COPD).
- Acute respiratory conditions such as pneumonia, pulmonary embolism, large pleural effusions.
- Pulmonary oedema (a collection of fluid in the lungs).
- Right to left cardiac shunt, e.g. Eisenmenger syndrome.
- Abnormal haemoglobin, giving inadequate oxygen uptake in the lungs.
- A condition known as polycythaemia (abnormal increase in the number of red blood cells) may present with central cyanosis.

Peripheral cyanosis Peripheral cyanosis affects the extremities and the skin around the lips but not the mucous membranes, and is indicative of impaired cardiac output (Vickers and Power 1999). Causes include:

- Reduced cardiac output, e.g. heart failure, hypovolaemia.
- Vasoconstriction, e.g. due to cold, Raynaud's phenomenon.
- Arterial obstruction, e.g. thrombosis or atheroma.
- Venous obstruction, e.g. iliofemoral deep vein thrombosis, can produce a painful blue leg (phlegmasia cerulea dolens).

Jaundice

Jaundice is a yellow discoloration of the skin and whites of the eyes caused by abnormally high levels of bilirubin (bile pigmentation) in the bloodstream as a result of liver disease. This condition is not usually directly linked to cardiovascular disease but may be observed as a secondary finding and should be documented and passed on to a senior colleague.

You can find other essential information to guide your visual assessment of the patient's mental condition and respiratory effort in the other sections of this book. This section will guide you in assimilating all the information to make your decision about the patient's condition.

Context

 When to perform a visual assessment

Visual assessment skills are an essential component of all nursing care and should be used continuously in conjunction with objective assessment of the patient's condition. Specific examples are:

- As part of the assessment process when patients are admitted to your clinical area.
- Before, during, and after a treatment or procedure.
- When the patient's general physical condition changes.
- As part of assessing airway, breathing, and circulation in an emergency.

Alternative interventions

To support what you see, ensure that you have checked:

- Blood pressure.
- Pulse rate and rhythm.
- Temperature.
- Respiratory rate.

As a result of your observations it may be appropriate and necessary for other tests and investigations to be undertaken, such as:

- An electrocardiogram (ECG) recording.
- Measurement of the oxygen saturation of the blood.
- Venous or arterial blood sampling and analysis.
- Chest X-ray.
- Blood cultures.
- Sputum culture.
- Further imaging (e.g. VQ scan/CTPA/echocardiogram).

Potential problems

There are no specific problems associated with this observation except failing to act on information gained. It is safer to ask for a second opinion than ignore subtle changes in the patient's condition. If in doubt, *ask*!

Indications for assistance

As with all skills and interventions, it is crucial that you work within your competency (Nursing and Midwifery Council (NMC) 2008).

- Call for urgent assistance if the patient's condition requires emergency cardiopulmonary resuscitation.
- Ask a senior colleague to asses the patient if you are not certain of the significance of your findings.

Interpreting observations

In order to understand and realize the clinical significance of your observations, you must be familiar with the extremes of normal. General inspection can yield many signs that may indicate the presence of heart disease, heart failure, or deterioration of the patient's cardiac condition.

Please note that many forms of heart disease are associated with unique signs, and this text can only offer an overview of general clinical signs. It is therefore recommended that students of advanced practice, or nurses working in specialist clinical areas such as cardiothoracic or intensive therapy, should consult a textbook on cardiology for details and examples of these. Some useful key texts and websites are listed at the end of the section.

Normal findings

- The patient should look well and show no sign of distress.
- A normal patient is mentally alert and aware of their surroundings, taking an interest in what is happening around them.
- Normal breathing should be quiet, cyclical, and smooth, i.e. require no effort.
- The patient's colour should be consistent with their ethnic origin, and mucous membranes should look pink.

- The patient should be neither hot nor cold and their skin should be dry to the touch, i.e. not sweating or clammy.
- There should be no signs of cyanosis, either centrally or in the periphery.
- The nail beds should be uniformly pink when testing capillary refill time, i.e. a quick return to normal colour that takes less than 2 seconds when pressure is lifted from the nail bed. Brisk refilling of the capillary bed from white to pink indicates good peripheral perfusion, and therefore good hydration of the patient and

Abnormal findings

- The patient may look unwell, lethargic, exhausted, and breathless in the presence of reduced cardiac output or congestive heart failure.
- Breathlessness may be subtle, occurring only when moving about (decreased exercise tolerance) and not when at rest in an ambulatory patient. Patients who are bedbound may experience breathlessness when lying flat (supine) but not when sitting up (recumbent); this is known as orthopnoea. Patients with long-standing cardiac conditions will often voluntarily reduce an activity that provokes breathlessness, and asking about

their exercise tolerance and changes in this can give clues as to the extent of the breathlessness they experience.

- The patient may be vague or confused, which could be due to severe hypoxaemia, or greatly reduced cardiac output leading to decreased cerebral perfusion.
- Patients who are restless and agitated may be experiencing pain, e.g. from myocardial infarction or pulmonary embolism.
- Central cyanosis may be of cardiac or pulmonary origin.

- Pallor may be due to anaemia, or reduced cardiac output causing poor perfusion of the peripheries.

- Slow capillary refilling at the nail bed (i.e. >2 seconds) is a sign of vasoconstriction and poor peripheral perfusion.

- Clubbing of the fingernails can indicate lung disease but not chronic obstructive airways disease (Myer and Farquhar 2001). If this sign is seen in patients with COPD, an underlying cause such as bronchiectasis or carcinoma of the lung should be considered. Other causes may be heart conditions, e.g. subacute bacterial endocarditis, or gastrointestinal disease, e.g. Crohn's disease.

- Facial changes, for example:
  - Malar flush (redness around cheeks) – mitral stenosis.
  - Xanthomata (yellowish deposits of lipids around eyes) – hyperlipidaemia.
  - Corneal arcus (a creamy ring around the cornea) – age or hyperlipidaemia.
  - Proptosis (forward projection or displacement of the eyeball). A sign associated with Graves' disease (a cause of hyperthyroidism), which may also cause atrial fibrillation.

- Nicotine staining on the fingers suggests that the patient is a smoker and therefore will have associated increased risk of CVD.

adequate cardiac output.

Remember: visual assessment is an ongoing assessment of the patient and their condition, and as such differs from other skills in that it does not have an end. Rather than looking at the patient for a single assessment, it is vital to monitor *changes* in their condition over time.

Special considerations

Patients with established cardiac disease will modify their behaviour and activity to accommodate their condition, so changes will need to be assessed not only in consideration of normal parameters but also taking into account what is normal for that patient. For example, patients with heart failure will describe feeling breathless; you will therefore need to ask 'Are you more breathless than usual?' or 'Has your breathing changed?'

When looking for signs of pallor in darker-skinned patients, look at palms of hands and soles of feet to see the underlying skin colour more easily.

When working in the community, it may be some time since you last saw the patient. Do they look different? Has their demeanour changed since the last time you saw them? Is the room warm or cold? Is there evidence of self-neglect? Your decision-making will be influenced not only by your observations but by the home situation, e.g. do they live alone, when will they next have a carer at the house, etc. In hospital, where a patient is under close observation, a 'watch and wait' approach can be adopted in certain scenarios; this is not always possible in the home, where you might be the only person seeing them that day or even that week.

Procedure: general observations of the cardiac patient

A plethora of information can be gathered merely by looking at the patient. As you approach the patient you can make a general judgement on their physical and mental condition (see *General observations* below) and then support this with a structured, systematic visual assessment. Findings from your general observations and your systematic visual assessment will need to be supplemented by objective clinical data. These three integral aspects of assessment can be thought of as the three points of a triangle, as shown in **Figure 6.1**.

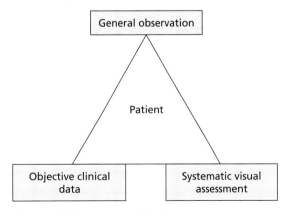

Figure 6.1 The assessment triangle.

General observations

- Determine the patient's apparent current state of health.
- Is the patient overweight? Cachexic?
- How are they positioned? Sitting in a chair or in bed?
- Is the patient restless or quiet?
- Is the patient dressed or in nightclothes?
- Do they look frail or robust?
- Look around the bed space; have they a jug for water? Is it full or empty?
- Are there vomit bowls by the bed?
- Is there monitoring equipment attached to the patient, intravenous infusions, or advisory signs such as 'nil by mouth'?
- Ask yourself: What is my general impression of this patient's condition?

Facial expression

This is an external indicator of state of mind, e.g. it is possible to see signs of pain, anxiety, sadness, tiredness.

Does the patient appear to be:

- Alert?
- Distressed?
- Anxious?
- Irritable?
- Exhausted?

Note that facial expressions such as grimacing, biting of lips, or screwing up eyes can be signs of pain (Williams 2002).

Posture

The position the patient adopts, either in bed or sitting in a chair, will again give clues to their physical and emotional well-being.

- Does the patient appear to be comfortable, restless, or agitated?
- Are they sitting? Curled into the foetal position? Lying supine?

Procedure: visual assessment of the cardiac patient

Preparation

Prepare the patient

- Introduce yourself to the patient before you begin the observation.
- Ensure that the patient is comfortable and lying in a semi-recumbent position on the bed. Note: in a patient's home, this may not always be possible and you may need to improvise.
- Ensure the patient's privacy and dignity is maintained by drawing curtains around the bed (or at the windows in the home).
- Assist the patient as necessary to remove any clothing in order to allow clear visual assessment.

Step-by-step guide to visual assessment of the cardiac patient

Step	Rationale
1 Introduce yourself, confirm the patient's identity, explain the procedure, and obtain consent.	To identify the patient correctly and gain informed consent.
2 Asses level of consciousness – AVPU: Alert Responds to Voice Responds to Pain Unresponsive.	Neurological assessment is an indicator of health status. See Section 8.1.

3 Look at patient's hands.
Are they warm or cold?
Dry or moist palms?
Are there splinter haemorrhages?
Is there clubbing of the fingernails? (Adam and Osborne 2005)

The temperature of the hands gives an indication of the patient's temperature and peripheral circulation.
Moist palms can be a sign of pain.
Multiple tiny, longitudinal subungual haemorrhages in the nails can be seen in **bacterial endocarditis**. However, they are also often found in people who haven't got anything wrong with them.
Clubbing is a phenomenon where the angle of the nail bed is lost in chronic respiratory conditions. The mechanism of its cause is not fully known (see **Figure 6.2**).

4 Assess capillary refill time. Gently press on nail bed, observe blanching, and look for the return of colour once pressure lifted. Should take <2 seconds.

A longer capillary refill time can be indicative of reduced cardiac output.
If longer, check radial pulse to ensure blood supply to hand.

5 Observe the skin.
Ask the patient if they have noticed any changes in the colour of the skin.
Examine and compare skin in symmetrical areas. Note:

- General facial flushing.
- Any increase in or loss of pigmentation.
- Any rashes.
- Erythema.
- Cyanosis.
- Jaundice.
- Pallor.
- Signs of dehydration (dry and lacking elasticity), cardiovascular insufficiency (e.g. hypoxia), or underlying pathology (e.g. hepatitis or signs of infection).

Patients or relatives are often aware of any changes and they will know what is 'normal' for them.
Flushing can be from anxiety or as result of peripheral dilatation of the blood vessels of the face associated with pyrexia.
See *Interpreting observations* section.

6 Observe for any signs of:

- Haemorrhage.
- Petechiae.
- Bruising.
- Haematomas.
- Is the skin dry or moist?
- Is the patient sweating (diaphoresis)?

Spontaneous haemorrhage can indicate a bleeding disorder.
Petechiae can signify infection or underlying pathology such as vasculitis, thrombocytopenia, or some malignancies.
Petechiae, bruising, and haematomas on the skin give clinical clues as to possible underlying pathology such as bleeding disorders. Note some medications can cause petechiae, e.g. warfarin, aspirin.
The skin can be moist ('clammy') with pain or when the patient is in shock.

continued overleaf

7	Ask the patient to pull down the lower eyelids gently and inspect the depth of colour of the conjunctiva on the anterior rim (should be red). This should be matched with the fleshy colour of the posterior aspect of the palpebral conjunctiva (Sheth *et al.* 1997). Observe the colour of the sclera.	Some people do not like to have their eyes touched. The sclera should be clear and white; a yellow tinge can indicate jaundice while redness could be infection or signs of acute red eye.
8	Ask them to poke out the tongue and lift it up. Inspect the condition of the mouth for signs of dental decay and caries.	Dark ruddiness on the underside of the tongue shows central cyanosis. Poor dental hygiene can lead to serious infective conditions of the heart, e.g. subacute endocarditis as the pathogens travel in the bloodstream.
9	Look at the patient's feet, ankles, lower arms, and sacral area for signs of oedema. Further assessment is made by palpation of the area using three fingers over a bony surface for 5 seconds and releasing.	Oedema can be an indicator of poor cardiac function and can be a new clinical finding or show deterioration of a pre-existing condition. Poor venous return leads to pooling of fluid in the extremities due to gravity.
10	Observe the patient's respiratory effort. Increased effort can be seen in flaring of the nostrils and elevation of the sternoclamastoid muscles. Are they using accessory muscles of respiration? Does the rate and quality of the breathing appear normal?	Changes in respiratory effort are early indicators of cardiovascular insufficiency, continued deterioration of the patient's condition, and possible collapse.
11	Subjectively, does the patient look well? Do they look comfortable?	Signs of discomfort (grimacing, etc.) may indicate that further intervention is needed (e.g. analgesia). A subjective impression of the patient's state can often be the first sign of deterioration and may precipitate further measurement of vital signs.

(a) Normal finger

160°

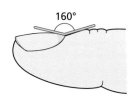

(b) Clubbed finger

>180°

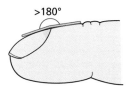

Figure 6.2 Clubbing of the fingernail.

Following the procedures

Check objective clinical data to support your visual assessment of the patient's condition and compare these to the previous documented measurements. Measure and record the following and any other significant signs.

- Pulse rate and rhythm (see Section 6.2)
- Blood pressure (see Section 6.3)
- Respiratory rate and depth (see Section 7.1)
- Temperature

Ensure that you act immediately if you believe the patient's condition is unstable, and instigate any local resuscitation procedures.

Report your findings to the appropriate clinician. Continue frequent observation, document findings, and follow the policies within your clinical area and the NMC guidelines (NMC 2008).

Recognizing patient deterioration

Repeat the four questions discussed in the background to the skill:

- Has the patient's colour changed?

- Has the patient's mental condition altered; are they agitated?

- Are there any changes, even marginal ones, in their vital signs?

- Is the patient complaining of 'just not feeling right'?

(Whitehead *et al.* 2002)

Reflection and evaluation

When your observation of the patient is over, think about the following questions:

1 Did I address the four key questions that can aid my assessment of the patient?

2 Did I accurately assess the patient's condition?

3 Did my visual assessment concur with the objective clinical data?

4 Did I act appropriately on the information I gained? If not, why not? What should I have done? What will I do next time?

5 Am I beginning to develop an intuitive ability when observing patients? Is it useful? Why and how?

Further learning opportunities

Continue to develop your observational skills and reflect on your actions using your chosen model of reflection. Spend time wherever possible with experienced clinicians; ask them about how they make their clinical decisions, what informs their practice, and why. Follow this up with reading textbooks and journals to support what you have been told. Each time you see a new sign or a patient describes a symptom, spend time to link them together. An accurate assessment of a patient's condition is the sum of all clinical findings: observed (visual assessment); actual (objective clinical data); and perceived (what the patient is telling you).

Reminders

- To carry out a visual assessment, you must undress the patient as necessary or you will miss signs.
- A visual assessment alone will not give you the whole picture; use it in conjunction with other objective assessments.

Patient scenarios

1 You are visiting Mrs A at home to redress a small venous ulcer on her leg. She is an elderly lady with heart failure, and you saw her 2 days ago when she 'was her usual self'. When you arrive today she is in bed, looks pale, is breathless when speaking to you, and has swollen legs. What do you think may be wrong with her? What should you do?

2 During the evening drug round, you observe that Mr B is sweaty, pale, clammy, and complaining of a tight pain in his chest. What is your immediate action?

3 Mrs C has heart failure and is in hospital for stabilization of her condition. Her daughter has asked you to come to see her because she has developed a blue tinge around her lips. What do you say to her daughter to explain what is happening to Mrs C?

Website

http://www.oxfordtextbooks.co.uk/orc/
endacott

You may find it helpful to work through our short online quiz and additional scenarios intended to help you to develop and apply the skills in this chapter.

References

Adam SK and Osborne S (2005). *Critical care nursing. Science and practice*, 2nd edition. Oxford University Press, Oxford.

Christensen M and Hewitt-Taylor J (2006). Defining the expert ICU nurse. *Intensive and Critical Care Nursing*, **22**(5), 301–7.

Davies MK, Gibbs CR, and Lip GYH (2000). ABC of heart failure Investigation. *BMJ*, **320**(7230), 297–300.

Myer KA and Farquhar DR (2001). The rational clinical examination: does this patient have clubbing? *JAMA*, **286**(3), 341–7.

NMC (2008). *Standards of conduct, performance and ethics for nurses and midwives*. NMC, London.

NMC (2008). *Standards for medicine management*. NMC, London.

Resuscitation Council UK (2008). *Resuscitation guidelines*. Resuscitation Council UK, London.

Sheth TS, Choudhry NK, Bowes M, and Detsky AS (1997). The relation of conjunctival pallor to the presence of anaemia. *Journal of General Internal Medicine*, **12**, 102–6. [online] **http://www.jr2.ox.ac.uk/bandolier/band45/b45-6.html** accessed 14/04/08.

Talley NJ and O'Connor S (2005). *Clinical examination: a systematic guide to physical diagnosis*, 5th edition. Churchill Livingstone, Australia.

Vickers MD and Power I (1999). *Medicine for anaesthetists*, 4th edition. Blackwell Science, Oxford.

Whitehead MA, Puthucheary Z, and Rhodes A (2002). The recognition of a sick patient. *Clinical Medicine*, **2**(2), 95–8.

Williams AC de C (2002). Facial expression of pain: an evolutionary account. *Behavioural and Brain Sciences*, **25**(4), 439–88.

Useful further reading and websites

An interactive website run by an independent technology company that is not affiliated with any medical or drug organization: **http://www.wrongdiagnosis.com**

This site contains interesting articles and images on cyanosis: **http://www.emedicine.com/med/topic3002.htm**

Online text book covering all aspects of medicine: **http://www.merck.com/mmpe/print/sec05/ch045/ch045a.html**

Cardiology explained in simple language with useful tables and diagrams: **http://www.ncbi.nlm.nih.gov/books/bv.fcgi?indexed=google&rid=cardio.chapter.10**

Clinical examination systematically explained: **http://www.clinicalexam.com**

Standards and advice sheets on record keeping **http://www.nmc-UK.org/aSection.aspx?SectionID=11.**

(A) **Answers to patient scenarios**

1 Pallor, dyspnoea, and oedema are all signs of heart failure and would indicate possible right-sided heart failure and progression of her disease (Davies *et al.* 2000). You should measure her pulse rate, respiratory rate, and blood pressure, and make a full visual assessment, looking for signs of deterioration in her condition or new signs that she may have some other presenting problem such as a chest infection. You would specifically ask about chest pain. You need to ensure that she is comfortable and safe and not in danger of having a cardiac event. You would call her GP to request a home visit that day. You would inform the GP of your clinical findings in order for them to make an informed decision as to the urgency of the visit.

2
- *Call for help*.
- Close and lock the drug trolley (NMC 2004).
- Assess the patient using ABCDE guidelines (Resuscitation Council UK 2008).

3 Measure and record Mrs C's pulse rate, respiratory rate, and pulse oximetry. Report any deterioration to the shift leader. Explain to her daughter that Mrs C's heart has to work very hard to pump the blood around her body and to her lungs to collect oxygen. The blue tinge is called cyanosis and means that there is not enough oxygen in her blood at the moment. If she has been prescribed oxygen you can administer this as per the drug sheet. Give mother and daughter the opportunity to ask you questions; if you cannot answer them fully, ask a more senior member of staff to talk to them.

6.2 Measuring and recording the pulse

Definition

The **pulse** is the expansion and recoil of the artery, which occurs as a result of the contraction of the left ventricle (Blows 2001). **Palpating** (examining by touch) the pulse is one of the most commonly performed procedures in health assessment. It is a simple, non-invasive procedure for assessing the rate, rhythm, and volume (sometimes also referred to as amplitude) of the blood being pumped through the arteries. By palpating the pulse we can get an indication of the heart rate, heart rhythm, and blood pressure (BP).

It is important to remember that:

- The purpose of palpating a pulse is to assess the cardiovascular system. This includes information about the heart rate, rhythm, and BP. All of these observations should be made while palpating a pulse.
- The cardiovascular and respiratory systems are inextricably linked. This must be taken into account when interpreting any observation. For example a patient with **hypoxia** (low levels of oxygen) may have a tachycardia (fast heart rate) to compensate, so it would be worthwhile measuring their oxygen saturation.
- The pulse is often measured in a limb. As well as giving information about the heart rate, rhythm, and blood pressure, the pulse is also giving an indication of the blood supply to the limb itself. Some conditions, such as **atherosclerosis** (hardening and narrowing of the arteries), trauma, and surgery, may affect the blood supply to the limb. Palpating the pulse is an important part of assessing the blood supply to the limb.
- There are alternative methods of measuring the heart rate, rhythm, BP, and blood supply to limbs, some of which will be covered in other chapters. When using these alternative methods, take a thorough approach and double-check the results by palpating a pulse.
- Palpating the pulse is the first step in the skill of measuring blood pressure, so practise and master the skill of palpating the pulses first.

Prior knowledge

Before attempting to measure a pulse, make sure you are familiar with:

1 Anatomy and physiology of the heart, blood vessels, and blood.
2 Cardiac cycle.
3 Cardiac conduction system.
4 Factors influencing heart rate.
5 Factors influencing heart rhythm.
6 Factors influencing blood pressure.
7 Pathophysiology of some common cardiovascular diseases and conditions (myocardial infarction, heart failure, atrial fibrillation, hypertension, shock, atherosclerosis, thrombosis/embolism, anaemia).

Palpating the pulse is an important part of a patient's health assessment. It is essential that you understand the possible cause of changes in the pulse, as this will guide your actions. Reviewing the areas above will help.

Background

The rate, rhythm, and volume of the pulse give an indication of the heart rate and rhythm, and the blood pressure. To be able to interpret your findings by palpating the pulse, you need to understand the function of the cardiovascular system.

Pulse rate

Each time the left ventricle of the heart contracts, a pressure wave moves along the arterial vessels and can be felt as a pulse (Blows 2001). The pulse rate (PR) gives an indication of the heart rate (HR) and is recorded in beats per minute (bpm or b/min). Therefore, if you palpate a pulse point for 1 minute and feel 72 pulsations, you will record a HR 72 bpm or PR 72 bpm.

The HR and PR measurements will sometimes differ (see *Pulse rhythm* section). Some clinicians argue that when you measure the pulse you should write PR, and when you measure the heart rate you should write HR. Check local policy to ascertain what is acceptable.

The normal resting HR for an adult is 60–100 bpm but will vary with age, level of fitness, and health status (Tortora and Derrickson 2006). The HR is determined by the auto-rhythmic cells of the cardiac conductive system and is also influenced by the autonomic nervous system, drugs (Blows 2001), hormones, and electrolytes (Marieb and Hoehn 2007).

Bradycardia (HR below 60 bpm) is a concern because a slow heart rate will mean a reduced **cardiac output** (amount of blood pumped from the ventricle per minute). The effect is inadequate amounts of blood being transported to the tissues to meet the demand for oxygen and nutrients (Marieb and Hoehn 2007).

Table 6.1 The pulse rhythm indicates the heart rhythm

Description of pulse	How the pulse feels during palpation (– pause, ^ pulse)	Possible heart rhythm
Regularly regular	—— ^ —— ^ — ^ — ^ —— ^ — ^ ——	sinus rhythm
Regularly irregular	—— ^ ^ —— ^ ^ — ^ ^ — ^ ^ ——	bigeminy
Irregularly irregular	—— ^ ^ — ^ —— ^ ^ ^ — ^ ——	atrial fibrillation

Tachycardia (HR above 100 bpm) is useful for increasing cardiac output when the tissues have a higher demand for oxygen and nutrients, for example during exercise or pyrexia (high body temperature). However, tachycardia is of concern when the rate is so fast that less time is spent in diastole (phase of cardiac cycle when heart muscle is relaxed); this is when the chambers fill with blood (Blows 2001). If the chambers are not adequately filled, there is insufficient stretch created to facilitate the elastic recoil of the heart. This results in a reduced cardiac output (Tortora and Derrickson 2006).

In addition, the heart muscle itself relies on blood supplied from the coronary arteries, which only fill during diastole (Tortora and Derrickson 2006). When diastole is too brief the heart muscle will not receive an adequate blood supply, leading to cardiac ischaemia (reduced blood supply), which in turn leads to cell dysfunction and damage.

The 60–100 bpm range is a rough guideline to the normal range for the heart rate. You may find that a young, fit person has a normal resting pulse rate of less than 60 bpm, or an elderly person in poor health has a normal resting pulse rate of more than 100 bpm. You must consider when measuring the pulse rate what is normal for that individual. If their pulse rate is not normal (for them), ask yourself what the possible causes are, as this will guide your actions. Take a moment to consider the factors that control heart rate and the conditions that may increase or decrease it.

Pulse rhythm

The heart rhythm is instigated by the cardiac conduction system and results in the phases of the cardiac cycle (Blows 2001). The pulse rhythm is an indication of the heart rhythm and can feel regularly regular, regularly irregular, or irregularly irregular (see **Table 6.1**).

The normal heart rhythm is regularly regular. This means that the ventricles contract at regular intervals of equal timing (as with sinus rhythm). Therefore, the pulse feels the same, emerging at regular intervals of equal timing. If the heart rhythm is regularly irregular (as with bigeminy), the pulse will feel regularly irregular. If the heart rhythm is irregularly irregular (as with atrial fibrillation), the pulse will feel irregularly irregular.

In some circumstances a ventricular contraction may not be powerful enough to create the pressure to produce a palpable pulse (e.g. heart failure and premature ventricular contractions). This will be discovered if the pulse is palpated at the same time as cardiac conduction is being monitored (by electrocardiogram) or the heart sounds are being auscultated (listened to through a stethoscope).

Pulse volume

The volume or strength of the pulse gives an indication of the force the blood is exerting on the walls of the artery (blood pressure) as long as there is no obstruction, disease, or injury to the artery in which the pulse is being palpated. The strength of the pulse is normally described in terms of absent, weak, normal, increased, or bounding (Beverage *et al.* 2005). For an explanation of these findings, see the *Interpreting readings* section.

It has been suggested that the presence or absence of a pulse can give an indication of the systolic blood pressure. For example, if a pulse is palpable in the radial artery, the systolic blood pressure can be estimated at a minimum of 80 mmHg. If the pulse is palpable in the carotid artery but not the radial artery, the systolic blood pressure can be estimated to be a minimum of 60 mmHg.

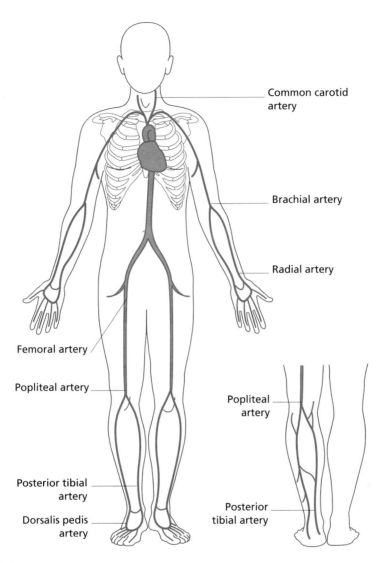

Figure 6.3 Pulse points.

This 'rule of thumb' method is a guide for the swift assessment of a patient's cardiovascular status but is not based on evidence. A study by Deaken and Low (2000) demonstrated that these guidelines overestimate the systolic blood pressure in the majority of cases.

Location of pulse points

A pulse can be palpated when the artery is near the surface of the skin (Blows 2001). There are a number of sites where a pulse can be palpated (see **Figure** 6.3). The most easily assessable of these is the radial artery.

Pulse points are located centrally or peripherally. The central pulses are those closest to the heart (carotid and femoral); the peripheral pulses are those further away from the heart in the limbs, radial, brachial, dorsalis pedis, posterior tibial, and popliteal (see **Figure** 6.4). The central and peripheral pulses feel different because of the size of the artery and strength of the pulse. Feel the difference in yourself by palpating your central and peripheral pulses.

The pulse is considered to be one of the four 'vital signs' of life (the others being respiratory rate, blood pressure, and temperature) because it is a fundamental indication of health status. The presence of a pulse indicates that the

(a)   (b)

(c)   (d)

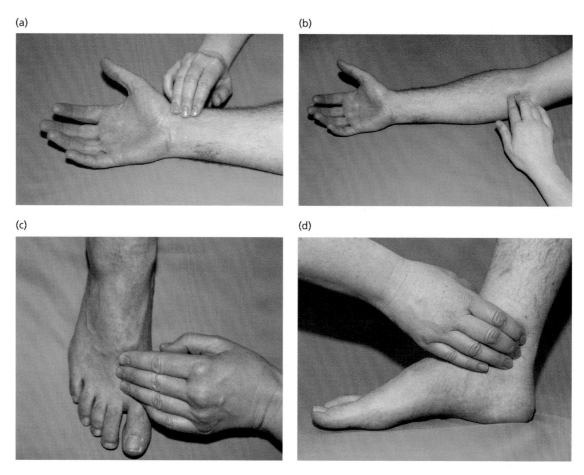

Figure 6.4 Taking a pulse at common peripheral pulse points: (a) radial pulse; (b) brachial pulse; (c) dorsalis pedalis pulse; (d) posterior tibial pulse.

heart is carrying out the essential function of moving blood around the body to perfuse the tissues. This function is vital to sustain life.

Context

 When to take a pulse

- On the patient's admission to your health care facility or service.
- Before, during, and after a treatment or procedure.
- When the patient's general physical condition changes.
- According to local policy.
- As part of assessing airway, breathing, and circulation in an emergency.

 When not to take a pulse

If the priority is airway and breathing during an emergency situation.

Alternative interventions

The pulse can be palpated to determine the heart rate, rhythm, and blood pressure, and assess the blood flow to a limb, but there are also some alternative methods. The heart rate and rhythm can be listened to using a stethoscope (auscultation) or recorded by an **electrocardiograph** (ECG). Using a pulse oximeter to measure oxygen saturations will also give the heart rate. The pulse can be listened to with the aid of a Doppler and the blood pressure can be measured using a sphygmomanometer.

If you have problems palpating a peripheral pulse then try a more central pulse. For example, if you cannot palpate the radial pulse, try the brachial. If you are unable to palpate the brachial pulse, try the carotid pulse. If you are unable to palpate the radial or brachial pulse or these pulses are too weak to enable you to count the rate accurately, this could indicate that the blood pressure is very low or there is some arterial obstruction in that limb. You could also compare the pulse in both arms. You *must* report any of these findings to a senior colleague immediately.

Hwu *et al.* (2000) in their review of the literature note that the length of time over which the radial pulse should be measured varies between sources. You could measure for 10 seconds and multiply by six to calculate the heart rate per minute, or for 15 seconds and multiply by four, and so on. You might also be instructed to count the first pulse as 1 or 0. In their study of 640 subjects, Hwu *et al.* found the accuracy of measuring the pulse for 15 or 30 seconds, counting the first beat as 1, was as reliable as measuring the pulse for 60 seconds in those with a heart rate below 100 bpm and without arrhythmia (abnormal heart rhythm).

It is recommended here that you count your first pulse as 1 and measure for 60 seconds until you become competent at the skill of assessing the rate, rhythm, and strength of a pulse in a shorter time. It is also recommended that you always measure for 60 seconds when the rate is greater than 100 bpm or there is an arrhythmia.

In some cases, assessment of the pulse alone will not give an accurate indication of the heart rate. If the heart rate is fast and/or irregular, as with atrial fibrillation, this requires measurement of the apex beat (Jevon *et al.* 2000). The apex beat is auscultated in the midclavicular line of the fifth intercostal space (see Figure 6.3). Measuring the apex beat and the radial pulse simultaneously by two health care workers can identify a difference between the heart rate and pulse rate. If the apex beat is higher than the pulse rate this suggests the heart is not contracting hard enough to create a pulse with every beat and is called an apex–radial pulse deficit.

Potential problems

If you press too hard on a pulse point you will obliterate the pulse and prevent blood flow. For this reason you should never palpate both carotid pulses at the same time. This will cause discomfort and potential harm to the patient. Be firm but gentle.

Table 6.2 Interpreting the findings from palpating a pulse

Finding	Interpretation
Unable to palpate a central or peripheral pulse.	The heart is not beating. Seek urgent help and if the patient is unresponsive commence basic life support.
Can palpate a central pulse but not a peripheral pulse.	Blood pressure is very low. *Seek urgent help.*
The peripheral pulse is weak but the central pulse is normal.	Blood pressure is low. *Seek urgent help.*
Can palpate a pulse in one limb but pulse is absent in the opposite limb.	Artery to affected limb is occluded or damaged. *Seek urgent help.*
Pulse rate is 60–100 bpm.	Normal pulse rate *but* interpretation will depend on: ■ How the patient looks and feels. ■ The physical and psychological state of the patient. ■ How this pulse rate compares with previous readings. ■ How this pulse rate compares with other vital signs.

Table 6.2 (*continued*)

Finding	Interpretation
Pulse rate is 50–60 bpm.	Bradycardia *but* this may be a normal pulse rate and interpretation will depend on: ■ How the patient looks and feels. ■ The physical and psychological state of the patient. ■ How this pulse rate compares with previous readings. ■ How this pulse rate compares with other vital signs.
Pulse rate is below 50 bpm	Bradycardia *but* this may be a normal pulse rate and interpretation will depend on: ■ How the patient looks and feels. ■ The physical and psychological state of the patient. ■ How this pulse rate compares with previous readings. ■ How this pulse rate compares with other vital signs. Some possible causes are: ■ Sick sinus syndrome. ■ Heart block. ■ Heart failure. ■ Drugs (beta-blockers, digoxin). ■ Hypothyroidism. ■ Hypoglycaemia. ■ Hypothermia. ■ Raised intracranial pressure. ■ Malnourishment.
Pulse rate 100–110 bpm.	Tachycardia *but* this may be a normal pulse rate and interpretation will depend on: ■ How the patient looks and feels. ■ The physical and psychological state of the patient. ■ How this pulse rate compares with previous readings. ■ How this pulse rate compares with other vital signs.
Pulse rate above 110 bpm.	Tachycardia – some possible causes are: ■ Recent exercise or exertion. ■ Fever. ■ Anxiety. ■ Pain. ■ Hypotension. ■ Myocardial infarction. ■ Heart failure. ■ Ischaemic heart disease. ■ Sick sinus syndrome. ■ Respiratory failure. ■ Drugs (nicotine, caffeine, cocaine, adrenaline). ■ Hyperthyroidism. ■ Anaemia.
Heart rate increases in inspiration and slows on expiration.	Sinus arrhythmia. This is a normal finding in young adults.

Table 6.2 (*continued*)

Finding	Interpretation
Pulse rhythm regularly regular.	Normal heart rhythm *but* must be considered along with rate and strength.
Pulse rhythm regularly irregular.	Regularly irregular heart rhythm *but* interpretation will depend on: ■ How the patient looks and feels. ■ How this pulse rhythm compares with previous readings. Some possible causes: ■ Regular premature atrial or ventricular contractions. ■ Heart block. ■ Sinus arrhythmia (normal in young adult).
Pulse rhythm irregularly irregular.	Irregularly irregular heart rhythm *but* interpretation will depend on: ■ How the patient looks and feels. ■ How this pulse rhythm compares with previous readings. Some possible causes: ■ Irregularly irregular premature atrial contractions such as atrial fibrillation. ■ Irregularly irregular premature ventricular contractions.
Pulse normal volume.	Normal cardiac output and systemic vascular resistance.
Pulse bounding.	High cardiac output and/or increased systemic vascular resistance. Some possible causes: ■ High blood pressure. ■ Fluid overload. ■ Physical exertion. ■ Early stage of septic shock. ■ Anxiety. ■ Hypercapnia (high carbon dioxide). ■ Fever. ■ Anaemia. ■ Pregnancy.
Pulse weak.	Reduced cardiac output and/or decreased systemic vascular resistance. Some possible causes: ■ Low blood pressure. ■ Hypovolaemia. ■ Heart failure.
Pulse is weak on inspiration and normal strength on expiration (pulsus paradoxus).	Cardiac output is affected by breathing. Some possible causes: ■ Lung disease (asthma). ■ Cardiac tamponade. ■ Pneumothorax. ■ Pericarditis.
Strength of pulse changes from beat to beat (pulsus alternans).	Cardiac output changes from beat to beat. Possible cause: heart failure.

Indications for assistance

If you are unable to locate a pulse or accurately assess the rate, rhythm, and strength (but are sure the patient is not in need of **cardiopulmonary resuscitation**), ask for assistance from a senior colleague.

Interpreting readings

When interpreting the findings from palpating a pulse, ask yourself these questions first:

- Am I attempting to palpate a pulse in the correct location?
- Am I pressing too hard and obliterating the pulse?
- Am I not pressing hard enough?
- Do I need to consider another pulse point because there is too much adipose tissue/oedema over this pulse point?

Special considerations

If the patient has excess adipose tissue or oedema over the pulse point then palpating the pulse may be difficult. Attempt to palpate the pulse at an alternative point.

Procedure

Preparation

Preparing yourself

Wash your hands and, if applicable, put on any other protective equipment that may be required (i.e. apron, gloves).

Preparing the equipment

You will need a watch with a second hand and a pen with black ink. The pulse rate should be recorded on a chart or in the clinical notes along with date, time, and your signature. Check your local policy.

Step-by-step guide to measuring a radial pulse

▶ Step	Rationale
1 Introduce yourself, confirm the patient's identity, explain the procedure, and obtain consent.	To identify patient correctly and gain informed consent.
2 Encourage the patient to remain quiet, relaxed, and still during the procedure.	To enable accurate measurement of a resting pulse.
3 The patient should be sitting or lying and rested after any physical activity or psychological upset (*However, in an emergency assessing the pulse must not be delayed*).	To gain an accurate recording of the heart rate at rest.
4 Their arm should be relaxed and supported on the bed or arm of the chair.	To help the patient's arm stay still and provide comfort.
5 Using your index, middle, and ring finger, feel for the pulse on the palmar aspect of the wrist, away from midline and towards thumb (see Figure 6.4a). Using your thumb is not recommended, as it has a pulse and this may lead to a misinterpretation.	This is the normal location of the radial artery. Using three fingers covers a larger surface area and therefore the pulse is more likely to be felt.

6	Palpation should be gentle but firm, using the pads rather than tips of your fingers.	The pads are more sensitive and will cover a larger surface area. Too much pressure will obliterate the pulse, too little may mean that the pulse cannot be felt or is misinterpreted as weak.
7	Feel for the rate, rhythm, and volume of the pulse.	To enable assessment of rate, rhythm, and volume of pulse.
8	Count the number of pulsations for 1 minute.	This will give you an indication of the heart rate.
9	Record the heart rate, rhythm, and strength of pulse.	Recording the rate, rhythm, and strength of pulse will give an indication of the patient's physical status at that time and will enable assessment of change.

Following the procedure

Explain the findings to the patient to aid understanding.

Recognizing patient deterioration

The pulse is one of the four 'vital signs' of life because it is a fundamental indication of health status. The presence of a pulse indicates that the heart is carrying out the essential function of moving blood around the body to perfuse the tissues. This function is life sustaining; therefore, any sign that it is starting to deteriorate should be reported to a senior colleague immediately. Signs of deterioration may be:

- Unable to palpate a pulse.

- The pulse rate, rhythm, or volume are abnormal or have changed.

- The patient is feeling and/or looking unwell.

Reflection and evaluation

When you have undertaken a pulse measurement, think about the following questions:

1 Were you able to find the pulse, and what was it about this patient and this situation that helped or hindered you?

2 Did you assess all three aspects of the pulse (rate, rhythm, and volume) and how did you record your findings?

3 Did your estimation of blood pressure from palpating the pulse reflect the sphygmomanometer blood pressure?

4 Were your findings as you expected for this patient's age, physical, and psychological condition?

Further learning opportunities

At the next available opportunity, try this:

- Palpate the pulses in different pulse points, noting the difference in volume.

- Measure your pulse during exercise and then after 5 minutes' rest. What is the difference in rate and strength?

Reminders

Don't forget to:

- Palpate for rate, rhythm, and volume of the pulse.

- Consider the best method of measuring a patient's pulse, for example, measuring the radial pulse and apical beat with atrial fibrillation.

- Compare the pulse in left and right when assessing limb perfusion.

Patient scenarios

1 Patient A reports that she feels unwell. You are unable to palpate her radial pulse in her left arm. What will be your next action to assess this patient's heart rate, rhythm, and blood pressure?

2 Patient B has returned from theatre after having surgery on his left femoral artery. The surgeon has

asked you to continue to assess the perfusion to his left leg. How will you do this?

3 Patient C has a pulse rate of 58 bpm. What information do you need to determine if this is normal?

Website

 http://www.oxfordtextbooks.co.uk/orc/ endacott

You may find it helpful to work through our short online quiz and additional scenarios intended to help you to develop and apply the skills in this chapter.

References

Beverage D, Mayer BH, Schaeffer L, and Thompson G, eds (2005). *Assessment made incredibly easy!* 3rd edition. Lippincott Williams and Wilkins, Philadelphia.

Blows WT (2001). *The biological basis of nursing: clinical observations*. Routledge, Taylor and Francis Group, London.

Deaken CD and Low JL (2000). Accuracy of the advanced trauma life support guidelines for predicting systolic blood pressure using carotid, femoral, and radial pulses: observational study. *British Journal of Medicine*, **321**, 673–4.

Hwu Y, Coates VE, and Lin F (2000). A study of the effectiveness of different measuring times and counting methods of human radial pulse rates. *Journal of Clinical Nursing*, **9**, 146–52.

Jevon P, Ewens B, and Lowe R (2000). Measuring the apex and radial pulse. *Nursing Times*, **96**(50), 43–4.

Marieb EN and Hoehn K (2007). *Human anatomy and physiology*, 7th edition. Pearson Benjamin Cummings, San Francisco.

Tortora G and Derrickson B (2006). *Principles of anatomy and physiology*, 11th edition. John Wiley and Sons Inc, New York.

Useful further reading and websites

Woodrow P (2003). Assessing pulse in older people. *Nursing Older People*, **15**(6), 38–40.

Website for *Principles of anatomy and physiology* by Tortora and Derrickson, giving you access to the tools and resources available for this text: **http://bcs.wiley.com/he-bcs/Books? action=index&bcsId=2287&itemId=0471689343**

Medline Plus, a US health information site, includes an encyclopaedia that gives details about this skill with diagrams: **http://www.nlm.nih.gov/medlineplus/ ency/article/003399.htm**

 Answers to patient scenarios

1 Attempt to palpate the carotid pulse as this is a more central pulse and should be more easily palpated. Any abnormalities you detect must be immediately reported to a senior colleague.

2 Palpate the dorsalis pedis for pulse presence and strength. Observe the colour, warmth, and capillary refill time of the skin on the leg.

3 Health status, age, medications being taken, previous pulse rate measurements.

6.3 **Measuring and recording blood pressure**

Definition

Blood pressure (BP) is the pressure exerted on the walls of blood vessels by the blood inside them. This pressure is created by the pumping action of the heart, resistance to the blood flow by the vessels themselves, and the viscosity (thickness) of the blood (Blows 2001).

Blood pressure can be measured either directly, using an invasive technique via an intra-arterial catheter, or indirectly, using a non-invasive instrument called a sphygmomanometer (meaning pulse pressure meter). Intra-arterial catheters are used in specialized settings such as critical care, so will not be covered in this section.

It is important to remember that:

- Palpating the pulse, particularly the radial and brachial, is essential to the skill of measuring the blood pressure, so master this first.
- The blood pressure may be the last vital sign to show signs of deterioration, so always consider the blood pressure in relation to other findings.
- It must be recognized that the blood pressure is a variable haemodynamic (blood movement) phenomenon, and is influenced by many factors

including age, sex, ethnicity, circadian rhythms (time of day), exercise, sleep, pain, emotion, temperature, body position, bladder distension, eating, tobacco, alcohol, and drugs (Beevers *et al.* 2001a). These influencing factors need to be considered when interpreting a blood pressure measurement.

- Many errors related to the process of measuring the blood pressure are possible, such as wrong size cuff, inadequately maintained equipment, and poor technique by the health care worker. It is important that these errors are minimized to avoid incorrect measurements and the patient's condition being treated inappropriately.

Prior knowledge

Before attempting this procedure, make sure you are familiar with:

1 Anatomy and physiology of the cardiovascular system.
2 Cardiac cycle.
3 Cardiac conductive system.
4 Factors influencing the blood pressure such as stroke volume (SV), preload, contractility, afterload, cardiac output (CO), and systemic vascular resistance (SVR).
5 The mechanisms that control the blood pressure.
6 **Pathophysiology** of some common cardiovascular conditions (myocardial infarction, heart failure, hypertension, shock, atherosclerosis, peripheral vascular disease).

Measuring the blood pressure is an important part of the patient's health assessment. It is essential that you understand the possible causes of change in the blood pressure, as this will guide your actions. Reviewing the areas above will help.

Background

The blood pressure is considered to be one of the four 'vital signs' of life (the others being respiratory rate, pulse, and temperature) because it is a fundamental indication of health status. An adequate blood pressure indicates that the heart is carrying out the essential function of moving blood around the body to perfuse the tissues. This function is vital to sustain life.

What is blood pressure?

Blood pressure is the pressure exerted on the walls of the blood vessels by the blood inside them. It results from a combination of **cardiac output** (CO) and **systemic vascular resistance** (SVR).

$$CO \times SVR = BP$$

Cardiac output

The healthy adult heart pumps or ejects approximately 5 litres of blood per minute from each ventricle – this is referred to as the cardiac output (CO) (Marieb and Hoehn 2007). With each heartbeat, approximately 70 ml is ejected from each ventricle into the pulmonary and systemic circulation – this is called the stroke volume (SV). You can calculate cardiac output by multiplying the stroke volume by the heart rate.

$$SV \times HR = CO$$

$$70 \text{ ml} \times 75 \text{ bpm} = 5250 \text{ ml}$$

A change in heart rate and/or stroke volume will lead to change in cardiac output. There are three factors that affect stroke volume: preload, contractility, and afterload (Tortora and Derrickson 2006).

Preload To pump effectively, the heart needs to receive an adequate volume of blood – this is called preload. Adequate preload will stretch the heart muscle and increase the force of recoil. This is known as Frank–Starling's Law of the Heart (Tortora and Derrickson 2006). If the blood volume entering the heart is insufficient, the heart muscle will not be stretched enough to produce adequate recoil and stroke volume will be reduced.

Contractility Contractility is the force with which the heart muscle contracts and is affected by the sympathetic nervous system, hormones, electrolytes, and drugs (Tortora and Derrickson 2006). Reduced contractility will lead to a reduced stroke volume. An increase in contractility will lead to an increase in stroke volume, as long as there is adequate blood volume.

Afterload The pressure in the **aorta** and pulmonary artery is called afterload, and is determined by the blood volume and resistance of the vascular system. If afterload is optimal, the heart will be able to eject a sufficient stoke volume with each contraction. If afterload is higher than the pressure created by the contraction of the ventricle, then stoke volume will be reduced.

Systemic vascular resistance

Systemic vascular resistance is the opposing force to blood flow from the heart. It is created by blood vessel size, blood vessel length, and blood viscosity (Tortora and Derrickson 2006). By constricting and dilating the vessels, systemic vascular resistance can be increased or decreased.

As cardiac output and systemic vascular resistance produce the blood pressure, any changes in these forces will affect blood pressure, and consequently perfusion of the tissues.

Control of blood pressure

The blood pressure is regulated by a variety of factors that affect blood volume, blood vessel diameter, heart rate, contractility, and blood flow.

Baroreceptors (pressure-sensitive nerves) detect stretch in the aorta, internal carotid arteries, and other large arteries in the neck and chest. If they detect a reduction in pressure, nerve impulses stimulate the cardiovascular centre of the brain to increase heart rate, increase contractility, and vasoconstrict blood vessels (Tortora and Derrickson 2006).

Chemoreceptors monitor blood hydrogen, carbon dioxide, and oxygen levels, and are located in the aorta and carotid sinus. They also provide sensory input to the cardiovascular centre of the brain. A severe decrease in oxygen or increase in hydrogen or carbon dioxide will stimulate an increase in heart rate and vasoconstriction (Tortora and Derrickson 2006).

It is also worthwhile noting that the cardiovascular centre receives input from the cerebral cortex, limbic system, and hypothalamus. Therefore, the blood pressure can be influenced by the emotional state and body temperature (Tortora and Derrickson 2006).

A number of hormones affect the blood pressure:

- Angiotensin II – causes vasoconstriction and stimulates the release of aldosterone, which increases blood volume by reabsorbing water from filtrate in the kidneys.

- Atrial natriuretic peptide (ANP) – released when the atrium is overstretched. Causes vasodilatation and promotes loss of water in the urine to reduce blood volume.

- Adrenaline and noradrenaline – produced by the adrenal cortex. They cause an increase in heart rate and contractility. Vasoconstriction occurs in the vessels supplying the abdomen and skin but vasodilatation occurs in the vessels supplying the cardiac and skeletal muscles (Tortora and Derrickson 2006).

- Antidiuretic hormone (ADH) – produced in the hypothalamus and released by the posterior pituitary gland in response to the osmotic pressure (concentration of solutes) of the blood. The release of ADH decreases urine output and causes vasoconstriction.

In the capillary bed, physical changes such as temperature and blood volume will instigate changes in the diameter of the vessels (Tortora and Derrickson 2006). For example, blood vessels in the skin will vasodilate in the heat to increase heat loss, and vasoconstrict in the cold to conserve heat. In addition, the blood vessels will vasoconstrict when blood volume is low to increase blood flow to the vital organs.

A number of cells in the blood and blood vessels release chemicals that lead to vasodilatation and vasoconstriction (Tortora and Derrickson 2006). For example, histamine, which is stored in white blood cells, is released during the inflammatory response and can lead to local or generalized vasodilatation.

How blood pressure is recorded

Blood pressure is recorded in **millimetres of mercury** (mmHg). Two values are given with a blood pressure measurement, and expressed, for example, as 'one hundred and fourteen *over* seventy six'.

The 114 mmHg is the pressure in the artery when the left ventricle is in systole (contracted) and is called the systolic blood pressure (SBP). The 76 mmHg is the pressure in the artery when the left ventricle is in **diastole** (relaxed) and is called the diastolic blood pressure (DBP).

You might assume that the DBP would go down to 0 mmHg but the elastic recoil action of the aorta acts like

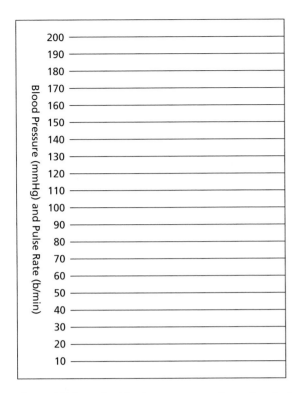

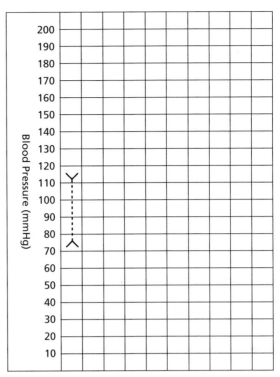

Figure 6.5 Recording blood pressure on an observation chart.

a pump during diastole (Blows 2001). The difference between the SBP and the DBP is called the pulse pressure, which in the previous example would be 38 mmHg (114 − 76 = 38).

This blood pressure reading would be recorded on an observation chart as shown in **Figure 6.5**.

Changes in blood pressure

The function of blood pressure is to provide adequate perfusion to all the cells of the body. A low blood pressure (**hypotension**) will lead to hypoperfusion, resulting in dysfunction, damage, and eventually death of the tissues. High blood pressure (**hypertension**) causes damage to the blood vessels and organs.

Hypertension

There are two main types of hypertension, primary (sometimes called essential) and secondary. Ninety-five per cent of cases of hypertension are primary, while 5% of cases are secondary (Feather 2006).

Although primary hypertension has no known cause, there are some identifiable risk factors for developing the disease: age, diabetes, ethnic origin, family history of high blood pressure, being overweight, high salt intake, not eating fruit and vegetables, not taking exercise, and excessive alcohol intake.

Secondary hypertension can be caused by renal disease, endocrine disorders, and pre-eclampsia in pregnancy. Consistently high blood pressure is of concern because of the damage it causes to the blood vessels, heart, brain, and kidneys. This in turn leads to the risk of myocardial infarction, heart failure, peripheral vascular disease, stroke, renal failure, and eye conditions.

Hypertension is often known as the 'silent killer' because it is asymptomatic (has no symptoms). It affects 40% of the adult population in the UK (Feather 2006).

Accelerated or malignant hypertension is a very high blood pressure (e.g. >180/>110 mmHg) that causes organ damage over weeks rather than years. It requires urgent treatment as the eyes, kidneys, and brain are at risk of permanent damage. The risk factors associated with accelerated hypertension are being male, of black ethnic origin, a smoker, and already having secondary hypertension (Willacy 2007).

Hypotension

Hypotension is an abnormally low blood pressure. Hypotension is of concern because without sufficient blood pressure, the tissues and organs are not perfused with the oxygen and nutrients needed to sustain life. The kidneys are particularly vulnerable and will fail with prolonged hypoperfusion (Woodrow 2000).

The causes of hypotension are related to blood volume, cardiac output, and systemic vascular resistance. The possible causes of acute hypotension are shock, drugs and medications, cardiac arrhythmias, heart valve dysfunction, cardiac tamponade, and pulmonary embolism. The other signs and symptoms associated with hypoperfusion may be tachypnoea, tachycardia, peripheral shutdown, dizziness, syncope (fainting), reduced urine output, nausea, and thirst.

Brief periods of hypotension after changing position, for example from sitting to standing, can lead to dizziness, blurred vision, and syncope, particularly in the elderly. This is called postural hypotension. To help diagnose postural hypertension, the blood pressure is first taken when the patient is lying or sitting, then again when they are standing.

Pulse pressure

The normal pulse pressure is 40 mmHg. Pulse pressure can widen because the systolic blood pressure becomes higher and/or the diastolic blood pressure becomes lower. Pulse pressure is narrowed when the systolic blood pressure becomes lower and/or diastolic blood pressure becomes higher. The systolic blood pressure is an indication of the stroke volume and the speed with which it is ejected from the ventricle. The diastolic blood pressure is an indication of systemic vascular resistance.

Conditions such as hypovolaemia will narrow the pulse pressure because of the reduced stroke volume and increased systemic vascular resistance caused by vasoconstriction. Conditions such as fever will widen the pulse pressure because of the increased stroke volume and reduced systemic vascular resistance caused by vasodilatation. Atherosclerosis and ageing increase the systolic blood pressure because of a stiffening of the arteries, which widens the pulse pressure (Woods *et al.* 2000).

How blood pressure is measured

The equipment used to measure blood pressure non-invasively and indirectly is called a sphygmomanometer, often referred to in short as a sphygmometer or sphyg. A common feature is that it occludes (stops blood flow) in an artery of the arm or leg with an inflatable bladder in a cuff. This enables measurement of the blood pressure by auscultation of the pulse (listening with a stethoscope) or oscillometry of the pulse (detecting movement) (Beevers *et al.* 2001a). Devices that require auscultation are manual, and those that use oscillometry are automated. There are advantages and disadvantages with each system.

Mercury and aneroid sphygmomanometers

The mercury sphygmomanometer (see **Figure 6.6**) is often referred to as the 'gold standard' of non-invasive blood pressure measurement, because of its accuracy when used correctly. However, concerns over the use of mercury, a toxic substance (Netea and Thien 2004), and its potential to contaminate the environment when disposed of (Feather 2001) has led to a reduction in its use (Beevers *et al.* 2001b).

In the mercury sphygmomanometer, an inflatable bladder is connected to a reservoir of mercury. As the bladder is inflated with air from the hand bulb, the pressure is represented by the height of the mercury in a gauged column. The mercury sphygmomanometer indirectly measures the blood pressure by measuring the pressure required in the bladder to occlude blood flow to the arm or leg. The health care worker observes the level

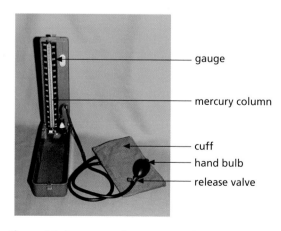

Figure 6.6 A mercury sphygmomanometer.

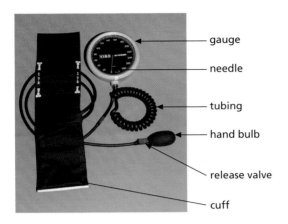

- gauge
- needle
- tubing
- hand bulb
- release valve
- cuff

Figure 6.7 An aneroid sphygmomanometer.

of the mercury as the bladder is inflated and deflated to get the blood pressure readings.

The aneroid (liquid free) sphygmomanometer (see **Figure 6.7**) works using bellows and levers (Beevers *et al.* 2001b). As with the mercury sphygmomanometer, the bladder is inflated with air from the hand bulb but the pressure is usually measured by observing a needle on a gauged dial. The aneroid sphygmomanometer is less accurate than the mercury sphygmomanometer and loses accuracy with the bumps and knocks of everyday use, leading to an underestimation of blood pressure (O'Brien *et al.* 2003).

Auscultation of Korotkoff sounds

Both the mercury and aneroid sphygmomanometer require the health care worker to auscultate the Korotkoff sounds (sounds made by the blood flow in the artery). As the bladder is deflated, the blood flow returns. This can be heard by placing a stethoscope over the artery just below the bladder. Dr Nikolai Korotkoff first described these sounds in 1905 and identified five phases. The sounds are described in a variety of ways in the published literature, which can at times be confusing and conflicting (see the variety of descriptions of phase 3 in **Table 6.3**).

For simplicity it is often suggested that the first tap you hear (start of phase 1) as the bladder is deflating is the systolic blood pressure. When the tapping stops (phase 5)

Table 6.3 The Korotkoff sounds

Phases of the Korotkoff sounds	Description of the sound of each phase
Phase 1 (start of phase 1 indicates the SBP)	■ Faint, repetitive, clear tapping (Beevers *et al.* 2001b). ■ Clear tapping (Hinkley and Walker 2005). ■ Sharp 'thud' (Dougherty and Lister 2008).
Phase 2	■ Sounds soften and acquire a swishing quality (Beevers *et al.* 2001b). ■ Muffled, swishing sounds (Hinkley and Walker 2005). ■ Blowing or swishing sound (Dougherty and Lister 2008). In some people the sound may disappear altogether here, creating an auscultatory gap.
Phase 3	■ Return of sharper sounds, which becomes crisper to regain or even exceed intensity of phase 1 (Beevers *et al.* 2001b). ■ Sounds become louder and more distinct (Hinkley and Walker 2005). ■ A softer thud than phase 1 (Dougherty and Lister 2008).
Phase 4 (start of phase 4 indicates DBP if the Korotkoff sounds can still be heard when the cuff is fully deflated).	■ Distinct abrupt muffling of sounds which become soft and blowing in quality (Beevers *et al.* 2001b). ■ Muffling of sound with soft, blowing quality (Hinkley and Walker 2005). ■ A softer blowing sound that disappears (Dougherty and Lister 2008).
Phase 5 (start of phase 5 indicates the DBP).	■ Point at which all sounds disappear (Beevers *et al.* 2001b). ■ Sound disappears completely (Hinkley and Walker 2005). ■ Silence (Dougherty and Lister 2008).

this is the diastolic blood pressure. However, this may lead to inaccuracies because the Korotkoff sounds can disappear and return in phase 2, causing an **auscultatory gap** (period with no sound), or may continue until the cuff is fully deflated.

It is important that the true systolic blood pressure is measured, rather than the returning sound at the end of the auscultatory gap. To ensure the bladder is inflated beyond the auscultatory gap, the health care worker palpates the pulse while inflating the bladder. When the pulse disappears, this is the **estimated systolic blood pressure**, and is beyond the auscultatory gap.

In some patients the Korotkoff sounds can be heard even when the cuff is fully deflated, meaning phase 4 does not end. To gain a measure of the diastolic blood pressure in these patients, it is recommended that the diastolic measure is taken at the start of phase 4 (Beevers *et al.* 2001a), rather than at the start of phase 5. This clearly means that you will need to be able to identify phase 4 sounds. Phase 4 sounds can be heard for the last 10 mmHg (or 5 seconds) as the cuff is deflating, but it is usually less than 5 mmHg (O'Brien *et al.* 2003). To listen to Korotkoff sounds, log onto the British Hypertension Society's website and have a go at the interactive exercise (**http://www.abdn.ac.uk/medical/bhs/tutorial/tutorial.htm**).

It is worthwhile noting that there will sometimes be faint single taps while the bladder is deflating before the phase 1 Korotkoff sounds commence. However, it is the first of the two consecutive taps that indicates the systolic blood pressure.

Research has shown that there are some inherent inaccuracies in using the auscultation technique (Beevers *et al.* 2001b). O'Brien (2003) proposes that these errors arise from the patient, equipment, and health care worker. Rose (1965 cited by O'Brien *et al.* 2003) classified the health care worker error into:

- Systematic error – the health care worker is unable to hear or correctly interpret the Korotkoff sounds.
- Terminal digit preference – the health care worker rounds the measurement up or down to the nearest 5 or 10 mmHg.
- Bias – the health care worker adjusts the pressure to meet their preconceived notion of what the blood pressure should be.

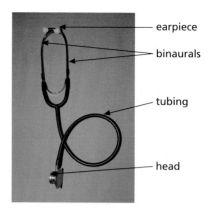

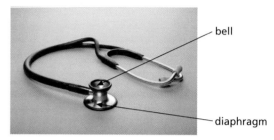

Figure 6.8 A double-headed stethoscope.
Danie/Loursclle/istock.com/

The aneroid sphygmomanometer is replacing the mercury sphygmomanometer on the assumption that it is equally accurate because it uses the auscultatory technique (O'Brien *et al.* 2003). But because the aneroid sphygmomanometer does require the use of the auscultation technique, it is subject to the same inherent inaccuracies (Beevers *et al.* 2001b).

In order to carry out auscultation you will need to use a stethoscope. There are generally two types. One has a diaphragm and a bell in the head (see **Figure 6.8**), the other just a diaphragm. The bell is for listening to low-pitched sounds and the diaphragm for high-pitched sounds. The Korotkoff sounds are low pitched but the use of the diaphragm is often recommended because it covers a larger surface area and requires less precise placement. It is recommended that you become proficient at locating the brachial pulse and use a stethoscope with a bell when it is available.

The stethoscope head and tubes should be free from obstruction during auscultation. Any contact with the cuff, tubes of the sphygmomanometer, clothing, or the patient's arm is amplified and may distract from the Korotkoff sounds.

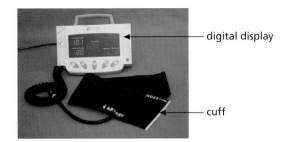

digital display

cuff

Figure 6.9 An automated oscillometry sphygmomanometer.

Oscillometry

Automated oscillometry sphygmomanometers (see **Figure 6.9**) use a sensor in the cuff that detects pulsations in the artery. It then calculates the blood pressure using an algorithm held secret by the manufacturers (Braam and Thien 2005). It will not work if the pulse is too weak to be detected by the sensor.

There is evidence that some automated devices overestimate blood pressure measurements compared with the mercury sphygmomanometer (Jones *et al*. 1996), and underestimate blood pressure compared with invasive monitoring (Bur *et al*. 2000). Myers (2006) found that the use of an automated device gave lower readings when compared with a mercury sphygmomanometer but suggests that this may be because the use of an automated device reduces white-coat hypertension (higher blood pressure as a result of the anxiety experienced when consulting a health care professional).

Braam and Thien (2005) found that oscillometry is more inaccurate in patients with high blood pressure. But this could be explained by an increased variability of blood pressure in patients with hypertension. It has also been suggested that oscillometry cannot be reliably used on patients with arrhythmias (O'Brien *et al*. 2003) and it has been found to underestimate the blood pressure in pre-eclamptic patients (Quinn 1994).

An advantage of the automated oscillometry sphygmomanometer is its ease of use and it eliminates many of the errors associated with auscultating the Korotkoff sounds. O'Brien *et al*. (2003) have called for the development of more accurate automated devices in light of the inherent inaccuracy of the auscultatory technique.

Clearly there is a need to be competent using both manual and automated devices, which will require practice and understanding.

Sources of error

The literature advocates a variety of steps in the procedure to eliminate factors that may lead to an inaccurate reading. McAlister and Straus (2001) carried out an evidence-based review of the factors and found that talking, acute exposure to cold, recent ingestion of alcohol, incorrect arm position, and incorrect cuff size are the factors that affect a reading by more than 5 mmHg.

It is often recommended that patients rest for 5 minutes before a measurement. However, there is no evidence for an optimal time (Netea and Thien 2004). Some patients may require longer if you are to get a true reading of their resting blood pressure.

There is evidence to both support and refute the idea that crossing the legs raises the blood pressure (Eser *et al*. 2007). It is therefore recommended that the patient has their legs uncrossed.

There is controversy in the literature as to which arm should be used. Some studies, but not all, have demonstrated a significant difference between arms (O'Brien *et al*. 1997 cited in Beevers *et al*. 2001a). It is recommended here that you measure the blood pressure in both arms for comparison on an initial assessment.

Netea and Thien (2004) cite evidence that smoking, eating, and consuming alcohol and caffeine can increase the blood pressure. They recommend that these activities should be avoided for at least 1 hour before measurement but do not provide supporting evidence for this time period.

Bladder and cuff size

The inflatable bladder applies pressure over the artery to occlude blood flow. It is contained within a cuff that holds the bladder in place. It is important that the correct bladder size is used to occlude the artery. If the bladder is too small the blood pressure measurement will be overestimated; too large and it will be underestimated.

Many cuffs now have the bladder as an integral part and conveniently have size indicators printed on the cuff. These guidelines must be followed to ensure an accurate reading. If, however, you are using a bladder and cuff that does not have a size indicator, you will need to remember that the bladder must encircle at least 80% of the circumference of the upper arm but no more than 100%. The width of the bladder must be at least 40% of the circumference of the upper arm.

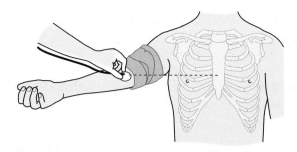

Figure 6.10 Correct arm height for reading blood pressure when the patient is sitting. The brachial pulse point should be level with the mid sternum.

Arm position

The level of the heart is generally considered to be from the mid to inferior end of the sternum. Aim to have the brachial pulse point level with the mid sternum when the patient is sitting (see **Figure 6.10**).

When the patient is **supine** (lying on their back) or semi-recumbent, the height of the heart is taken from the phlebostatic axis (the estimated location of the right atrium). It is found by drawing an imaginary line from the fourth intercostal space to an intersection with the midaxillary line. Aim to have the brachial pulse point level with the phlebostatic axis (see **Figure 6.11**).

Avoid measuring the blood pressure of a patient lying on their side, as one arm will be below the level of the heart, giving a falsely high reading, and the other will be above the heart, giving a falsely low reading.

One- or two-inflation technique

There are two techniques for measuring the blood pressure using a manual device. One requires the bladder to be inflated and deflated once, and the other requires the bladder to be inflated and deflated twice.

Using the two-inflation technique, the systolic blood pressure is estimated on the first inflation by palpating the pulse and observing the pressure at which it disappears. The bladder is then deflated and re-inflated for the Korotkoff sounds to be auscultated on the second deflation. The two-inflation technique is recommended by the British Hypertension Society and can be viewed on their website (**http://www.bhsoc.org/how_to_measure_blood_pressure.stm**).

Using the one-inflation technique, the systolic blood pressure is estimated on inflation by palpating the pulse and the Korotkoff sounds are auscultated on deflation.

The two-inflation technique is widely recommended but there are suggestions that venous engorgement may occur between readings, leading to inaccuracy. Studies by Koehler *et al.* (2004) and Yarows *et al.* (2001) found no evidence of significant differences in consecutive readings, but Jones *et al.* (2006) found that the two-inflation technique showed a significantly lower diastolic blood pressure when compared with the one-inflation technique. They hypothesize that this is the result of vasodilatation, caused by the occlusion of the brachial artery during the first inflation. Because the one-inflation technique is a shorter procedure but does not compromise the

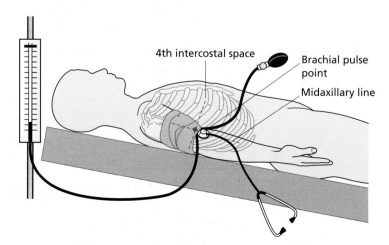

Figure 6.11 Correct arm position for reading blood pressure when the patient is semi-recumbent or supine. The brachial pulse point should be level with the plebostatic axis.

objective of gaining an accurate reading, it is the one described in this chapter.

Context

 When to measure blood pressure

There are a number of situations in which you will be required to measure a patient's blood pressure, and these situations will require different preparation.

If you are in a primary care setting screening for hypertension, then the measurement will need to be taken while eliminating factors that will increase the resting blood pressure. This may require adjustment to the time, place, and circumstances in which the blood pressure is measured.

If you are in an acute or emergency care setting then measuring the blood pressure should not be delayed but the health care worker must be mindful of factors that may increase or decrease the blood pressure.

Blood pressure is measured:

- Usually on the patient's admission to a health care facility or service.
- Before, during, and after some treatments or procedures.
- When the patient's general physical condition changes.
- According to local or national policy.

 When not to measure blood pressure

If the priority is assessing airway, breathing, and circulation in an emergency situation.

There are contraindications to measuring a blood pressure in a particular limb. If any of the following conditions are present, use an alternative limb.

- Lymphoedema or general swelling.
- Paralysis.
- Fistula for dialysis.
- Arterial or venous blood flow disruption.
- Recent surgery or trauma.
- After mastectomy.
- Intravenous device.

Box 6.1 Classification of hypertension

Systolic blood pressure *and/or* diastolic blood pressure (mmHg) of:

	Systolic	Diastolic
Mild	140–159	90–99
Moderate	160–179	100–109
Severe	>180	>110

Interpreting readings

Hypertension

The classification of hypertension given by the British Hypertension Society (Williams *et al.* 2004) is shown in **Box 6.1**.

Blood pressure varies greatly in individuals but it is a persistent blood pressure of above 140/90 mmHg that is considered hypertension (NICE 2006). In order to establish that the blood pressure is persistently above 140/90 mmHg it should be measured on more than one occasion, and factors that cause variability in the blood pressure should be taken into account, such as 'white-coat' hypertension (Beevers *et al.* 2001a).

Hypotension

Classification varies depending on the normal blood pressure for that person, but hypotension is often considered to be a systolic blood pressure lower than 90 mmHg.

Special considerations

- During pregnancy the woman must have her blood pressure monitored for signs of pre-eclampsia (pregnancy-induced hypertension). Quinn (1994) found that an automated blood pressure monitor underestimated pregnant women's blood pressure by as much as 30 mmHg. It is recommended, therefore, that the manual method is used by a skilled practitioner to avoid underdetection of this potentially harmful condition.

- Some automated devices overinflate the cuff (Hinkley and Walker 2005), causing the patient pain and bruising. It is recommended, particularly if there are going to be frequent recordings, that the manual method is used on the elderly or frail.

- It has not yet been established if the oscillometric or auscultatory methods differ in accuracy in obese patients, but the correct bladder size is essential to give an accurate reading (O'Brien 2003).

Procedure

Preparation

Preparing yourself

- Wash your hands and if necessary put on any personal protective equipment that may be required (i.e. apron, gloves).
- Be familiar with the patient's past medical history.

Preparing the patient

If appropriate:

- Allow the patient adequate time to be fully rested.
- You will need to gain access to the upper arm so roll up the sleeve. If the sleeve is tight around the arm, remove the garment.
- The patient's legs should be uncrossed.

Preparing the equipment

Before carrying out the procedure you should (if appropriate):

- Have the room warm and quiet.
- Have an observation chart and pen with black ink ready to record your results.
- Check the sphygmomanometer has been serviced and calibrated within the period stipulated by local policy (usually indicated by a label attached to the equipment).
- Check the equipment is clean and intact.
- Test the mercury sphygmomanometer by closing the valve and inflating the bladder. The level of

the mercury should remain still when the bladder is inflated and the valve is closed. The level of the mercury should move smoothly down when the valve is opened and sit at zero when the bladder is fully deflated.

- Test the aneroid sphygmomanometer by closing the valve and inflating the bladder. The needle should remain still when the bladder is inflated and the valve is closed. The needle should move smoothly round the dial when the valve is opened and sit at zero when the bladder is fully deflated.
- The mercury or aneroid sphygmomanometer will need to be at your eye level during the reading, so find a suitable surface.
- When using an automated device, check the power supply cable is intact before use and follow the manufacturer's guidelines.
- Have the correct bladder and cuff size available.

Caution: Because the mercury sphygmomanometer contains mercury (a toxic metal), care needs to be taken with this equipment. If the sphygmomanometer is dropped or broken seek help immediately, as specific health and safety precautions need to be followed.

To measure the blood pressure with a mercury or aneroid sphygmomanometer you will need a stethoscope.

- Check that the tubing and diaphragm are not damaged and the stethoscope is clean.
- Check the stethoscope by placing the earpieces in your ears, gently tapping the diaphragm, and listening for adequate volume.

Step-by-step guide to measuring blood pressure using a mercury or aneroid sphygmomanometer

If using an automated oscillometry sphygmomanometer, follow the first six steps in the table below and then refer to the manufacturer's guidelines.

Step		Rationale
1	Introduce yourself, confirm the patient's identity, explain the procedure, and obtain consent.	To identify the patient correctly and gain informed consent.
2	Inspect the arms for signs that measuring the BP in that limb is contraindicated. Ask the patient if they know of any reason why you should not measure the BP in a particular limb.	Occluding arterial or venous blood flow may cause harm in some circumstances.
3	Locate the brachial pulse in the antecubital fossa. (Note this is easiest when the patient's arm is extended or slightly hyperextended.)	To aid correct placement of bladder and head of stethoscope.
4	Place the centre of the bladder or artery marker indicated on the cuff two fingers width above the brachial pulse point.	Correct position for occluding the brachial artery.
5	Secure the cuff snugly around the arm.	Preventing movement of the bladder.
6	Guide or assist your patient's arm into the correct supported position – level with the heart and relaxed.	Correct position for accurate measurement.
7	Ask the patient not to speak while you carry out the rest of the procedure.	Speaking may raise their BP and impede your ability to hear the Korotkoff sounds.
8	Place the stethoscope in your ears. Have the head of the stethoscope in easy reach.	To enable quick placement of the stethoscope head on the brachial pulse point when ready to deflate the cuff, to minimize patient discomfort.
9	Palpate the brachial pulse while inflating the bladder (the valve needs to be closed – turned fully clockwise).	To enable estimation of the SBP.
10	Look at the level of the mercury column or dial while you inflate the bladder.	To enable measurement of the estimated SBP.
11	When you can no longer feel the brachial pulse you have reached the **estimated SBP** and need to inflate the bladder for another 30 mmHg. (Note: if the radial pulse is easier to palpate then you can use it as an alternative.)	This means you can be confident you have inflated the cuff beyond the auscultatory gap.

continued overleaf

12	Stop palpating the brachial pulse and place the bell of the stethoscope over the brachial pulse point (this is the uncomfortable part for the patient so try to be swift).	To enable you to ausculate the Korotkoff sounds.
13	Open the valve very slightly by turning it anticlockwise. The mercury column or needle on the dial will start to drop. You are aiming for it to drop at 2 mmHg per second.	This will enable you to measure to the nearest 2 mmHg.
14	Listen for the first two consecutive taps of the Korotkoff sounds and note the point on the mercury column or dial.	To obtain an accurate reading of the SBP to the nearest 2 mmHg.
15	As the column of mercury/needle continues to drop, note the point at which the phase 4 sounds start (just in case phase 4 does not end) and when phase 5 starts.	To obtain an accurate reading of the DBP to the nearest 2 mmHg.
16	Continue to allow the bladder to deflate at 2 mmHg per second for the next 20 mmHg, then allow complete deflation.	To be sure you are not in the auscultatory gap.
17	Record the BP measurement along with date, time, right or left arm. It may also be necessary to document the patient's position, i.e. lying, sitting, or standing.	To enable assessment of the patient's health status.

Following the procedure

- Explain the findings to the patient to aid understanding.
- Clean equipment and store safely to avoid cross-infection and ensure health and safety.

Recognizing patient deterioration

It is important to inform a senior member of staff if patients are found to be hypertensive or hypotensive. Hypotension leads to hypoperfusion, with signs such as:

- Tachypnoea.
- Tachycardia.
- Peripheral shutdown.
- Urine output less than 0.5 ml/kg/hour.
- Reduction in the patient's level of consciousness.

Reflection and evaluation

When you have undertaken a blood pressure measurement, think about the following questions:

1 Did the sphygmomanometer give the reading you expected for this patient, having palpated the pulse first?
2 Were you able to interpret the reading in light of the patient's condition?
3 Did you have a choice of equipment (manual and automated) from which to select the correct device for the patient?
4 Were you able to identify the start of phase 4 of the Korotkoff sounds?
5 Did you manage to support the patient's arm at heart level?

Further learning opportunities

At the next available opportunity have your blood pressure measured with both an automated and manual device.

- Which caused the most discomfort?
- Does it make a difference whether your arm is below or above heart level?

To listen to Korotkoff sounds and practise reading blood pressure, log onto the British Hypertension Society's website and have a go at the interactive exercise (**http://www.abdn.ac.uk/medical/bhs/tutorial/tutorial.htm**).

Reminders

- The accuracy of the reading will depend on the use of the correct technique and the quality of the equipment used.
- Have equipment serviced and calibrated according to local policy and when you suspect it is no long accurate or is damaged.
- Always check there are no contraindications to using a particular limb before taking a reading.

Patient scenarios

1 You have used an automated sphygmomanometer on patient A without checking his pulse first and it cannot give a reading. What might be the problem?

2 You are measuring patient B's blood pressure using a mercury sphygmomanometer. You can hear the Korotkoff sounds until the bladder is completely deflated and the mercury column is at zero. What will you do next?

3 You cannot find patient C's brachial pulse point in her left arm in order to measure her blood pressure using a manual sphygmomanometer. What will you do?

Website

 http://www.oxfordtextbooks.co.uk/orc/endacott

You may find it helpful to work through our short online quiz and additional scenarios intended to help you to develop and apply the skills in this chapter.

References

Beevers G, Lip GYH, and O'Brien E (2001a). ABC of hypertension. Blood pressure measurement. Part I – Sphygmomanometry: common factors to all techniques. *British Medical Journal*, **322**, 981–5.

Beevers G, Lip GYH, and O'Brien E (2001b). ABC of hypertension. Blood pressure measurement. Part II – Conventional sphygmomanometry: technique of auscultatory blood pressure measurement. *British Medical Journal*, **322**, 1043–7.

Blows WT (2001). *The biological basis of nursing: clinical observations*. Routledge, London.

Braam RL and Thien T (2005). Is the accuracy of blood pressure measuring devices underestimated at increasing blood pressure levels? *Blood Pressure Monitoring*, **10**, 283–9.

Bur A, Hirschl MM, Herkner H *et al.* (2000). Accuracy of oscillometric blood pressure measurement according to the relation between cuff size and upper-arm circumference in critically ill patients. *Critical Care Medicine*, **28**(2), 371–6.

Dougherty L and Lister S, eds (2008). *The Royal Marsden Hospital manual of clinical procedures*, 7th edition. Blackwell Publishing, Oxford.

Eser I, Khorshid L, Gunes UY, and Demir Y (2007). The effect of different body positions on blood pressure. *Journal of Clinical Nursing*, **16**(1), 137–40.

Feather C (2001). Equipment for blood pressure measurement. *Professional Nurse*, **16**(11), 1458–62.

Feather C (2006). A practical guide to reaching hypertension targets. *Practice Nurse*, **31**(11), 12–19.

Hinkley P and Walker S (2005). Measuring blood pressure. *Practice Nurse*, **29**(9), 54–61.

Jones D, Engelke MK, Brown ST, and Swanson M (1996). A comparison of two non-invasive methods of blood pressure measurement in the triage area. *Journal of Emergency Nursing*, **22**, 111–15.

Jones S, Simpson H, and Ahmed H (2006). A comparison of two methods of blood pressure measurement. *British Journal of Nursing*, **15**(17), 948–51.

Koehler NR, Poli de Figueiredo CE, and Mendes-Ribiero AC (2004). Time interval between pairs of arterial blood pressure measurements – does it matter? *American Journal of Hypertension*, **17**, 194–6.

Marieb EN and Hoehn K (2007). *Human anatomy and physiology*, 7th edition. Pearson Benjamin Cummings, San Francisco.

McAlister FA and Straus SF (2001). Measurement of blood pressure: an evidence based review. *British Medical Journal*, **322**, 908–11.

Myers MG (2006). Automated blood pressure measurement in routine clinical practice. *Blood Pressure Monitoring*, **11**, 59–62.

Netea RT and Thien T (2004). Blood pressure measurement: we should all do it better! *Netherlands Journal of Medicine*, **62**(8), 297–303.

National Institute for Health and Clinical Excellence (2006). *Hypertension: management of hypertension in adults in primary care*. London: NICE. [online] **http://guidance.nice.org.uk/CG34/niceguidance/pdf/English** accessed 17/12/08.

O'Brien E (2003). Demise of the mercury sphygmomanometer and the dawning of a new era in blood pressure measurement. *Blood Pressure Monitoring*, **8**, 19–21.

O'Brien E, Asmer R, Beilin L *et al.* (2003). European Society of Hypertension recommendations for conventional, ambulatory and home blood pressure measurement. *Journal of Hypertension*, **21**, 821–48.

Quinn M (1994). Automated blood pressure measurement devices: a potential source of morbidity in preeclampsia? *American Journal of Obstetrics and Gynaecology*, **170**, 1303–07.

Tortora GL and Derrickson B (2006). *Principles of anatomy and physiology*, 11th edition. Wiley, New York.

Willacy H (2007). *Accelerated hypertension*. PatientPlus [on-line] **http://www.patient.co.uk/showdoc/40000569/** accessed 17/12/08.

Williams B, Poulter NR, Brown MJ *et al.* (2004). British Hypertension Society guidelines for hypertension management (BHS-IV): summary. *British Medical Journal*, **328**, 634–40.

Woods SL, Sivarajan Froclicher ES, and Underhill Motzer S (2000). *Cardiac nursing*, 4th edition. Lippincott Williams and Wilkins, Philadelphia.

Woodrow P (2000). *Intensive care nursing: a framework for practice*. Routledge, London.

Yarows SA, Patel K, and Brook R (2001). Rapid oscillometric blood pressure measurement compared to conventional oscillometric measurement. *Blood Pressure Monitoring*, **6**(3), 145–47.

Useful further reading and websites

The British Hypertension Society website has many useful resources and plenty of information about the condition and its management: **http://www.bhsoc.org/default.stm**

 Answers to patient scenarios

1 The patient has a weak or irregular pulse and you will need to use a manual device to attempt to gain a reading.

2 Record when you heard the start of phase 4 of the Korotkoff sounds as the diastolic blood pressure.

3 Palpate for a radial pulse in the left arm to determine its presence if you have not already done so when measuring the pulse. If you can palpate a radial pulse then the brachial should also be present. Try fully extending or hyperextending the left arm, as long as this causes the person no distress. Start palpating from the midline of the antecubital fossa and work your fingers medially. Make sure you are not pressing too hard or being too gentle. If you are still unable to locate a brachial pulse in the left arm try locating it in the right arm. If unable to locate either, ask for help from an experienced colleague.

6.4 Measuring and recording capillary refill time

Definition

Capillary refill time (CRT) is a non-invasive test used to gain a rapid 'snapshot' assessment of adequate tissue perfusion in a patient. Capillary refill is the rate at which blood refills empty capillaries after they have been emptied by external pressure. The subsequent recorded filling time may offer vital clues about a patient's cardiovascular status. The importance of CRT is based on the assumption that skin perfusion is a valid indicator of peripheral and central vascular status.

Other recognized names for the CRT test include subcutaneous venous plexus filling time, subpapillary plexus filling time, capillary fill time, and capillary return test. The extensive use of CRT has occurred despite an absence of sound research evidence to substantiate its effectiveness, and its popularity may be due to the fact that the test is easily conducted and doesn't require expensive pieces of equipment.

It is important to remember that:

- Capillary refilling time is a measurement of the time required to reperfuse the skin, and therefore an indirect measurement of the actual perfusion of that part of the body. It is not a single diagnostic test for any specific illness, injury, or disease, and should only be used in conjunction with other methods of examination and assessment.
- Factors such as patient's age, prescribed pharmacological vasodilators or constrictors, low body temperatures, and cold environments may affect the refilling time and make the clinical findings unreliable as a diagnostic tool. In addition, the presence of health factors such as arteriosclerosis, circulation-based anomalies (e.g. Raynaud's phenomenon), and the presence of neurogenic shock can all give unreliable results and render CRT a less valuable tool in the evaluation of circulatory adequacy (National Association of Emergency Medical Technicians 2006). A prolonged CRT should be interpreted in parallel with other circulatory parameters (Evans and Tippins 2007).

Prior knowledge

Before using the CRT test, make sure you are familiar with:

- Cardiovascular anatomy and physiology.
- Pathophysiology of common illnesses and injuries (e.g. clinical shock, dehydration, etc.).
- Mechanism of oxygen transport to the tissues.

Review of these three areas will assist you in understanding the relevance of CRT.

Background

Tissue survival is not only dependent on nutrients but also requires a constant supply of oxygen, delivered via the respiratory and cardiovascular systems (see Table 7.2, Section 7.2, for the four-stage journey of oxygen from the atmosphere to the tissues). Tissue perfusion is reliant on adequate blood pressure in the aorta, which in turn is determined by cardiac output and peripheral resistance. Cardiac output itself (the volume of blood ejected from the left ventricle in 1 minute) is a product of heart rate and stroke volume.

CRT measures the function of the vascular system and the adequacy of oxygen delivery to the distal parts of the body, notably the peripheral extremities. When hypoperfusion develops, the body 'shuts down' circulation to the extremities (parts of the body furthest from the heart) first and restores it last. This is because the skin is not a priority when oxygen demand is high and oxygenated blood is diverted to vital organs. This is known as the adrenergic response or 'fight or flight' syndrome and is used as a compensatory mechanism to maintain oxygen delivery to the body organs that need it the most. Peripheral vasoconstriction is initiated and the redirection of blood flow is often referred to as central shunting (Evans and Tippins 2007). Evaluation of CRT may provide early indication that hypoperfusion is developing.

Primarily used in the assessment of paediatric patients, CRT is thought to be most reliable in children younger than 12 years of age (Sanders 2006). Refill time in adults is not considered as accurate due to differences in circulation caused by medications and various other factors. However, CRT is widely and traditionally used as a measure of a patient's **peripheral perfusion**. One of the earliest descriptions of its use dates back to 1924, when Buerger described the assessment of vascular disease by skin blanching and measuring the time taken for skin colour to return (Klupp and Keenan 2007).

CRT can be measured from peripheral locations such as a nail bed (nail plate), the fleshy part of a distal phalanx, or the fleshy eminence at the base of the thumb (see **Figure 6.12**). For central CRT, location sites such as the patient's forehead and sternum can be used (see **Figure 6.13**).

Context

 When to perform a CRT test

This skill can be performed as a rapid assessment method for evaluating a patient's circulation. CRT may be used as an indicator for conditions such as:

- Clinical shock (such as hypovolaemia)
- Heart failure
- Dehydration
- Arterial disruption from soft tissue damage or fractures
- Hypothermia
- Peripheral vascular disease (arteriosclerosis)

(a)

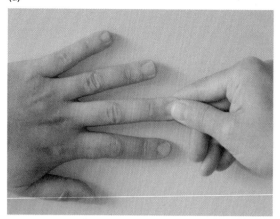

(b)

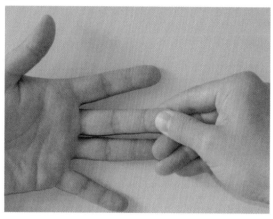

(c)

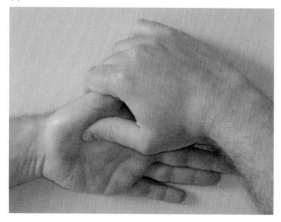

Figure 6.12 Peripheral locations to measure CRT: (a) nail bed; (b) fleshy part of a distal phalanx; (c) fleshy eminence at the base of the thumb.

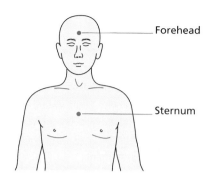

Figure 6.13 Central locations of CRT points (sternum and forehead).

This is not an exhaustive list, but it includes all conditions that manifest poor perfusion and subsequently reduce capillary refill time.

CRT is also commonly used as part of the criteria for 'sieving' patients (a primary triaging method used in major incidents), which is the preferred alternative method to taking a pulse (Advanced Life Support Group 2002). This is thought to be because measuring CRT is faster than a timed pulse assessment and, when there are large numbers of patients to triage, time is of the essence. However, environmental factors may affect the readings (i.e. if it is cold).

When not to perform a CRT

Hodgetts *et al.* (1998) identified practical problems with measuring CRT in adverse lighting conditions. This makes it difficult to detect the colour of blood returning to the capillary bed and so CRT is unreliable in certain out-of-hospital circumstances.

Additional interventions

Additional interventions may include systematic observation, pulse, blood pressure, respiratory rate, etc. depending on patient presentation.

In fact, recent research evidence indicates that inter-rater reliability and validity of CRT is increasingly being brought into question. Cruse (2004) conducted a literature review of relevant articles on CRT and concluded that CRT in isolation does not provide sufficient information about a patient's cardiovascular status, and that other haemo-dynamic variables are needed for a general bedside assessment. An evaluation of CRT by Klupp and Keenan (2007) found that both intra- and inter-tester comparisons produced clinically significant error and that the use of CRT for assessment of microvascular and macrovascular disease states of the lower limb should also be questioned.

Potential problems

CRT is a quick and easy technique, but results can be inaccurate or misleading when the patient is in poorly lit situations or is cold or peripherally shut down. If you are taking a CRT in a cold environment, measure your own CRT to establish a 'normal' baseline and compare this to the patient's. Remember also that different skin pigmentations indicate the need to observe normal skin colour for the patient prior to the test.

Indications for assistance

If CRT is outside of normal parameters (see Interpreting readings box) then assistance should be requested, particularly where there are additional signs and symptoms of inadequate circulation and impaired cardiovascular function, e.g. abnormal respiratory rates, cyanosis, abnormal pulses, hypotension, thirst, or diaphoretic skin.

Interpreting readings

Capillary refill time	Interpretation
<2 seconds	Patient appears to have normal perfusion.
>2 seconds	Possible causes to consider may be: ■ Shock. ■ Dehydration. ■ Arterial disruption. ■ Hypothermia. ■ Peripheral vascular disease.

Procedure: taking a peripheral CRT

Preparation

There is no risk associated with CRT and the test requires no preparation in order to conduct it. However, you should explain to the patient why you need to perform it and that they may feel minor discomfort where pressure is applied. Remember to apply infection control measures by washing hands prior to patient contact and if necessary wear examination gloves.

Step-by-step guide to taking a peripheral CRT

Step	Rationale
1 Introduce yourself, confirm the patient's identity, explain the procedure, and obtain consent.	To identify the patient correctly and gain informed consent.
2 Clean hands prior to conducting the procedure using the recommended local practice method of hand washing. If necessary, wear examination gloves before touching the patient.	Infection control measures.
3 Locate position for CRT. CRT can be measured by applying gentle pressure to a nail bed of a digit or the pad of a distal phalanx (see **Figure 6.14**). Alternatively, you can use the soft prominence at the base of the thumb.	A vascular area is needed to observe a distinct colour change.

continued overleaf

4 Where possible any extremity used should always be positioned at approximately the same level as the patient's heart when conducting the test.

This will ensure the assessment of arteriolar capillary and not venous stasis refill (Jevon 2007). Incorrect limb placement may cause venous drainage/engorgement.

5 Explain to the patient that they may feel minor discomfort caused by gentle pressure.

So the patient can prepare themselves for mild discomfort.

6 If using the patient's nail bed, inspect for nail varnish. This can either be removed prior to the procedure or a different position can be used.

Nail varnish would obscure any colour changes.

7 Blanch the skin/nail bed by firmly pressing with your thumb on the area for five seconds (see Figure 6.14a).

Pressure forces blood from the capillaries (Resuscitation Council UK 2006).

8 Release the pressure. Immediately confirm that the site has been blanched by the pressure and observe the time it takes for normal colour to return to the skin/nail bed (or the same colour as the surrounding skin) (see Figure 6.4b and c). Jevon (2007) suggests a useful way of doing this is to count 'one thousand, two thousand, three thousand' and so on – with each number equating to one second.

To observe the return and resupply of blood to the area.

9 Note the CRT in seconds. Document the findings within the patient notes by annotating whether the CRT is <2 seconds or >2 seconds. It is sometimes useful to record the actual time (i.e. 1 second, 3 seconds, 5 seconds, etc.). Also record the site or sites from which these readings were obtained.

A delay in the return of blood of >2 seconds to the compressed vascular area may indicate underlying circulatory compromise.

10 Analyse results. Capillary refill should be prompt (<2 seconds) suggesting adequate skin perfusion. A slow CRT (>2 seconds) suggests inadequate skin perfusion.

Abnormally slow CRT may be indicative of:
- Dehydration.
- Shock.
- Peripheral vascular disease (PVD).
- Hypothermia.
- Arterial disruption.

11 Wash your hands using Ayliffe method and dispose of examination gloves appropriately.

Maintain infection control measures.

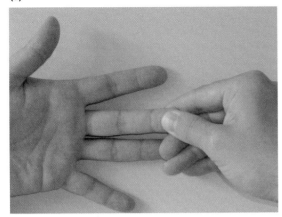

(a)

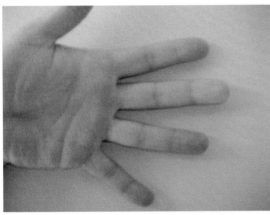

(b)

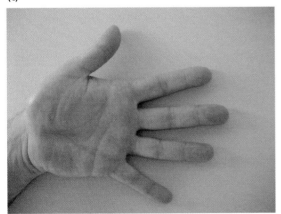

(c)

Figure 6.14 How to measure CRT: (a) apply gentle pressure to the digit; (b) observe the time it takes for blanching to return to normal colour; (c) normal colour returns to digit.

Following the procedure

It is important that other signs, symptoms, and tests are conducted to assess the status of the patient's cardiovascular function. If there is cause for concern, ask for help or advice.

Recognizing patient deterioration

For patients with prolonged CRT, additional measurements can be taken on the opposite limb for comparison of timings. This is useful if the hypoperfusion is localized to one side of the body.

If prolonged CRT is encountered on both limbs, then measure a central CRT on the sternum or the forehead to investigate the extent of the hypoperfusion further.

Use other methods of cardiovascular assessment to corroborate your findings. Remember that CRT on its own is not a definitive test but an early indicator. Use it in the context of the other tests and with the information from previous observations. Seek help from senior members of staff where necessary.

Reflection and evaluation

When you have undertaken a CRT test, think about the following:

- Consider all the factors that may produce an abnormal CRT.
- Think about whether you need to take another CRT on another location of the body to compare against the first reading.
- Did you use CRT in conjunction with other diagnostic assessment to identify an underlying cause?
- Remember that different skin pigmentations indicate the need to observe normal skin colour for the patient prior to the test, or to observe return to the same colour as the surrounding skin.

Further learning opportunities

- Practise CRT on different locations of the body and be familiar with optimal sites for different age groups.
- Measure your own CRT in a cold environment and see how a change in ambient temperature can affect a previously normal refill time.

Reminders

Remember always to interpret a prolonged CRT in context with other cardiovascular measurements and the environment.

 Patient scenarios

1 Patient A has been brought into the Accident and Emergency department of your hospital with a head injury after being found by paramedics. He has spent the night on the floor in his kitchen following a fall and has been unable to get up. He appears confused and his skin is pale and cold to the touch. CRT is recorded as >2 seconds. What are the potential causes of this reading and what factors should you consider that may affect the validity of the reading?

2 Patient B has been admitted to hospital with a fracture to the tibia. On examination you find that distal to the fracture site her skin looks pale and cyanosed. What location would you select for taking a CRT and what other observations would you need to confirm your findings?

Website

 http://www.oxfordtextbooks.co.uk/orc/ endacott

You may find it helpful to work through our short online quiz and additional scenarios intended to help you to develop and apply the skills in this chapter.

References

Advanced Life Support Group (2002). *Major incident medical management and support: the practical approach at scene*, 2nd edition. BMJ Publishing Group, London.

Cruse L (2004). Psychological measures in intensive care, *Paediatric Nursing*, **16**(9), 14–7.

Evans C and Tippins E (2007). *The foundations of emergency care*. McGraw-Hill, Maidenhead.

Hodgetts TJ, Hall J, Maconochie I, and Smart C (1998). Paediatric triage tape. *Pre-Hospital Immediate Care*, **2**, 155–9.

Jevon P (2007). Measuring capillary refill time. *Nursing Times*, **103**(12), 26–7.

Klupp NL and Keenan A (2007). An evaluation of the reliability and validity of capillary refill time test. *The Foot*, **17**(1) 15–20.

National Association of Emergency Medical Technicians (2006). *PHTLS: Prehospital Trauma Life Support*, 6th edition. Mosby/JEMS, Missouri.

Resuscitation Council UK (2006). *Advanced life support*, 6th edition. Resuscitation Council UK, London.

Sanders MJ (2006). *Mosby's paramedic textbook*. Mosby, Missouri.

Useful further reading and websites

Advanced Life Support Group (2005). *Pre-hospital paediatric life support*, 2nd Edition. Blackwell Publishing, London.

http://www.nda.ox.ac.uk/wfsa/html/u10/ u1002_02.htm

 Answers to patient scenarios

1 The patient may be hypothermic having spent the night on the floor, or he may have underlying clinical shock as a result of the trauma. Alternatively, he may be dehydrated or have pre-existing heart failure prior to the fall. Hence the importance of conducting a comprehensive patient examination and history, to rule out other injuries and illnesses apart from the obvious.

2 Obtaining a CRT measurement distal to the injury is useful, to obtain an indication of arterial or circulatory damage caused by the fracture. This should then be compared to a CRT measurement on the opposite (unaffected) limb. This will then determine if any abnormal CRT is local to that fractured limb or is widespread as a result of clinical shock. Other observations should include taking the peripheral pulse distal to the fracture.

6.5 **ECG monitoring**

Definition

An **electrocardiogram** (ECG) is a recording of the electrical activity of the heart, which is shown as an electrical waveform on the ECG trace. ECG monitoring is a valuable

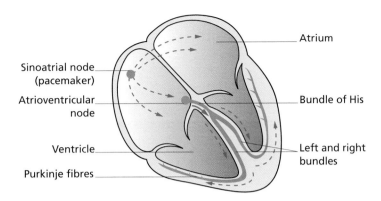

Figure 6.15 Electrical conduction through the heart.

diagnostic tool in medicine and is essential in recognizing cardiac arrhythmias. It can also alert nursing staff to changes in the patient's condition, and can assist with diagnostic decisions (Jevon 2003).

It is important to remember that:

- ECG monitoring must be meticulously undertaken. Potential consequences of poor technique include misinterpretation of cardiac arrhythmias, mistaken diagnosis, wasted investigations, and patient mismanagement. Electrode placement may vary, so check local policies prior to performing the skill.
- When a cardiac arrhythmia occurs, the ECG trace recorded by a single-lead cardiac monitor is not always sufficient to enable accurate interpretation of the rhythm. A 12-lead ECG should therefore be recorded wherever possible (Resuscitation Council UK 2006) (see Section 6.13, *Performing a 12-lead electrocardiogram*).

Prior knowledge

Before attempting ECG monitoring, make sure you are familiar with:

1 Anatomy and physiology of the heart.
2 The pathology of common cardiac conditions, e.g. myocardial infarction/ischaemia, ventricular hypertrophy, arrhythmias.

Background

Normal electrical conduction (cell depolarization) through the heart (see **Figure** 6.15) starts at the sinoatrial (SA) node, also known as the 'pacemaker'. A wave of electrical conduction spreads across the atria generating the 'P wave' on an ECG.

This is followed by a slowed rate of conduction through the atrioventricular (AV) node, down the bundle of His and into the right and left ventricles through Purkinje fibres. On an ECG recording this is translated as a straight section (an isoelectric line) representing the delay in transmission through the AV node, followed by a QRS wave depicting left and right ventricular contraction.

Finally the conducting system and ventricular myocardium recover by repolarization, which is depicted as a T wave on the ECG. This normal full sequence is known as sinus rhythm (see **Figure** 6.16 for an illustration of the wave sequence).

Context

 When to perform ECG monitoring

Reasons to monitor the ECG include:

- Patients with chest pain.
- Patients with suspected myocardial infarction.
- Patients with palpitations.
- Patients with a history of syncope.
- Shocked patients.

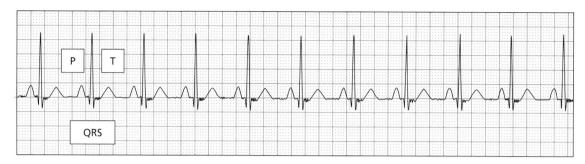

Figure 6.16 A normal ECG. The P wave represents the contraction that starts in the atrium. The QRS wave represents the ventricles contracting. The T wave represents ventricular recovery.

- Patients with bradycardia/tachycardia.
- Patients in heart failure.
- During cardiopulmonary resuscitation (CPR).

Additional (and alternative) interventions

While ECG monitoring, it may also be necessary to:

- Take a pulse (see Section 6.2) for:
  - cardiac output (carotid pulse)
  - volume (central and peripheral pulses)
  - rate and rhythm (to ensure they match the monitor).
- Listen to the heart (auscultation – see Section 6.14) for heart sounds.

Common features of a cardiac monitor

Common features of an oscilloscope or cardiac monitor include:

- A screen for displaying the ECG trace – usually fitted with a switch to adjust the level of brightness.
- Heart rate counter – calculates the heart rate by counting the QRS complexes.
- Monitor alarms – alarms can be set to alert at specified heart rates and in more advanced machines can alert for specific ECG changes.
- A lead select switch – adjusted to select the preferred monitoring lead, e.g. Lead II.
- ECG gain – changes the size of the ECG complex.
- ECG printing – for printing records (very useful for diagnosis of arrhythmias).
  (Jevon 2003)

Alternative methods of ECG recording

Monitoring through defibrillation paddles It is possible to monitor the ECG through most manual defibrillation machines. Paddles should be placed on defibrillation pads on the right sternal margin below the clavicle and in the anterior axial line at the fifth intercostal space. This procedure is only suitable for a 'quick look' (Resuscitation Council UK 2006).

Self-adhesive defibrillation and monitoring pads Some defibrillators also enable the use of selfadhesive electrode pads, which should be placed as for defibrillation paddles. This is a more effective system of monitoring than defibrillation paddles.

Five ECG cable system In the *Procedure* section we describe the three ECG cable system; however, cardiac monitoring using a five ECG cable system is increasing in popularity. The system has the advantage of being able to monitor different ECG leads at the same time. This is very useful for the analysis of cardiac arrhythmias as it provides alternative views of the waveform (Jevon 2003).

Standard positioning for the five ECG electrodes is (note: colour coding systems may differ):

- RA (red ECG cable) – right shoulder.
- LA (yellow ECG cable) – left shoulder.
- RL (black ECG cable) – right lower thorax/hip region.
- LL (green ECG cable) – left lower thorax/hip region.
- White ECG cable – on the chest in the desired position, usually V1 (fourth intercostal space just right of the sternum). This is known as modified chest lead V1 (MCL1) (see Box 6.2) (adapted from Jacobson 2000).

Box 6.2 MCL1

Modified chest lead V1 (MCL1) enables differentiation between ventricular ectopic beats and aberrantly conducted supraventricular beats, and clearly demonstrates the P wave (Jowett and Thompson 2003). MCL1 can be viewed using the ECG electrode position described for the five ECG cable monitoring system or with a modified ECG electrode position for using a three ECG cable system (see *Procedure* section).

Telemetry Telemetry is a method of monitoring the ECG while the patient is mobilizing. ECG electrodes are connected to a small portable transmitter, which the patient carries in a pouch on their clothing. Radio signals are transmitted to a central console (e.g. at the nurses' station in a coronary care unit) and any cardiac arrhythmias can be identified without restricting the patient to their bed (Jevon 2003). The advantage of this system is that monitored beds can be freed up and patients can be mobilized early, yet still benefit from close cardiac monitoring (Jowett 1997).

Ambulatory cardiac monitoring (24-hour tape) Ambulatory cardiac monitoring records an ECG over a 24-hour period, identifying transient ECG disturbances with any associated symptoms (Hampton 2003), for example ischaemic changes, the effectiveness of anti-arrhythmic drug therapy, and the frequency of arrhythmias.

The patient continues their daily activities while keeping a diary, logging, for example, dizziness, palpitations, pain, and syncope. An 'event marker' button may be available on some machines for patients to press at the onset of symptoms.

Exercise testing Exercise stress testing is usually used for diagnosis of patients with suspected coronary artery disease. It helps to evaluate the efficacy of medical therapy, assess disability, and select patients for cardiac transplantation (Woods *et al*. 2000).

The main aims of exercise testing are:

- Chest pain assessment.
- Prognosis assessment.
- Exercise-related symptom assessment.
  (Jowett and Thompson 2003)

Severe coronary artery disease may be diagnosed dependent on the blood pressure response, exercise time, and the degree of ST segment shift (Jowett and Thompson 2003). Exercise testing may be contraindicated for a number of reasons including recent myocardial infarction, unstable angina, arrhythmias, aortic stenosis, myocarditis or pericarditis, and heart failure (Jowett and Thompson 2003). Resuscitation facilities must always be available during testing as life-threatening arrhythmias can occur.

Indications for assistance

Call for help immediately if there is no detectable pulse and/or significant ECG abnormalities (see **Figure 6.17**). If you have problems monitoring and recording an ECG, refer to your technical department for advice.

Interpreting readings

Some basic arrhythmias are identified in Figure 6.17. The reader should refer to a text on ECG analysis for a full explanation (e.g. Resuscitation Council UK 2006 or Hampton 2003).

Special considerations

There may be normal changes to the ECG reading in, for example:

- Children.
- Black people.
- Tall people.
- Obese people.
- Athletes.
- Pregnancy.

Hampton (2003)

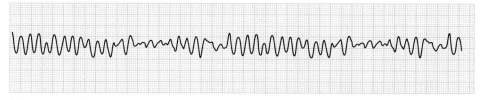

(a) Ventricular fibrillation: the patient is in cardiac arrest and requires immediate defibrillation.

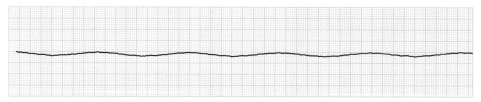

(b) Asystole: the patient is in cardiac arrest and requires resuscitation procedures.

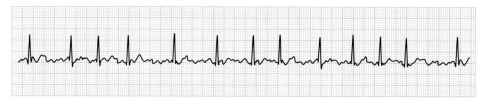

(c) Atrial fibrillation: treat the primary cause and/or give prescribed medication, e.g. digoxin, to control ventricular rate.

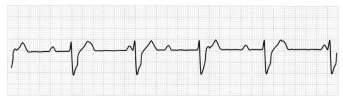

(d) Complete heart block (third degree): treatment depends on symptoms but is likely to include cardiac pacing.

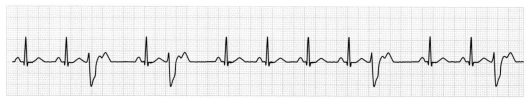

(e) Sinus rhythm with ventricular ectopics: treatment depends on the frequency of the ectopics (a few may be normal) and may require correction of underlying cause, e.g. hyperkalaemia and hypoxia.

Figure 6.17 ECG arrhythmias.

The procedure

Preparation

Prepare yourself
Consider how you will position the ECG electrodes using the three ECG cable system.

The standard positioning of ECG electrodes when using a three ECG cable monitoring system is shown in **Figure 6.18** and described below (note: colour coding systems may differ). This position ensures that the chest remains clear should resuscitation and defibrillation be required (Resuscitation Council UK 2006).

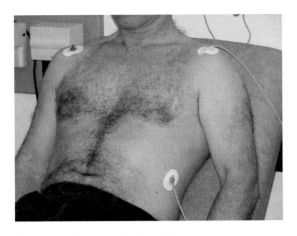

Figure 6.18 Three ECG leads positioning.

- RA (red ECG cable) – right shoulder.
- LA (yellow ECG cable) – left shoulder.
- RL/LL (black or green ECG cable) – left abdominal or lower left chest wall.

Lead II (set on the monitor's lead select switch) tends to be the standard monitoring lead as it provides a good recording of atrial (P waves) and ventricular activity (QRS waves), enabling cardiac arrhythmias to be identified.

Alternative forms of monitoring include MCL1 (modified chest lead 1, i.e. V1 – see Box 6.2) (Jowett and Thompson 2003). The positioning of ECG electrodes is:

- RL/LL (black or green ECG cable) – right shoulder.
- RA (red ECG cable) – left shoulder.
- LA (yellow ECG cable) – fourth intercostal space, just to the right of the sternum, i.e. corresponding to V1.

Prepare the patient

Where possible, the ECG machine is best placed to the patient's left side to facilitate optimum lead placement. Positioning of the electrodes will be influenced by the needs of the patient (e.g. consideration of skin lesions and injuries), equipment availability, manufacturer's recommendations, and local protocol. Applicable positioning will ensure accurate information is obtained (Jacobson 2000).

Prepare the equipment

Prepare the following equipment:

- Skin cleansers (e.g. alcohol wipes).
- Razor.
- Gauze pads.
- ECG electrodes.
- ECG cables.
- ECG monitor.

Step-by-step guide to establishing ECG monitoring

 Step | **Rationale**

Step	Rationale
1 Introduce yourself, confirm the patient's identity, explain the procedure, and obtain consent.	To identify the patient correctly and gain informed consent.
2 For greasy skin, clean with a mild soap or an alcohol wipe. If the patient is sweating profusely, apply a small amount of tincture benzoin to the skin and leave it to dry (Jowett 1997).	To ensure electrodes stick to the skin and that there is good electrical contact.
3 Shave dense hair.	To ensure better contact and to reduce discomfort when removing electrodes (Resuscitation Council UK 2006 and Society for Cardiological Science and Technology 2006).
4 Rub the skin gently with some gauze.	Mild abrasion of the skin reduces impedance between the skin and electrode (Jowett 1997).

continued overleaf

5	Check the ECG electrodes have not passed their expiry date.	Electrodes can dry out, reducing their effectiveness.
6	Expose the gel disc by removing the protective backing from electrodes.	To enable the electrode to be stuck to the skin.
7	Following locally agreed protocols, place the ECG electrodes onto the patient's chest, ensuring that they lie flat. Point electrodes with an offset connector in the direction of the electrodes (to absorb tugs). Ensure leads do not track across the patient's chest (see Figure 6.18).	To ensure applicable monitoring and to ensure the chest is kept clear of leads in case resuscitation is required.
8	Smooth down the adhesive area using a circular motion but avoiding the gel disc (Thompson 1997).	Pressure on the gel disc may cause damage, reducing conductivity.
9	Attach the correct ECG cables to the electrodes. Note: if 'snap on' cables with central stud electrodes are in use, they must be connected prior to application to the skin.	To ensure monitoring is correct and that there is no damage to the electrode.
10	Turn on the monitor, selecting the required monitoring ECG lead (e.g. Lead II).	To commence monitoring in the applicable lead.
11	Check that the ECG trace is clear, rectifying any problems (see troubleshooting section).	To ensure that the ECG is clearly displayed.
12	Set the alarms applicable to the patient's condition and complying with local protocol.	To ensure patient safety.
13	Secure ECG cables appropriately.	To reduce pull on ECG electrodes.
14	Position the cardiac monitor so that it can be seen by health care staff.	To ensure monitor is clearly visible.
15	Record the commencement of monitoring and the cardiac rhythm in the patient's notes.	To ensure accurate record keeping.
16	Observe the electrode sites regularly and change electrodes and their position (approximately every 3 days) (Adam and Osborne 2005).	To identify signs of skin irritation/allergy and to ensure electrodes remain moist.

(Adapted from Jevon 2003)

Following the procedure

Report any abnormalities to a senior member of staff. Monitoring problems and their resolution are discussed below.

ECG monitoring problems and troubleshooting

(Adapted from Jevon 2003)

'Flat line' ECG trace

- Check the patient – do they require resuscitation?
- Check to see if an appropriate ECG monitoring lead has been selected (e.g. Lead II).
- Check the ECG gain. Has the ECG machine's automatic gain setting been over-ridden by a low setting?
- Are the cables correctly connected to the ECG electrodes?
- Are the ECG cables broken or not plugged into the monitor?

Poor quality ECG trace

- Check the connections.
- Check the brightness display.
- Are the ECG electrodes 'in date', moist, and correctly attached (Perez 1996)?

Movement artefact

Movement artefact is usually caused by patient movement, often during respiration (Moule and Albarran 2005). Reducing cable movement or changing electrode positions may help (Jowett 1997). Patients with a rigor (tremor) should be reassured and kept warm where applicable.

Wandering ECG baseline

A wandering ECG baseline may be caused by patient movement, but where there is a sudden break in the signal it is often due to a loose electrode or a damaged lead. Try repositioning the electrodes over clean, dry skin or if necessary replacing the leads.

Electrical interference

Electrical interference can cause disruption to the ECG trace. Remove the source of the interference where possible.

Small ECG complexes

If the display appears to be too small, try repositioning the electrodes and check that the gain and monitoring lead have been selected correctly. Note, however, that ECG complexes can be reduced in size where there is a pericardial effusion, hypothyroidism, or obesity.

Incorrect heart rate display

If you suspect that the heart rate display is inaccurate, check pulses and auscultate the heart (see Sections 6.2 and 6.14). Heart rate displays can be displayed incorrectly when the ECG complexes are too small, or where large T waves, interference, and muscle movement become confused with QRS complexes. This may be due to electrical interference, poor electrode contact, or incorrect lead settings or gain.

False alarms

False alarms can be due to incorrect settings or poor electrode connections. These should be corrected immediately to ensure patient safety and to alleviate patient anxiety.

Skin irritation

Electrode sites should be examined regularly for redness, erythema, and itching. If irritation occurs, change the electrode site (Adam and Osborne 2005), or if applicable use hypoallergenic ECG electrodes (Thompson 1997).

Recognizing patient deterioration

- Observe the patient and the ECG for changes.
- Treat cardiac arrest and associated rhythms immediately.
- Identify known (and unknown) arrhythmias and report to senior members of staff.

NOTE: a normal rhythm on the ECG monitor does not necessarily mean that the patient has a cardiac output. In pulseless electrical activity (PEA) cardiac arrests, a normal rhythm may be seen but the patient may not have a pulse, so do not rely solely on ECG monitoring.

Reflection and evaluation

When you have established ECG monitoring, consider the following questions:

- Did the ECG recording match your observations of the patient and their basic parameters (e.g. pulse rate)?
- Did you understand the need for an ECG and the procedure for attaching a monitor?
- Were you able to interpret the ECG rhythm?

Further learning opportunities

You may wish to improve your skills by:

- Attaching the leads in different positions to see how the trace is altered.
- Printing off ECG rhythms you are unsure of and checking them in a textbook (e.g. Hampton 2003). Discuss your findings with colleagues.

Reminders

Don't forget to:

- Adequately prepare the skin prior to electrode placement.
- Use 'in date', moist electrodes.
- Position electrodes as per locally agreed protocol.
- Set cardiac monitoring alarms to the patient's clinical condition.
- Ensure the ECG trace is accurate.
- Report any arrhythmias immediately.

Patient scenarios

1 After commencing ECG monitoring on Mr Smith, you notice that only a straight line is displayed on the monitor. What would you do?
2 The heart rate indicator on the ECG displays 80, but the patient is unconscious and appears to be lifeless. What would you do?

Website

 http://www.oxfordtextbooks.co.uk/orc/ endacott

You may find it helpful to work through our short online quiz and additional scenarios intended to help you to develop and apply the skills in this chapter.

References

Adam SK and Osborne S (2005). *Critical care nursing. Science and practice.* Oxford University Press, Oxford.

Hampton JR (2003). *The ECG in practice.* Churchill Livingstone, London.

Jacobson C (2000). Optimum bedside cardiac monitoring. *Progress in Cardiovascular Nursing*, **15**(4), 134–7.

Jevon P (2003). *ECGs for nurses.* Blackwell Publishing, Oxford.

Jowett NI (1997). *Cardiovascular monitoring.* Whurr Publishers Ltd, London.

Jowett NI and Thompson DR (2003). *Comprehensive coronary care*, 3rd edition. Bailliere Tindall, London.

Moule P and Albarran J, eds (2005). *Practical resuscitation: recognition and response.* Blackwell Publishing, Oxford.

Perez A (1996). Cardiac monitoring: mastering the essentials. *Registered Nurse*, **59**(8), 32–9.

Resuscitation Council UK (2005). *Resuscitation guidelines 2005.* Resuscitation Council UK, London.

Resuscitation Council UK (2006). *Advanced life support*, 5th edition. Resuscitation Council UK, London.

Society for Cardiological Science and Technology (2006). *Clinical guidelines by consensus. Recording a standard 12-lead electrocardiogram. An approved methodology.* British Cardiovascular Society, UK.

Thompson P (1997). *Coronary care manual.* Churchill Livingstone, London.

Woods SL, Sivarajan Froelicher ES, and Underhill Motzer S (2000). *Cardiac nursing*, 4th edition. Lippincott Williams and Wilkins, Philadelphia.

Useful further reading and websites

Hampton JR (2003). *The ECG made easy.* Churchill Livingstone, London.

Gardiner J (2005). *The ECG: what does it tell?* Nelson Thornes, Cheltenham.

Answers to patients scenarios

1

- Check that the patient is alive.
- Check that the correct monitoring lead is selected (usually Lead II).
- Check that the ECG gain (size) is set correctly (not too low).
- Check that the ECG leads are connected to the electrodes on the patient.

2

- Request immediate help (and resuscitation status if unknown).

- Assess the patient's vital signs, following basic life support guidelines (Resuscitation Council UK 2005).
- Commence CPR as required.

(NB treat the patient, not the monitor.)

6.6 **Assessing and recording fluid balance**

Definition

Fluid balance is the maintenance of the correct amount of fluid in the body. Fluid balance can alter with disease and illness. Body fluids are regulated by fluid intake, hormonal controls, and fluid output (Potter and Perry 2001).

It is important to remember that:

- Visual observation can give a good indication of the patient's hydration status.
- A patient's condition can fluctuate rapidly and it is essential to monitor vulnerable patients closely.

Prior knowledge

Before attempting this skill, make sure you are familiar with:

1 Cellular anatomy.
2 Movement of fluids within the body – intracellular and extracellular compartments.

Background

In order to monitor a patient's fluid balance it is essential to understand how fluid in the body is stored and what happens within a normal individual, as well as what the clinical signs of a fluid imbalance are.

Water moves freely between the intracellular and extracellular compartments of the body, delivering oxygen and nutrients to tissues while removing waste products such as carbon dioxide and metabolic acids, resulting in a very fine balance being maintained. Fluid, whether from a cup of tea or an intravenous infusion, transfers into interstitial and then intracellular fluid compartments.

Typically most water loss is in urine, with the kidneys being able to increase or decrease urine volume to maintain total body fluid balance. This is regulated by hormones, especially antidiuretic hormone (ADH).

Fluid balance between compartments varies, both in health and in ill health. In health, body water volume is mainly affected by the amount of body fat. Fat repels water, whereas muscle contains relatively large amounts of water. Generally, obese people have fewer stores of water than muscular people. In ill health or impaired function of body systems (especially the kidneys), fluid imbalances can result in complications for other organs.

Oedema is the presence of excessive extravascular fluid, which may be interstitial or intracellular, or both. Many acute and chronic diseases, such as heart failure, cause interstitial oedema, which may also be caused by excessive IV fluid administration. This is seen clinically with patients often presenting with swollen ankles or pulmonary oedema with dyspnoea.

Intracellular oedema is not easy to detect but causes more problems. Damage to the sodium–potassium pump system causes sodium to move into the cell, drawing water in with it, increasing the cell volume. This places excessive pressure on the already damaged cell membrane, ultimately resulting in cell death. If enough cells are affected, widespread cell death and organ failure will result (Woodrow 2002).

In contrast, dehydration occurs when water loss exceeds water intake and the body is in negative balance. It can occur as a result of haemorrhage, hypovolaemia, severe burns, prolonged bouts of diarrhoea and vomiting, profuse sweating, or diuretic abuse. In addition to water loss there may be an electrolyte disturbance, which can affect the normal functioning of the nervous system, heart, and kidneys. This accounts for some of the clinical signs of acute dehydration such as confusion, hallucinations, seizures, renal damage, coma, and eventually cardiovascular collapse and death (Longmore *et al.* 2004).

There are two types of dehydration – hyponatraemic and hypernatraemic.

Hypernatraemic dehydration is one of the simplest chemical disorders, arising usually when water intake is less than is needed to maintain balance. This is possible only for a limited period and can quickly be overwhelming. The renal tubules control this by passing out very concentrated urine. The high salt content of the extracellular fluid draws water out of the cells in order to compensate and the initial response is thirst to try and increase water intake. Often there is little change in the blood pressure or plasma sodium level due to this compensatory response. In severe hypernatraemia there can be mental confusion, hallucinations, and a dangerous reduction in renal blood flow. It is this type of dehydration to which older people are more vulnerable (Iggulden 1999).

Hyponatraemic dehydration occurs as a result of excessive fluid loss through trauma, burns, surgical intervention, or excessive diarrhoea and/or vomiting. It usually results in salt depletion as well as water depletion. Thirst is not usually experienced, **skin turgor** is poor, eyes rapidly look sunken, and the tongue is dry. The accompanying signs are those of shock and the disturbance may cause nausea and vomiting (Iggulden 1999).

Small but still significant amounts of body water are lost though other means, which are difficult to measure. This is known as insensible loss. The main sources of this loss are through perspiration, breathing, and faeces. It is important to consider loss from other sources such as from a **colostomy** or **ileostomy**. Normally insensible loss is estimated to be 500 ml (Tortora and Grabowski 2003) but there are factors that may increase or decrease insensible loss:

- Pyrexia (due to increasing perspiration)
- Diarrhoea/constipation
- Tachypnoea
- Breathing dry air or unhumidified oxygen

During ill health fluid loss from this source is thought to increase to 1 litre, especially if febrile, and it is estimated that in fever insensible losses increase by 100 ml/day/°C rise (Chapelhow and Crouch 2007). Although calculating these losses is difficult, this increased insensible loss can explain, or contribute to, dehydration.

Once a patient is assessed as being at risk of a fluid imbalance, close monitoring and observation of the patient is essential to observe for an improvement or deterioration. It is important to ensure that all documentation is comprehensively completed to allow accurate analysis of the data to be made. A study by Chung *et al.* in 2002 showed that of 250 patients, 50% had a fluid balance chart yet 32% of these were incomplete or inaccurate, thereby making the information useless. Common errors that render fluid balance charts unreliable according to Iggulden (1999) are:

- Failure to communicate with staff, clients, and their family.
- Tendency to guess at amounts, which over time increases the error margin considerably.
- Forgetting to record amounts when attempting to attend to several things at once.
- Assuming that the contents of an empty container have been drunk by the client.
- Attempting to standardize estimates of amount of loss from incontinence, diarrhoea, vomiting, or wound exudates.
- Lack of calibrated containers to record small amounts.

Context

One of the difficulties is knowing when to start, interpret, and stop the use of a fluid chart. This section tries to provide some guidance.

 ### When to use a fluid chart

For many organizations the administration of intravenous fluids dictates the need for a fluid chart. In addition, however, it should be used for those patients:

- Whose fluid intake is restricted.
- Whose urine output requires observation.
- Who are regularly vomiting or have drainage (e.g. surgical, gastric, colostomy) that requires monitoring.

 ### When not to use a fluid chart

- When there are no signs of fluid imbalance (bloods and physical appearance normal).
- Patient is catheterized but this is longstanding with no acute issues (check local policy).
- Fluid balance can be recorded by another method such as daily weighing.

Interpreting readings

When recording a patient's fluid balance it is essential to know what you are looking for in order to identify the potential areas of concern. Completing a fluid chart is not sufficient truly to manage the care of the patient effectively, as it is essential to have a good understanding of the underlying conditions that make a patient at risk of a fluid imbalance. A number of other assessments such as measurement of CRT, pulse, blood pressure, and full clinical examination make up a complete assessment of fluid balance. Fluid charts are an important factor in that assessment, but are not sufficient by themselves.

It is essential that a detailed medical and nursing assessment is performed that includes a patient history, physical examination, clinical observation, and the interpretation of laboratory results. (For information on blood results, see the Further reading section.)

Special considerations

Fluid balance should be continually monitored for patients who have already shown signs of fluid imbalance. Other patients at risk, for example patients who are critically ill or post-surgical, should be closely monitored. Fluid output recorded as 'passed urine + + +' or 'up to toilet' does not provide a clear indication of the amount of urine passed and results in total balance calculations not being possible.

As with most conditions, the ageing process has an effect on the body's ability to cope. The ability of the kidneys to fine-tune decreases with age, so that by the age of 80 a person's renal function is half of what it was when they were 40 (Holman *et al*. 2005). In the absence of disease it usually remains adequate to remove body waste, but, combined with other factors such as having less muscle and more fat, they may be at greater risk.

The prevalence of acute and chronic diseases in older people, such as chronic heart failure, makes them more susceptible to fluid imbalances. In addition to the physiological changes, physical limitations such as immobility or arthritis may discourage the elderly from getting drinks or **micturating** (Woodrow 2002). Experiencing ailments such as nocturia or incontinence may result in the individual restricting their fluid intake, which may result in not only dehydration but further problems such as urinary infection.

A patient's history should include information on their pre-morbid medical and physical well-being. A detailed account of the patient's normal and current fluid intake and output should be obtained to highlight the likelihood of a fluid problem. There are many factors that make a

patient vulnerable to fluid imbalance and the most common of these are listed in **Table 6.4**. While this is adapted from an article published in 1999, the principles remain unchanged.

Procedure: assessing fluid balance

Preparation

A clinical assessment of the patient should be carried out, in addition to recording vital observations such as blood pressure, pulse, respiration, and temperature. The patient's physical appearance should be noted, with particular attention being paid to the condition of the skin, tongue, and face (see **Table 6.5**).

Procedure: recording fluid balance

This will vary with different organizations, with some charting when a jug of water is removed while others measure each volume of fluid intake at the time it is taken. It is essential, however, to clarify that the patient has consumed the glass of water and not a visitor (this happens surprisingly often). Another great variation between organizations is how intravenous fluids are recorded on the fluid chart. Typically this is either calculated hourly or when the bag is completed; again, referral to local policy is required. Examples can be seen on charts 1 and 2.

Both charts are correct but it is essential to have a consistent approach in documentation in order to ensure accuracy.

(The intake and output totals have been completed on the charts but the column totals have been left blank. Why not practise totalling these to ensure you make the totals the same?)

While fluid charts can detect poor fluid balance, it is essential to act on this information and be aware of what is known as the cumulative total. This provides a more accurate picture of the patient's fluid status over a period of days. It is essential to calculate these correctly, as often some days will provide a total balance that is positive while other days they will give a negative total.

Chart 1

Time	Input		Total	Output			Total
	Oral	IVI		Drain (stomach)	Vomit	Urine	
16.00		125				30	
17.00	50	125		70		45	
18.00		125				40	
19.00		125				35	
20.00		125			300	70	
21.00	150	125		50		60	
22.00		125				50	
23.00		125				30	
24.00		125				200	
Total	Input total +1325			Output total −980			+345

Chart 2

Time	Input		Total	Output			Total
	Oral	IVI		Drain (stomach)	Vomit	Urine	
16.00		Bf 500				30/30	
17.00	50/50			70/70		45/75	
18.00						40/115	
19.00		1000/8 hours	500			35/150	
20.00					300	70/220	
21.00	150/200			50/120		60/280	
22.00						50/330	
23.00						30/360	
24.00			625			200/560	
Total	Input total +1325			Output total −980			+345

Example:

Date	Total balance (ml)	Cumulative total (ml)
1 Feb 2009	+1500	+1500
2 Feb	−900	+400
3 Feb	+300	+700

A fluid balance of minus 1000 ml may not be important on its own, but if the patient is post-operative and over the previous week the fluid balance reached minus 7000 ml, this is of concern. If the same figures are for a patient being treated with heart failure then this should be seen as a positive improvement. Understanding the rationale for the fluid balance recording is essential.

Procedure: daily weighing

If this is performed it is essential to record the weight using the same scales, at the same time of day, wearing similar clothes. Typically just after a wash in the morning is the favoured time. The best method to record this is using simple graph paper as it shows a visual

Table 6.4 Factors that increase the risk of fluid imbalance

Mobility	People with limited mobility may be at risk as they may not be able to meet their own hydration needs. Consider whether the patient is able to reach a drink or walk to the bathroom.
Digestion	People with physical symptoms that affect the gastric tract such as vomiting and diarrhoea are more susceptible to dehydration. Symptoms can be caused by the condition itself (e.g. irritable bowel syndrome) or the treatment (e.g. antibiotics).
Incontinence	Patients may make a conscious decision to limit fluid intake to manage continence problems. The volume of urine passed is difficult to assess and simple signs of dehydration such as urine colour are difficult to obtain.
Age or general well-being	There may be an accumulation of risks with older age and multiple problems. The treatment, such as multiple medications, can also exacerbate the risk of dehydration.
Polypharmacy	Many medications, in particular diuretics, alter fluid balance. Many effects are positive; however, some result in over- or under-diuresis. Some medications such as antibiotics cause nausea, resulting in a patient not wanting to eat or drink and becoming dehydrated as a result.
Acute illness – there are many different diseases or conditions making a patient vulnerable to fluid imbalance	
Infection	Increased fluid loss due to increased insensible loss.
Diarrhoea	The intestinal tract contains large amounts of sodium and water, which can result in major losses to the body if diarrhoea interferes with normal reabsorption.
Fractures	There may be obvious blood loss or there may be invisible fluid shift from the damaged area into the extracellular space where it tends to remain.
Burns	This loss occurs typically in full thickness and partial thickness burns or burns over more than 20–25% of the body surface area. Plasma moves from the circulating fluid to the extracellular space.
Ruptured organs or organ lesions	Fluid goes into the extracellular space making it effectively unavailable to the circulation.
Chemotherapy/ pancreatitis/dialysis	Normal equilibrium is altered. Control is dependent on regular analysis of blood results.
Dysphagia	Having an altered swallow often results in patients not taking in enough oral fluids and becoming dehydrated. Those who have artificial feeding such as nasogastric or percutaneous endoscopic gastrostomy (PEG) require close monitoring for signs of dehydration and hypernatraemia.

Adapted from Iggulden (1999).

Table 6.5 Assessing fluid balance

Tongue	If dehydrated the tongue will be smaller and more furrowed than normal. With sodium excess, however, the tongue becomes red and swollen.
Skin	Severe dehydration causes the skin to be pale and cool. If hyponatraemic/septic it may be flushed.
Face	In dehydration the face appears pinched and eyes sunken, but only in the very advanced stage.
Pulse	In dehydration this will be more rapid and weaker in volume.
Blood pressure	There may be no significant change in early stages of hyponatraemic water depletion. A falling BP and clinical signs of shock in dehydration will occur due to excessive loss. Postural hypotension, where BP falls on standing or sitting, may be a result of a drug side effect. It is also a reliable early sign of hypovolaemia (Chapelhow and Crouch 2007).
Fever	A raised temperature will result in an increased metabolic rate, increased insensible loss, and the need for increased water intake.
Urine output	Colour and volume of urine can give a good indication of hydration status, as well as underlying urine infection.
Respiration	Hyperventilation increases insensible fluid losses and this should be taken into account for rehydration. Oxygen therapy, unless on humidified oxygen, can significantly enhance insensible loss.
Conscious level	If drowsy or unconscious the patient is unable to drink.
Neck and hand veins	Central venous pressure is a measurement of pressure on the right atrium of the heart and is a good indicator of the amount of fluid contained within the body. Without a central line this can be estimated by looking at the veins in the hand. These will be flat in a person lying flat, indicating poor plasma volume (Iggulden 1999).
Mental status	Sudden changes such as disorientation, confusion, hallucinations, or personality changes may be indicative of electrolyte disturbance or hypovolaemia. Generally, confused patients tend to drink less and depression can contribute to a lack of motivation to drink. It is important also to obtain a full history regarding alcohol dependency – for example it may be that sudden deterioration following admission into hospital is associated with withdrawal from alcohol and be unrelated to the reason for admission.
Body appearance	The general well-being of the patient is a good indication of fluid loss or gain. Looking at a patient's body, in particular the extremities such as the feet and ankles, can reveal signs of peripheral oedema. If it is severe this swelling may be as high as the thighs. Gently pressing the skin with your finger will leave an indentation and occasionally the legs will 'weep' clear serous fluid. A more generalized swelling can indicate low albumin, which in turn affects fluid absorption; this tends to be associated with poor dietary intake or liver problems and should be investigated. If a person's skin appears loose then this could indicate recent dehydration (Woodrow 2002).
Body weight	Weight change is a good indicator of water gains and losses if carried out under the same conditions each day. Weight and fluid balance alters during the menstrual cycle, typically with weight increasing just before and during menstruation. It is also important to get an accurate history from the patient – weight loss or gain may be intentional and not an indication of a medical problem!

representation of weight gain or loss. It is also good practice to show on the chart the alteration of medications to help understand the effect of the drugs.

Following the procedures

If a positive balance is recorded, the patient should be assessed for indicators of fluid overload and any signs of pulmonary or peripheral oedema. If a deficit is identified then treatment is required, which does not necessarily have to be invasive such as intravenous rehydration. It is possible that early dehydration can be treated conservatively, and hospitalization, for example, could be avoided. Steps to take may include:

- Client and family education and discussion about fluid intake and output (this may include advice on continence or mobility if this is thought to be affecting oral intake).
- Instigation of a monitoring regime for people at risk (such as training the patient to observe urine colour).
- Encouragement of early resumption of diet and fluids as soon as possible post-operatively (see local guidelines for specific time delays).
- Evaluation of effectiveness of feeding aids, or referral to appropriate professional (speech therapist or occupational therapist) who will have access to many different feeding cups to assist those who are unsteady or have an altered swallow. The dietician can advise on fortified supplements if needed.
- Provision of a range of drinks and beverages with well-understood nutritional properties.
- Giving prescribed antiemetics if nausea or vomiting are occurring.
- Evaluation of effectiveness of tube feeding, ensuring adequate hydration following feed. This should include the fluids given during medication administration.
- Consideration should be given within the team if oral fluid intake is not sufficient for the initiation of artificial supplementation. This may be by subcutaneous therapy (**hypodermoclysis**) rather than intravenous rehydration, which can provide a low volume of fluids with a lower associated risk of infection.
- Frequent mouth care is an important comfort measure, particularly for those unable to take oral fluids (McNicholl *et al.* 2006).

Recognizing patient deterioration

Take appropriate action where the:

- Urine output is less frequent and more concentrated.
- The patient appears drowsier or confused, which may be as a result of abnormal electrolyte levels. This will often result in a further deterioration due to a decreased oral intake as the consciousness level reduces.
- The patient is short of breath on minimal exertion, which may be due to excessive fluid within the system and is often associated with swollen extremities.

Reflection and evaluation

When reflecting on the task of fluid balance it is important to consider the basics of nursing care such as mouth care and drinks being available within reach, as well as the accurate numeracy skills involved in calculating an individual's cumulative balance.

It is important to ensure that all patients under your care are able to reach their drinks (bearing in mind additional problems such as visual or motor weaknesses), all intake and output is accurately recorded (rather than estimated), and during observations or washing a patient, signs of an imbalance are observed, reported, and documented. Early identification of a problem is essential and it should be noted that Hodgkinson *et al.* (2003) reported that hospitalized older people suffering from dehydration had a mortality rate of 45%.

It is essential to consider the needs of your patient at all times and the key role of the nurse, regardless of qualification, is to act as the patient's advocate. If at any time you have concerns regarding decisions on management of fluids, this needs to be discussed with your mentor, ward manager, or medical team.

Further learning opportunities

- Assess each of your patients and consider their need for fluid balance observation, regardless of whether they are already on a fluid balance chart.
- Ensure that the patient and family are aware of the rationale behind fluid monitoring and allow them to be involved.

- Ensure that all staff know the volume of typical glasses and cups used so that accurate recording occurs. You may find it useful to measure accurately the volume of the cups, mugs, and glasses in regular use if this has not already been done in your clinical area (remember to fill only to the usual level, not to the brim). You may find it useful to make a poster showing the volume held in a typical cup or glass in your area and place it in the kitchen or where the fluid charts are kept.

Reminders

Don't forget to:

- Document your findings of clinical change in condition in the nursing or medical paperwork (check your local policy) and any fluid intake or output on the fluid chart.
- Update the care plan if you have changed or altered a patient's planned care.
- Check if the patient is on a fluid chart before you dispose of any body waste (this may be vomit, stoma, or from a drain, as well as urine).

Q Patient scenario questions

1 You are totalling the fluid charts at midnight. Patient A has received 1000 ml of fluids via IVI and 1750 ml via oral route but you are unable to calculate the urine output volume, as 'OTT' (out to toilet) has been documented regularly. When you hand over this patient's care, what will you discuss about the chart with your colleagues?

2 Patient B has had a stroke affecting her right arm; her swallow has also been affected, resulting in her needing thickened fluids. You are concerned that she is becoming dehydrated. What could you do to minimize this?

3 Patient C is 25 years old and has come into day surgery to have a wisdom tooth extraction performed. She asks if she will require a 'drip'. What would you tell her?

Website

 http://www.oxfordtextbooks.co.uk/orc/ endacott

You may find it helpful to work through our short online quiz and additional scenarios intended to help you to develop and apply the skills in this chapter.

References

Chapelhow C and Crouch S (2007). Applying numeracy skills in clinical practice: fluid balance. *Nursing Standard*, **21**(27), 49–56.

Chung L, Chong S, and French P (2002). The efficiency of fluid balance charting: an evidence-based management project. *Journal of Nursing Management*, **10**, 103–13.

Hodgkinson B, Evans D, and Wood J (2003). Maintaining oral hydration in older patients: a systematic review. *International journal of Nursing Practice*, **9**(3), 19–28.

Holman C, Roberts S, and Nicol M (2005). Practice Update: Clinical skills with older people: promoting adequate hydration in older people. *Nursing Older People*, **17**(4), 31–2.

Iggulden H (1999). Dehydration and electrolyte disturbance. *Nursing Standard*, **13**(19), 48–56.

Longmore M, Wilkinson I, and Rajagopalan S (2004). *Oxford handbook of clinical medicine*, 6th edition. Oxford University Press, Oxford.

McNicholl M, Dunne K, Garvey A, Sharkey R, and Bradley A (2006). Using the Liverpool Care Pathway for a dying patient. *Nursing Standard*, **20**(38), 46–50.

Potter PA and Perry AG (2001). *Fundamentals of nursing*. Mosby, St Louis.

Tortora GJ and Grabowski SR (2003). *Principles of anatomy and physiology*, 10th edition. Wiley, New York.

Woodrow P (2002). Assessing fluid balance in older people: fluid needs. *Nursing Older People*, **14**(9), 31–2.

Useful further reading and websites

Doherty B and Coote S (2004). Fluid-balance monitoring as part of track and trigger. *Nursing Times*, **102**(45), 28–9.

Doherty B and Foudy C (2005). Homeostasis, Part 4: fluid imbalance. *Nursing Times*, **102**(17), 22–3.

Woodrow P (2003). Assessing fluid balance in older people: fluid replacement. *Nursing Older People*, **14**(10), 29–30.

A Answers to patient scenarios

1 This fluid chart does not allow an accurate balance to be recorded. A decision is required about:

- Is an IVI still required?
- Should urine output be measured? If so can the patient use a bottle or jug and record it themselves?
- Is a fluid chart still required? Assessment of their clinical condition, reason for admission, and analysis of blood results should be done.

2 This patient is at high risk of dehydration due to not being able to reach her glass. Having thickened fluids also results in them appearing less appetizing. There may also be a possibility of having a cognitive or visual problem as a result of the stroke.

Methods to minimize a problem may be to:

- Ensure that drinks are offered regularly and offer squash/cordial rather than plain water.
- Record urine output in addition to oral intake, observing for concentration as an early indicator of dehydration.
- Consider the need for fluid supplementation such as intravenous or subcutaneous until her swallowing has improved. This could be done during the evening/night so as not to affect her rehabilitation.
- If a nasogastric tube is in place, water boluses can be given via this route to supplement oral intake (ensure these are also recorded on the fluid chart).

3 Local policy will determine this; however, a fit person who was drinking well prior to admission and whose procedure is short is not likely to require fluid replacement. Explain that the body can compensate well for short periods of no fluid intake and you will be recording her blood pressure and pulse, and monitoring how her body is coping. Reassurance is essential as it is highly probable that this is the first hospital procedure received and she is likely to be very anxious.

6.7 **Administering intravenous fluids**

Definition

The giving of a fluid with a volume of more than 100 ml directly into a **vein**. It can be either by small volume over a short time (bolus) or by intermittent or continuous infusion.

It is important to remember that:

- Intravenous fluids may be given for a variety of reasons, the most common being to replace blood or other fluids lost through surgery, trauma, diarrhoea, vomiting, or being unable to drink.
- The use of intravenous fluids should be taken seriously as they are associated with complications, which could ultimately be fatal. Many of the complications can be avoided or reduced when practitioners have underpinning knowledge.
- Your ability to carry out this skill will depend on your local Trust policy. It is essential to be aware of this before carrying out any procedure.
- You will carry out this skill under direct supervision at all times, with the supervising registered practitioner taking full responsibility for the clinical procedure.
- It is vital in the management of intravenous therapy that prevention of complications or early detection is held in high regard.
- You should be able to demonstrate safe, evidencebased practice, having due regard for the patient's safety and your level of competence.
- You should of course demonstrate a sound knowledge of any drug's actions, side effects, and contraindications before administering.
- Always remember the five 'Rs' of drug administration:
  - Right patient
  - Right drug
  - Right route
  - Right dose
  - Right time

(Clayton 1987)

Prior knowledge

Before attempting to administer intravenous fluids, make sure you are familiar with:

1 Understanding and applying the concepts of consent, accountability, negligence, malpractice, and vicarious liability.

2 The NMC *Code of conduct* (2008b) assists practitioners in understanding their responsibilities.

3 Specific knowledge related to each drug – see 5.1, *Principles of drug administration*.

4   Anaphylaxis and its emergency management.

5   Normal serum values.

6   The mechanisms for understanding homeostasis.

7   Cellular anatomy.

8   Principles of cellular movement.

In addition to having an understanding of the fluids to be infused, nurses also need to:

9   Be familiar with the nursing care of patients with intravenous infusions, including assessment of condition of vein and cannula (see Section 6.11), awareness and interpretation of a treatment plan, and equipment used (such as infusion pumps).

Background

Section 6.6 on recording fluid balance discussed the importance of maintaining equilibrium for fluid balance and how water is stored in different compartments – intracellular and extracellular. It is important to have a good understanding of the normal processes of cellular activity to enable the full implications of acute and chronic conditions to be understood. In summary:

- Electrolytes are essential for the smooth running of cells, with sodium and potassium being the most abundant.
- There are different classes of fluids, colloids and crystalloids, and their use is dependent on the rationale for fluid administration.
- Water movement within the body is due to osmotic pressure, where it moves from an area of low concentration (hypotonic) to an area of higher concentration (hypertonic).

When the balance between intracellular and extracellular water levels is not met and adjustments such as increasing oral intake are not sufficient, artificial intervention via intravenous fluids is often required. It is essential also to address the underlying cause of the imbalance, such as bleeding or vomiting, because until the causative factor is identified and managed, fluid replacement and stability will not result.

Sodium is the main plasma (and interstitial) cation with normal levels of 135–145 mmol/litre. It is important in maintaining irritability and conduction of nerve and muscle tissue and assists with acid–base balance

(Woodrow 2003). If sodium levels rise slightly the osmotic pressure of serum increases, which in turn stimulates the thirst centre to release antidiuretic hormone (ADH). This conserves water, thus diluting the sodium (Woodrow 2003).

Ninety-eight per cent of potassium is found in the intracellular fluid (Hand 2001) – 140 mmol/litre compared with a serum potassium level of 3.5–4.5 mmol/litre (Woodrow 2003). This strong concentration difference between the intracellular and extracellular compartments helps to determine the resting potential of nerve and muscle cells (Hand 2001); any alteration to potassium levels therefore affects neuromuscular and cardiac function. Potassium is routinely excreted in urine but in some situations, such as with diabetes or the use of diuretics, excessive potassium loss may occur, triggering abnormal cardiac rhythms or myocardial infarction.

Severe hyperkalaemia (serum levels of 7–8 mmol/litre) can be fatal due to cardiac effects, so early treatment is essential. It is typically managed by administration of intravenous glucose and insulin, or calcium gluconate or chloride. These drugs transfer serum potassium rapidly into cells and out of the plasma, thereby reducing high potassium levels. Over time, however, it may transfer back into the plasma, so a drug called calcium resonium is sometimes used. This binds with the potassium and enables it to be excreted from the body, via the bowel (Woodrow 2003). Alternatively, some diuretics may be used to excrete potassium via the kidneys.

Signs of raised potassium are ECG changes and tingling and numbness in the extremities. Signs of low potassium are malaise, loss of strength in skeletal and smooth muscle, muscle cramps, and postural hypotension.

Intravenous fluids can be classified in several ways and the choice of fluid used is often dependent on two main factors – the volume of the loss that has occurred and which solutes need to be replaced (Diehl-Oplinger and Kaminski 2004).

Crystalloids

Crystalloid solutions mimic the body's extracellular fluid, with the most common crystalloid being 0.9% sodium chloride (Diehl-Oplinger and Kaminski 2004). It diffuses through the capillary walls that separate plasma from interstitial fluids and expands both intravascular and extravascular fluid volume. Crystalloids move quickly within the body and, after 20 to 40 minutes, only one-fifth of normal saline remains intravascularly (Haljamae and Lindgren 2000 cited in Woodrow 2003).

Another commonly used crystalloid is 5% dextrose. In 5% glucose the constituents are only glucose and water but the calorific value is poor, with each litre only containing 170 kCal (Hand 2001). It is a common misbelief that intravenous fluids provide energy as well as hydration but this is rarely the case, and the patient's nutritional needs must be considered.

The side effect of using crystalloids is that they can result in volume overload, electrolyte disturbances, heart failure, pulmonary oedema, interstitial oedema, and acute respiratory distress (Diehl-Oplinger and Kaminski 2004).

Colloids

Colloids, by contrast, contain undissolved particles such as protein, sugar, and starch molecules that are too large to pass through capillary walls (Diehl-Oplinger and Kaminski 2004). In theory these large molecules result in the colloid remaining longer intravascularly, therefore sustaining blood pressure for longer (Woodrow 2003). In addition the colloid solution draws fluid from interstitial and intracellular spaces, increasing intravascular volume. The degree of osmotic pull that a colloid exerts depends on its particle concentration.

While colloid solutions may help to maintain blood pressure, they do not improve the ability of the blood to perform its primary task of carrying oxygen around the body and waste products to the lungs, so a blood transfusion may also be required (Docherty 2002). Although synthetic colloids such as Gelofusin® and Haemaccel® give an initial favourable result of improving blood pressure and urine output, some research has found that they also leaked from the intravascular space into tissues, creating pulmonary problems and more hypotension (Alderson *et al.* 2000).

There has been considerable debate over which fluid type to use, crystalloid or colloid, in fluid resuscitation. A Cochrane review in 1997 by Perel and Roberts found that there was no evidence that colloids were more effective than crystalloids in reducing mortality in the critically ill or injured. This view was supported by Schierhout and

Roberts (1998). The general accepted practice continues to be the use of initial infusions of crystalloids followed by the administration of colloids when large volumes are necessary, but check your local policy for more specific guidance.

Osmotic pressure and fluid tonicity

Fluid moves between the fluid compartments via osmosis, so providing cell stability. Water moves from an area of low concentration (hypotonic) to an area of higher concentration (hypertonic) and the amount of pressure depends on the ratio between the concentration of ions in the infused solution and the concentration of ions in cell fluid (Rosenthal 2006).

Isotonic fluids have the same tonicity as plasma and are typically 280–300 mOsm/litre. When an isotonic fluid is infused, water moves neither into nor out of cells as they have the same concentration. These fluids are given to expand circulating volume and replace actual fluid loss without changing plasma electrolyte concentration (Rosenthal 2006). Common isotonic fluids are 0.9% sodium chloride or lactated Ringer's solution. These fluids are used when a patient's fluid loss is a result of vomiting or diarrhoea or in patients with surgical fluid loss (Diehl-Oplinger and Kaminski 2004). Due to the volume expanding nature, it is essential to monitor for fluid overload.

Hypotonic fluids (<280 mOsm/litre), such as 0.45% sodium chloride, have a lower concentration of particles than plasma, so when administered they put more water in the serum than is found inside cells. Water therefore moves into the cells, causing them to swell.

Hypotonic fluids are rarely administered and must be given with expert guidance; however, they may be given to those patients whose sodium intake must be restricted. Monitoring is needed as too much hypotonic fluid can result in intravascular fluid depletion, hypotension, cellular oedema, and tissue damage (Diehl-Oplinger and Kaminski 2004). In addition, these solutions have the potential to cause sudden fluid shift from blood vessels into cells, so can cause cardiovascular collapse from intravascular fluid depletion and increased intracranial pressure from fluid shift into brain cells. It is important therefore that these fluids are not given to those already at risk of increased intracranial pressure, such as with stroke, head trauma, and neurosurgery (Rosenthal 2006).

Hypertonic fluids (>300 mOsm/litre), such as 3% or 5% sodium chloride, have greater tonicity than fluid in the extracellular compartment so they exert more osmotic pressure, resulting in these solutions drawing fluid from the intracellular to the extracellular compartment, causing cells to shrink and relieving cellular oedema (Diehl-Oplinger and Kaminski 2004). In this situation water moves out of cells in an attempt to dilute the infusate, having the knock-on effect of shrinking the cells. Again, these are rarely given, and must be administered with expert supervision.

Hypertonic solutions are used to help re-establish the equilibrium in electrolyte and acid–base imbalances, and include electrolyte replacement solutions and parenteral nutritional solutions. When the cells shrink at the cannula site, however, the basement membrane of the vein's lining is exposed, increasing the risk of phlebitis and infiltration (Rosenthal 2006). It is for this reason that all fluids with osmolarity of >600 mOsm/litre should be given through a central venous catheter to allow for greater dilution. This includes solutions with more than 10% dextrose and high electrolyte concentrations.

Administration of intravenous fluids has changed considerably over the past decades from a comparatively simple procedure relying on gravity to the use of complex, multichannel electronic pumps. Often these pumps are used without a full understanding of how they work, and Campbell (2001) reported that 400 people die or are seriously injured each year in adverse events involving medical devices in the UK, with the Medical Devices Agency identifying that one of the most serious types of medication error involves the use of infusion pumps.

The advantage of using an infusion control device for IV drugs and additives is that it ensures efficient, accurate, and convenient delivery. Due to a lack of available pumps this is often not possible, and priority should be given to those with cardiac or renal disease, the very young or old, and infusions that need to be given over a very accurate time range (Workman 1999). It is important to check your local policy regarding the criteria of pump usage locally. What is essential, however, is that when using an infusion pump you are fully aware of how the equipment works and what to do if there is a problem. If there is a knowledge gap then assistance should be sought before setting up the device (Murray and Glenister 2001).

It is essential to remember that administration of wrong concentrations or types of fluid can be fatal

(Johnston *et al*. 2004) and errors in rate of administration can cause clinical complications such as heart failure or volume depletion. In a study by Han *et al*. (2005), observation of 687 administrations found 126 errors; of these 79.3% were wrong administration rate.

Context

When to administer IV fluids

Intravenous fluids may be given for a variety of reasons, the most common being to replace blood or other fluids lost through surgery, trauma, diarrhoea, or vomiting (Rosenthal 2006).

Untreated hypovolaemia can quickly advance into hypovolaemic shock (Diehl-Oplinger and Kaminski 2004). Signs of this in the mild stage may be increased anxiety, increased capillary refill time (see Section 6.4), and cool extremities. As the effect of volume loss increases, so do the clinical signs, including increased heart rate and respiratory rate and decreased urine output. It is not until the condition is more severe that hypotension is evident, and often at this stage there is altered mental status, ultimately resulting in a comatose state (Diehl-Oplinger and Kaminski 2004).

Other reasons for using intravenous fluids are:

- Maintaining fluid balance when nil by mouth (NBM).
- Correcting electrolyte imbalances, such as potassium, by either supplementation or the giving of a drug to aid its excretion.
- Providing a medium for administering medications and nutritional support.
- Drug administration – some drugs cannot be given via the gastrointestinal route due to molecule size or presence of gastric fluid (Dougherty 2002). In addition, some drugs require rapid receipt by the target site, and the quickest method for this is intravenously. The cardiac drug adenosine is an example of this, as the half-life is very short (10 seconds *in vivo*) and it needs to be administered rapidly in order to inhibit the AV node and calcium channels in the heart when treating cardiac arrhythmias.

Some methods to monitor the need for intravenous fluids are:

- Vital signs – blood pressure, pulse.
- Fluid intake and output measurements.
- Daily weight.
- Skin turgor – elasticity of skin.
- Jugular vein filling.
- Central venous pressure measurements.
- Arterial blood gas analysis.
- Serum electrolyte levels.
- Urinary specific gravity.

When not to administer fluids intravenously

Intravenous fluids are not always required and their use involves risks, e.g. infection control issues with cannulation. Always consider the underlying cause and the rationale for administering fluids. It is important that urine output, blood pressure and pulse, and blood results are regularly assessed to evaluate:

- Need for continued intravenous fluid administration.
- That the correct fluid is being administered.
- That the correct rate of fluid is being administered.

It is essential that the patient is willing to receive the fluid. It is a vital role of the nurse, regardless of experience, to be the patient's advocate and to ensure that consent is obtained and any concerns are voiced to the nurse in charge, medical team, or mentor at the earliest opportunity.

Alternative interventions

Before commencing intravenous fluids, it is important to consider two factors:

- Input – Is the need for fluids due to dehydration? Could this be rectified by encouraging oral intake, use of subcutaneous fluids, or bolus fluid administration via a nasogastric tube?
- Output – Is the patient unable to pass urine and this is giving an inaccurate fluid balance? Always check urine output and examine if the bladder is enlarged. It may be necessary to consider catheterizing the patient.

It is possible that fluid balance cannot be achieved using intravenous fluid correction alone and that high strength drugs are required. This can be more accurate, but invasive, often requiring monitoring via a central venous catheter. See Section 6.12 for more information.

Additional expertise or resources

When assessing the need for intervention, it is essential that you are able to:

- Interpret a fluid balance chart.
- Palpate for a bladder or consider using a bladder scan to assess if there is residual urine, and if necessary insert a catheter (ensuring additional skills and training are obtained – check your local policy).

If intravenous fluids are required, skills are needed in:

- Connection and changing of fluid bags.
- Use of an intravenous fluid pump, and knowledge of the local policy when a pump is indicated.

Potential problems

Intravenous fluids are drugs, and adverse reactions may occur, so recognition and treatment of these are essential. This will typically be the usual signs of anaphylaxis: sweating, pallor, increased pulse. Additionally, complications such as **phlebitis** of the cannulation site may occur, so regular checking of this is essential (see Section 6.11 on cannula care). Recognition, management, and reporting of an administration error such as infusion completed too quickly or slowly are essential.

Other potential complications and treatments:

- Circulatory overload – stop drug administration and inform doctor.
- Chemical phlebitis – incorrect method of administration, rate, concentration, or volume, vascular irritation and thrombophlebitis, systemic toxicity and type of fluid – stop administration, remove cannula, and observe site.
- Infiltration (inadvertent administration of non-vesicant drugs or fluid into surrounding tissues due to cannula dislodgement) – remove cannula.
- Pulmonary embolism and air embolus.
- Physical or chemical incompatibility/interaction.
- Bacterial phlebitis (inflammation of the intima of the vein associated with a bacterial infection) – remove

cannula, elevate, monitor temperature, swab site for microscopy, culture and sensitivity, inform doctor.

- Anaphylaxis – follow local anaphylaxis policy.
- Speed shock – a systemic reaction that occurs when a substance that is foreign to the body is rapidly introduced. As a result, syncope, shock, and cardiac arrest may follow.
- Bleeding/haematoma – uncontrolled bleeding at venepuncture site.
- Ecchymosis – infiltration of blood into tissues.

Interpreting readings

It is essential to be aware of the potential complications associated with fluid administration and observe for it at all times. Typically a normal reaction would be an improvement in a patient's condition. This may be sudden, such as replacement following rapid loss due to trauma, or gradual, as with resolving low potassium due to vomiting. Circulatory overload is a major disadvantage of intravenous fluid administration and while the use of gauges and infusion pumps have assisted in the correct rate of infusion, it is essential that all staff are aware of the clinical signs of overload:

- Flushed face.
- Headache.
- Congestion.
- Tightness in chest.

If overload is suspected it is important to:

- Stop infusion and inform doctor.
- Provide symptomatic relief – sit patient upright, provide oxygen (as per local policy), monitor pulse and respiration rate.
- Reassure the patient.
- Identify cause in order to prevent a reoccurrence.

Specific observations

The frequency of observations such as blood pressure recording will depend on the patient's general condition and local policy. The importance of visual assessment should not be underestimated – observing the fluid drip rate, the cannula site, and, more importantly, the patient's general condition (skin turgor, colour, and general well-being).

Special considerations

As with most treatment options, it is important to consider the disadvantages as well as the advantages of IV fluids. Direct access into the vein is not without complications, with infection and irritation of the vein being of concern. Drug incompatibilities also occur and these may be in a variety of forms:

- **Physical** – a visible reaction such as colour change, haze, turbidity, precipitate, or gas formation.
- **Chemical** – the chemical degradation of the drug, which might not be visible.
- **Therapeutic** – occurs within the patient, where there are overlapping effects of drugs administered concurrently. This may not be evident until the patient's response is evaluated (Dougherty 2002).

In addition to the drug effects, consideration of the patient is important. For example:

- **Age** – with the young and elderly the response to fluids can be very dramatic and organs such as the kidneys and heart are potentially very sensitive, so close monitoring is essential.
- **Location** – if undertaking this skill in the patient's home, remember that the patient and family should be aware of the signs of phlebitis and have clear guidelines about when the infusion should be stopped.

- **Chronic illness** – always consider the patient as a whole, as underlying conditions such as diabetes or heart disease will increase their susceptibility to only minor fluctuations in fluid volume. Rheumatoid arthritis sufferers may have complications from the cannula rather than the fluid, but this can still have considerable implications. Also remember that patients with renal failure, particularly dialysis patients, are very susceptible to fluid overload.

- **Other conditions** – if the patient is pregnant, remember that the normal fluid balance shift is altered, so closer observation is essential in order to observe for complications. Menstrual cycle, time of day, and the time from the last meal can all affect weight and should be taken into consideration if fluids are prescribed in response to a weight change.

- **Infection control risks** – the cannula site is a well-recognized risk of infection, but any additive to the infusion, such as potassium, increases the likelihood of infection.

Procedure

Preparation

Prepare the equipment

- Patient's prescription chart.
- Fluid chart or local equivalent.
- The prescribed intravenous infusion fluid (ensure checked in accordance with local policy).
- Personal protective equipment as required by local policy – gloves or alcohol gel.
- Infusion line.
- Drip stand.

Step-by-step guide to administering IV fluids

 Step   Rationale

	Step	Rationale
1	Collect infusion fluid, checking expiry date and looking carefully for signs of potential contamination. Cloudiness, discoloration, or particles in the fluid can indicate contamination. If in doubt contact pharmacy department for clarification – most fluids are clear, while some, in particular some antibiotics, are a straw colour.	To avoid administering potentially harmful fluids.
2	Check prescription chart taking care to confirm the correct name, date, and that the prescription is signed. Check the prescription against the patient's identity band (see **Figure 6.19**).	Intravenous fluids are a medication and the principles for administration of medicines as set by the NMC (2008a) should be followed.
3	Observe cannula site (see **Section 6.11**).	It is essential not to commence an infusion if there are concerns regarding the patency of the cannula.
4	Introduce yourself, confirm the patient's identity, explain the procedure, and obtain consent.	To identify the patient correctly and gain informed consent. Patients can perceive that IV therapy is frightening and an indication that they are very ill, and therefore may be anxious. It is essential to explain the length of therapy, reasons for it, what to expect, and when to call for assistance. Pain and discomfort should not be acceptable and complaints should be taken seriously and investigated.
5	Ensure all equipment is available, including an infusion device if being used.	It is important not to leave the patient mid-procedure.
6	Wash and dry hands.	As per local infection control protocol. It is essential to check with your local policy but some organizations recommend a clean technique and that 'gloves should be used when performing infusion procedures' (RCN 2003). However, the *Royal Marsden* (Dougherty and Lister 2008), like many organizations, recommends you 'wash hands thoroughly using bactericidal soap and water or bactericidal alcohol hand rub'.

continued overleaf

Step-by-step guide to administering IV fluids

7	Carefully open fluid packaging and place the infusion bag on a clean surface.	Reduces damage to the infusion and allows it to be stored with minimal risk of contamination.
8	Open appropriate giving set. Unwind the tube to ensure that it is not twisted or damaged. Be careful not to let either end trail to the floor or touch the bed or other furniture.	Awareness of cost implication and waste. Infection control precautions. If the ends of the infusion line do become contaminated it is important to start the procedure again using a new infusion line.
9	Turn off the roller clamp by moving it to the bottom of the chamber (see Figure 6.20).	This stops the fluid flowing through the set and creating air bubbles. Air bubbles as small as 100 microlitres could be hazardous so it is essential to take time over priming the line, and turning off the clamp to allow the chamber to be filled aids this (Venn 2004). If an infusion bag is dropped or shaken it becomes agitated so it is important to wait until the fluid has settled before continuing.
10	Remove spike cover, ensuring that you do not touch the exposed spike (see **Figure 6.20**).	To maintain infection control precautions using a 'non-touch technique'.
11	Remove the protector from the infusion fluid.	To maintain infection control precautions using a 'non-touch technique'.
12	Without touching either end, pierce the infusion bag with the giving set, ensuring that it is securely inserted (see Figure 6.20).	To maintain infection control precautions using a 'non-touch technique'.
13	Squeeze the chamber to enable it to be half-filled with the infusion fluid (see **Figure 6.21**).	Enables fluid to pass through the set with minimal risk of air bubbles. Only filling halfway allows the 'drips' to be seen clearly when the infusion is running.
14	Slowly open the clamp allowing the fluid to fill the giving set (see Figure 6.21).	Controlled filling of the giving set.
15	When the giving set line is totally full of fluid, turn the clamp to the down position.	Stops fluid from being lost and ensures all the air is removed.
16	Connect the giving set to the cannula. Depending on local policy you may need additional training to enable you to do this, so check first.	Allows the infusion to begin.
17	If not using an infusion pump, adjust the rate of the infusion by calculating the drips within the chamber using the guide for calculation rates on page 258.	Ensures that the infusion will be given over the prescribed time.
18	Check infusion rate, cannula site, and condition of patient regularly. This may be required hourly or more frequently depending on their condition and infusion type.	Infection control and documentation as per local policy.

19	Document on fluid chart and ensure fluid prescription signed and batch number documented as appropriate.	Documentation as per local and NMC guidelines.
20	Document, according to local policy, the date and time of a new infusion line.	Infection control. Pratt *et al.* (2007) state that most infusion sets for intravenous fluids should be changed every 72 hours, but it is essential to check your local policy.
21	Inform patient what to expect and what not to do, such as adjust infusion rate.	Enables patient to feel informed and gain control and understanding of their care.

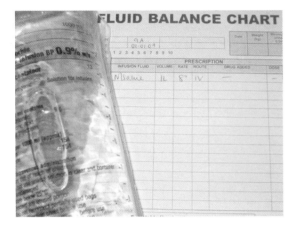

Figure 6.19 Check the prescription against the fluid. Note the expiry date and ensure the fluid is clear and the protective cover is intact.

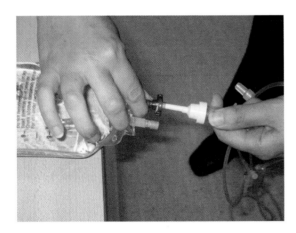

Figure 6.20 Turn off the roller clamp and carefully insert the spike into the infusion bag, taking care not to touch the unprotected ends.

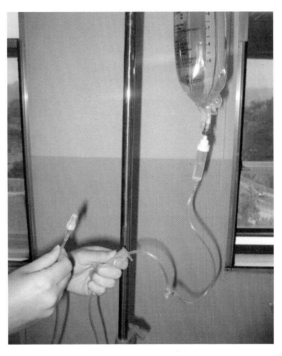

Figure 6.21 Squeeze the chamber. Allow it to fill half full and slowly open the roller clamp until the fluid reaches the end of the giving set.

If using an infusion pump:

- Open the pump door and insert the giving set line.
- Set the infusion rate and volume according to the operation manual.
- Ensure power supply is on.
- Have a good working knowledge of alarm settings, maintenance, etc.

Depending on local policy you may need to have additional training to enable you to do this, so check first to ensure that patient safety is maintained.

Following the procedure

After the fluids have been safely commenced, it is important to observe regularly, considering:

- Reassessing your patient regarding the need for IV hydration and considering the underlying cause.
- Ensuring your patient is aware of the rationale and feels involved.
- Checking your patient, observing the rate of infusion and condition of the patient. This will also include ensuring further prescriptions being available, especially at the weekend and overnight. There should also be a medical plan for what to do if blood pressure or urine output drops further.
- Observing the fluid rate and ensuring running to time. The rate will vary when not in a pump if the patient changes position, especially if cannulated in the inner aspect of the elbow.

Calculation rates

There is a simple formula that is used to determine the drop rate:

$$\frac{\text{Volume (ml)}}{\text{Time (hours)}} \times \frac{\text{drops per ml}}{60 \text{ (minutes)}}$$

Drop rate for a standard administration set is 20 drops of fluid per ml, while blood sets allow 15 drops per ml.
E.g. a 1 litre infusion prescribed over 8 hours equates to:

$$\frac{1000}{8} \times \frac{20}{60} = 41.6 \text{ drops per minute.}$$

Recognizing patient deterioration

It is essential to observe your patient for signs of:

- Allergic reaction.
- Circulatory overload.
- Peripheral irritation/infection.
- Positive outcomes of hydration, e.g. via observations or urine output.

Reflection and evaluation

When you have administered intravenous fluids, think about the following questions:

- Is the fluid replacement still required?
- Have I told the patient what is happening, why, and what they should expect?
- Is this intervention still the best for the patient?
- Have potential complications, such as infection, been taken into consideration and checked for?
- Have I handed over to colleagues the rationale, risks, and management options when discussing the fluid?

Further learning opportunities

- Practise assessing your patients regarding the need for IV hydration and consider the underlying causes.
- Always check your patient by observing the rate of infusion and their condition. This will also include ensuring further prescriptions being available, especially at the weekend and overnight. There should also be a medical plan for what to do if blood pressure or urine output drops further.

Reminders

- Complications of IV fluids may be systemic and local:
  - Circulatory overload.
  - Speed shock.
  - Pharmaceutical problems.
  - Embolism.
  - Allergic reaction (Hyde 2002).
- Observe the infusion bag as there can be physical or chemical interactions.
- Inform patient what you are doing.
- Check the infusion rate, cannula site, and condition of patient regularly.
- Document on fluid chart and fluid prescription.
- If using an infusion pump you need to know how the equipment works and what to do if there is a problem.

Patient scenarios

1 A patient has been admitted for routine surgery and has been prescribed a litre of normal saline infusion over 6 hours. You have checked the local policy and an infusion pump is not required. What is the drip rate that you need to set the giving set to?

2 You have taken over the care of a patient with an intravenous fluid infusion in progress. The patient has been in for 4 days and there is no clear documentation to indicate when the giving set was last changed. What do you do?

3 One of your patients has just been treated for hypovolaemia with three 500 ml bags of Gelofusine® and now has a litre of normal saline in progress. The patient now feels better. How frequently should you perform the observations?

4 You are managing a patient who has an infusion running into a cannula in the right antecubital fossa. Every time she bends her arm to take a drink, the rate of the infusion alters, meaning maintaining an accurate drip rate is difficult. What can you do to help in this situation?

Website

 http://www.oxfordtextbooks.co.uk/orc/endacott

You may find it helpful to work through our short online quiz and additional scenarios intended to help you to develop and apply the skills in this chapter.

References

Alderson P, Schierhout G, Roberts I, and Bunn F (2000). *Colloids versus crystalloids for fluid resuscitation in critically ill patients (Cochrane review)*. Cochrane Database System Review, Issue 4.

Campbell K (2001). Vincristine fatalities: lessons to be learnt. *Nursing Times*, **97**(26), 39–40.

Clayton M (1987). The right way to prevent medicines errors. *Registered Nurse*, **50**, 30–1.

Diehl-Oplinger L and Kaminski MF (2004). Choosing the right fluid to counter hypovolaemic shock. *Nursing*, **34**(3), 52–4.

Docherty B (2002). Nursing considerations for fluid management in hypovolaemia. *Professional Nurse*, **17**(9), 545–9.

Dougherty L (2002). Delivery of intravenous therapy. *Nursing Standard*, **16**(16), 45–52.

Dougherty L and Lister S, eds (2008). *The Royal Marsden Hospital manual of clinical nursing procedures*, 7th edition. Blackwell Publishing, Oxford.

Han PY, Coombes ID, and Green B (2005). Factors predictive of intravenous fluid administration errors in Australian surgical care wards. *Quality and Safety in Health Care*, **14**, 170–84.

Hand H (2001). The use of intravenous therapy. *Nursing Standard*, **15**(43), 47–52.

Hyde L (2002). Legal and professional aspects of intravenous therapy. *Nursing Standard*, **16**(26), 39–42.

Johnston R, Boiteau P, Charlebois K, Long S, and David U (2004). Responding to tragic error: lessons from Foothills Medical Centre. *CMAJ*, **170**, 1659–60.

Murray W and Glenister H (2001). How to use medical devices safely. *Nursing Times*, **97**(43), 36–8.

Nursing and Midwifery Council (2008a). *Standards for medicines management*. NMC, London [online] **http://www.nmc-uk.org** accessed 26/08/08.

Nursing and Midwifery Council (2008b). *The Code: Standards of conduct, performance and ethics for nurses and midwives*. NMC, London [online] **http://www.nmc-uk.org** accessed 26/08/08.

Perel P and Roberts I (2007). Colloids versus crystalloids for fluid resuscitation in critically ill patients. *Cochrane Database of Systematic Reviews*, Issue 4. Art. No. CD000567.

Pratt RJ, Pellowe C, and Wilson JA (2007). National Evidence-based guidelines for preventing healthcare-associated infections in NHS hospitals in England. *Journal of Hospital Infection*, **655**(Suppl), S1–S64.

Royal College Nursing (2003). *Standards for infusion therapy. RCN IV therapy forum*. Royal College of Nursing, London.

Rosenthal K (2006). Intravenous Fluids: the whys and wherefores. *Nursing*, **36**(7), 26–7.

Schierhout G and Roberts I (1998). Fluid resuscitation with colloid or crystalloid solutions in critically ill patients: a systematic review of randomized trials. *BMJ*, **316**, 916–64.

Venn C (2004). SUHT peripheral infusion therapy and intravenous drug administration. Self directed learning package [online] **http://www.suht.soton.ac.uk/clinicalskills/Docs/Adult%20Peripheral%20version4.pdf** accessed 26/08/08.

Woodrow P (2003). Assessing fluid balance in older people: fluid replacement. *Nursing Older People*, **14**(10), 29–30.

Workman B (1999). Peripheral intravenous therapy management. *Emergency Nurse*, **7**(9), 31–9.

Useful further reading and websites

Brogben B (2004). Current practice in administration of parenteral nutrition: venous access. *British Journal Nursing*, **13**(18), 1068–73.

Edwards S (2001). Regulation of water, sodium and potassium: implications from practice. *Nursing Standard*, **15**(22), 36–42.

Platt S and Wade P (2001). Intravenous fluids: the options. *Professional Nurse*, **18**(1), 47.

National evidence-based guidelines for preventing hospital-acquired infections: **http://www.epic. tvu.ac.uk**

Extravasation website: **http://www. extravasation.org.uk/home.html**

British National Formulary: **http://www.bnf.org**

 Answers to patient scenarios

1 $\dfrac{1000}{6} \times \dfrac{20}{60} = 55.55$ drops per minute.

2 Check all the appropriate documentation – nursing paperwork, fluid paperwork, etc. If still unclear, the giving set should be changed at the earliest opportunity in order to minimize infection rates. Ensure that this is clearly documented.

3 It is essential to establish the reason for a low circulating volume as this may reoccur if not identified. There is evidence that there is a delayed hypotension effect with Gelofusine® that may occur several hours after the event, so recording the BP and pulse should continue. The frequency will depend on their overall early warning score but if the infusion should be checked hourly this is a good baseline to observe the patient. If in doubt, ask a member of the medical or senior nursing staff how frequently the observations are needed. Also discuss with the patient the signs and symptoms of hypovolaemia so that they are able to call for help if they feel unwell.

4 Consider whether infusion is still required as she's now taking fluids. If still required, consider movement of cannula to non-dominant arm or a more peripheral location. In the past a splint may have been used to reduce elbow movement but this practice is not recommended and should be avoided.

6.8 **Administering blood transfusions**

Definition

A blood transfusion is a procedure that involves the administration of prepared, compatible donor blood (or blood component) directly into the recipient patient's circulatory system via an intravenous route. It is always performed using aseptic techniques and should always follow local hospital blood transfusion policy. The blood may be whole blood or a component of blood, prescribed and ordered by a medical practitioner.

It is important to remember that:

- There are risks associated with blood transfusions. Avoidable mistakes can result in serious or fatal consequences. Complications are largely associated with human error, failure to comply with hospital policy, or most commonly the failure of the nurse to recognize adverse reactions during transfusions and respond with appropriate interventions (Wilkinson and Wilkinson 2001, Gallacher 2004, Hainsworth 2004). Remember always to check the identity of the patient to ensure that the right patient is receiving the right blood product. Photo identification cards have been developed for patients who regularly receive blood transfusions as outpatients or day cases. They are increasingly being used as a sustainable and cost-effective alternative to wristbands (National Patient Safety Agency (NPSA) 2006).

- Hospitals should have their own policy and procedural steps in place for safe blood transfusion (British Committee for Standards in Haematology 1999). It is important that all practitioners responsible for administering blood transfusions familiarize themselves with these policies and are personally accountable for reviewing their practice, minimizing risk of untoward events, investigating problems as they arise, and ensuring that they respond to changes in the light of best evidence, in order to minimize active errors (Wilkinson and Wilkinson 2001).

Prior knowledge

Before administering blood transfusions, make sure you are familiar with:

1 Intravenous therapy.
2 Aseptic techniques.
3 Blood compatibility.
4 Blood components (erythrocytes, platelets, and plasma).
5 Pathophysiological changes that occur during an incompatible blood transfusion.
6 Hospital policy relating to blood transfusions.

Review of these six areas will assist you in understanding the relevance of administering blood components.

Background

Blood transfusions are an important intervention conducted within nursing practice. Blood is made up of a mixture of 55% plasma (the majority of which is water) and 45% formed elements (red blood cells, white blood cells, and platelets) – see **Figure 6.22** for an overview.

Over 3.4 million blood components are transfused every year in the UK (Royal College of Nursing (RCN) 2004) and these transfusions not only save lives, but also enable patients to improve their quality of life by correcting clinical abnormalities in a range of conditions (Hainsworth 2004). Transfusion therapy can replace blood volume following exsanguination, maintain circulatory blood volume during and after surgical intervention, or restore deficiencies in the blood's oxygen-carrying capacity by increasing haemoglobin levels that have been affected by blood disorders such as anaemia.

Nurses can be responsible, through delegation, for the administration procedures of blood components and it is of utmost importance that they are thorough and methodical in all the tasks associated with the process (British Committee for Standards in Haematology 1999). These responsibilities include:

● Explaining the procedures to the patient.
● The completion of the request form.
● Taking a sample for pre-transfusion testing.
● Collection of blood from the blood bank.
● Checking patients' details.
● Administering the transfusion.
● Assessing the clinical condition of patients receiving the therapy.

Currently, prescribing of blood components is conducted by doctors, but a recent study has suggested that the development of non-medical prescribing may also allow nurses to adopt this role in the future (Pirie and Green 2007).

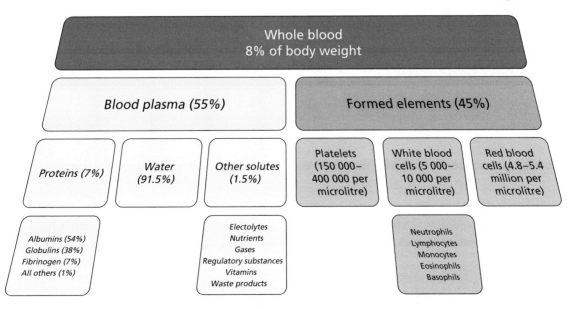

Figure 6.22 Blood components.

A haemovigilance programme, the UK Serious Hazards of Transfusion Scheme (SHOT), has been gathering and surveying any reported data provided voluntarily from NHS and independent hospitals. By collating information on the serious adverse effects of transfusion, safety standards are being improved. The vast majority of reporting highlights human error as a main cause of unexpected death or morbidity in transfusions, either through the prescription and ordering of the blood product (SHOT 2006) or through misidentification and poor monitoring procedures at the patient's bedside (Parris and Grant-Casey 2007).

Two EU Directives, 2002/98/EC and 2005/61/EC, have been introduced into UK law through the Blood Safety and Quality Regulations (Medicines and Healthcare Products Regulatory Agency 2005). These regulations set standards for quality and safety in the collection, testing, processing, storage, and distribution of human blood and blood components. Aspects of the regulations apply to 'blood establishments' (the UK Blood Services) and hospital blood banks.

Most notably, there is now a legal requirement for all blood to be monitored from donor to recipient (i.e. to have traceability in a regulated way) and for the records of recipient blood transfusions to be kept for 30 years (by either an electronic or paper method). It is essential that you are aware of the method used in your practice and follow local policy for documentation. The regulations also require that from 2005, all serious adverse events or serious adverse reactions must be reported to the Medicines and Healthcare Products Regulatory Agency (MHRA) by blood establishments and hospital blood banks/transfusion teams.

A recent initiative that offers a range of short- and long-term strategies for safer blood transfusions has evolved from a collaboration between the NPSA, the Chief Medical Officer's National Blood Transfusion Committee, and SHOT (NPSA 2006). From May 2007, all NHS and independent sector organizations in England and Wales responsible for administering blood transfusions should:

- Have an action plan for competency-based training and assessment of all staff involved in blood transfusions. All staff must undergo a direct observational assessment and be deemed competent.

- Have a policy stipulating that the final identity check must be done next to the patient by matching the blood pack with the patient's wristband (or identity band/photo ID card).
- Formally risk assess their local transfusion procedures and explore the feasibility of using:
  - Bar codes or electronic identification/tracking systems for patients, samples, and blood components.
  - Photo ID cards for those undergoing regular transfusions.
  - A labelling system of matching samples and blood for transfusion to the patient concerned.

Best practice within hospitals now includes the employment of a transfusion practitioner, such as a specialist nurse or biomedical scientist (SHOT 2003, Hainsworth 2004, RCN 2004, Parris and Grant-Casey 2007). These practitioners work closely with lead consultants in blood transfusion and local blood bank managers and support clinical teams in the safe and effective use of blood. One of their main roles is to encourage education and increasing clinical competency in the skill of giving a blood transfusion.

Blood groups

Cross-matching of a patient's blood is essential prior to transfusion as it contains various antigens that can affect how compatible one person's blood is with another. The surfaces of erythrocytes have a genetically determined mixture of **glycoproteins** and **glycolipids** that act as antigens and are called isoantigens or **agglutinogens**. Blood is categorized into different blood groups according to specific combinations of these. There are more than 24 genetically determined blood groups and more than 100 isoantigens that can be detected on the surface of an erythrocyte (Tortora and Grabowski 2000).

Within this section, for the purposes of transfusion, blood can be sectioned into four main types based on the presence or absence of antigens and **antibodies** – ABO blood groups and the Rhesus factor. For further reading you may wish to investigate other blood groups, which include the Lewis, Kidd, Kell, and Duffy systems.

The four **blood types** of the ABO blood groups are determined by whether an individual's erythrocytes carry

Table 6.6 ABO blood types

Antigen on RBC	Antibody developed	Antibody attacks/destroys	Compatible blood
A	Anti-B	Blood type B and AB	A, O
A and B (AB)	None	None	A, B, AB, O
B	Anti-A	Blood type A and AB	B, O
O (neither)	Anti-A and Anti-B	Blood type A, B, and AB	O

the A antigen, the B antigen, both A and B antigens, or no antigens at all (Hearnshaw 2004). From infancy, during normal growth, individuals develop antibodies against the A or B antigens that are not present in their blood; these will aggressively bind to 'incompatible' red blood cells (RBCs) and attack and destroy them – see Table 6.6 (McClelland 2007).

Blood type AB has both A and B antigens on the red cells. Therefore, patients with this blood type do not develop antibodies against either of these antigens. Patients with blood type AB are called universal recipients, as they can receive donor blood types A, B, AB, and O without having an ABO reaction.

Conversely, patients with blood type O have no antigens on their RBCs but carry antibodies to both antigen A and antigen B within their plasma. This type is known as the universal donor, because it can be transfused into patients of blood types A, B, and AB safely; however, patients with blood type O can only receive donor blood type O. The donor blood type O does contain a certain amount of antibody A and antibody B, but they are diluted within the recipient's blood and normally cause no adverse reactions.

The Rhesus blood group is named after discovery of the antigen in the blood of the Rhesus monkey. Individuals whose RBCs have the Rhesus (Rh) antigen are designated RhD+ (Rh positive) and those who lack the antigen are RhD− (Rh negative). Usually, plasma does not contain anti-Rhesus antibodies. However, if a RhD− person receives a RhD+ blood transfusion, it causes sensitization within the recipient and their immune system begins to develop anti-Rh antibodies that will remain in their blood. In any subsequent transfusion of RhD+ blood, haemolysis of the donated blood occurs.

Haemolytic disease of the newborn (HDN) can occur when a pregnant woman who is RhD− is carrying a RhD+ foetus (the antigen having been inherited from the father). Problems arise when a small amount of foetal blood leaks across the placenta into the maternal bloodstream from a first pregnancy, thus creating anti-Rh antibodies in the mother. A second pregnancy with a Rh+ foetus will cause a haemolytic reaction when maternal blood crosses the placenta into the foetal blood. RhD− females or those whose blood group is unknown (and who are of child-bearing potential) should always be given RhD− blood to avoid stimulation of anti-Rh antibodies.

If an incompatible blood type is given to a recipient, the RBCs in the donor blood will be attacked and destroyed by the antibodies present in the patient's blood plasma. This causes an immunological response known as an acute haemolytic reaction (Tortora and Grabowski 2000, Gillespie and Hillyer 2001):

1 Plasma proteins of the complement family are activated, causing intravascular haemolysis (RBCs become leaky and then burst or rupture). The liberated haemoglobin now freely released into the plasma may cause kidney damage.

2 The kinin system produces bradykinin, which increases capillary permeability, dilates arterioles, and eventually results in systemic hypotension.

3 The coagulation system is activated and initiates the intrinsic blood clotting cascade, causing small clots and thrombi that can be fatal.

Ideally, patients should receive the same blood group as their own, confirmed by a cross-match. In emergencies this may not be available, so plasma volume expanders (e.g. Haemaccel) or blood type O (universal donor) may be transfused.

Other considerations

Blood must be stored at 4°C to avoid damage to the cells. If the storage temperature is too high, then there is a tendency for bacterial growth to occur in the blood. If the temperature is too low, then cell breakdown may occur as RBCs become damaged through freezing (Atterbury and Wilkinson 2000).

The findings from an audit conducted by Stevenson (2007) suggest that giving blood transfusions to patients at night may put them at greater risk than those receiving transfusions during the day. Results from this study indicated that poor or infrequent observational data were being obtained in 40% of those transfused at night. This may be due to lower staff to patient ratios, reluctance to perform observations on sleeping patients, poor lighting, or because patients were located in side rooms away from the main nursing station. Where possible, it is advisable to attempt to transfuse patients in daylight hours unless there is an urgent medical need for overnight transfusion.

Although blood transfusion therapy is becoming increasingly used in modern medicine, there are patients who may not wish to receive blood or blood components due to personal preference or religious beliefs, such as Jehovah's Witnesses. An ethical dilemma may be faced by health care professionals when a refusal to accept bloods is given by the patient or their family. When this occurs, the doctor should discuss the risks associated with refusal as well as the potential alternatives (Doyle 2002).

Hearnshaw (2004) advocates the importance of fully explaining the transfusion procedure to the patient in order to obtain their informed consent and cooperation throughout the whole process. Written consent for a blood transfusion is not a legal requirement in the UK (Gallacher 2004, Hainsworth 2004); however, the Department of Health's *Good practice in consent implementation guide* (2001) states that all patients have a right to decide what happens to their own bodies, and the patient's religious, cultural, and ethical concerns must be honoured. The patient should always be given sufficient information to enable them to decide. Risks and benefits should be discussed, and if alternatives to transfusion are available (and the patient is eligible) they should be fully explained to the patient or their representative. Royal College of Nursing (2004) guidance recommends the use of patient information leaflets available from the Blood Transfusion Service or from local health services (see Box 6.3 and the section below).

Alternatives to blood product transfusions

Autologous blood donation

This is where blood is taken periodically from the patient for some time prior to surgery, stored, and then used if necessary during or after surgery.

Pre-operative iron therapy

Peri-operative anaemia is a common condition among surgical patients and it is one of the chief prognostic factors for peri-operative blood transfusion. Anaemia is a reduced blood haemoglobin concentration and is common in chronic kidney disease (CKD). Pre-operative anaemia can be corrected before elective surgery. To maintain or accelerate erythropoiesis (the process by which RBCs are produced), effective management can be achieved through the use of genetically engineered erythropoiesis-stimulating agents (ESAs), an adequate level of iron, and folate and vitamin B12. Oral administration is often the preferred route for iron supplementation; however, the pre-operative use of intravenous iron might also be considered when time to surgery is too short for oral administration (Muñoz *et al.* 2005, 2008).

Intra-operative cell salvage

Sometimes known as autologous blood salvage, this is a clinical procedure that involves recovering blood lost during surgery and then reinfusing it back into the patient. It is often used in cardiac surgery.

Post-operative cell salvage (POCS)

This involves the collection of blood from surgical drains followed by reinfusion, with or without a wash cycle. POCS is used, for example, in orthopaedic surgery and in recovery areas after surgery.

Volume expanders

When a patient has lost a lot of body fluids but does not need RBCs or other blood cells, volume expanders may be

Box 6.3 Potential risks of blood transfusions

- Haemolytic reactions (fatal acute reactions estimated at one case per 250 000–1 100 000 units).
- ABO incompatibility following administrative errors.
- Allergic and anaphylactic reactions.
- Circulatory overload causing pulmonary oedema.
- Delayed transfusion reactions (3–10 days) due to antibodies to minor red cell antigens that were not detected by the pre-transfusion antibody assay (reported incidence ranges from 1 case per 2000–11 000 units).
- Transmission of viral infections such as HIV (risk of contracting HIV from a unit of blood ranges from 1 case in every 1.4 million units to one case in every 11 million units), hepatitis B (risk estimated at 1 case per 6000–320 000 units transfused), or hepatitis C (risk of contracting hepatitis C from a unit of blood ranges from 1 case in every 1.2 million units to 1 case in every 13 million units transfused).
- Transmission of a human prion disease, the commonest being the sporadic form of Creutzfeldt–Jakob disease (sCJD). A study by Hewitt (2006) has identified three occurrences, from three different donor/recipient pairs, in which a recipient of a transfusion (obtained from a 'vCJD' donor) has developed infection with vCJD. Because of the small size of the total at-risk recipient population, and the

background mortality rate for vCJD in the general UK population (0.24 per million per annum), the study provides strong evidence that vCJD can be transmitted from person to person through blood transfusion, which has had important connotations for national and international public health policy.
- Parasitic infections, most commonly transfusion transmitted malaria (risk of incidence 1 case per 4 million units). However, in countries where malaria is endemic, the risk sharply increases to 1 in 3.
- Bacterial contamination of blood components, such as *Yersinia enterocolitica* in packed red cells, and *Staphylococcus aureus*, *Staphylococcus epidermis*, *Klebsiella pneumoniae*, and *Serratia marcescens* in platelet concentrates. Risk of sepsis following platelet transfusion is estimated to be 1 case per 2000–3000 transfusions.
- Transfusion-related acute lung injury (1 case per 5000 transfusions).
- Transfusion-related immunomodulation.
- Febrile response to donor leukocyte or platelet contaminants.
- Graft versus host reactions (this usually occurs in immunocompromised patients and is commonly fatal following its onset 2–4 weeks after transfusion).

(Kaplan and Maerz 2007)

administered to avert or treat shock caused by fluid loss. Common volume expanders are Gelofusine®, normal saline, and lactated Ringer's solution (saline plus additional additives).

Context

 When to administer a blood transfusion

The procedure is initiated by a medical practitioner who prescribes the blood transfusion. An intravenous route, separate from all other infusions, is established in the patient by an appropriately qualified person. You may be asked to provide assistance with the IV cannulation (see Section 6.7). A dedicated IV site prevents contamination of the blood by other infusion fluids, which may be incompatible with the blood product (e.g. dextrose can cause clumping of RBCs).

Non-sterile gloves and an apron should be worn throughout the procedure to prevent contamination with body fluids and to maintain good infection control.

 When not to administer a blood transfusion

If there is any cause for concern during any part of the checking procedure for compatibility, or patient refusal, the transfusion should not be initiated. Medical staff and the blood bank should be informed immediately. The compatibility form and the blood unit should then be returned to the blood bank at the earliest opportunity.

Procedure

Whole blood is now rarely used, and the majority of transfusions are RBCs. The transfusions of other blood components (e.g. platelets) have very different requirements for transfusion. For this text, the procedure covers the administration of RBCs.

For ease of reference the procedure for administering a transfusion of RBCs has been separated into 'mini-procedures' of:

1 Obtaining and labelling a blood sample for cross-matching.
2 Withdrawal of blood from the blood bank.
3 Checking at the bedside prior to transfusion of blood.

Note: a framework document (Pirie and Green 2006) has been developed to assist health care professionals working in the community to ensure that transfusion practice in the primary care setting meets all the contemporary recommended requirements. The document outlines personnel, training, transport, equipment, and the practices required for delivering a blood transfusion service to the patient in the 'out-of-hospital' setting.

Good practice procedure for obtaining and labelling a blood sample for cross-matching is covered by Gallacher (2004), Hainsworth (2004), Hearnshaw (2004), and the RCN (2004). It is recommended that you obtain a blood sample from only one patient at a time. This will help to reduce the risk of error in labelling. Being accurate in this requires strict concentration, which may be difficult when working under pressure. The environment in which the sample is obtained must also allow adequate working space.

Step-by-step guide to obtaining and labelling a blood sample for cross-matching

Step	Rationale
1 Introduce yourself and positively identify the patient by verbally asking for their full name and date of birth, using open questions.	This encourages communication with the patient and assists with the verification process.
2 Check that these details match those on the patient's identity wristband and sample request form.	This confirms that you have the right patient. Unconscious patients or those with comprehension or communication difficulties should have a unique identification number and their gender as minimum patient identifiers on a wristband. Ask another member of staff, carer, or relative to verify this.
3 Brief the patient on the procedure and obtain consent.	The patient's autonomy, privacy, and self-esteem must be maintained at all times.
4 Prepare yourself (e.g. appropriate hand washing and use of aprons and examination gloves).	It is a strict requirement that you follow both your hospital infection control policy and blood transfusion policy when taking blood samples.
5 Collect and assemble the required equipment.	So everything is ready and to hand when you begin the procedure.
6 Select an appropriate vein from which to obtain the sample.	Blood should not be taken from an arm that is currently being infused as it may result in a diluted sample being sent for analysis. Use the patient's other arm.
7 Collect the required amount of blood into the sample tube.	To provide the sample.

8	Correctly label the sample tube. This should be done immediately after the blood has been collected and before you leave the patient. Record the patient's date of birth, gender, identification number, and the date. Correct spelling is essential. Do not write the details on the sample tube in advance of drawing the blood. Sign the sample tube as the person drawing the sample.	To avoid identification errors. Pre-labelling is one of the biggest causes of patient identification error leading to fatal transfusions.
9	Ensure that the patient details on the sample tube are recorded on the request form. This will also include a valid reason for transfusion, past transfusion history, and any special requirements.	Giving information pertinent to the prospective transfusion.
10	Safely dispose of contaminated or used items from the procedure and wash hands.	Local infection control policy must be followed at all times.
11	Ensure that the patient is comfortable.	To maintain patient comfort.
12	Send the sample to the hospital transfusion laboratory (HTL). Remember to include the request, date, and time.	So the sample can be analysed.

Step-by-step guide to withdrawing blood from the blood bank

Step		Rationale
1	Obtain the prescribed unit of blood product from the blood bank one unit at a time, immediately before use.	Blood must be maintained at the correct temperature until its use. The transfusion itself should be completed within 4 hours of its removal to reduce blood deterioration.
2	Check the information on the label of the blood container (see **Figure 6.23**) against the appropriate documentation and complete the documentation of withdrawal for the Blood Transfusion Service and the patient's medical records. The person collecting should document the date and time and sign the blood fridge register or electronic release system.	To ensure that the correct blood is used.
3	Inform the person who requested the blood product as soon as it is delivered.	So that the transfusion can commence as soon as possible.

(RCN 2004)

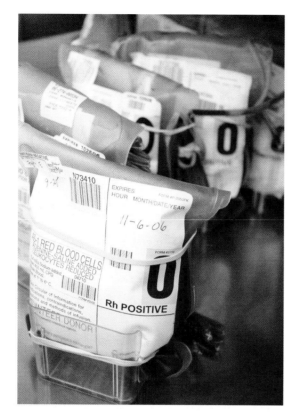

Figure 6.23 Blood bag and label, courtesy of Jill Davis/istock.com

Procedure: checking at the bedside prior to transfusion of blood

(Hearnshaw 2004, RCN 2004)

Preparation

Transfusion should commence as quickly as possible after the blood has arrived in the clinical area (British Committee for Standards in Haematology 1999). McClelland (2007) recommends that an RBC unit that has been out of cold temperature storage (CTS) for longer than 30 minutes should not be accepted back into stock by the blood bank, unless there is a validated local procedure to ensure that any unit returned to blood bank stock is suitable for transfusion. Once the unit is out of CTS, the risk of bacterial proliferation increases with time,

especially in warm ambient temperature. Transfusion of the unit should be completed within 4 hours after its removal from the CTS.

All patients receiving blood components must be wearing an identification name band, and it is paramount that corroboration of the right therapy to the right patient is conducted at the bedside by at least one Registered Nurse or doctor (British Committee for Standards in Haematology 1999) or following the protocol within hospital policy. The patient should be positively identified if they are capable of responding by verbal communication.

The following identification check should be carried out without interruption to avoid error. If interrupted, you must start again.

1 All patients undergoing transfusion should have an identification wristband (or photo ID card) displaying their gender, date of birth, and identification number. These should be clearly marked. The details on the wristband must then be finally checked against the blood compatibility label on the blood pack, and conducted at the patient's side (NPSA 2006). Recent SHOT data indicate that over-reliance on compatibility forms and checking those against patient notes has been a significant contributory factor to ABO-incompatible transfusions.

2 The blood group and unit number of blood must be identical to those on the blood transfusion compatibility form. The blood group on the blood unit must be compatible (not necessarily identical) as indicated on the compatibility label on the blood pack. Where the blood is not identical, a specific comment should have been made on the compatibility form.

3 The unit must be checked for alignment with any special requirement on the prescription chart (such as for gamma-irradiated blood). When nursing haematology or renal patients and the immunocompromised, special care should be taken, especially with regards to the CMV (cytomegalovirus) status, use of irradiated blood, and potential risk of sensitization. A second check with medical staff is appropriate before administration to the patient, especially if the patient is being nursed on a non-renal/haematology ward.

4 The unit must be checked to ensure that it has not passed its expiry date and shows no sign of leakage, unusual colour, or haemolysis.

5   The person conducting the checks must sign the blood transfusion compatibility form and prescription chart.

6   If there is any cause for concern during any part of the checking procedure, the unit should not be transfused and the blood bank should be informed. The compatibility form and the blood unit should be returned to the blood bank.

This process should be followed with each component administered.

Preparing the patient

Explain the procedure to the patient so they fully comprehend the transfusion process. This allows them to give consent, or opt out of the treatment.

Baseline observations of the patient should then be taken. These should be conducted just prior to administration, in order to monitor for adverse effects during the transfusion. They must include the patient's temperature, pulse, respirations, and blood pressure. Vital signs should be measured and recorded before the start of each unit of blood or blood component, and at the end of each transfusion episode. They should be noted separately from routine observations as well as clearly dated to facilitate easier retrieval of information later, if necessary. Routine observations should be continued on unconscious patients in operating theatres and intensive care.

Observations of the patient should follow local hospital policy; however, contemporary literature advises the assessment periods and durations as follows:

- Serious adverse reactions usually occur within the first 15-minute period and so continual observation during that time is vital (Parris and Grant-Casey 2007), especially for an unconscious patient who is unable to communicate (Gallacher 2004).
- Thereafter, monitor their temperature and pulse every 15 minutes for the first hour of transfusion.
- Then continue to record their pulse, respirations, blood pressure, temperature, and urinary output every hour for the duration of the transfusion.
- If any abnormal findings are observed, such as an increase in temperature, a tachycardia, or a drop in blood pressure, stop the transfusion and report the incident to medical staff immediately to allow prompt interventions to be initiated at the earliest opportunity.

- Accurately record the quantity of blood product administered, as any adverse effects may be related to the quantity given. As a guide, one unit of whole blood is 500 ml and one unit of concentrated RBCs is 300 ml.

Organize the environment and help the patient into a position that will be most comfortable for them to accept the transfusion. As the procedure may continue over a considerable period of time, the patient should be in an area where they can be readily observed throughout the procedure and have a means of alerting ward staff if they experience any adverse effects.

Confirm blood product is suitable for the patient by checking that the blood component has been prescribed appropriately, its expiry date has not been passed, and there are no signs of leakage, discoloration, clumping, or clouding on visual inspection. Do not proceed until any discrepancies have been resolved.

Preparing the equipment

Throughout the transfusion process, the patient's autonomy, privacy, and self-esteem must be maintained at all times. The environment in which the transfusion is conducted must have adequate working space and be in a position where the patient can be adequately observed. Ensure that the procedure for checking that the blood product is the one intended for that patient is followed (see previous section on procedure for checking at the bedside).

It is a strict requirement that you follow both your hospital transfusion policy and infection control policy when administering blood components. This means appropriate hand washing and use of aprons and examination gloves. Collect and assemble the required equipment by connecting the blood bag to the administration set and to the patient.

Blood components should be given via a sterile blood giving set that has a 170 microgram filter (Atterbury and Wilkinson 2000). The giving set should be primed first by:

- Closing the clamp on the giving set.
- Pulling off the tabs to expose the outlet port and inserting the spike into the blood component pack outlet.
- Inverting the bag and the giving set, so that the giving set is pointing upwards.

- Opening the clamp and squeezing the blood up through the first chamber and a third of the way into the second chamber.

- Re-inverting the bag, hanging it up, and running through as normal so that blood continues to the end of the line.

Step-by-step guide to transfusion

Step	Rationale
1 Begin the transfusion of blood. Use the rate determined by the medical practitioner. Regulate the roller clamp to adjust the input to the prescribed rate.	So that the patient receives the blood at the correct rate.
2 Ensure observations are made throughout the transfusion process. Refer to hospital policy on the frequency of observations.	To monitor for any adverse effects. To ensure that professional obligations are met.
3 Ensure that the patient remains comfortable throughout the duration of the therapy.	To maintain patient comfort.

Following the procedure

Clarify that the patient is comfortable and discuss the importance of reporting any ill effects or experiences post-administration. Don't forget to dispose of any used equipment appropriately and safely to prevent transmission of infection. Empty blood bags should be kept on the ward or returned to the blood transfusion department – but follow local hospital policy. Document the transfusion in the medical records, and note any after-effects or abnormal findings.

Recognizing patient deterioration

The nurse should be aware of the signs and symptoms of acute transfusion reactions, such as:

- A significant rise in the patient's temperature (>1°C).
- Shivering.
- Flushing.
- Urticaria (or signs of a rash on the patient's chest or abdomen).
- Itching.
- Vomiting and diarrhoea.
- Chest or abdominal pain.
- Oedema of the eyes or face.
- Pain or inflammation at or near transfusion site.
- Shortness of breath.
- Tachycardia.
- Headache.
- Rigor.
- Severe backache or loin pain.
- Circulatory failure or shock.
- Hypotension/Hypertension.
- General malaise or anxiety.

NB if the patient feels unwell or shows signs of a reaction then stop the transfusion immediately and call the doctor. Take and record temperature, pulse, blood pressure, respiration rate, and oxygen saturation readings. Recheck the identity of the recipient against the details on the pack and compatibility report to ensure correct blood has been given to the patient.

Reflection and evaluation

When you have undertaken a blood transfusion, think about the following questions:

1 Did you remember all of the checking procedure to ensure the safe transfusion of blood components?
2 Would you be able to explain alternative treatments if a patient refused to receive blood transfusion therapy?

Further learning opportunities

At the next available opportunity:

- Observe a blood transfusion being given and assist with the regular observational assessments.
- Talk with the patient about their experiences of receiving a blood transfusion.
- Find out if you have a transfusion practitioner in your hospital and contact them for further information.

Reminders

- As a final check at the patient's bedside, details on the patient's wristband should always be checked against the blood transfusion and the blood compatibility label on the blood pack. If there is any cause for concern during any part of the checking procedure, the unit should not be transfused and the blood bank should be informed.
- Follow your local transfusion and infection control policies when administering blood components.
- Observe the patient throughout the transfusion process to monitor for any adverse effects.

Patient scenarios

1 You have been asked to perform the baseline observations on a patient prior to a blood transfusion. What observations do you include?
2 During the blood transfusion process, the intravenous line becomes disconnected from the patient, causing a significant spillage of blood on and around the patient. What actions should you take?
3 As you are about to commence a blood transfusion, the patient suddenly informs you that they have changed their mind and now refuse to accept treatment. What should you do?

Website

 http://www.oxfordtextbooks.co.uk/orc/ endacott

You may find it helpful to work through our short online quiz and additional scenarios intended to help you to develop and apply the skills in this chapter.

References

Atterbury C and Wilkinson J (2000). Blood transfusion. *Nursing Standard*, **14**(34), 47–52.

British Committee for Standards in Haematology (1999). The administration of blood and blood components and the management of transfused patients. *Transfusion Medicine*, **9**, 227–38.

Department of Health (2001). *Good practice in consent implementation guide: consent to examination or treatment*. Health Service Circular 2001/023, London.

Directive 2002/98/EC of the European Parliament and of the Council (2003). Setting standards of quality and safety for the collection, testing, processing, storage and distribution of human blood and blood components and amending Directive 2001/83/EC. *Official Journal of the European Union*.

Directive 2005/61/EC of the European Parliament and of the Council (2005). Implementing Directive 2002/98/EC as regards traceability requirements and notification of serious adverse reactions and events. *Official Journal of the European Union*.

Doyle DJ (2002). Blood transfusions and the Jehovah's Witness patient. *American Journal of Therapeutics*, **9**, 417–24.

Gallacher R (2004). Using guidance to prevent errors when giving blood transfusions. *Nursing Times*, **100**(43), 34.

Gillespie TW and Hillyer CD (2001). Granulocytes. In CD Hillyer, KL Hillyer, L Jefferies, F Strobl, LE Silberstein, eds. *Handbook of transfusion medicine*, pp. 63–7. Academic Press, San Diego, CA.

Hainsworth T (2004). Guidance for preventing errors in administering blood transfusions. *Nursing Times*, **100**(27), 30–1.

Hearnshaw K (2004). Understanding the blood group system and blood transfusions. *Nursing Times*, **100**(45), 38–41.

Hewitt P (2006). vCJD and blood transfusion in the United Kingdom. *Transfusion Clinique et Biologique*, **13**(5), 312–16.

Kaplan LJ and Maerz LL (2007). *Transfusion and autotransfusion* [online] **http://www. emedicine.com/med/topic3215.htm#section~ References** accessed 10/04/08.

McClelland DBL (2007). *Handbook of transfusion medicine*, 4th edition. The Stationery Office, London.

Medicines and Healthcare Products Regulatory Agency (2005). *SABRE – a user guide. UK blood safety and quality regulations 2005 – implementation of the EU blood safety directive*. MHRA, London.

Muñoz M, Breymann C, García-Erce JA, Gómez-Ramírez S, Comin J, and Bisbe E (2008). Efficacy and safety of intravenous iron therapy as an alternative/adjunct to allogeneic blood transfusion. *Vox Sanguinis*, **94**(3), 172–83.

Muñoz M, Garcia-Erce JA, Cuenca J, Izuel M, Martinez A, and Solano VM (2005). Is there a role for perioperative intravenous iron therapy in orthopaedic and trauma surgery? Clinical experience in major lower limb surgery. *Transfusion Alternatives in Transfusion Medicine*, 8, 58–67.

National Patient Safety Agency (2006). *Safer practice notice (14) right patient, right blood. Advice for safer blood transfusions* [online] **http://www. npsa.nhs.uk/patientsafety/alerts-and- directives/notices/blood-transfusions/** accessed 10/04/08.

Parris E and Grant-Casey J (2007). Promoting safer blood transfusion practice in hospital. *Nursing Standard*, **21**(41), 35–8.

Pirie E and Green J (2006). Framework for the safe delivery of a blood transfusion service. *Journal of Community Nursing*, **20**(3) [online] **http://www. jcn.co.uk/journal.asp?MonthNum=03&YearNum= 2006&Type=backissue&ArticleID=903** accessed 26/08/08.

Pirie E and Green J (2007). Should nurses prescribe blood components? *Nursing Standard*, **21**(39), 35–41.

Royal College of Nursing (2004). *Right blood, right patient, right time*. RCN, London.

Stevenson T (2007). The safe administration of blood transfusions at night. *Nursing Times*, **103**(5), 33–4.

The UK Serious Hazards of Transfusion (2003). *Annual Report 2001–2002*. SHOT, Manchester.

The UK Serious Hazards of Transfusion (2006). *Annual Report 2006*. SHOT, London.

Tortora GJ and Grabowski SR (2000). *Principles of anatomy and physiology*, 9th edition. John Wiley and Sons, New York.

Wilkinson J and Wilkinson C (2001). Administrations of blood transfusions to adults in general hospital settings: a review of the literature. *Journal of Clinical Nursing*, **10**(2), 161–70.

Useful further reading and websites

The Scottish Blood Service have developed an e-learning package that is available to all NHS hospitals in the UK and is promoted by all UK Blood Services: **http://www.learnbloodtransfusion.org.uk**

This DH website incorporates a blood transfusion toolkit and has useful links to contemporary guidance: **http://www.transfusionguidelines.org.uk/ index.asp?Publication=BBT&Section= 22&pageid=315**

North Bristol NHS Trust has produced a blood transfusion training workbook with a good selection of multiple choice questions to enhance underpinning knowledge: **http://www.transfusionguidelines.org.uk/docs/ pdfs/rtc-sw_edu_assess_workbook.pdf**

The National Blood Service has good information on blood and blood stocks in the UK: **http://www.blood.co.uk/pages/e13basic.html**

There is a very good DVD called 'The strange case of Penny Allison' available from: **http://hospital.blood.co.uk/library/pdf/ PennyAorderForm2–3.pdf**

Website with information about blood types and an interactive game to ensure you know blood type compatibility: **http://nobelprize.org/educational_ games/medicine/landsteiner/readmore.html**

Ⓐ Answers to patient scenarios

1 In order to monitor for adverse effects during the transfusion, you must include the patient's temperature, pulse, respirations, and blood pressure. Depending on local policy these will normally be recorded before the start of each unit of blood or blood component, 15 minutes after transfusion has commenced, at hourly intervals during the transfusion, and at the end of each transfusion episode. They should be noted separately from routine observations as well as clearly dated to facilitate easier retrieval of information later.

2 Stop the transfusion immediately and secure the patient's cannula by recapping it (to avoid the

patient losing blood through it). Remember that when dealing with any blood spillages you must be wearing appropriate personal protective equipment, use recommended cleaning products, and dispose of all clinical waste safely (according to local hospital infection control policy). Clean the patient and environment. The incident must be noted in the patient's notes and reported to a doctor. Depending on how much spillage occurred, further units may need to be reordered and prescribed. Throughout the process, ensure that the patient is not displaying any adverse effects and reassure them to remove any anxiety the incident may have caused.

3 Initially, calmly ask the patient about their concerns and reasons for their decision. Sometimes there may be a simple reason or doubt that may be resolved by clarifying certain issues. If the patient still refuses to accept treatment, then the doctor should be informed in order to discuss the risks associated with that refusal as well as the potential alternatives (Doyle 2002). The Department of Health's *Good practice in consent implementation guide* (2001) states that all patients have a right to decide what happens to their own bodies, and their religious, cultural, and ethical concerns must be honoured. If the blood unit remains sealed, return it to the blood bank.

6.9 **Cardiopulmonary resuscitation (CPR)**

Definition

In the event of cardiac arrest, cardio (heart) pulmonary (lung) resuscitation (revive) (CPR) is the method employed to deliver oxygenated blood to the vital organs of the body in order to prevent, or reduce, tissue damage.

It is important to remember that:

- Prevention of cardiac arrest is the main goal.
- Survival from in-hospital cardiac arrest is poor (Nolan *et al*. 2006).
- Clinical observations will give early warning signs of deterioration.

- A 'Do not attempt resuscitation' (DNAR) order may be in place.

Prior knowledge

Before undertaking CPR, make sure you are familiar with:

- Cardiovascular anatomy and physiology.
- Respiratory anatomy and physiology.

Understanding the mechanism by which the body is supplied with oxygenated blood will aid an understanding of the skills required to perform CPR, and also interpretation of clinical observations that may give warning of a patient at risk of cardiac or respiratory arrest.

Background

Survival from in-hospital cardiorespiratory arrest is poor, so prevention of arrest is the goal. Patients often exhibit clinical signs of deterioration prior to cardiac arrest, which can be picked up by simple, routine monitoring of respiratory rate, pulse, and blood pressure (McGaughey *et al*. 2007). Hospital staff should be alert to the signs and act early to prevent arrest wherever possible. Early warning scores give guidance on calling for help such as the critical outreach or medical emergency team. Staff in the community should contact the patient's GP or the national emergency number (e.g. 999 in the UK) if the patient is *in extremis*.

Some patients may have a valid DNAR order or have made an advance directive (living will) stating they do not wish to receive CPR. It is essential you are aware of the resuscitation status of the patients for whom you are caring. However, ***if in doubt start CPR*** as brain damage is likely within 3–5 minutes of arrest without quality CPR.

CPR forms the second link of the well-recognized chain of survival (**Box 6.4**), revised in 2005 (Nolan 2006).

Box 6.4 Chain of survival

1 Early recognition and call for help – to prevent cardiac arrest.
2 Early **CPR** – to buy time.
3 Early defibrillation – to restart the heart.
4 Post-resuscitation care – to restore quality of life.

When a person has a cardiorespiratory arrest, the heart stops working as an effective pump and oxygenated blood is not circulated around the body. Within a few minutes irreversible brain damage will occur. Causes include ischaemic heart disease, pulmonary embolus, respiratory depression, airway obstruction, trauma, electrolyte disturbances, and hypothermia.

Various methods of reviving people have been experimented with over the years. The combination of rescue breaths together with chest compressions, used today, was introduced in the 1960s (American Heart Association 2008). The method has been revised over the decades as evidence of efficacy is reviewed. The core components remain the same; that of creating a blood flow by compressing the patient's chest and providing oxygen by ventilating their lungs.

The International Liaison Committee on Resuscitation (ILCOR) was created in 1993, its remit being to review the available literature and make recommendations for treatment (Nolan 2005). The most recent UK guide-line changes were issued in November 2005 – based on the evidence available, once cardiorespiratory arrest has been confirmed, 30 chest compressions should be delivered followed by two rescue breaths. There are minor international variations in procedure, so familiarize yourself with those that apply to your country of employment. What follows are the UK guidelines.

CPR can be performed by anyone physically able to deliver it. You should be familiar with current resuscitation guidelines and have attended a practical workshop to practise the skills. It is well recognized that skills deteriorate over time (Hamilton 2005), so attending a practical refresher at least annually is essential.

In the UK there is no 'Good Samaritan' law; however, nurses have a duty of care to their patients and should be prepared to perform CPR when required. The following statement from the UK Resuscitation Council (2000) makes clear the legal position for health care staff:

> *Members of the health-care professions who attempt resuscitation will be expected to employ the highest professional standard of care, compatible with their position in the health service and with their level of training. Their level of competence will be judged on an objective basis and they could therefore be held liable if that standard of care falls below that to be expected of a reasonably competent health professional of the same qualifications and experience. Therefore, provided resuscitation procedures are performed correctly and in accordance with current guidelines, it is unlikely that a successful claim could be brought. Liability is only likely to arise if procedures are carried out incorrectly and with disregard to accepted practice and guidelines.*

Chest compressions are a key element in survival, providing blood flow not only to the brain but also to the heart. Interruptions to chest compressions have an unfavourable effect on survival and should therefore be kept to a minimum (Eftestol *et al.* 2002).

ABCDE assessment of the casualty

A systematic assessment of anyone in apparent distress is vital to ensure the correct action is taken as soon as possible. The ABCDE approach covers this requirement (see **Table 6.7**) (see also Sections 8.1 and 8.2).

Table 6.7 The ABCDE approach

Step	Assessment
A	**Airway** – is it patent, can you hear them breathe (talk)? Does the patient exhibit signs of airway obstruction such as stridor?
B	**Breathing** – can you see them breathing? Is their chest moving in a normal manner? Are breath sounds normal? Is there any deviation of the trachea from the midline of the neck?
C	**Circulation** – can you feel a pulse? Is it regular? Is it of good volume? Is the patient warm? What is their capillary refill time?
D	**Disability** – what is their neurological status using **AVPU** or Glasgow Coma Scale? Is there any obvious deviation from normal perceived behaviour? What is the patient's blood glucose level?
E	**Exposure** – make a full examination of the patient, assessing for signs such as haemorrhage, rash, etc.

Context

CPR should be started immediately on any patient in confirmed cardiorespiratory arrest, i.e. **apnoeic** and pulseless, unless the patient is known to have a valid DNAR order or resuscitative efforts would be futile, e.g. if the patient is in rigor mortis or has sustained an injury incompatible with life.

Indications for assistance

If after using the ABCDE approach you have identified a patient is compromised in any of A, B, C, or D, you must call for assistance. The nature of the assistance will depend on whether the patient is *in extremis*.

With cardiac or peri-arrest in hospital (see **Figure 6.24**), call or send someone to telephone for the resuscitation team and trolley. The equipment available will vary locally; you should be familiar with the trolley nearest to your workplace.

With cardiac or peri-arrest out of hospital (see **Figure 6.25**), telephone for the emergency services giving full details of the problem. Equipment available will vary dependent on the location. As with in-hospital staff, you should know what equipment is available in the places you work. The emergency services, based on the information given, will assess what equipment to send with the medical assistance.

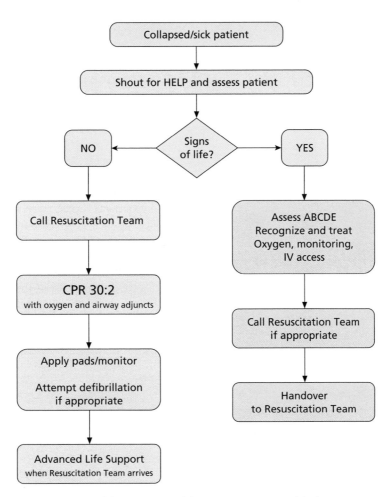

Figure 6.24 In-hospital resuscitation guidelines, courtesy of the Resuscitation Council (UK).

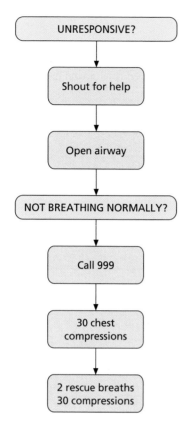

Figure 6.25 Basic life support guidelines, courtesy of Resuscitation Council (UK).

Hospital call systems

Ensure you are familiar with the cardiac arrest call system in your place of work and the emergency telephone number in your country of residence. There has been harmonization of emergency numbers in UK hospitals, and 2222 is now recognized as the cardiac arrest number, but in some settings it may be simply a 999 or 911 call.

NB some clinical areas, e.g. CCU, ICU, and A&E, may have staff trained to manage the cardiac arrest without calling the hospital arrest team. You should check the procedure in the place where you work and where available ensure that you are familiar with bedside emergency alarm systems.

Special considerations

Resuscitation outside the hospital setting presents a challenge as there may be less equipment and fewer people. Staff should be provided with pocket masks (or face shields) but mouth-to-mouth ventilation may have to be considered. There have been a few reports of cross-infection from mouth-to-mouth ventilation with diseases such as TB and severe acute respiratory syndrome (SARS), but no reports involving hepatitis B or HIV (Nolan *et al.* 2006). Care should always be taken if blood is present as there may be a risk of contracting blood-borne diseases such as hepatitis B.

Cardiac arrest and emergency situations can be hazardous since there is a tendency to hurry and not follow safe practice. Be alert to potential hazards, e.g. sharps, body fluids, manual handling issues (Resuscitation Council (UK) 2001). Wear a pair of gloves as a minimum. Ensure your own personal safety and that of those around you (i.e. other patients and members of staff) at all times.

Pregnancy involves not one casualty but two, and positioning the casualty effectively to prevent compromising the CPR attempt is important. Beyond 20 weeks gestation, the weight of the foetus when a woman is supine reduces blood return via the inferior vena cava. Therefore, if a pregnant woman requires CPR, she should be tilted to the left at an angle of approximately 12.5–15° to reduce aortocaval compression (Bamber and Dresner 2003, Kinsella 2003). This can be achieved by positioning a wedge or suitable alternative under the right hip (Morris and Stacey 2003).

Laryngectomy patients cannot be ventilated via the mouth or nasal route but require ventilation via the stoma in their neck. Ensure the stoma is patent and not blocked by a mucus plug.

Patients may collapse in confined areas, e.g. lavatories or cars. CPR in these circumstances will be problematic. Assistance will be needed to move the patient; there may be special equipment that can be used. You should consider your own safety at all times and not risk injury due to poor manual handling.

Step-by-step guide to CPR

▶ Step   Rationale

	Step	Rationale
1	Approach the patient after checking it is safe to do so.	There may be some chemical, electrical, or physical hazard present that caused the patient's collapse in the first place.
2	Check the patient for response and signs of life.	To exclude patients who may be asleep or resting.
3	If the patient is unresponsive, call for help.	To ensure you have someone to send for appropriate medical treatment ASAP.
4	Open the patient's mouth to assess for foreign material.	The mouth needs to be clear to ensure the airway remains patent (dentures, if well fitting, may be left in place).
5	Open the airway by tilting the head back and lifting the jaw with your fingertips.	If someone is unconscious, the tongue falls back and obstructs the airway. This manoeuvre lifts the tongue from the pharynx (see **Figure 6.26**).
6	Assess for normal respirations by looking for chest movement, listening for breath sounds, and feeling for exhaled air on your cheek. *If trained and experienced*, simultaneously assess for a carotid pulse.	Having opened the airway the patient may now start to breathe. However, do not mistake gasps/agonal respirations (which may occur in up to 55% of cardiac arrests, Eisenberg 2006) for normal breathing. Assessing carotid pulses requires experience.
7	In the absence of any normal respirations, call the arrest team/paramedics.	Additional experienced help is required as soon as possible, together with equipment such as a defibrillator. If you are alone this call needs to be made before you start CPR.
8	With the patient on a firm, flat surface, start CPR.	A soft, yielding mattress will reduce the effectiveness of chest compressions. Supine position will aid blood flow to the brain.
9	Place the heel of one hand in the centre of the patient's chest on the sternum. Put your other hand on top, keeping your fingers clear of the ribs.	Avoid pressing on the ribs to reduce the risk of rib fractures.
10	Position yourself so that your shoulders are over the patient's chest. This may require placing a knee on the bed or adjusting the height of the bed/trolley. Keeping your arms straight with elbows locked, press down vertically on the patient's chest (see **Figure 6.27**).	This position allows for effective chest compressions and helps reduce back strain for the rescuer.

continued overleaf

11	Aim to push down about 4–5 cm (the pressure required to achieve this will vary according to the size of the patient). Without lifting your hands off the chest, release the pressure fully.	Compression and release are equally important since this is how the blood is circulated.
12	Repeat, giving 30 compressions at a rate of 100/minute (should take approx. 18 seconds). Do not 'bounce' or move your hands around; compressions should be delivered smoothly.	Compressions deliver blood to both the brain and heart and should not be interrupted for more than 10 seconds.
13	Give two rescue breaths (see **Boxes 6.5 and 6.6** for technique). Each breath should be enough to create a visible chest rise. As soon as oxygen is available it should be attached to the pocket mask at a rate of 15 litres/min.	To deliver oxygen to the patient. Forceful ventilation and high tidal volumes should be avoided as this is likely to cause inflation of the stomach, which increases the chance of regurgitation and pulmonary aspiration.
14	Do not make more than two attempts at rescue breaths each cycle. If the chest does not rise then on the next attempt ensure that the airway is properly open using the head tilt, chin lift, or jaw thrust manoeuvre, and ensure a good seal has been achieved.	To ensure oxygen is being delivered to the patient.
15	In certain situations it may not be possible or advisable to use mouth-to-mouth, e.g. when dealing with a patient who has taken certain poisons such as cyanide (Health and Safety Executive 2007). In these circumstances endeavour to maintain a patent airway and deliver chest compressions only.	To maintain your own safety.
16	Repeat the chest compressions and rescue breaths at a ratio of 30:2 until further help arrives or you become exhausted.	Continuation of seamless chest compressions and rescue breaths gives the patient the best possible chance of survival while awaiting more advanced medical intervention. Chest compressions, correctly delivered, are tiring, so where possible rescuers should alternate every 2 minutes.

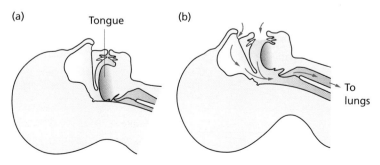

Figure 6.26 Closed and open airway.

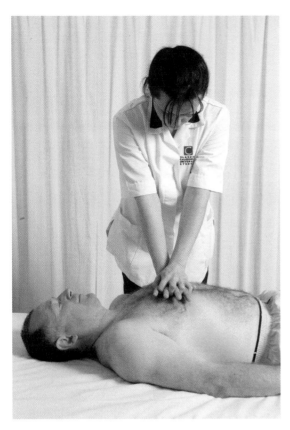

Figure 6.27 Position for chest compressions. The heel of one hand is on the sternum, the other hand is on top, the shoulders are over the patient's chest, and arms are straight with locked elbows.

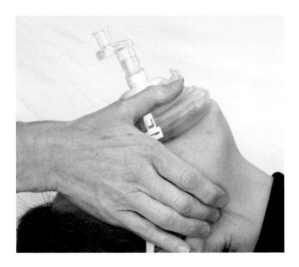

Figure 6.28 How to position a mask on a patient.

Box 6.5 Mouth-to-mouth

- Open the patient's airway as before, using a head tilt and chin lift.
- Pinch the patient's nose with your thumb and forefinger.
- Take a breath.
- Cover the patient's mouth entirely with your mouth, ensuring a good seal, and blow in.
- The patient's chest should rise.
- Lift your head clear.
- Allow the chest to fall and repeat once.
- Each breath should take approximately 1 second.

Box 6.6 Mouth-to-mask

Mouth-to-mask is more easily achieved by positioning yourself at the patient's head when working with a second person who is delivering the chest compressions.

- Open the mask, attach the one-way valve (and oxygen if available at 10 litres/min).
- Position the mask over the patient's nose and mouth (see **Figure 6.28**) and hold in place using your thumbs.
- Apply a jaw thrust with your fingers and press the mask onto the patient's face. (A jaw thrust is achieved by placing your fingers on the angle of the jaw and lifting upwards.)
- Blow through the valve, watching to see the chest rise.
- Allow the chest to fall and repeat once.
- Each breath should take approximately 1 second.
- Immediately resume 30 chest compressions followed by two rescue breaths.
- Continue 30:2 until further assistance arrives.
- Attach oxygen at 10 litres/min as soon as it is available.

Use of airway adjuncts

In a patient who requires resuscitation, use of an oropharyngeal airway helps maintain a patent airway as it keeps the tongue clear of the pharynx. The correct size of airway (see **Figure 6.29**) is the vertical distance between the incisors and the angle of the jaw. Insert it upside down to the back of the hard palate and then rotate 180°.

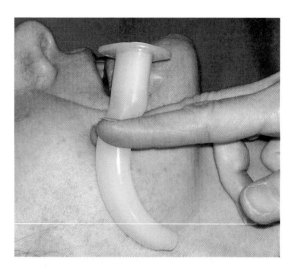

Figure 6.29 Selecting an oropharyngeal airway of the correct size. The length should equal the vertical distance between the incisors and the angle of the jaw.

- The patient's family/next of kin need to be informed.
- Nurses should also consider whether a critical incident report should be completed.
- Emergency equipment needs to be checked and replenished.
- Staff involved in the arrest may well benefit from having some time to reflect and a chance to talk over the event.

Recognizing patient deterioration

If the resuscitation attempt is successful, it is important to observe the patient closely in case of deterioration, as the reason for the cardiac arrest may still be present. Monitor the patient's vital signs (respirations, oxygen saturation, pulse, and blood pressure) and neurological status, observing for any untoward signs.

Bag valve mask ventilation requires two people and is not covered in this book (see Resuscitation Council (UK) 2005: 46).

Following the procedure

- Once the emergency team attends, various advanced life support measures may be instituted, e.g. defibrillation, intubation, administration of drugs, etc. During the resuscitation attempt, chest compressions remain a core, essential component and should be maintained with minimal interruptions.
- Safety of staff/helpers is paramount, so attention to the possibility of discarded sharps needs to be borne in mind and observed for.
- Following CPR where patients regain a circulation and are for full active care, they require monitoring in a high dependency area.
- In some cases patients may regain an output but the decision is taken that further interventions would not be appropriate. The patient and family (if present) require considerate end of life care.
- Most resuscitation attempts result in the death of the patient and nurses need to be familiar with the correct procedure for managing a death (refer to Section 3.4).

Reflection and evaluation

When you have undertaken CPR, think about the following:

- Did you give good quality chest compressions using the correct technique?
- Were you able to ventilate the patient effectively?
- Did help arrive promptly?
- Was all the equipment readily available?
- Reflect on the event and consider whether it went smoothly or if things could be improved.

Further learning opportunities

- Attend a national accredited resuscitation course as appropriate to your level of training.
- Consider arranging a resuscitation skills training session for your work area. Discuss with senior staff.

Reminders

- Know the emergency procedures and equipment where you work.
- Attend at least annual basic life support refresher sessions.
- Compression:breath ratio – 30:2.
- Compression rate – 100/min.

Patient scenarios

1 Mr J is admitted to a medical assessment unit with chest pain, and a 12-lead ECG is requested. As this is being prepared, Mr J stops talking and slumps in the bed. He is unresponsive and apnoeic with no signs of life. Two nurses are present. What should they do?

2 Mrs B is receiving treatment in her home from the district nurse for a diabetic foot ulcer. She says she hasn't been feeling well that morning and collapses on the sitting room floor. Her husband is in the next room. What do you do?

Website

http://www.oxfordtextbooks.co.uk/orc/endacott

You may find it helpful to work through our short online quiz and additional scenarios intended to help you to develop and apply the skills in this chapter.

References

American Heart Association (2008). *History of CPR* [online] **http://www.americanheart.org/presenter.jhtml?identifier=3012990** accessed 26/08/08.

Bamber JH and Dresner M (2003). Aortocaval compression in pregnancy: the effect of changing the degree and direction of lateral tilt on maternal cardiac output. *Anesthesia and Analgesia*, **97**, 256–8.

Eftestol T, Sunde K, and Steen PA (2002). Effects of interrupting precordial compressions on the calculated probability of defibrillation success during out of hospital cardiac arrest. *Circulation*, **105**(19), 2270.

Eisenberg MS (2006). Incidence and significance of gasping or agonal respirations in cardiac arrest patients. *Current Opinion in Critical Care*, **12**(3), 204–6.

Hamilton R (2005). Nurses' knowledge and skill retention following cardiopulmonary resuscitation training: a review of the literature. *Journal of Advanced Nursing*, **51**(3), 288–98.

Health and Safety Executive (2007). *Cyanide poisoning – New recommendations on first aid treatment*, updated 12/05/08 [online] **http://www.hse.gov.uk/pubns/misc076.htm** accessed 26/08/08.

Kinsella SM (2003). Lateral tilt for pregnant women: why 15 degrees? *Anaesthesia*, **58**, 835–6.

McGaughey J, Alderdice F, Fowler R, Kapila A, Mayhew A, and Moutray M (2007). Outreach and Early Warning Systems (EWS) for the prevention of Intensive Care admission and death of critically ill adult patients on general hospital wards. *The Cochrane Collaboration, Cochrane Reviews*. July 18.

Morris and Stacey (2003). Resuscitation in pregnancy. *British Medical Journal*, **327**, 1277–9.

Nolan (2005). European Resuscitation Council guidelines for resuscitation 2005: introduction. *Resuscitation*, **67**(Suppl 1), S3–6.

Nolan J (2006). The chain of survival. *Resuscitation*, **71**(3), 270–1.

Nolan J, Soar J, Lockey A *et al.*, eds (2006) *Advanced life support*, 5th edition. Resuscitation Council (UK), London: 130–3.

Resuscitation Council (UK) (2000). *The legal status of those who attempt resuscitation* [online] **http://www.resus.org.uk/pages/legal.htm** accessed 26/08/08.

Resuscitation Council (UK) (2001). *Guidance for safer handling during resuscitation in hospital* [online] **http://www.resus.org.uk/pages/safehand.pdf** accessed 26/08/08.

Resuscitation Council (UK) (2005). *Advanced life support manual*, 5th edition. Resuscitation Council (UK), London.

Useful further reading and websites

Resuscitation Council UK website: **http://www.resus.org.uk**

Advanced Life Support Group website: **http://www.alsg.org**

European Resuscitation Council website: **http://www.erc.edu**

American Heart Association website: **http://www.americanheart.org**

Australian Resuscitation Council website: **http://www.resus.org.au**

New Zealand Resuscitation Council website: **http://www.nzrc.org.nz**

South African Resuscitation Council website: **http://www.resuscitationcouncil.co.za**

Up-to-date articles on evidence-based medicine: **http://www.Bestbets.org**

Answers to patient scenarios

1 One nurse puts the bed flat and starts chest compressions while the other ensures a call for the cardiac arrest team goes out and returns with emergency equipment. Using a pocket mask with additional oxygen attached, two rescue breaths are given. CPR is delivered by the two nurses using a ratio of 30 compressions to two rescue breaths. Once the arrest team arrive, the nurses assist as directed by the team leader.

2 Ensuring personal safety, assess responsiveness of Mrs B and shout for help. Check mouth and open airway by tilting head back. Assess breathing and (if confident) carotid pulse. If no breathing or pulse, send Mr B to call for an emergency ambulance, stating that it is a cardiac arrest.

   Start chest compressions and after 30 compressions deliver two rescue breaths using a pocket mask. Repeat the process using a ratio of 30:2 until the paramedics arrive. They will take over – give assistance as directed.

6.10 **Venepuncture**

This is an advanced skill. You *must* check whether you can assist with or undertake this skill, in line with local policy.

Definition

Venepuncture is the introduction of a needle into a vein in order to obtain a blood sample for haematological, biochemical, or bacteriological analysis and/or monitor levels of blood components.

It is important to remember that:

Laboratory test results are only as good as the specimen, and the specimen is only as good as the method by which it is collected, handled, and processed. It is imperative therefore that you are aware of the correct procedures and follow them accordingly. Blood tests are probably the most commonly used diagnostic aid in the care and evaluation of patients.

Prior knowledge

Before attempting venepuncture, make sure you are familiar with:

1 Cardiovascular anatomy and physiology, especially the structure of a blood vessel.
2 Factors influencing venous circulation.
3 Infection control policy.
4 Needlestick injury policy.

Background

The structure of veins

All blood vessels (with the exception of the capillary) have a similar construction. There are three layers to the vessel wall and the individual variations between the vessels are determined by the location and the function of each vessel. The layers of the blood vessels are shown in **Figure 6.30**.

Tunica intima

This is the inner layer and consists of flattened endothelial cells that are arranged longitudinally along the vessel. Endothelium facilitates blood flow along the vessel, preventing the adhesion of blood cells to the vessel wall. Trauma to the vessel can roughen the endothelial lining and encourage platelets to adhere to the vessel wall. This can result in thrombus formation and the inflammatory process of phlebitis.

One feature of veins, not seen in the arterial system, is the presence of valves. Valves are semi-lunar folds of endothelium and their function is to assist the blood flow back to the heart. Valves occur more frequently at

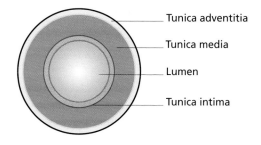

Figure 6.30 Structure of a blood vessel wall.

junctions of veins and can sometimes be seen as small bulges in the vessel. Valves can interfere with the withdrawal of blood and the advancement of cannulae, and should be avoided.

Tunica media

This is the middle layer and consists of smooth muscle and elastic tissue. Veins have less smooth muscle and elastic tissue than arteries and as a result are more prone to collapse if venous pressure is low. This layer also contains nerve fibres that make the vessel sensitive to changes in temperature, and spasm of the vessel can be induced by chemical or mechanical irritation. Vessel spasm can impede blood flow and cause pain; this can often be relieved by heat.

Tunica adventitia

This is the outer layer and consists of fibrous connective tissue, collagen, and nerve fibres, which surround and support the vessels. The nerve fibres are mainly from the sympathetic nervous system and the impulses keep the vessel in a state of tonus, allowing it to constrict and dilate as physiologically required.

Venepuncture site selection

Patient anxiety about venepuncture may result in vasoconstriction (Thurgate and Heppell 2005). Anxiety causes an increase in circulating adrenaline, causing increased vasoconstriction. A calm and confident approach to venepuncture with an adequate explanation of the procedure may help to reduce anxiety before site selection.

To perfect the technique of venepuncture, it is essential that the person undertaking it has a good understanding of the anatomy and physiology of arteries, veins, and associated nerves. The superficial veins of the arm are usually chosen for venepuncture, namely the basilic, cephalic, and medial cubital veins in the antecubital fossa (see **Figure 6.31)** (Tortora and Grabowski 2003).

Although the larger and fuller median cubital and cephalic veins of the arm are used most frequently, the basilic vein on the dorsum of the arm or dorsal hand veins are also acceptable for venepuncture (see Figure 6.33). Foot veins are a last resort because of the higher probabil-

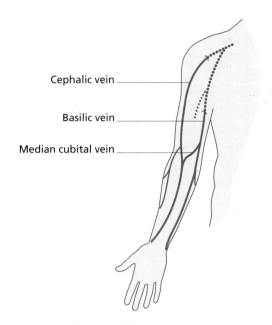

Figure 6.31 The veins of the arm.

ity of complications, and should be used only by medical staff or appropriately trained health care professionals (Harris and Walker 2005).

Inspect and note any signs of infection, bruising, or phlebitis. Palpate and trace the path of veins with the index finger. Thrombosed veins lack resilience, feel cord-like, and roll easily. The healthy vein feels soft, bouncy, and will refill when pressed (Lavery and Ingram 2005). In comparison arteries pulsate, are more elastic, and have a thick wall; these need to be avoided.

Certain areas are to be avoided when choosing a site:

- Extensive scars from burns and surgery – it is difficult to puncture the scar tissue and obtain a specimen.
- The arm on the side of a previous mastectomy – test results may be affected because of lymphoedema.
- Haematoma – may cause erroneous test results. If another site is not available, collect the specimen distal to the haematoma.
- Intravenous therapy (IV)/blood transfusions – fluid may dilute the specimen, so collect from the opposite arm if possible. Otherwise, satisfactory samples may be drawn from below the IV site by following these procedures:
  - Turn off the IV for at least 2 minutes before venepuncture.

- Apply the tourniquet below the IV site. Select a vein other than the one with the IV.
- Perform the venepuncture.
- Oedematous extremities – tissue fluid accumulation alters test results (Dougherty 2002).
- Areas of previous venepunctures should be avoided as they can result in pain from repeated trauma to the vein (RCN 2003).

Blood collection tubes

Blood collection tubes are glass or plastic tubes sealed with a partial vacuum inside by rubber stoppers. For safety reasons, plastic tubes tend to be the most common. The air pressure inside the tube is negative, i.e. less than in the normal environment. After inserting the longer needle into the vein, the tube is then inserted into the holder so that the shorter needle pierces the stopper. The difference in pressure between the inside of the tube and the vein causes blood to fill the tube. The tubes are available in various sizes for adult and paediatric phlebotomies. Adult tubes have volumes of 5, 7, 10, and 15 ml and paediatric tubes are available in volumes of 2, 3, and 4 ml.

Different blood tests require different types of blood specimen. For instance, some specimens require the addition of an **anticoagulant** in the tube. The anticoagulant prevents blood from clotting. It is of critical importance that you understand which type of tube to use for each test ordered.

In the vacuum blood collection system, the anticoagulants are already in the tubes in the precise amounts needed to mix with the amount of blood that will fill the tube. The colour of the stopper on each tube indicates what, if any, anticoagulant the tube contains. It is important to fill each tube completely so that the proportion of blood to chemical additive is correct, otherwise the test results may not be accurate or the specimen will be rejected and will need to be recollected.

Order of draw

Blood collection tubes must be drawn in a specific order to avoid cross-contamination of additives between tubes. The recommended order of draw for plastic vacutainer tubes is:

1 Blood culture bottle or tube (yellow or yellow-black top).
2 Coagulation tube (light blue top). If a routine coagulation assay is the only test ordered, then a single light blue top tube may be drawn. If there is concern over contamination by tissue fluids or thromboplastins, then you may draw a non-additive tube first (see below), and then a coagulation tube.
3 Non-additive tube (red top).
4 Additive tubes in this order:
   - SST (red-grey or gold top). Contains a gel separator and clot activator.
   - Sodium heparin (dark green top).
   - PST (light green top). Contains lithium heparin anticoagulant and a gel separator.
   - EDTA (lavender top).
   - ACDA or ACDB (pale yellow top). Contains acid citrate dextrose.
   - Oxalate/fluoride (light grey top).

Note: tube colours may differ internationally. Tubes with additives must be thoroughly mixed. Erroneous test results may be obtained when the blood is not thoroughly mixed with the additive.

Safety procedures

When handling the body fluids of patients, it is important to follow safety and infection control procedures (Schramm and Hannan 2006).

Protect yourself

Practise universal precautions:

- Wear gloves and an apron when handling blood/ body fluids.
- Wash hands frequently.
- Dispose of items in appropriate containers.
- Dispose of needles immediately upon removal from the patient's vein. Do not bend, break, recap, or resheath needles to avoid accidental needle puncture or splashing of contents (The Health Protection Agency 2005).

Protect the patient

- Place blood collection equipment away from patients.

- Practise hygiene for the patient's protection. When wearing gloves, change them between patients and wash your hands frequently. Always wear an apron.
- Record the patient's name and ID number.

Context

 When to perform venepuncture

Only perform venepuncture when a blood sample is needed for diagnostic purposes or to monitor therapeutic blood levels, and this information is vital to the patient's well-being and treatment.

 When not to perform venepuncture

If not requested by a senior colleague. Requests should preferably be in writing; however, some situations will necessitate a verbal request.

Alternative interventions

Winged infusion sets or 'butterflies' as they are routinely known are used for performing venepuncture on very small veins, often seen in children and in the geriatric population. Butterfly needles used for phlebotomy are usually 21-, 23-, or 25-gauge with lengths of $^1/_2$–$^3/_4$ inch. Plastic attachments to the needle that resemble butterfly wings are used for holding the needle during insertion. A butterfly set may be attached to a vacutainer needle adaptor.

Potential problems

Arterial stab
If an artery has been punctured, the blood will be bright red and the container may fill quickly (see **Figure 6.32f**). Should this occur, the needle should be removed quickly and firm pressure applied for more than 5 minutes or until the bleeding stops. In order to prevent this, be sure you are familiar with sites of arteries and veins and take your time selecting the vein prior to the procedure (Scales 2008).

Haematoma
A collection of blood in the subcutaneous tissue caused by blood being forced out of the vein under increased pressure. This occurs if the needle has gone through or

'nicked' the vein or because the tourniquet was not removed prior to removing the needle (Cox and Roper 2005). If you see a haematoma form under the skin adjacent to the puncture site (see **Figure 6.32e**), release the tourniquet immediately, apply the swab, withdraw the needle, and apply firm pressure for 2 minutes until the bleeding stops to avoid bruising.

Haemoconcentration
Increase in the proportion of red blood cells in blood, usually due to a reduction in the volume of plasma; the absolute number of red blood cells remains unchanged. Haemoconcentration results in increased blood viscosity. It is caused by dehydration and may be artificially induced by:

- Using the tourniquet for too long (it should not be in place for any more than 1 minute).
- Excessive rubbing, pressing, pinching, or gripping of the site.
- Patients who have either sclerosed veins (Lavery and Ingram 2005) or have had IV therapy over extensive periods will have higher propensity to haemoconcentration in their blood.

During haemoconcentration, large molecules (e.g. proteins), coagulation factors, and cells accumulate disproportionately. Specimens drawn from haemoconcentrated veins may not reflect the patient's real status.

Incomplete collection or no blood obtained
This can happen for a number of reasons and can be easily remedied:

- Adjust the position of the needle, slowly moving it forwards or backwards (maybe you or the patient moved a fraction and you're not quite there but incredibly close). If this is unsuccessful, withdraw the needle slightly (you may have gone a little too far). If neither of these approaches work, double-check the angle that you used (Cox and Roper 2005) – see **Figure 6.32a, b**, and **c**.
- Check your equipment – is the tourniquet too tight or too loose? Is the needle or vacuum device faulty?
- Sometimes veins move, particularly in elderly patients. Prior to the procedure, push the vein from side to side; does it move easily? Try to anchor it with your finger (Cox and Roper 2005).

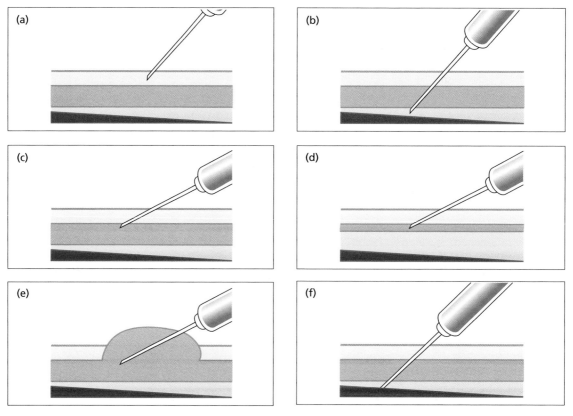

Figure 6.32 Common problems during venepuncture. (a) **Incomplete vein penetration**. The needle has not reached the lumen. It needs to be moved further forward. (b) **Penetration is too deep**. The needle has penetrated beyond the lumen. It needs to be moved backward. (c) **Incorrect angle of penetration**. The bevel is against the vein's wall. Adjust the angle of the needle. (d) **Collapsed vein**. (i) Resecure the tourniquet to increase venous filling. (ii) Remove the needle and draw from another vein. (e) **Formation of a haematoma**. Release the tourniquet immediately and withdraw the needle. Apply firm pressure. (f) **Arterial puncture**. The blood is bright red, signifying it is arterial, not venous. Apply firm pressure for at least 5 minutes.

- Try again – remove the tourniquet, swab the site, dispose of the needle, double-check everything, and start again.
- Remember to relax; anxiety will not help. If you find it difficult to get blood, ask a senior colleague if you can watch them do it.

Nerve injury

This happens when the needle hits a vein and the patient may feel intense pain. This is particularly likely in the antecubital fossa, where the median nerve runs close to the brachial artery. Should you damage a nerve during the procedure, withdraw the needle, swab the site, document the event, and seek assistance from a senior colleague. To prevent this, revisit your anatomy and identify sites where nerves are close to major veins and arteries (Scales 2008).

Indications for assistance

- If you cannot locate a suitable vein because the patient's condition is deteriorating, call for help from a senior colleague.
- No more than *two* attempts should be made to obtain a sample as this will cause the patient unnecessary discomfort and distress. Ask a senior colleague to obtain the sample for you.

Special considerations

- *Therapeutic drug monitoring*: different pharmacological agents have patterns of administration, body distribution, metabolism, and elimination that affect the drug concentration as measured in the blood. Many drugs will have 'peak' and 'trough' levels that vary according to dosage levels and intervals. Check for timing instructions for drawing the appropriate samples.

- *Effects of exercise:* muscular activity has both transient and longer-lasting effects. The creatine kinase (CK), aspartate aminotransferase (AST), lactate dehydrogenase (LDH), and platelet count may increase.

- *Age, gender, weight, and pregnancy* have an influence on laboratory testing. Normal reference ranges need to be noted.

- If the patient is in *shock or dehydrated* there will be poor superficial peripheral access. It may be necessary to wait until fluid therapy has taken place.

- *Syncope (fainting)* may occur with venepuncture, especially if the patient has a needle phobia. Patients will show signs of agitation, pallor, and sweating.

Remove the needle and tourniquet, cover site, and lie patient down.

- *Location:* ensure you have all the equipment necessary to carry out the procedure. If you are working in the patient's home, find a suitable location to ensure their comfort and ensure the procedure can be carried out safely. Place used equipment in appropriate containers and remove from patient's home.

- Needlestick injury: regardless of the disease process or infection control status of the patient, be careful not to stick yourself or others with a used needle. If an accidental needlestick injury does happen, ***immediately***:
  - Go to the sink, turn on the water, and bleed the site well by alternating squeezing and releasing the area around the site.
  - Do this for approximately 3–5 minutes.
  - Afterwards scrub the site with an alcohol swab.
  - Follow with a thorough hand washing.
  - Report it to your supervisor immediately.
  - Fill out an accident report form.
  - Report to staff occupational health.

Procedure

Preparation

Prepare yourself

Ensure you understand all the equipment necessary and the rationale for use. Wash your hands using the Ayliffe technique (Ayliffe *et al.* 2000). Always follow professional guidelines and recognize limitations (NMC 2008).

Prepare the patient

The procedure should be fully explained to the patient.

Prepare the equipment

Select the appropriate blood sample bottles according to investigations ordered. Select the correct needle size for the patient's age and condition.

Step-by-step guide to venepuncture

Step	Rationale
1 Introduce yourself, confirm the patient's identity, explain the procedure, and obtain consent.	To identify the patient correctly and gain informed consent.
2 Determine the patient's preferred site for the procedure based on their previous experience.	To involve the patient actively in their care. To acquaint the nurse with the patient's medical history and factors that may influence choice of vein.
3 Allow the patient to ask any questions and discuss the procedure.	Anxiety results in vasoconstriction; if the patient is relaxed their veins will be dilated.
4 Double-check the identity of the patient against the requisition form.	To ensure the sample is taken from the correct patient.
5 Assemble equipment for procedure, checking blood testing tubes are correct against requisition form.	To ensure the correct blood investigations are performed and equipment is not damaged.
6 Ensure adequate lighting, ventilation, and privacy.	To ensure both patient and nurse are comfortable and can see the task in hand.
7 Wash hands using a bactericidal soap and water or bactericidal alcohol hand rub, and dry thoroughly. Put on gloves.	To minimize the risk of health care-associated infection. Gloves will protect against blood spillage but not needlestick injury.
8 Push the tube into the needle adaptor by twisting clockwise.	To open system.
9 Support the chosen limb.	To ensure patient comfort and facilitate venous access.
10 Apply the tourniquet to the upper arm.	Increases venous pressure to facilitate vein identification and entry.
11 Ensure tourniquet does not obstruct arterial blood flow. Check for arterial pulse.	Prolonged pressure may lead to venospasm, tortuous vein, pain, and haematoma.
12 Observe and palpate the vein.	To identify its place among other structures, i.e. arteries and tendons.
13 If needed to encourage venous filling further, consider: ■ Gently tapping vein. ■ Allowing arm to hang down. ■ Asking patient to clench/unclench hand.	To aid venous filling.
14 Inspect the device carefully.	To detect faulty equipment and ensure needle is sharp with no barbs.

15	With the patient's arm in a downward position, align the needle with the vein. Anchor the vein by applying manual traction on the skin a few centimetres below the proposed insertion site.	To immobilize the vein and provide counter-tension, which will facilitate a smoother needle entry.
16	With the bevel of the needle upward, insert the needle at an angle of 15–30° into the vein. A sensation of resistance will be felt followed by the needle entering the vein.	To facilitate a successful, pain-free venepuncture.
17	Advance the needle a further 1–2 mm into the vein (Lavery and Ingram 2005).	To stabilize the needle and prevent it becoming dislodged while collecting sample.
18	Ensure the needle is held firmly in place.	To prevent any movement of the needle.
19	Secure the blood collection tube onto the needle by twisting clockwise.	To allow blood to enter the bottle. To ensure the system is closed.
20	Subsequent samples may be taken by this technique until final sample is taken and removed.	To aid blood sampling procedure.
21	Release the tourniquet.	To aid normal blood flow in the arm.
22	Place a low-linting swab over the needle site, remove the needle from the vein fully, and place in sharps box.	To prevent pain when removing needle. To prevent needlestick injuries.
23	Apply digital pressure directly over the puncture site for 1–2 minutes. Do not allow the patient to bend arm.	To prevent leakage and haematoma formation.
24	Once puncture site has sealed, cover with an adhesive plaster (or hypoallergenic dressing if patient has an allergy).	To prevent leakage of blood until healing is complete.
25	Ensure the patient is comfortable. Explain how long results will take.	To alleviate any anxieties and keep patient informed of care.
26	Discard waste, making sure it is placed in the correct containers. Remove gloves and wash hands.	To ensure safe disposal and prevent any needlestick injuries.
27	Label the bottles with patient details, checking details against patient's notes.	To ensure blood samples are labelled correctly.
28	Send blood samples to the appropriate laboratories.	To ensure samples reach intended destination and are analysed.

Following the procedure

Ensure that the patient informs a staff member if the venepuncture site starts to bleed or if they feel uncomfortable. Record the date, time, and site of venepuncture and tests undertaken in the patient's notes, as well as any adverse incidences, i.e. if patient's anxiety level was high.

Recognizing patient deterioration

If the patient is on blood-thinning medication, there is potential for prolonged bleeding after the procedure. You must stay with the patient until bleeding has stopped and leave the patient with access to a call bell so they can call for help if bleeding recommences. Cover the puncture site with a low-linting swab and apply gentle pressure until bleeding has stopped.

Reflection and evaluation

When you have undertaken venepuncture with a patient, think about the following questions:

1 How did you feel about the procedure?
2 Could you palpate the patient's veins? Did they feel how you expected them to?
3 Were you able to answer the patient's questions?
4 If you failed to hit the vein, how would you do it differently next time?

Further learning opportunities

Practise the skill at every opportunity. Many hospitals now have access to clinical skills facilities where rubber arms are available for venepuncture practice.

Reminders

- Do not label the sample tubes in advance in case venepuncture is unsuccessful and the tubes are mistakenly used for another patient.
- The best veins are usually found at the front of the elbow, in the antecubital fossa. These veins are less mobile, easier to puncture, and less painful than veins in the hand or lower arm.

- The tourniquet should not be applied for longer than 1 minute before collecting the blood specimen. Prolonged use will cause intravascular fluid to leak into the tissues and may affect the accuracy of the blood test.
- If you use a skin-cleansing agent it is usually alcohol based and must be allowed to dry completely before proceeding. Any residual alcohol causes pain for the patient and may damage the cells and affect the blood specimen (Nicol *et al.* 2004).

 Patient scenarios

1 An elderly gentleman (patient A) is admitted to hospital with nausea and vomiting. He is frail and looks dehydrated. Routine bloods have been requested. What factors would you consider before taking the sample?
2 You are requested to take a sample of blood from patient B to ascertain his therapeutic digoxin levels. What should you consider?
3 Patient C is very anxious and upset about having to have a blood sample taken. What steps can you take to alleviate their anxiety?

Website

 http://www.oxfordtextbooks.co.uk/orc/ endacott

You may find it helpful to work through our short online quiz and additional scenarios intended to help you to develop and apply the skills in this chapter.

References

Ayliffe GAJ, Fraise AP, Geddes AM, and Mitchell K (2000). *Control of hospital infection. A practical handbook*, 4th edition. Arnold, London.

Cox NLT and Roper TA (2005). *Clinical skills: Oxford core text*. Oxford University Press, Oxford.

Dougherty L (2002). Delivery of intravenous therapy. *Nursing Standard*, **16**(16), 45–52.

Harris S and Walker S (2005). Venepuncture. *Practice Nurse*, **29**(5), 16–26.

Health Protection Agency (2005). *Eye of the needle*. HPA, London.

Lavery I and Ingram P (2005). Venepuncture: best practice. *Nursing Standard*, **19**(49), 55–65.

Nicol M, Bavin C, Bedford-Turner S, Cronin P, and Rawlings-Anderson K (2004). *Essential nursing skills*, 2nd edition. Mosby, Edinburgh.

Nursing and Midwifery Council (2008). *The Code: standards of conduct, performance and ethics for nurses and midwives*. NMC, London.

Royal College of Nursing (2003). *Standards for IV therapy*. RCN, London.

Scales K (2008). A practical guide to venepuncture and blood sampling. *Nursing Standard*, **22**(29), 29–36.

Schramm M and Hannan C (2006). HCAIs can be minimised through effective teamwork. *British Journal of Nursing*, **15**(16), 844–5.

Thurgate C and Heppell S (2005). Needlephobia – changing venepuncture practice in ambulatory care. *Paediatric Nursing*, **17**(19), 15–18.

Tortora GJ and Grabowski SR (2003). *Principles of anatomy and physiology*, 10th edition. Wiley, New York.

Useful further reading and websites

Collins M (2006). A structured learning programme for venepuncture and cannulation. *Nursing Standard*, **20**(26), 34–40.

Gower A (2006). Venepuncture. *Nursing Standard*, **21**(3), 67–8.

Phillips S, Collins M, and Dougherty L (2008). *Venepuncture and cannulation: essential clinical skills for nurses*. Blackwell Publishing, UK.

(A) Answers to patient scenarios

1 A patient who is dehydrated will have less circulating volume. This will affect blood test results and make it more difficult to obtain the sample. If bloods are routine, consider hydrating the patient before obtaining the sample.

2 It is necessary for the sample to be taken at certain times both before the digoxin is given and after. Always read guidelines as results will be skewed by incorrect testing intervals.

3 Ascertain patient's previous experience, approach in a calm and confident manner, explain procedure fully including why tests are necessary, consider diversion therapy while undertaking skill.

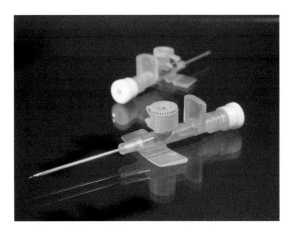

Figure 6.33 BD Venflon IV cannula, printed with permission of BD Medical.

6.11 **Intravenous cannulation care and removal** (A)

This is an advanced skill. You *must* check whether you can assist with or undertake this skill, in line with local policy.

Definition

Intravenous cannulation is a surgical procedure involving insertion of a flexible catheter into a blood vessel (arterial or venous) using a cannula (from Latin 'little reed'; plural cannulae) such as a Venflon (see **Figure 6.33**). Venous cannulation is used to administer:

- Prescribed intravenous fluid.
- Prescribed blood products.
- Prescribed intravenous drugs.
- Dyes or contrast media for radiographic examinations.

It is important to remember that:

Cannulation is an invasive procedure and as such should be carried out under aseptic conditions to reduce the risk of iatrogenic bacteraemia and sepsis. Ensure that you follow infection control procedures as you may be exposed to the patient's blood while you carry out the procedure. Blood spills should be cleaned up promptly and contaminated equipment disposed of as per local policy.

Prior knowledge

Before attempting cannulation care, make sure you are familiar with:

1 Cardiovascular anatomy and physiology, especially the structure of a blood vessel.
2 The equipment necessary to carry out the procedure.
3 Factors influencing venous circulation.
4 Infection control policy.
5 Needlestick injury policy.

Background

It is essential that anyone undertaking cannulation has a good understanding of the anatomy and physiology of arteries, veins, and associated nerves. The metacarpal veins and the dorsal venous arch at the back of the hand (see **Figure 6.34**) or the superficial veins of the wrist or lower arm such as the cephalic or basilic veins (see Figure 6.31, Section 6.10) are normally chosen for short-term infusions (Scales 2005).

The structure of veins

See Section 6.10 on venepuncture for a description of the structure of veins.

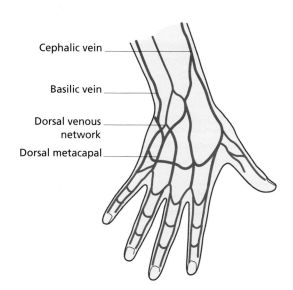

Figure 6.34 Veins of the hand.

(Labels in figure: Cephalic vein, Basilic vein, Dorsal venous network, Dorsal metacapal)

Selection of site of cannulation and size of cannula

In selecting a site for cannulation or the size of the cannula, it is important to consider:

● What is the cannula to be used for?
● How quickly does the fluid need to be infused?
● How long is the cannula to be left in the site?

Different types of fluid will require different sized cannulae. An infusion of antibiotics or normal saline in a stable patient may not necessitate as large a diameter cannula as an infusion of blood products.

The size of the cannula also depends on the condition of the patient and on how fast fluids need to be replaced (see **Table 6.8**). In haemodynamically unstable patients in the emergency setting, where urgent fluid replacement is needed to maintain blood pressure, a fast infusion rate is necessary; the most important thing here is the diameter of the cannula.

When selecting a catheter, consider the patient's condition and the type of solution you'll be running through

Table 6.8 Catheter sizes

Size		Length		Flow rate (ml/min)
Gauge	Ø (mm)	Inches	mm	
24	0.7	3/4	19	22
22	0.9	1	25	36
20	1.1	1	25	65
20	1.1	1 1/4	33	61
18	1.3	1 1/4	33	103
18	1.3	1 3/4	45	96
17	1.5	1 3/4	45	128
16	1.7	2	50	196
14	2.2	2	50	343

the catheter. Using the smallest-gauge catheter in the largest vein possible will reduce the mechanical and chemical irritation to the vein wall. Keep these general guidelines in mind:

- 24- to 22-gauge for children and elderly patients.
- 24- to 20-gauge for medical patients and post-operative surgical patients.
- 18-gauge for surgical patients and for rapid blood administration. Blood can be infused through smaller gauge catheters, but the flow rate will be slower.
- 14- to 16-gauge for trauma patients and those requiring large volumes of fluid rapidly.

Patient comfort is of utmost importance when deciding on the site of cannulation. The duration of cannulation must also be taken into consideration, e.g. is it needed for day case surgery or does the patient require fluids over a longer period of time? Cannula tips tend to cause irritation of the veins, leading to thrombophlebitis, and excessive movement at the tip of the cannula exacerbates this problem. Therefore, be careful not to site a cannula tip over a moving joint.

Inspect the arm, noting any signs of:

- Local skin infection, *erythema* (redness), swelling, heat, discharge, or pain.
- Bruising or discoloration of the skin (ranging from bluish black to yellow).
- Phlebitis (inflammation of a vein).

Palpate and trace the path of veins with the index finger. The healthy vein feels soft, bouncy, and will refill when pressed. Thrombosed veins lack resilience, feel cord-like, and roll easily. Arteries pulsate, are more elastic, and have a thick wall (Lavery and Ingram 2005).

Areas to avoid when choosing a site

- Extensive scars from burns or surgery – it is difficult to puncture the scar tissue.
- Oedematous extremities.
- Areas of previous cannulation, as they can cause pain due to repeated trauma to the vein (RCN 2003).
- The bend at the patient's elbow or wrist, as this will cause the patient discomfort and irritate the vein.

Context

When to IV cannulate

Inserting a cannula is an invasive procedure that carries potential risk to the patient. You must ensure there is a clinical need for the procedure, for example fluid replacement therapy, drug administration, infusion of blood products, or diagnostic procedures.

When not to IV cannulate

When clinical need cannot be identified.

Alternative interventions

If a patient is dehydrated you need to establish why and treat accordingly, e.g. by encouraging oral fluids.

Potential problems

Needlestick injury

Follow the procedure in Section 6.10 for needlestick injuries.

Superficial phlebitis

Phlebitis is an inflammation of the vein that may occur where a peripheral intravenous line has started. The surrounding area may be sore and tender along the vein:

- There is usually a slow onset of a tender, red area along the superficial veins on the skin.
- A long, thin, red area may be seen as the inflammation follows a superficial vein.
- This area may feel hard, warm, and tender. The skin around the vein may be itchy and swollen.
- The area may begin to throb or burn.
- A low-grade fever may occur.
- If an infection is present, symptoms may include redness, fever, pain, swelling, or breakdown of the skin.

Extravasation

Extravasation is the accidental administration of IV-infused medicinal drugs into the surrounding tissue, by either leakage (e.g. because of brittle veins in very elderly patients) or direct exposure (e.g. because the needle has punctured the vein and the infusion has gone directly into the arm tissue). Extravasation of medicinal drugs during IV therapy is a side effect that can and must be avoided.

In mild cases, extravasation can cause pain, reddening, and irritation on the arm with the infusion needle. Severe damage may cause tissue necrosis. In extreme cases, it even can lead to loss of an arm.

Infection control

When in potential contact with a patient's body fluids, it is essential to follow safety and infection control procedures to avoid problems (Schramm and Hannan 2006).

Protect yourself

Practise universal precautions:

- Wear gloves and an apron when handling blood/ body fluids.
- Wash hands frequently.
- Dispose of items in appropriate containers.
- Dispose of needles immediately upon removal from the patient's vein. Do not bend, break, recap, or resheath needles to avoid accidental needle puncture or splashing of contents (The Health Protection Agency 2005).

Protect the patient

- Place cannula equipment away from patients.
- Practise hygiene for the patient's protection. When wearing gloves, change them between patients and wash your hands frequently. Always wear an apron.

Indications for assistance

- If you cannot locate a suitable vein because the patient's condition is deteriorating, call for help from a senior colleague.
- No more than two attempts should be made to cannulate a vein as this will cause the patient unnecessary discomfort and distress.

> **Special considerations**
>
> - Extreme patient anxiety about the procedure may result in vasoconstriction (Thurgate and Heppell 2005). Anxiety causes an increase in circulating adrenaline, causing increased vasoconstriction. A calm and confident approach with an adequate explanation of the procedure may help to reduce anxiety.
>
> - If the patient is in shock or dehydrated, there will be poor superficial peripheral access.

Procedure: insertion of a cannula

Preparation

Confirm with senior colleagues and patient's notes that a cannula needs inserting.

Prepare yourself

Wash your hands and, if applicable, put on protective equipment (i.e. apron, gloves). Ensure you understand all the equipment needed and the rationale for use. Always follow professional guidelines and recognize limitations (NMC 2008).

Prepare the patient

Explain what you propose to do and why, and gain the patient's consent. Encourage the patient to remain quiet, relaxed, and still during the procedure.

Prepare the equipment

Ensure all equipment is in date and in sealed packaging. Select the correct size of cannula for the patient's age, reason for insertion, and condition. Equipment needed includes:

- Gloves
- Tourniquet
- Alcohol wipes
- Cannula
- Sterile gauze
- Sharps container
- Cannula dressing
- 5 ml syringes
- Ampoule of sodium chloride 0.9%

Step-by-step guide to inserting a cannula

	Step	Rationale
1	Introduce yourself, confirm the patient's identity, explain the procedure, and obtain consent.	To identify the patient correctly and gain informed consent.
2	Determine the patient's preferred site for the procedure, which may be related to their medical history.	To involve the patient actively in their care. To confirm the patient's medical history and factors that may influence choice of vein.
3	Assemble equipment for procedure.	To ensure that all equipment is available before procedure commences.
4	Ensure adequate lighting, ventilation, and privacy.	To ensure both the patient and nurse are comfortable and can see the task in hand.
5	Wash hands using a bactericidal soap and water or bactericidal alcohol hand rub, and dry thoroughly. Put on gloves.	To minimize the risk of health care-associated infection. Gloves will protect against blood spillage but not needlestick injury.
6	Support the chosen limb, which will normally be the patient's non-dominant arm.	To ensure patient comfort and facilitate venous access.
7	Apply the tourniquet to the upper arm, 5–10 cm above proposed site of cannulation.	Increases venous pressure to facilitate vein identification and entry.
8	Ensure tourniquet does not obstruct arterial blood flow; check for arterial pulse.	Prolonged pressure may lead to venospasm, tortuous vein, pain, and haematoma.
9	Observe and palpate the vein.	To identify its place among other structures, i.e. arteries and tendons.
10	If required, further encourage venous filling by: ■ Gently tapping vein. ■ Allowing the arm to hang down. ■ Asking the patient to clench/unclench hand.	To aid venous filling.
11	Clean the patient's skin using an appropriate alcohol-based wipe (Pellowe *et al.* 2004) and allow to dry thoroughly. Do not repalpate the vein.	To minimize the risk of infection.
12	Inspect the cannula device carefully. Hold the cannula in your dominant hand.	To detect faulty equipment and ensure cannula needle is sharp with no barbs.
13	With the patient's arm in a downward position, align the needle with the vein. Anchor the vein by applying manual traction on the skin a few centimetres below the proposed insertion site.	To immobilize the vein and provide counter-tension, which will facilitate a smoother needle entry.

continued overleaf

14	With the bevel of the needle upward, insert the needle at an angle of 20–30° into the vein. A sensation of resistance will be felt on entering the vein, as well as a flashback of blood. Stop advancing the needle.	To facilitate a successful, pain-free cannulation, as the cutting edge on the bevel will cleanly insert through the skin.
15	Holding the needle part of the cannula, slide the cannula off the needle and into the vein with the other hand.	To stabilize the needle and prevent it from going through the vein. To insert cannula into vein.
16	Hold the cannula in place. Release the tourniquet.	To ensure cannula is secure. To aid normal blood flow in the arm.
17	Place some sterile gauze under the end of the cannula.	To contain any drops of blood during removal of needle.
18	Apply pressure to the vein at the insertion site.	To minimize blood flow.
19	Remove the needle and immediately insert the (injectable) cap. Place needle in sharps box.	To prevent blood loss and seal end of cannula. To prevent any needlestick injuries.
20	Cover with a sterile see-through cannula dressing or hypoallergenic dressing if patient has an allergy.	To fix the cannula *in situ*. So cannula site can be observed without removing dressing.
21	Flush the cannula with 5 ml of 0.9% sodium chloride.	To ensure patency.
22	Ensure the patient is comfortable. Keep patient informed of care.	To maintain patient comfort and alleviate any anxieties.
23	Discard waste, making sure it is placed in the correct containers. Remove gloves and wash hands.	To ensure safe disposal.
24	Document date and time of insertion of cannula in patient's notes.	To ensure staff will be aware of the length of time cannula has been *in situ* (Biswas 2007).

Following the procedure

Explain any restrictions to mobility to the patient and stress the need to protect the cannula site. Instruct them to report any swelling, redness, or pain. To ensure patency, the cannula should be flushed every 12 hours with 5 ml of 0.9% saline (RCN 2003).

Polyurethane cannulae may remain *in situ* for 96 hours provided there is no evidence of phlebitis (Centers for Disease Control and Prevention (CDC) 2002). A phlebitis scale (see Table 6.9) should be used to assess the cannula site (RCN 2003).

Care of cannula

Care of puncture sites and IV equipment are of key importance in the prevention of infection. The following measures should be incorporated into the management of all IV cannulae:

- Hand washing is paramount when handling cannulae or equipment.
- The insertion site should be inspected each time the cannula is used for signs of infection/ extravasations.

Table 6.9 Phlebitis scale

Observations	Score	Judgement
IV site appears healthy.	0	No signs of phlebitis. Observe cannula.
One of the following is evident: ■ Slight pain near IV site. ■ Slight redness near IV site.	1	Possibly first signs of phlebitis. Observe cannula.
Two of the following are evident: ■ Pain at IV site. ■ Erythema. ■ Swelling.	2	Early stage of phlebitis. Resite cannula.
All the following are evident: ■ Pain along the path of the cannula. ■ Erythema. ■ Induration.	3	Medium stage of phlebitis. Resite cannula. Consider treatment.
All the following are evident and extensive: ■ Pain along the path of the cannula. ■ Erythema. ■ Induration. ■ Palpable venous cord.	4	Advanced stage of phlebitis or early stage of thrombophlebitis. Resite cannula. Consider treatment.
All the following are evident and extensive: ■ Pain along the path of the cannula. ■ Erythema. ■ Induration. ■ Palpable venous cord. ■ Pyrexia.	5	Advanced stage thrombophlebitis. Resite cannula. Initiate treatment.

(RCN 2003)

- All connections should be checked for tightness.
- Wet or soiled dressings should be changed.

Use a phlebitis scale to ensure any changes are picked up and dealt with quickly (see **Table 6.9**).

Procedure: removal of a cannula

Preparation

Confirm with senior colleague and patient's notes that cannula needs removing.

Prepare yourself

Wash your hands and, if applicable, put on any protective equipment required (i.e. apron, gloves). Ensure you understand all the equipment needed and the rationale for use. Always follow professional guidelines and recognize limitations (NMC 2008).

Prepare the patient

Explain what you propose to do and why, and gain the patient's consent. Encourage the patient to remain quiet, relaxed, and still during the procedure.

Prepare the equipment

Ensure that it is in date and in sealed packaging. Equipment needed includes:

- Gloves.
- Sterile gauze.
- Tape.
- Sharps container.

Step-by-step guide to removing cannula

▶ Step	Rationale
1 Introduce yourself, confirm the patient's identity, explain the procedure, and obtain consent.	To identify the patient correctly and gain informed consent.
2 Put on gloves.	To prevent cross-infection.
3 Loosen securing dressing from around the cannula.	To aid easy removal of cannula.
4 Place sterile gauze over the cannula insertion site.	To protect the cannula exit site from extrinsic contamination while a scab forms.
5 Withdraw the cannula and apply firm pressure over the gauze/cannulation site (1 minute is usually sufficient).	To cease the venous blood flow, and prevent leakage of blood from the cannula exit site.
6 Secure the gauze in place with tape.	To hold the gauze in place.
7 Discard cannula into sharps bin and remaining waste into a suitable waste bag.	To prevent cross-infection.

Following the procedure

Ensure that the patient informs a staff member if the cannulation site starts to bleed or if they feel uncomfortable. Record the date, time, and site of cannulation in the patient's notes, as well as any adverse events or reactions.

Recognizing patient deterioration

Closely observe all patients following insertion or removal of a cannula for the following:

- **Haematoma** is a collection of blood formed following leakage of blood from the vein into the tissues surrounding the insertion site. It may occur as a result of failure to puncture the vein properly during cannula insertion.

- **Infiltration** (or 'tissuing') occurs when the infusate enters the subcutaneous tissue rather than the vein.

- **Thromboembolism** occurs when a blood clot on the catheter or vein wall becomes detached and is carried by the venous flow to the heart and pulmonary circulation.

- Air embolism is a possible hazard during all forms of IV therapy; however, in peripheral cannulation it is extremely rare. The risk is reduced by ensuring that adequate peripheral pressure is maintained by appropriate use of the tournequet.

- Phlebitis is an inflammation of the vein and can be due to chemical or mechanical irritation, or infection. A thrombus can form in association with the inflammation, resulting in thrombophlebitis. Of all the factors affecting the development of phlebitis (such as catheter size, venepuncture site, etc.), the duration of the cannulation and the type of fluids administered are the most important.

Reflection and evaluation

When you have undertaken the cannulation procedure, consider the following:

1   How did you feel about the procedure?
2   Could you palpate the patient's veins? Did they feel how you expected them to?
3   Were you able to answer the patient's questions?
4   If you failed to hit the vein, how would you do it differently next time?

Further learning opportunities

Practise the skill at every opportunity. Many hospitals now have access to clinical skills facilities where simulated arms are available for cannulation practice.

Reminders

- If a skin-cleansing agent is used, it is usually alcohol-based and must be allowed to dry completely before proceeding as residual alcohol may cause pain and irritation.
- Remember, cannulation is an invasive procedure; always ensure it is necessary.
- Inspect cannula site for any redness, swelling, or pain using a phlebitis scale.

Ⓠ Patient scenarios

1   Mrs Kabila has been admitted into hospital for a routine operation. You have been asked to insert a cannula. What do you need to take into consideration when choosing the cannula size?
2   John is complaining that his arm is hurting. You observe that the cannula site and just above is red and inflamed. His next dose of antibiotics is due now. What would you do?
3   You are still new to inserting cannulae and are learning to perfect the technique. You are called urgently to a cardiac arrest and are asked to insert a cannula. What would you do?

Website

  http://www.oxfordtextbooks.co.uk/orc/ endacott

You may find it helpful to work through our short online quiz and additional scenarios intended to help you to develop and apply the skills in this chapter.

References

Biswas J (2007). Clinical audit documenting insertion date of peripheral intravenous cannulae. *British Journal of Nursing*, **16**(5), 281–3.

Centers for Disease Control and Prevention (2002). Guidelines for the prevention of intravascular catheter related infections. *MMWR Recommendations and Reports*, **51**(RR-10), 1–29.

Health Protection Agency (2005). *Eye of the needle*. HPA, London.

Lavery I and Ingram P (2005). Venepuncture: best practice. *Nursing Standard*, **19**(49), 55–65.

Nursing and Midwifery Council (2008). *The Code: standards of conduct, performance and ethics for nurses and midwives*. NMC, London.

Pellowe C, Pratt R, Loveday H, Harper P, Robinson N, and Jones S (2004). The epic project. Updating the evidence base for national evidence-based guidelines for preventing healthcare associated infections in NHS hospitals in England: a report with recommendations. *Journal of Hospital Infection*, **5**(6), 10–16.

Royal College of Nursing (2003). *Standards for IV therapy*. RCN, London.

Scales K (2005). Vascular access: a guide to peripheral venous cannulation. *Nursing Standard*, **19**(49), 48–52.

Schramm M and Hannan C (2006). HCAIs can be minimised through effective teamwork. *British Journal of Nursing*, **15**(16), 844–5.

Thurgate C and Heppell S (2005). Needlephobia – changing venepuncture practice in ambulatory care. *Paediatric Nursing*, **17**(19), 15–18.

Useful further reading and websites

Blows WT (2001). *The biological basis of nursing: clinical observations*. Routledge, Taylor and Francis Group, London.

Collins M (2006). A structured learning programme for venepuncture and cannulation. *Nursing Standard*, **20**(26), 34–40.

Phillips S, Collins M, and Dougherty L (2008). *Venepuncture and cannulation: essential clinical skills for nurses*. Blackwell Publishing, UK.

Answers to patient scenarios

1 You need to establish what type of operation Mrs Kabila is having. Will she require fluid replacement, blood products, or antibiotic therapy? All have a bearing on the size of cannula required. Also make sure the cannula is away from the operation site.

2 The cannula should be removed and a new cannula inserted into the opposite arm. Only then can the antibiotics be given.

3 As you are still learning about cannulation, it would be better for both you and the patient if you decline and ask someone with more experience. It is an emergency and a cannula is needed quickly.

6.12 Insertion, monitoring, care, and removal of a central venous catheter Ⓐ

This is an advanced skill. You *must* check whether you can assist with or undertake this skill, in line with local policy.

Definition

A **central venous catheter** (CVC) is a hollow, flexible tube inserted directly into a large vein. It allows the administration of drugs, and blood can be withdrawn and pressure measurements made through it.

It is important to remember that:

You are expected to work within your own competency and adhere to institutional and professional policies and guidelines. Some of the information in this section will cover skills you cannot perform as a student or without post-registration training but that you may observe.

Prior knowledge

Before attempting to use the skills outlined in this section, make sure you are familiar with:

1 The anatomy of the veins commonly used for CVC placement and the associated anatomical structures – see for example Tortora and Derrickson (2005).

2 Review the physiology and anatomy of the cardiovascular system. (For a good revision session, see **http://www.ecme.com/**.)

3 Aseptic technique (see Section 4.1). Maintain strict hygiene and use of personal protective equipment throughout the following procedures.

4 Awareness of the signs of common complications associated with the procedure, and immediate actions required.

5 Your scope of practice in the administration of intravenous fluids (see Section 6.7). It is your responsibility to make yourself aware of, and follow, local policies and guidelines.

Background

Central venous catheters, often referred to as 'central lines', are increasingly used both in critical care areas and on general wards (Polderman and Girbes 2002b).

Central venous catheterization is a highly invasive procedure. About 15% of patients experience complications associated with the insertion, maintenance, or removal of CVCs (Taylor and Palagiri 2007). These complications may be mechanical or due to a catheter-related infection. Haematoma, pneumothorax, and arterial puncture are the most common mechanical complications of central venous catheterization (Taylor and Palagiri 2007). Studies suggest that using strict sterile technique during CVC insertion followed by high standards of aseptic care when accessing the catheter minimizes catheter-related infections (Deshpande *et al.* 2005). Nursing staff have a role in enforcing these standards, e.g. by challenging unacceptable practice.

Positioning CVCs

Choice of position for placement of a CVC is generally determined by the person performing the procedure, usually a medical practitioner. This should be decided in line with manufacturer's guidelines and organizational policies, and the individual patient assessment. Common central sites are the subclavian vein lying under the clavicle, which carries blood from the arm back to the heart, and the internal or external jugular veins in the neck, which carry blood from the head back to the heart (see **Figure 6.35**). The catheter tip sits close to the right side of

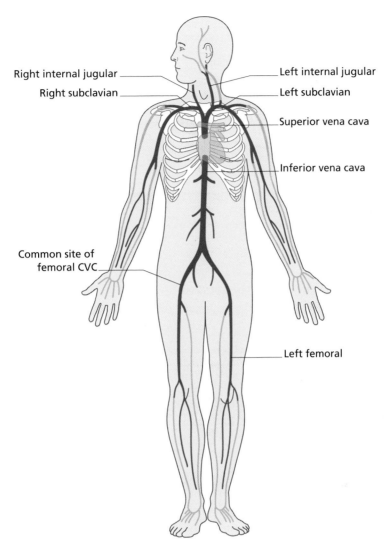

Figure 6.35 Common sites for placement of central venous catheters.

the heart, in the superior vena cava (SVC). When the femoral vein in the groin is used, the catheter tip lies in the inferior vena cava (IVC).

Deep veins run close to arteries, which may be accidentally punctured during catheter insertion. For example, the femoral vein runs next to the femoral artery and the subclavian vein lies next to the subclavian artery. It is important to review the anatomy of the veins commonly used for CVC placement, and nearby structures. This will help you to recognize any complications. For example, the lung may be accidentally punctured when a catheter is placed via a subclavian or neck vein.

If the subclavian or jugular sites are to be cannulated, the patient is ideally placed in the Trendelenberg position, where the legs are higher than the head (see **Figure 6.36**). This has two benefits:

1 The position causes the veins in the neck to fill with blood and become more visible, making them easier to cannulate.
2 In normal respiration, a negative pressure is generated in the chest during inspiration, which moves air into the lungs. This can also entrain air into the vein during the procedure, with potentially fatal consequences

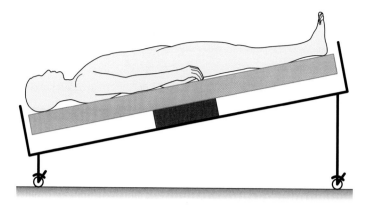

Figure 6.36 The Trendelenberg position. The patient's legs should be higher than their head.

(McGee and Gould 2003). The Trendelenberg position increases intra-thoracic pressure, reducing the risk of air embolism.

There are various types of CVC. These include skin-tunnelled catheters and ports suitable for longer-term use, and non-tunnelled single and multilumen catheters (Bishop *et al.* 2007). Indirect access to central veins can be gained from peripheral sites, such as the antecubital fossa in the forearm, with a peripherally inserted central venous catheter (PICC).

A modified Seldinger technique is commonly used for catheter placement. This involves feeding a guidewire into the vein through an introducer needle and syringe. The catheter is then threaded over the guidewire into the vein, and the wire is then removed (Duffy and Sair 2007). Passage of the guidewire into the right side of the heart can cause **cardiac arrhythmias**, which are usually transient. The introduction procedure carries a slight risk of arterial or ventricular perforation, and cardiac tamponade (Soni *et al.* 2000).

The traditional landmark method involves using anatomical 'landmarks' as a guide to positioning the catheter (McGee and Gould 2003). The use of an **ultrasound** device to locate the vein when siting most CVCs is recommended (National Institute for Health and Clinical Excellence (NICE) 2002).

Risks of CVC use

The less experience the practitioner has in performing the procedure, the greater the risk of complications (Taylor and Palagiri 2007). A patient who has a **coagulopathy** has an increased risk of haemorrhage. Although this is not an absolute contraindication to catheter insertion, the subclavian vein is the site least able to be compressed to stop bleeding, so another site may have to be chosen (Taylor and Palagiri 2007).

A CVC puts the patient at significant risk of developing a catheter-associated bloodstream infection. It is important to record the patient's temperature regularly, at least daily, and to suspect a catheter-related infection in any patient with a CVC who shows signs of infection that cannot be accounted for by another source. Strict aseptic technique *must* be used for catheter site care and all episodes of accessing the system. Aseptic technique (see Section 4.1) includes hand washing, alcohol-based hand decontamination, and the use of either clean gloves and a no-touch technique, or sterile gloves, as dictated by local policy. The use of a sterile, transparent, semi-permeable polyurethane dressing is recommended to cover the site of a CVC (RCN 2005).

During catheter placement the nurse's role includes assisting the trained operator to ensure safe practice and high standards of asepsis and see that suitable checks are made before the catheter is inserted. They must ensure patient comfort and dignity, observe for signs of complications or distress, and offer support and reassurance. Following placement, they should ensure correct checks are performed prior to catheter use. The nurse may be responsible for continuing care of the catheter, including patient or carer education.

Context

 ## When to insert a CVC

Indications for central venous catheterization:

- To gain intravenous access when peripheral access is poor.
- To allow administration of a number of incompatible solutions through a multilumen catheter.
- To allow the administration of a **vesicant**, irritating, or hypertonic solution, which would cause tissue damage if given through a peripheral cannula. For example, administration of parenteral nutrition, vasoactive drugs, or chemotherapy.
- To allow for the insertion of a transvenous cardiac pacing catheter.
- To enable measurement of central venous pressure (CVP), and assessment of 'fluid responsiveness' (Vincent and Weil 2006).
- Early goal-directed therapy in a septic patient involves targeted central venous pressures (Rhodes and Bennett 2004, Antonelli *et al.* 2007). To find out more, see **http://www.survivingsepsis.com**.
- To allow access and return of blood during renal replacement therapy.

 ## When not to insert a CVC

- Carotid endarectomy in ipsilateral (same) side, large tricuspid valve vegetation.
- When appropriate monitoring cannot be provided.
- Where adequate asepsis cannot be maintained.

Cautions

Coagulopathy is a relative risk, while thrombocytopenia (low platelets) holds a greater risk for bleeding (Mumtaz *et al.* 2000). The decision to proceed depends on urgency. CVC placement in patients with disorders of homeostasis should only be performed by a skilled practitioner.

Alternative interventions

- Can a medication be given by an alternative route, for example by the oral or rectal route?
- Would a peripheral cannula, midline, or peripherally inserted central catheter (PICC) provide adequate intravenous access?

Potential problems

Central venous cannulation is a highly invasive procedure with a number of associated problems, for example:

- Cardiac arrhythmias
- Arterial and/or ventricular perforation
- Cardiac tamponade
- Arterial cannulation
- Nerve damage
- Local and systemic infection
- Haematoma
- Pneumothorax
- Air embolus

(NICE 2002)

Indications for assistance

The nurse should request assistance if any problems are identified and/or if they are in doubt about CVC line insertion, monitoring, care or removal.

Interpreting readings

1 Cardiac output is the product of **stroke volume** multiplied by heart rate. Stroke volume is influenced by preload, contractility, and afterload (see Section 6.6). Preload is the degree of tension placed on the resting myocardial fibres at end-diastole just before the onset of systole. The main factor influencing preload is the venous return to the heart.

2 Within limits, in the normal heart, the greater the tension or length of stretch of the myocardial fibres, the stronger the contraction. This relationship is referred to as Frank–Starling's Law of the Heart. It must be remembered that cardiac filling pressure, as reflected in central venous pressure (CVP), is a measurement of *pressure* not *volume*, and may not always reflect

continued overleaf

cardiac preload. Therefore CVP readings should be interpreted with caution (Vincent and Weil 2006).

3 Remember that dynamic changes are more important than single measurements. A change in CVP in response to a fluid bolus should be interpreted with other physiological parameters such as heart rate, blood pressure, neurological responsiveness, and respiratory function. For an accurate reading, the patient should be in the supine position and the manometer zero position should be aligned with the patient's right atrium, the 'phlebostatic axis' (Soni *et al.* 2000). External landmarks are used to locate this position (see Figure 6.38a). For further reading see Tortora and Derrickson (2005) and Vincent and Weil (2006).

4 CVP can be measured via a fluid-filled manometer, with typical pressures around 5–10 cmH$_2$O (Mayer *et al.* 2002). Alternatively a pressurized transducer system attached to a monitor is often used in critical care areas, with normal values around 0–9 mmHg (Soni *et al.* 2000). Note that 1 mmHg is equivalent to 1.36 cmH$_2$O. A mean pressure value is usually recorded. Dynamic changes are more important than absolute values, as they reflect the response to treatment.

5 Whichever method is used to measure CVP, certain rules typically apply. The distal lumen (the lumen nearest to the tip of the catheter) is usually used for pressure measurement, while the other lumens are used for fluid or drug administration. When CVP measurement is used to direct fluid management, it is important that the patient's position is consistent for sequential readings. Any change in CVP in response to a fluid bolus should be interpreted along with other physiological parameters such as heart rate, blood pressure, neurological responsiveness, and respiratory function.

Factors that increase central venous pressure

6 A high CVP can be an indicator of hypervolaemia. Causes can include the administration of too much

intravenous fluid or poor renal function, reducing the kidneys' ability to keep the body in balance by producing appropriate volumes of urine. Left or right side heart failure, mitral regurgitation, pulmonary hypertension, cardiac tamponade, and chronic obstructive pulmonary disease (COPD) are all causes of raised CVP readings. Anything that raises abdominal pressure can also increase CVP (Soni *et al.* 2000), such as positive pressure ventilation (a breathing machine) and high levels of positive end expiratory pressure (PEEP), a form of respiratory support.

Factors that decrease central venous pressure

7 **Hypovolaemia** is a decreased or inadequate circulating blood volume. The patient may have been unwell for some time and so may not have taken in enough fluids. Other causes may include fluid loss, for example through bleeding, or diarrhoea and vomiting. A *relative* hypovolaemia occurs with the redistribution of fluid within the body associated with shock. Causes can include the vasodilatation associated with sepsis, anaphylaxis, or spinal shock (Soni *et al.* 2000).

Special considerations

8 Some patient groups may not tolerate lying head down. The Trendelenberg position is contraindicated in patients with raised intracranial pressure, because the position causes obstruction of the blood returning from the brain (Hickey 2003). This increases cerebral blood volume and in turn causes an increase in the pressures within the head (Rosenthal *et al.* 1997). Other patient groups who may not tolerate lying head down include those with acute or chronic respiratory problems, or pregnant women.

9 The risk of pneumothorax associated with CVC insertion is increased in patients with COPD, and in mechanically ventilated patients receiving large tidal volumes due to hyperinflation of the lungs (Taylor and Palagiri 2007).

Procedure: insertion of a CVC

Preparation

Prepare the patient

Consent is normally gained by the person performing the procedure (NMC 2004), who in most cases will be either a doctor or a specialist nurse.

A trained assistant is required to help with the procedure, usually a nurse. The procedure must be performed with full aseptic technique (Polderman and Girbes 2002b, McGee and Gould 2003, Duffy and Sair 2007, Pratt *et al.* 2007) – see Section 4.1.

Explain to the patient that during the procedure and immediately after, it will be necessary to monitor their electrocardiography (ECG), pulse oximetry, respirations, and pulse (Taylor and Palagiri 2007).

Prepare the equipment

Note: this is a complex, advanced procedure. Follow local guidance for the authority to perform this procedure and seek guidance and assistance as required.

You will need a lines trolley with:

- Appropriate CVC introduction kit – consider age/ route/purpose. Catheters are often impregnated with an antimicrobial, which may cause a reaction in a small number of patients. Check if the patient has any known allergies.
- Sterile mask, gown, gloves, and surgical mask, large sterile drapes, and gauze swabs. Insertion of a central line must be performed using full aseptic technique.
- 2% chlorhexidine gluconate in 70% isopropyl alcohol (Adams and Elliot 2007, Pratt *et al.* 2007) if no allergy. Check manufacturer's recommendations and local policy. The chlorhexidine solution must be allowed to dry.
- Sterile 0.9% sodium chloride for injection. Used to flush catheter lumens.
- Local anaesthetic, needle, and syringe. To provide pain relief.

- Scalpel blade with handle. For skin puncture.
- Sutures and needle holder. To secure the line.
- Sharps container. For safe disposal of sharps.
- Ultrasound machine. To reduce the risk of inserting the catheter into an artery (NICE 2002).
- ECG, blood pressure, and pulse oximetry monitoring equipment. To allow the detection of cardiac arrhythmias and respiratory function.
- Transparent, sterile, semi-permeable dressing. To cover catheter site.

If the line is to be transduced, prime the transducer set following manufacturer's guidelines and connect to a suitable monitor. (The sterile flush solution, usually 0.9% sodium chloride, is then placed in a pressure bag inflated to 300 mmHg; check prescription and local guidelines.) The CVP flush port is usually transduced with a line marked blue to distinguish it from the arterial flush line, which is marked red. This is to reduce the risk of drugs accidentally being given into an arterial line.

Check that all connections are secure and that all ports are capped. Check that there are no air bubbles in the line. This will minimize the risk of introducing air into the monitoring system, which may affect the accuracy of readings and risk an air embolus to the patient.

Step-by-step guide to inserting the central venous catheter

Note that insertion of the CVC is only undertaken by a doctor or specially trained nurse ('the practitioner').

Step	Rationale
1 Introduce yourself, confirm the patient's identity, explain the procedure, and obtain consent. Note: an explanation is particularly important as the patient will be asked to turn their head away from the cannulation site for a neck or subclavian line. Surgical drapes may cover their face.	To identify the patient correctly and gain informed consent. To gain cooperation and reduce anxiety. Asking the patient to remain still and try not to touch anything will aid the procedure and help maintain the sterile field.
2 Position the patient. For catheters entering the chest, this is the head down Trendelenberg position (Figure 6.36). If the patient is unable to tolerate this, place supine with a small rolled-up towel under the shoulders. Expose the proposed catheter site.	To reduce the risk of air embolism and make neck veins more visible. Familiarize yourself with local manual handling policies. If manual handling slide sheets are used, local policy may involve removing the sheet before placing the patient head down to reduce the risk of sliding.

continued overleaf

3	Commence ECG and pulse oximetry monitoring. Check baseline blood pressure.	To allow early detection of arrhythmias or reduced oxygen saturation.
4	The practitioner puts on a mask and sterile gown, hat and gloves. Surgical drapes are used to provide a sterile field.	CVC line insertion is a sterile procedure.
5	The skin is cleaned with chlorhexidine solution and allowed to dry.	CVC line insertion is a sterile procedure.
6	The skin is infiltrated with local anaesthetic.	To minimize patient discomfort.
7	The CVC is placed percutaneously under ultrasound guidance, following the manufacturer's guidelines.	To minimize the risk of a misplaced catheter. Inadvertent arterial cannulation is usually apparent by pulsating blood, but in the shocked patient with a low blood pressure this may not be obvious.
8	If the CVC is properly positioned, it should be possible to aspirate blood from all lumens, which should then be flushed. If after three attempts the practitioner is unable to site the catheter, McGee and Gould (2003) suggest help should be sought from a more experienced clinician.	To minimize patient discomfort, anxiety, and risk.
9	It is important that the primary fixation point, which is an integral part of the line, is secured immediately (Medicines and Healthcare Products Regulatory Agency 2007). The catheter should be sutured in position using primary and secondary fixation points.	The secondary clamp and fastener are attached to the line during insertion and may not hold the catheter securely. If only the secondary clamp is sutured, there is a danger that any tension applied to the CVC will cause it to slide through the clamp, dislodging the catheter.
10	A sterile, transparent, semi-permeable polyurethane dressing is recommended (NICE 2002, Pratt *et al.* 2007).	To provide a barrier to bacteria while allowing the line to be inspected daily.
11	Connect distal CVC lumen to the primed transducer and zero to the monitoring system. Review the trace to ensure that a venous trace not arterial waveform is seen (Soni *et al.* 2000, Duffy and Sair 2007) – see Figure 6.37. Local policies may vary. If a transducer is not available, consider aspirating a sample for blood gas analysis (McGee and Gould 2003). Low arterial oxygen saturation and pressure may be present in a shocked patient (Duffy and Sair 2007).	It is essential to assess that the CVC is correctly sited in a great vein before use, as there is a risk that an artery may be cannulated inadvertently during the procedure. Introduction of drugs or air entering a catheter placed in an artery could have fatal consequences. A low pressure central venous pressure waveform will produce a distinctive trace which can be distinguished from a high pressure arterial waveform. If the patient has an arterial line *in situ* an arterial blood sample may be taken along with a blood sample from the newly placed catheter for blood gas analysis. There should be a marked difference in oxygen levels between the arterial and venous samples.

12 Following the insertion of a subclavian or jugular line, obtain a chest X-ray. The X-ray must be reviewed by a suitably trained practitioner to verify correct positioning. Confirmation of correct position should be documented in the patient's clinical notes, along with a record of the procedure and any complications encountered, and a date for review or removal.

The X-ray should reveal any **pneumothorax**, and ensure correct catheter position. The tip of the catheter should sit in the vena cava, outside the right atrium (Soni *et al.* 2000, Duffy and Sair 2007). It will not confirm if the CVC is in a vein or an artery.

Following the procedure

Make the patient comfortable; sit them up if safe to do so. Alert an appropriate person to any problems or unusual findings.

Checking the position before use

Pre-use position checks may vary with local policy, and are vital to avoid inadvertent infusion of drugs or parenteral nutrition into an artery, which can lead to severe morbidity or death. Normally the distal lumen is transduced, if monitoring equipment is available, and the trace checked for the characteristic central venous waveform (see **Figure 6.37**), or acceptable venous pressures.

Ensure that no drugs or fluids are infused through the device before the correct position has been verified by suitably qualified staff. Following the insertion of a neck or subclavian catheter, a chest X-ray should be performed to check for a pneumothorax and confirm the correct position of the catheter tip, which should lie in the lower third of the superior vena cava (RCN 2005).

A pneumothorax may occur immediately after CVC insertion, or may develop more slowly (Polderman and Girbes 2002a), and should be considered in any patient who has signs of respiratory distress following CVC insertion. A symptomatic pneumothorax is normally treated with a chest drain, which will allow the air to escape and the lung to reinflate.

A record of the procedure in the patient's clinical notes should include the date, anatomical location, and any complications encountered, plus length of catheter at insertion site to allow daily checks for catheter migration.

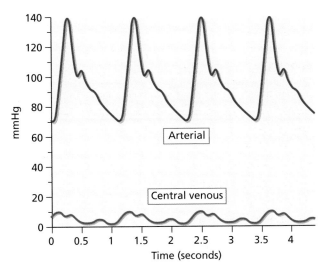

Figure 6.37 Shows an example of transduced arterial and venous waveforms. Notice the difference in pressures and shape. The higher arterial pressures are usually recorded as systolic and diastolic, for example 135/65 mmHg. Venous pressure is usually recorded as a mean. A pressure of 10/4 mmHg would be 10 + 4 + 4 divided by 3 = 6 mmHg. The monitor will normally do this calculation for you and display the mean figure automatically.

Procedure: measurement of central venous pressure

 ### When to measure CVP

- As part of routine patient observations.
- Before and after a fluid bolus, to assess fluid responsiveness (see Interpreting readings box earlier in the section).
- When requested to do so by senior staff.

The choice of method used to measure CVP will depend on the monitoring equipment available.

Preparation

Prepare yourself

Wash hands, put on apron. Maintain strict hand hygiene and use of personal protective equipment throughout procedure (see Section 4.1).

Prepare the patient

Explain the procedure to the patient.

Prepare the equipment

Gather and make yourself familiar with the equipment, including the transducer set and monitor, and a pressure bag and prescribed intravenous fluid for a continuous flush.

Step-by-step guide to transduced measurement of central venous pressure

Note: this procedure is complex and will vary dependent on the equipment available. An outline is set out below but local policy and manufacturer's guidelines should always be adhered to. Follow local guidance for the authority to perform this procedure and seek guidance and assistance as required. Student nurses will not normally be expected to perform this procedure.

Action	Rationale
1 Introduce yourself, confirm the patient's identity, explain the procedure, and obtain consent.	To identify the patient correctly and gain informed consent.
2 Place prescribed intravenous fluid usually 0.9% saline for the continuous flush in the pressure bag and prime the flush line and transducer to remove any air, following the manufacturer's instructions. Check all connections are tight.	To ensure no air is entrained into the system. Air is compressible so bubbles can distort the waveform. Use of a fluid containing glucose can potentially cause inaccuracy when sampling bloods.
3 Each lumen of a multilumen catheter will normally be marked by the manufacturer with lumen size and position. If a multilumen catheter is used, the transducer flush line is usually attached to the distal (tip) lumen of the CVC. Unclamp the line.	The distal lumen is usually the largest gauge lumen and is closest to the heart, although in theory other lumens can be used as long as they exit in the central venous system.
4 Attach the cable from the monitor to the transducer. Zero the transducer to air following the manufacturer's instructions.	The transducer should be zeroed to obtain accurate measurements.

5	Place the patient in a supine or semi-recumbent position (Woodrow 2006). Secure the transducer at the patient's phlebostatic axis point (midaxilla in line with the fourth intercostal space) or as local policy. An alternative site is the second intercostal space in line with the sternal edge, a point about 5 cm above the right atrium (Anderson 2003). Chart the mean CVP (and/or systolic and diastolic pressures as local policy) and zero reference point used.	To allow a consistent zero position to be used for subsequent readings, so that an accurate comparison can be made between sequential readings.
6	The transducer should be zeroed at the start of each shift. Check that: ■ The pressure bag is correctly inflated. ■ Adequate fluid remains in the flush bag.	To maintain patency of the line and to ensure accurate readings.
7	Record readings hourly, and before and after any intervention such as a fluid bolus, or as directed. The measurement is in mmHg.	To look for trends. To monitor patient response to fluid administration.

Table 6.10 Common problems with transduced central venous pressures

Problem	Possible cause	Prevention and intervention
An over-damped trace, which gives a false low systolic and high diastolic reading.	Inspect for blood or air bubbles in the transducer line, which may be compressed by the pressure wave and reduce the amplitude.	Take meticulous care when running through the transducer system to expel all air. If any air or blood is observed, this should be removed.
A flat line, despite changing the waveform scale displayed.	The transduced CVC line is kinked. Transducer has become disconnected. Catheter tip is resting against a vessel wall.	Check the line for any kinks and rectify. Check that the cable is still connected to the monitor and at the transducer. Ensure that the flush bag is not empty. Has the pressure bag deflated? Check for patency by aspirating and observing for free flow of blood.
A change in CVP measurement that cannot be explained clinically.	Improper position of the transducer: too high will give a false low reading, too low will give a false high reading.	Establish correct level of transducer before recording measurement, and after any change of patient position.
An inaccurate trace or unexpected reading.	Fluids running through the CVP measurement line.	Check that no fluids or drugs are running through the transduced line while recording a measurement.

Procedure: recording central venous pressure using a manometer

CVP is measured manually using a disposable single patient use glass or plastic vertical tube called a manometer attached to intravenous fluid. The manometer will give a reading in cmH$_2$O. Full aseptic technique should be used throughout the procedure.

Preparation

Prepare equipment

- Manometer attached to drip stand.
- Spirit level.
- Sterile intravenous fluid. Usually 500 ml of 0.9% sodium chloride solution, as prescribed.

Step-by-step guide to recording CVP using a manometer

Note: this is a complex, advanced procedure. Follow local guidance for the authority to perform this procedure, and seek guidance and assistance as required.

Step		Rationale
1	Introduce yourself, confirm the patient's identity, explain the procedure, and obtain consent.	To identify the patient correctly and gain informed consent.
2	Help the patient into a supine position, lying in either a flat or semi-recumbent position (Woodrow 2006).	Venous return may be reduced when in the upright position, and increased when lying flat.
3	Locate a point midaxilla in line with the fourth intercostal space, which is taken to be in line with the right atrium. Using the spirit level for accuracy, adjust the manometer height on the drip stand so that the zero point is in line with the level identified as the patient's phlebostatic axis. The second intercostal space in line with the sternal edge can be used as an alternative zero point, which is about 5 cm above the atrium (Anderson 2003) (see **Figure 6.38a**).	This approximates the level of the right atrium (the phlebostatic axis). If the alternative zero point is used, this should be recorded so that subsequent readings can be compared accurately.
4	Connect the bag of intravenous fluid, as prescribed, to a giving set. Then attach to a three-way tap attached to the manometer and an extension line. The line between the fluid bag and the patient connection line of the manometer set should be fully primed before connection to the patient (Figure 6.38a).	To flush the tubing and remove any air to avoid accidental venous air embolus.
5	Connect the fully primed extension line to the distal lumen of the CVC (Woodrow 2006). Take great care not to entrain any air. The in-line clamp on the CVC lumen should be used.	When a multilumen catheter is used, the distal lumen is used for CVP measurement (usually labelled by the manufacturer).

6	Briefly turn the three-way tap to allow flow between the fluid bag and the CVC port (Figure 6.38b).	To check that the fluid runs freely.
7	Turn the three-way tap off to the patient, and open to the manometer. Allow the fluid to run from the fluid bag into the manometer to 20–25 cm level (Figure 6.38c).	To prime the manometer. Check there are no bubbles, which could affect the reading.
8	Turn the three-way tap off to the flush bag, and open between the manometer and the patient (Figure 6.38d). Watch the fluid column fall until it stabilizes. Gentle fluctuation with the patient's respiration should be seen. Note the figure, which will be in cmH$_2$O.	This allows a direct fluid column to link the tip of the catheter sitting in the superior vena cava to the manometer, and reflects the pressure of venous blood as it enters the right atrium.
9	Turn the tap off to the manometer (Figure 6.38b). Any intravenous infusion can be restarted at the prescribed rate.	To continue prescribed infusion.
10	Record the CVP measurement on the patient's observation chart. Typical values are 0–12 cmH$_2$O (Soni *et al.* 2000).	To leave a record for other health professionals and to allow comparison with previous/later measurements.
11	Record the anatomical zero reference point used. Record patient position (e.g. 30° head up).	To allow a consistent zero position to be used for subsequent readings, enabling accurate comparison to be made between sequential readings.

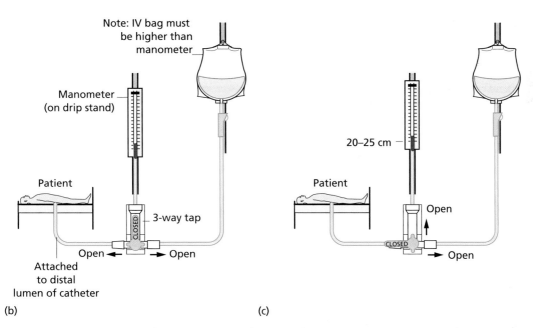

(b)　　　　　　　　　　　　　　　　　　(c)

Figure 6.38 The initial set-up of the manometer to perform central venous pressure measurement. Always remember to prime the manometer and line before attaching to the patient to avoid introducing air into the bloodstream. Connect to the distal lumen of the catheter. To obtain your CVC measurement turn the three-way tap as indicated so that the column of fluid is in direct contact with the patient via the CVC port. You will observe slight fluctuation with respiration. Note the position of the three-way taps: (**a**) Note that the zero point is in line with the phlebostatic axis (**b**) shows the tap open from fluid bag to patient to ensure flow; (**c**) fluid off to patient but able to fill manometer. Stop at about 20 cm.

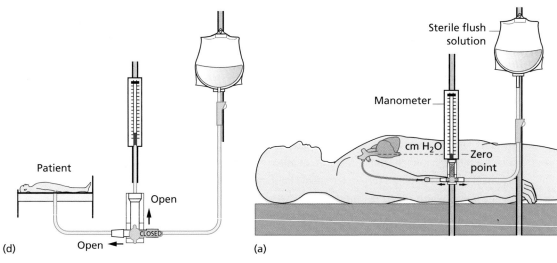

Figure 6.38 (*continued*)

Procedure: catheter care

Step-by-step guide to daily inspection of the catheter

Action	Rationale
1 Introduce yourself, confirm the patient's identity, explain the procedure, and obtain consent.	To identify the patient correctly and gain informed consent.
2 Consider daily: is CVC still required? The CVC should be removed as soon as no longer required, or if infection is suspected or confirmed, or another catheter-related problem exists (McGee and Gould 2003). Routine catheter replacement is not recommended (NICE 2002).	Central venous cannulation is a highly invasive procedure with a number of associated problems, so it should only be continued as long as absolutely necessary.
3 Inspect entry site. Check sutures are intact and secure. Check for catheter migration. Is insertion length the same as recorded? Look for clinical signs of infection – inflammation, erythema, exudate, discomfort, or pain at the entry site.	Discomfort, pain, swelling, or leakage at the entry site may indicate catheter migration. Any infection must be noticed and acted upon as soon as possible.

4	Check the dressing is secure. It should normally be changed at 7 days as long as it remains intact and there is no moisture under it (Pratt *et al.* 2007, NICE 2002). If indicated, change the dressing as described in the next section.	To maintain patient comfort and bacterial barrier with as little disruption to the site as possible.
5	The catheter lumens will need to be flushed regularly. Refer to local policy for frequency and choice of flush.	To maintain patency.
	A syringe no smaller than 10 ml is recommended (Conn 1993).	This size of syringe minimizes the risk of catheter rupture.
	A pulsated push-pause positive pressure should be used.	This causes turbulence in the catheter lumen, which helps to remove debris (RCN 2005).
	In a transduced line the pressurized flush bag provides a controlled continuous flush, typically giving a flow of 3 ml/hour. Heparinized saline solution or 0.9% saline is a common choice.	

Procedure: renewing the dressing of a central venous catheter

The procedure can take place in a treatment room or on the patient's bed with screening to maintain privacy and dignity. Maintain strict hand hygiene and use of personal protective equipment throughout procedure (see Section 4.1)

Preparation

Prepare equipment
Depending on local policy:

- Clean dressing trolley.
- Clean gloves and apron, and antibacterial hand rub.
- Sterile gauze and gloves, galley pot, dressing towel (or dressing pack containing these items), and waste bag.
- Cleaning solution: 2% chlorhexidine gluconate in 70% isopropyl alcohol, or as local policy and no allergy.
- Sterile, transparent, semi-permeable polyurethane dressing.

Step-by-step guide to renewing the dressing of a central venous catheter

Note: this is a complex, advanced procedure. Follow local guidance for the authority to perform this procedure, and seek guidance and assistance as required.

Step		Rationale
1	Introduce yourself, confirm the patient's identity, explain the procedure, and obtain consent.	To identify the patient correctly and gain informed consent.
2	Make the patient comfortable, ideally lying supine.	To allow easy access to the site.
3	Decontaminate hands. Open the dressing pack without contaminating, and arrange contents on the dressing trolley. This may be done with a hand inside the sterile waste bag. Pour chlorhexidine solution if used into the galley pot or open and tip sterile applicator onto sterile field.	To maintain asepsis.
4	Wearing clean gloves and apron, and taking great care not to dislodge the catheter, carefully remove and discard the old dressing. Do not use scissors. Discard gloves. Cleanse hands with alcohol scrub and allow to dry.	To minimize the risk of accidentally dislodging or cutting the catheter. To minimize risk of infection.
5	Don sterile gloves. The site should be cleaned with the chlorhexidine gluconate solution and allowed to dry, as long as this complies with the manufacturer's recommendations and local policy (NICE 2002, Pratt *et al.* 2007).	To minimize risk of infection.
6	Apply sterile, transparent, semi-permeable polyurethane dressing, which should be changed after 7 days, or when damaged or excessively moist (NICE 2002, Pratt *et al.* 2007). Sterile gauze secured with tape may be a better choice for a patient who has very moist or sweaty skin, or if there is bleeding or oozing at the catheter site. Gauze dressings should be changed when moist, loosened, or soiled. The continued need to use a gauze dressing should be assessed daily, and it should be replaced with a transparent semi-permeable dressing as soon as possible (Pratt *et al.* 2007).	To provide a barrier to bacteria. Benefits of the polyurethane dressing include being able to inspect the site without removing the dressing, and comfort for the patient.

Following the procedure

- Clear away and dispose of waste safely, and decontaminate hands.
- Make patient comfortable.
- Document procedure, including any complications and assessment of insertion site in the clinical record.

Procedure: drawing blood from a CVC

Blood should be drawn from a CVC when requested by a suitably qualified practitioner, and when it is accepted practice within local policy and guidelines. Strict aseptic technique and universal precautions should be observed and must be adhered to whenever a CVC is accessed (Department of Health 1998) (see Section 4.1).

No single method of obtaining blood samples from a CVC has been described. The following guidelines describe one suggested method. Guidelines may vary, so it is important to check. Local infection control policies in some areas may preclude this procedure as there is an infection risk (Gabriel *et al.* 2005).

Preparation

Prepare the equipment
Gather the equipment, ideally on a small dressing trolley:

- Apron and antibacterial hand rub for use before contact with patient and during procedure.
- Clean or sterile gloves, as dictated by local policy. Chlorhexidine 2% in alcohol wipe or solution to cleanse access port or needle-free access device, as directed by local policy.
- Sterile 0.9% sodium chloride for injection and 10 ml syringe.
- Injection tray, Vacutainer® system or syringe and appropriate blood sample bottles, and sterile obturator.

Step-by-step guide to drawing blood from a CVC

Note: this is a complex, advanced procedure. Follow local guidance for the authority to perform this procedure, and seek guidance and assistance as required.

Step	Rationale
1 Introduce yourself, confirm the patient's identity, explain the procedure, and obtain consent.	To identify the patient correctly and gain informed consent.
2 Wash hands and put on apron and gloves, following local infection control policies.	To minimize the risk of infection.
3 Temporarily stop and clamp any infusions running through the CVC. Ideally, select the proximal or largest bore lumen to draw blood.	To reduce the risk of any drugs or fluids running through other lumens being drawn back with the blood collected.
4 Clamp the line, remove obturator, and cleanse port or needle-free access device if used. Attach an empty syringe, unclamp, and slowly withdraw and discard 5–6 ml of blood. Clamp line and remove syringe, taking care not to allow any air to enter the catheter lumen.	To clear the lumen of residual fluid, in order to prevent haemodilution or contamination of the specimen. To minimize infection risk. Alternatively discard can be drawn into a spare blood tube and disposed of (see below). Replacement of discarded blood may introduce clots (RCN 2005). To avoid air embolus.

continued overleaf

5	Attach a Vacutainer® system or syringe, unclamp, and fill blood bottles in the order specified by the laboratory. Clamp line. If a syringe is used to draw blood, *do not* attach a needle to fill blood bottles. Remove rubber stopper from blood bottle, fill, and replace stopper. Caution: some samples may be contaminated by residue in the line (e.g. bloods for drug levels or coagulation studies) and may be inaccurate (RCN 2005).	To reduce the risk of accidental needlestick injury. (See Section 6.10.)
6	Attach a 10 ml syringe of 0.9% sodium chloride, unclamp, and flush. Check that the line is clear of blood. Reclamp.	It is recommended that a syringe no smaller than 10 ml is used to minimize the risk of catheter rupture (Conn 1993). To reduce the risk of clot formation.
7	Cleanse port and place a sterile obturator (bung) on the end of the catheter if used. Any infusions can now be restarted as appropriate.	To minimize infection risk. To continue prescribed infusion.
8	Carefully label and date the blood bottles immediately.	To allow correct identification.

Note: if the catheter is patent but there is no blood return, ask the patient to cough, take a deep breath, or change position.

Following the procedure

- Send the bloods to the labs promptly for accurate results.
- Check whose responsibility it is to obtain and act on the results.
- Remember that some samples, for example those for drug levels or coagulation studies, may be inaccurate due to contamination when taken from a CVC (RCN 2005).

Procedure: removal of a short-term non-tunnelled CVC

A CVC poses a significant risk of complication for the patient (McGee and Gould 2003). The device should be removed as soon as it is no longer required, or if there is a suspected or confirmed infection, or other catheter-related problem. A catheter-related infection should be suspected when there are signs and symptoms of infection in any patient with a CVC that are not accounted for by another source.

The risk of developing a catheter-related infection increases the longer a CVC remains *in situ* (McGee and Gould 2003). The removal procedure can take place in a treatment room or on the patient's bed, with screening to maintain privacy and dignity. CVC removal should be performed using full aseptic technique and universal precautions (see Section 4.1).

Preparation

Catheter removal must be performed on the order of a suitably qualified health care professional, and should be performed by someone with the correct knowledge, experience, and skills. Check that the patient's clotting is within normal limits before attempting the removal of a CVC. This is particularly important when the subclavian approach has been used, as it is difficult to compress the vein to stop any bleeding.

Prepare yourself

Before performing this procedure, make sure that you are familiar with:

- Aseptic technique and universal precautions (Section 4.1).
- Awareness of possible complications.
- Local policy and procedures.

Prepare the equipment

- Clean dressing trolley.
- Clean gloves and apron, and antibacterial hand cleanser.
- Sterile gauze and gloves, galley pot, dressing towel, and waste bag (or dressing pack containing these items). Cleaning solution: 2% chlorhexidine gluconate in 70% isopropyl alcohol, or as local policy.
- Stitch cutter or blade with handle.
- Sterile scissors and plain specimen pot if line tip is to be sent for culture, and sterile wound swab if there are concerns that line site is infected.
- Sterile gauze, hypoallergenic tape, and sterile occlusive dressing.
- Sharps container.

Step-by-step guide to removal of a short-term non-tunnelled CVC

Note: this is a complex, advanced procedure. Follow local guidance for the authority to perform this procedure, and seek guidance and assistance as required.

Step	Rationale
1 Introduce yourself, confirm the patient's identity, explain the procedure, and obtain consent. The explanation should include the need for the head down position during the procedure (Trendelenberg position, see Figure 6.36). The patient must also be taught the Valsalva manoeuvre (see **Box 6.7**).	To identify the patient correctly and gain informed consent and cooperation. The Trendelenberg position increases intra-thoracic pressure, reducing the risk of air embolism.
2 Make sure that there is someone nearby to give help if needed, and that the equipment has been gathered.	Prompt help needs to be available if problems are encountered.
3 Wash and dry hands. Don apron (or protective apparel as per local policy). Ensure that all infusions are switched off, clamp all lines, and put an obturator (deadender cap) on each port to occlude the ports.	Universal precautions must be followed to protect patient and health care worker. To reduce the risk of entraining air during removal, causing a venous air embolism. To avoid blood leaking from the catheter.
4 Open the dressing pack and arrange the contents on the trolley within the sterile field. This can be done using a hand inside the sterile waste bag. Attach the waste bag to the trolley. Pour chlorhexidine solution into the galley pot or open packet of chlorhexidine application device. If there is suspicion that the line access site is infected, open and tip the sterile wound swab on to sterile field.	Universal precautions and aseptic technique must be observed throughout the procedure to avoid contamination.

continued overleaf

5	Ideally the patient is placed in the supine, head down (Trendelenberg) position. Expose the catheter site. Inspect the dressing and insertion site.	The Trendelenberg position reduces the risk of air embolus (see Box 6.8).
6	Wearing clean gloves and apron, take down the dressing, being careful not to dislodge the line. If the site is red, swab the area before removing catheter. Discard gloves and dressing in waste bag. Decontaminate hands with antibacterial hand rub. Don sterile gloves. Cleanse the skin and allow to dry.	To avoid the catheter tip being contaminated during removal.
7	Carefully cut the sutures with the stitch cutter or blade and remove, taking great care not to cut or dislodge the CVC line. Dispose of all sharps appropriately following completion of the procedure.	To ensure safety of patient and health care worker.
8	Fold one sterile gauze square into four. Place this over the site where the line enters the skin.	To enable digital pressure to be applied directly over the exit site.
9	Ask the patient to take a deep breath and hold it in (the Valsalva manoeuvre). If unable to do this, it is important to remove the catheter during expiration (RCN 2005).	To reduce the risk of air embolism.
10	Holding the catheter near to the skin entry site, pull the catheter firmly and smoothly to remove, while applying firm digital pressure over the exit site with the gauze pad with your other hand. Tell the patient they can breathe normally once the line is removed. Maintain the pressure for several minutes until bleeding has stopped. If oozing continues, add extra gauze and continue to apply pressure.	To remove catheter and minimize bleeding.
11	Place the line on the sterile field. Inspect to make sure the catheter tip is intact (RCN 2005).	To avoid contamination of the line tip. To alert to catheter damage.
12	When bleeding has stopped, cover the site with a sterile occlusive dressing, which should remain *in situ* for 72 hours (RCN 2005).	To prevent contamination of the site, allow observation, and prevent air embolism, which may occur up to 72 hours following catheter removal (RCN 2005).
13	If the tip is to be sent for culture, cut the distal 5 cm off with sterile scissors and place in the sterile specimen pot. Label the pot with the patient's details, date, time, and contents.	To allow accurate investigation of the presence of pathogenic microorganisms by the laboratory.

Box 6.7 Teaching the patient to perform the Valsalva manoeuvre

A method to achieve a significant increase in intra-thoracic pressure is to ask the patient to perform the Valsalva manoeuvre. The patient will need to be able to cooperate and follow your directions. Ask them to take a deep breath, hold it in, and then to bear down for 10 seconds against a closed epiglottis, as if trying to open their bowels. This will raise the pressure within their chest above atmospheric pressure so that air will not be sucked in. The procedure may cause a brief, transient slowing of the pulse.

Note: the Valsalva manoeuvre is not suitable for patients with raised intracranial pressures. Increased intra-thoracic and intra-abdominal pressure impedes venous return from the brain, which causes a dangerous rise in intracranial pressure (Hickey 2003).

Following the procedure

- Make patient comfortable.
- Clear away equipment, dispose according to policy.
- Monitor for deterioration.

Recognizing patient deterioration

- After insertion of a CVC, observe for complications, e.g. pneumothorax and local or systemic infection.
- At all times, but especially after removal of the CVC, monitor the site and the patient for signs of bleeding, air embolus (see **Box 6.8**), dyspnoea, chest pain or cardiovascular collapse, agitation, or neurological deterioration.
- Ask the patient to alert staff if the CVC site becomes painful or if it begins to produce exudate.

Reflection and evaluation

When you have been involved in the care of a CVC, think about the following questions:

1 Are you able to differentiate between an arterial and central venous pressure waveform?
2 Do you feel able to perform the daily assessment of a CVC?
3 Were you able to perform and interpret CVP readings if appropriate?

Box 6.8 Venous air embolism

Venous air embolism is an uncommon but devastating complication of CVC breach or removal. Problems can occur when 20 ml or more of air enters a vein. More than 50 ml of air can lead to hypotension and cardiac arrhythmias, with possible lethal consequences. Signs include an increase in heart and respiratory rate and a reduction in level of consciousness, blood pressure, and oxygen saturations. A cardiac 'mill wheel' murmur may be heard over the precordium. Symptoms include dyspnoea, chest pain, agitation, and disorientation. A large air embolism can pass through the right atrium, right ventricle, and into the pulmonary artery, and can cause an airlock. This causes outflow obstruction, which may lead to cardiac arrest requiring cardiorespiratory resuscitation (see Section 6.9).

If an air embolism occurs or is suspected, clamp the line (if *in situ* – and below the breach if it has been cut) and place the patient in a head down position on their left side. The aim is to trap the air in the apex of the right ventricle, reducing the risk of ejection into the pulmonary artery and allowing right ventricular output to continue. One attempt may be made to aspirate the air through the catheter (McGee and Gould 2003). One hundred per cent oxygen should be administered through a face mask and urgent help sought immediately.

4 Are you confident changing a CVC dressing?
5 Do you feel able to explain the insertion procedure to the patient and family, including information on why a CVC may be indicated?
6 Consider the possible self-image implications of having a CVC for the patient, especially when sited in a neck vein.

Further learning opportunities

- Take the opportunity to observe or assist with the placement and care of a CVC.
- Familiarize yourself with local policies and procedures.

Reminders

Don't forget:

- To observe your patient for complications of CVC insertion, e.g. pneumothorax and infection.

- For sequential central venous pressure readings to be meaningful, they should be taken with the patient in the same position and zeroed at the same reference point.
- Discomfort, pain, swelling, or leakage at the entry site may indicate catheter migration.
- To monitor for signs of infection – fever, elevated (or very low) white cell count, tachycardia, and tachypnoea, in any patient with a CVC (see SCCM/ESICM/ACCP/ATS/SIS (2003) for definition of sepsis).
- Be cautious and careful when drawing blood from a CVC and label samples correctly.
- When removing a CVC, ensure that your patient has been briefed and that assistance is available.
- Follow local policy carefully with all aspects of CVC care.

Patient scenarios

1 A patient has just had a central venous catheter placed via the subclavian route. He is now anxious, restless, and short of breath, and is complaining of chest pain. What may be the problem?

2 Ms Rizvi was admitted to your ward following an emergency operation to remove her spleen 3 days ago. She suffered significant bleeding intra-operatively and had an internal jugular CVC inserted. She has made a good recovery and her observations are stable. She is mobilizing, taking oral fluid and diet, and is comfortable on regular oral analgesia and antibiotics. What should you consider on your daily catheter inspection?

Website

 http://www.oxfordtextbooks.co.uk/orc/endacott

You may find it helpful to work through our short online quiz and additional scenarios intended to help you to develop and apply the skills in this chapter.

References

Adams D and Elliott T (2007). IV nursing care. Skin antiseptics used prior to intravascular catheter insertion. *British Journal of Nursing*, **16**(5), 278–80.

Anderson ID, ed (2003). *Care of the critically ill surgical patient*, 2nd edition, Royal College of Surgeons. Hodder Arnold, London.

Antonelli M, Levy M, Andrews P *et al.* (2007). Hemodynamic monitoring in shock and implications for management. International Consensus Conference, Paris, France, 27–28 April 2006. *Intensive Care Medicine*, **33**(4), 575–90.

Bishop L, Dougherty L, Bodenham A *et al.* (2007). Guidelines on the insertion and management of central venous access devices in adults. *International Journal of Laboratory Hematology*, **29**, 261–78.

Conn C (1993). The importance of syringe size when using implanted vascular access devices. *Journal of Vascular Access Nursing*, **3**, 11–18.

Department of Health (1998). *Guidance for clinical health care workers: protection against infection with blood-borne viruses: recommendations of the Expert Advisory Group on AIDS and the Advisory Group on Hepatitis*. DH, London.

Deshpande KS, Hatem C, Ulrich HL *et al.* (2005). The incidence of infectious complications of central venous catheters at the subclavian, internal jugular and femoral sites in an intensive care population. *Critical Care Medicine*, **33**, 13–20.

Duffy M and Sair M (2007). Cannulation of central veins. *Anaesthesia and Intensive Care Medicine*, **8**(1), 17–20.

Gabriel J, Bravery K, Dougherty L, Kayley J, Malster M, and Scales K (2005). Vascular access: indications and implications for patient care. *Nursing Standard*, **19**(26), 45–54.

Hickey J (2003). *The clinical practice of neurological and neurosurgical nursing*, 5th edition. Lippincott, Williams and Wilkins, Philadelphia.

Mayer B, Eggenberger T, Folin S, and Robinson K, eds (2002). *Fluids and electrolytes made incredibly easy*, 2nd edition. Springhouse, Pennsylvania.

McGee D and Gould M (2003). Preventing complications of central venous catheterization. *New England Journal of Medicine*, **348**, 1123–33.

Medicines and Healthcare Products Regulatory Agency (2007). *Intravascular and epidural devices; top tips*. DH, London.

Mumtaz H, Williams V, Hauer-Jensen M *et al.* (2000). Central venous catheter placement in patients with disorders of hemostasis. *American Journal of Surgery*, **180**(6), 503–5.

National Institute for Health and Clinical Excellence (2002). *Guidance on the use of ultrasound locating* devices for placing central venous catheters. *Technology Appraisal Guidance No 49* [online] **http://www.nice.org.uk** accessed 28/08/08.

Nursing and Midwifery Council (2004). *The NMC code of professional conduct: standards for conduct, performance and ethics standards*. NMC, London.

Polderman K and Girbes A (2002a). Central venous catheter use. Part 1: mechanical complications. *Intensive Care Medicine*, **28**, 1–17.

Polderman K and Girbes A (2002b). Central venous catheter use. Part 2: infectious complications. *Intensive Care Medicine*, **28**, 18–28.

Pratt R, Pellowe C, Wilson J *et al.* (2007). Epic 2: national evidence-based guidelines for preventing healthcare-associated infections in NHS hospitals in England. *Journal of Hospital Infection*, **65**(Suppl 1), S1–64.

Rhodes A and Bennett E (2004). Early goal-directed therapy: an evidence based review. *Critical Care Medicine*, **32**(Suppl), S448–50.

Rosenthal R, Hiatt J, Phillipse E, Hewitt W, Demetriou, and Grode M (1997). Intracranial pressure effects of pneumoperitonium in a large animal model. *Surgical Endoscopy*, **11**(4), 376–80.

Royal College of Nursing (2005). *Royal College of Nursing IV Therapy Forum, standards for infusion therapy*. RCN, London. (Reprinted with minor amends 2007.)

SCCM/ESICM/ACCP/ATS/SIS (2003). 2001 SCCM/ESICM/ACCP/ATS/SIS International Sepsis Definitions Conference. *Crit Care Med*, **31**(4), 1250–6.

Soni N, Welch J, Colardyn F, and Billet E (2000). *Invasive haemodynamic monitoring*. Becton Dickinson UK, Oxford.

Taylor R and Palagiri A (2007). Central venous catheterization: concise definitive review. *Critical Care Medicine*, **35**(5), 1390–6.

Tortora GJ and Derrickson BH (2005). *Principles of anatomy and physiology*, 11th edition. John Wiley and Sons, Chichester.

Vincent J and Weil MH (2006). Fluid challenge revisited. *Critical Care Medicine*, **34**(5), 1333–7.

Woodrow P (2006). *Intensive care nursing: a framework for practice*, 2nd edition. Routledge, London.

Useful further reading and websites

eCME is an e-learning site sponsored by AstraZeneca that offers a useful interactive cardiovascular course: **http://www.ecme.com/** Note that registration is required (free).

 Answers to patient scenarios

1 Be alert for signs and symptoms of respiratory distress (tachypnoea, dyspnoea, decreased or absent breath sounds, nasal flaring, accessory muscle use, asymmetrical chest expansion, restlessness, and anxiety) following the insertion of a subclavian CVC, as this may indicate a pneumothorax. Tracheal deviation, hyper-resonance on auscultation, and circulatory collapse indicate a tension pneumothorax, a clinical emergency.

2 Is the CVC still required? A CVC puts the patient at significant risk of developing a catheter-related infection, so should be removed when no longer required.

6.13 **Performing a 12-lead electrocardiogram (ECG)**

This is an advanced skill. You *must* check whether you can assist with or undertake this skill, in line with local policy.

Definition

An ECG is a recording of the electrical activity of the heart. The 12-lead ECG (see **Figures 6.39** and **6.40**) is a graphic record of the electrical activity looking at the heart in three dimensions, performed using an electrocardiograph. It gives valuable diagnostic information about the condition of the myocardium or abnormal QRS complexes. The

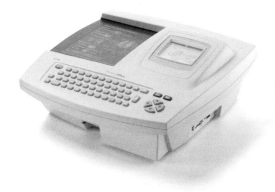

Figure 6.39 A 12–lead ECG machine.

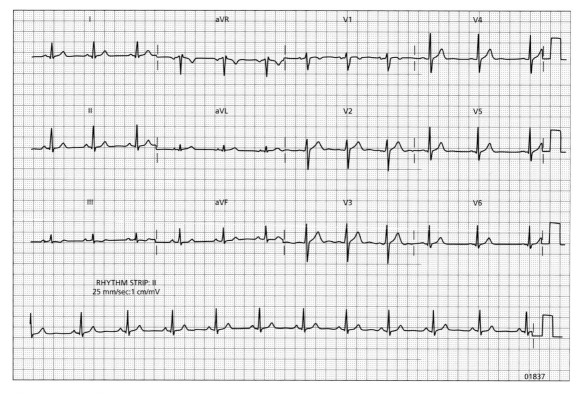

Figure 6.40 A 12–lead ECG with rhythm strip.

recording of an ECG is performed within a strict protocol to ensure standardization and reproducibility (SCST 2006).

It is important to remember that:

- Clarity with the explanation will help to reduce anxiety and ECG artefact.
- The patient requiring the ECG may deteriorate, so be alert to their condition.
- Accuracy in lead placement and order is essential for diagnostic quality as well as serial ECGs.

Prior knowledge

Before performing a 12-lead ECG, make sure you are familiar with:

1 Cardiovascular anatomy and physiology (especially location and function of structures involved in the cardiac cycle).

2 Basic understanding of the ECG (especially components of the electrical waveform with relevance to the mechanical events).

3 Awareness of coronary heart disease.

4 Awareness of the NMC *Code of conduct* (NMC 2004).

Background

Please also refer to Section 6.5 for a review of the cardiac cycle.

The cardiac cycle consists of three components: atrial systole, ventricular systole, and complete cardiac diastole. Each of these components is clearly identifiable on the ECG and has a normal range of duration outside of which it becomes pathological.

The 12 leads of the ECG look at the heart from two different planes. The limb leads look at the frontal plane of the heart as if the body were lying flat. The chest leads look at the heart in the transverse plane, allowing a view of the front and left side of the heart.

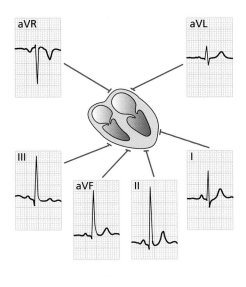

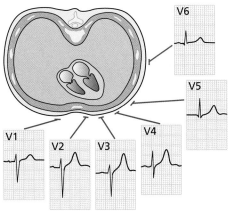

Figure 6.41 ECG angles of view (limb and chest).

The 12 leads of the ECG therefore look at the heart from different angles (see **Figure 6.41**):

- Leads II, III, and aVF look at the inferior surface.
- V1–V4 look at the anterior surface.
- Leads I, aVL, V5, and V6 look at the lateral surface.

None of the routine 12 leads look at the true posterior surface, although leads V7, V8, and V9 can be added to achieve this by continuing placement of electrodes around the back in the same plane.

Nursing staff performing a 12-lead ECG should be trained and assessed to a standard accepted by the employing Authority. Nursing staff performing a 12-lead ECG must also work within the scope of the applicable professional standards, e.g. NMC *Code of conduct* (NMC 2004). There is an increasing need for nurses and health care assistants to be able to perform extended roles in order to maximize patient care. Obtaining diagnostic data as soon as clinically indicated can obviously speed up treatment and therefore potentially reduce a patient's hospital stay.

Many areas throughout the UK are expanding the role of community nursing by taking ECG into the patient's home rather than bringing the patient to the hospital. The UK government is keen to encourage 'point of care' procedures to limit delays in the retrieval of diagnostic information.

Many health care authorities and organizations, e.g. NHS Trusts, are also expanding out-of-hospital diagnostics with the aid of telemedicine (Lancashire and South Cumbria Cardiac Network 2007). Community nurses are performing 12-lead ECG tests in the patient's home and sending the ECG via telephone to the GP or cardiology doctor for immediate interrogation. This system reduces diagnostic and treatment delay to a minimum while still having a health care professional on site to give the patient reassurance and immediate care.

Context

 When to perform a 12-lead ECG

This investigation is indicated in many circumstances to obtain diagnostic information, so the ability to perform it accurately is vital.

Reasons for performing a 12-lead ECG include:

- Baseline cardiac status prior to medical or surgical intervention.
- Chest pain of unknown aetiology.
- Myocardial ischaemia.
- Myocardial infarction.
- Electrolyte disturbances.
- Disturbances in cardiac rate and rhythm.
- Sudden collapse.
- Ventricular hypertrophy.
- Sudden deterioration in a patient's condition.

(This list is not exhaustive.)

 When not to perform a 12-lead ECG

During a resuscitation attempt it is important to visualize the ECG to establish which side of the resuscitation treatment algorithm needs to be followed. Under these circumstances, all that is required is an idea of rate and rhythm, and a 12-lead ECG would be unnecessary and inappropriate until the post-resuscitation period is reached.

Alternative interventions

Standard 3- and 5-lead ECG monitoring

An ECG monitor (3- or 5-lead) can be used to gain information on rate and rhythm but is usually inappropriate for a definitive diagnosis (see Section 6.5).

Community and the telemetric 12-lead ECG

Recent technological developments have enabled diagnostic data to be gathered in remote situations and sent via the telephone network (or satellite) to an appropriate specialist for interpretation. This has increased the potential for immediate treatment when previously the patient would have had to travel purely for the investigation. These developments have been rigorously tested in hostile environments such as in space exploration with the National Aeronautics and Space Administration (NASA) and Antarctica with the British Antarctic Survey Medical Unit (BASMU).

As the popularity of telemedicine has grown, so costs have fallen, enabling community medical care to benefit. Now a simple **telemetric** device can be purchased for under £500 (**http://www.broomwellhealthwatch. com**), enabling a patient's ECG to be taken at home or in the GP clinic and sent to a specialist for interpretation within minutes (Lancashire and South Cumbria Cardiac Network 2007).

Continuous ambulatory 12-lead ECG monitoring

Patients may sometimes experience symptoms that may be cardiac related but on investigation have a normal ECG. Continuous **ambulatory** 12-lead ECG monitoring is a method of obtaining a 12-lead ECG while the patient performs their normal daily activities. The advantage of obtaining an ECG recording over a 24-hour period is that any symptomatic period can be captured for analysis. Modern computer technology can interpret a 24-hour recording in a matter of minutes to identify disturbances in rate, rhythm, and complex, and the physician can then compare this against adverse symptoms described by the patient.

Potential problems

Patients with exceptionally dry skin can create an electrical conduction problem as the moisture content of gel electrodes may not be high enough to cope with the level of dryness. This may result in a poor connection reported as 'lead off' or as a wandering baseline. In cases such as these, meticulous skin preparation is required using spirit and an abrasive pad.

To assist in obtaining a quality trace, patients who have a tremor or are fidgety may benefit from sitting on their hands during the procedure.

Indications for assistance

- Patient deterioration.
- Abnormal ECG.
- Inability to obtain an ECG of diagnostic quality.

Interpreting readings

There is a basic order for interpreting an ECG (see below). For more in-depth information, consult, for example, *The ECG made easy* by Hampton (2003) – see further reading section.

Basic order for ECG interpretation:

1 What is the rate (see calculation methods below)?

2 What is the rhythm?

3 Is it regular?
 – Is it regularly irregular? – e.g. 2nd degree block Type 1 (Wenckebach).
 – Is it irregularly irregular? – e.g. atrial fibrillation.

4 Are the conduction intervals normal? (See Standard times of the ECG below.)

5 Is the cardiac axis normal?

6 Are the QRS complexes normal?

7 Are the ST segments and the T waves normal?

Calculating the heart rate on a rhythm strip

The 6 second tracing method
Count the number of 'R' waves that appear on a 6 second (30 large (5 mm) squares) rhythm strip and multiply by 10.
- e.g. 9 × 'R' waves in a 6 second strip would be 9 × 10 = **90 bpm**

The 300 method

Count the number of large (5 mm) squares between two 'R' waves and divide this into 300.

- e.g. 3.5 large (5 mm) squares between two 'R' waves would be 300/3.5 = **86 bpm**

The 1500 method

Count the number of small (1 mm) squares between two 'R' waves and divide this into 1500.

- e.g. 16 small (1 mm) squares between two 'R' waves would be 1500/16 = **94 bpm**

Standard times of the ECG (seconds)

(1 × small (1 mm) square = 0.04 seconds, 1 × large (5 mm) square = 0.2 seconds, 5 × large squares = 1 second.)

PR	0.12–0.20 seconds
ST	0.27–0.33 seconds
QT	0.35–0.42 seconds
QRS	0.08–0.11 seconds

Special considerations

Pregnancy

When performing a 12-lead ECG on someone who is in the third trimester of pregnancy, it is important to ensure they are not lying flat on their back as this may cause supine hypotensive syndrome (Bamber and Dresner 2003). This is caused by **aortocaval** compression and affects 10% of pregnant women, resulting in **hypotension** affecting the **cardiac output**. A wedge (blanket or other) should be placed under the right side to prevent the gravid uterus from pressing on the aorta and inferior vena cava. Bamber and Dresner (2003) demonstrated that tilting the patient to the left laterally up to 12.5° is tolerated well and avoids any detrimental effects on cardiac output. This is compared to the Resuscitation Council's printed advice of a 15° tilt (Kinsella 2003).

Dextrocardia and situs inversus

There are a small number of congenital anomalies affecting the cardiovascular system that can extend past childhood. Some of these will need to be taken into account when performing an ECG. Dextrocardia is a condition where the apex of the heart is on the right side of the chest instead of the left, and situs inversus is where the heart and lungs are reversed in the thorax making a mirror image on the wrong side of the thorax. In these rare cases the ECG lead positions will have to be mirrored on the opposite side of the chest to gain a meaningful recording. Technical dextrocardia can be produced by placing the limb leads on the wrong limbs, and is seen as a common error with inexperienced operators.

Procedure: recording a 12-lead ECG

Preparation

Prepare the patient

Prior to starting the procedure, the patient should be offered the opportunity to go to the toilet as complete relaxation is desirable. Obviously this may not be appropriate due to the patient's condition and degree of urgency of the ECG. The patient's general medical condition should be taken into account to reduce any extraneous effects on the ECG that may not be directly associated with it, such as muscle tremor, coughing, anxiety, etc.

The bed should be positioned at a comfortable height for the operator. Position the ECG machine on the patient's left-hand side for ease of chest lead location and preparation. The patient's dignity should be maintained by isolating them from the view of other patients and staff. A full explanation should be given about the procedure, with particular emphasis on the need to expose the chest for electrode placement.

Prepare the equipment

- An electrically in-date, tested 12-lead electrocardiograph (meeting or exceeding the requirements of the International Electro-technical Commission 2005) with sufficient paper.
- Disposable 12-ECG electrodes (meeting or exceeding the requirements of the Association for the Advancement of Medical Instrumentation 2000).
- Warm private environment.
- Patient bed/trolley wide enough to allow the arms to rest comfortably down by the sides.
- Skin preparation equipment (disposable shaving equipment, hand towels, abrasive tape, alcohol wipes).

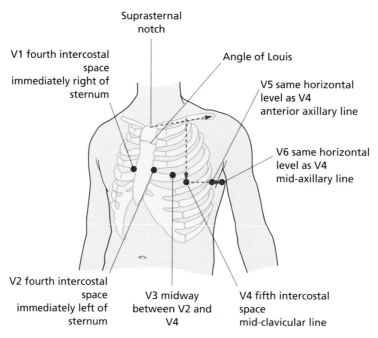

Suprasternal notch

V1 fourth intercostal space immediately right of sternum

Angle of Louis

V5 same horizontal level as V4 anterior axillary line

V6 same horizontal level as V4 mid-axillary line

V2 fourth intercostal space immediately left of sternum

V3 midway between V2 and V4

V4 fifth intercostal space mid-clavicular line

Figure 6.42 Chest landmarks.

There is a standard colour code for the lead wires in accordance with the International Electro-technical Commission (IEC) (European) recommendations, but this colour-coding may differ depending on the manufacturer.

The limb leads (and chest leads) are colour-coded by convention (Garvey 2006) and should be applied as described below. It is important that any deviation from the prescribed positions of the limb leads should be documented, as evidence suggests this can alter the ECG (Nelwan SP *et al.* 2001). Twelve views of the heart are obtained with the use of 10 leads. The limb leads provide six views of the heart (I, II, III, aVR, aVL, and aVF) from three of the limb leads (right arm, left arm, and left leg). The right leg limb lead provides the electrical ground, so it is important to pay particular attention to skin preparation for this lead.

It is also worth turning off all unnecessary electrical appliances prior to commencing the ECG as these may cause (50 Hz AC) interference, seen as a fine woolly line that reduces the clarity of the ECG.

Position of the limb leads

- Right arm limb lead (RA/red) – right forearm proximal to the wrist.
- Left arm limb lead (LA/yellow) – left forearm proximal to the wrist.

- Left leg limb lead (LL/green) – left lower leg proximal to the ankle.
- Right leg limb lead (RL/black) – right lower leg proximal to the ankle.

Locating intercostal spaces Location of the correct position for the chest (precordial) leads is relatively easy once certain anatomical landmarks are identified. First locate the suprasternal notch (see **Figure 6.42**) and move the fingers down a few centimetres until a ridge is felt; this is the angle of Louis or sternal angle. The second rib is contiguous with the sternal angle and the second intercostal space is below this. Palpate down from this point to find the third and fourth ribs and their corresponding intercostal spaces.

Another way to identify the correct intercostal space is to locate the clavicle (collar bone). The first rib felt below the clavicle is the second rib (the clavicle actually lies over the first rib and therefore it cannot normally be felt). Once this landmark is identified it is relatively simple to count down to the fourth intercostal space. Obesity can make this method slightly more challenging.

Position of the chest leads

- V1 (red/C1) – fourth intercostal space at the right sternal edge (where the rib meets the sternum).

- V2 (yellow/C2) – fourth intercostal space, left side of chest at the left sternal edge.
- V3 (green/C3) – midway between V2 and V4.
- V4 (brown/C4) – fifth intercostal space, left midclavicular line.
- V5 (black/C5) – anterior axillary line (at right angles to midclavicular line) on same horizontal line as V4.
- V6 (purple/C6) – midaxillary line (at right angles to midclavicular line) on same horizontal line as V4 and V5.

Hygiene requirements prior to an ECG being recorded are limited to skin preparation to ensure good electrode contact. Washing the area with soap and water may only be required if the patient is in a particularly dishevelled state. Normal skin preparation would include wiping the area of electrode placement with a spirit wipe and possibly abrading the area with a paper towel or preparatory skin abrasive.

Step-by-step guide to recording a 12-lead ECG

	Step	Rationale
1	Prepare the ECG machine. It should have an in-date electrical test and sufficient paper.	To ensure the machine is ready and working properly.
2	Introduce yourself, confirm the patient's identity, explain the procedure, and gain consent.	To identify the patient correctly and gain informed consent.
3	Ensure privacy for the patient and a suitable environment. The patient should be in a recumbent position (SCST 2006) if at all possible and it should be documented on the ECG if this is not possible.	It is important that the patient is warm and relaxed as skeletal muscle activity from movement or shivering can cause interference on the ECG.
4	Enter the patient's details in the machine (if applicable). Minimum data include the patient's name, hospital number, and date of birth.	These will be included on the ECG printout. Ensures the patient is correctly identified.
5	Ensure the date and time on the ECG machine are correct and the 1 mV calibration equals 10 mm.	This ensures the machine is ready for use and will display correct, valid information.
6	Ensure the paper speed is set to 25 mm/sec.	This is the standard speed (any deviation from this must be documented on the tracing).
7	Identify the electrode positions and prepare the skin. With female patients, the lateral chest leads (V4, V5, and V6) are placed beneath the left breast (Macfarlane *et al.* 2003).	To ensure good electrical contact.
8	Ensure the filter is turned off.	This maximizes the diagnostic potential of the recording. If the filter is required to reduce interference it must be documented on the recording (attach both recordings together in the notes).
9	Ensure the patient is relaxed and completely still.	To obtain a printout of the ECG without any artefact.
10	Press the record button.	To obtain a recording of the patient's ECG.

Following the procedure

Immediately after the ECG has been recorded it must be inspected to ensure quality for diagnosis. For example, are the leads on the correct limb (remember, in a normal ECG aVR is negative; downwards deflection) and in the correct order on the chest; is the baseline (isoelectric line) horizontal or is it wandering or sloping up or down; is there excessive interference (mains AC or patient movement)? If the impulse size is too large or too small the sensitivity button should be pressed and this action documented, whether 5 mm/mV or 20 mm/mV on the tracing.

The ECG must be labelled straight away unless this has already been done in the machine setup procedure, according to the protocol of the device. The minimum information required is patient name, date of birth, hospital number, date, time, location, and person recording ECG, as well as any special information such as reasons for recording (chest pain, post-thrombolysis therapy, etc.). If serial ECGs are required the same lead positions should be adopted each time.

It is important for the patient's well-being to be circumspect about discussing abnormal tracings in front of them until the ECG has been reviewed by a medical practitioner.

Recognizing patient deterioration

If while carrying out the procedure the ECG does not look typical, always check the condition of the patient; a quiet patient may be a patient in cardiac arrest!

Reflection and evaluation

When you have undertaken a 12-lead ECG with a patient, think about the following questions:

- Did the ECG give the reading you were expecting for that particular patient?
- Were you able to answer the patient's questions?
- Did your visual assessment of the patient alert you to any potential problems with using the 12-lead ECG machine?
- Were you able to interpret the reading in light of the patient's medical condition?

Further learning opportunities

- Familiarize yourself with a 12-lead ECG machine (individual machines may well have buttons in different places).
- Check how to replace paper in the machine.
- Observe a qualified person using the ECG machine to consolidate your learning.
- Enrol on a training course in ECG interpretation.

Reminders

- If the ECG looks odd, always check the condition of the patient.
- Always double-check your leads are on the correct sites.

Patient scenarios

1 You are attempting to record an ECG on an elderly, dehydrated patient. The ECG trace is wandering up and down and there appear to be a lot of extra erratic complexes. What might be the cause and what effect could this have on the patient?

2 There is a continuous straight flat line in V3 on the ECG trace but all the other leads appear satisfactory. What might the problem be?

3 You are trying to record an ECG but there is a thick baseline obscuring the fine detail of the ECG. What is the cause of this?

Website

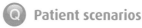 **http://www.oxfordtextbooks.co.uk/orc/ endacott**

You may find it helpful to work through our short online quiz and additional scenarios intended to help you to develop and apply the skills in this chapter.

References

Association for the Advancement of Medical Instrumentation (2000). *EC12–00: Disposable ECG Electrodes*. AAMI, Arlington, VA.

Bamber JH and Dresner M (2003). Aortocaval compression in pregnancy: the effect of changing the degree and direction of lateral tilt on maternal cardiac output. *Anesth Analg*, **97**, 256–8.

Garvey JL (2006). ECG techniques and technologies. *Emergency Medicine Clinics of North America*, **24**, 209–25.

International Electro-technical Commission (2005). *Medical electrical equipment Part 2–51: particular requirements for safety, including essential performance, of recording and analysing single channel and multichannel electrocardiographs. IEC 60601–2–51*. IEC, Geneva.

Kinsella SM (2003). Lateral tilt for pregnant women: why 15 degrees? *Anaesthesia*, **58**, 835–6.

Lancashire and South Cumbria Cardiac Network (2007). *Cardiac telemedicine in primary care. Delivering benefits for patients and the NHS in Lancashire and Cumbria. A report for commissioners*. NHS North West, UK.

Macfarlane PW, Colaco R, Stevens K, Reay P, Beckett C, and Aitchison T (2003). Precordial electrode placement in women. *Netherlands Heart Journal*, **11**, 118–22.

Nelwan SP, Meij SH, van Dam TB, and Kors JA (2001). Correction of ECG variations caused by body position changes and electrode placement during ST-T monitoring. *Journal of Electrocardiology*, **34**(Suppl), 213–16.

Nursing and Midwifery Council (2004). *NMC code of professional conduct: standards for conduct, performance and ethics*. NMC, London [online] **http://www.nmc-uk.org/aFrameDisplay.aspx? DocumentID=201** accessed 28/08/08.

SCST (2006). *Clinical Guidelines by Consensus. Recording a standard 12-lead electrocardiogram: an approved methodology*. The society for Cardiological Science and Technology [online] **http://www.scst.org.uk/docs/ Consensus_guideline_for_recording_a_12_lead_ ECG_2006.pdf** accessed 28/08/08.

Useful further reading and websites

Your local policy for performing a 12-lead ECG.

Hampton J (2003). *The ECG made easy*, 6th edition. Churchill Livingstone, Edinburgh.

Hampton J (2003). *The ECG in practice*, 4th edition. Churchill Livingstone, Edinburgh.

http://www.interactivephysiology.com/demo/ systems/buildframes.html?cardio/cardcycl/01

http://www.ecglibrary.com/ecghome.html

http://occawlonline.pearsoned.com/bookbind/ pubbooks/ehapplace/chapter0/deluxe.html

http://www.anaesthetist.com/icu/organs/heart/ ecg/Findex.htm

http://www.nmc-uk.org/aFrameDisplay.aspx? DocumentID=201

 Answers to patient scenarios

1 Quickly assess the patient's condition. If stable and normal, this problem is most probably caused by poor electrode to skin contact. The patient's skin will need to be prepared with spirit and a small abrasive pad to ensure optimal skin contact with minimal electrical resistance and artefact.

2 Loss of electrode contact. Inspect all the ECG electrodes – you're likely to find electrode V3 peeling or actually hanging off. Prepare the skin again with spirit and mild abrasion, and then record as quickly as possible after reattaching the leads.

3 This is caused by mains AC electrical interference (50 Hz). Turn off as many electrical items attached to the bed and patient as is safe. If this continues, switch the ECG 'filter' on but remember to document this fact on the ECG tracing and attach the unfiltered tracing to the notes too.

6.14 Cardiac auscultation for apical pulse and pulse deficit measurements

This is an advanced skill. You *must* check whether you can assist with or undertake this skill, in line with local policy.

Definition

Cardiac auscultation is the use of a stethoscope to listen to heart sounds as blood is pumped through it in the **cardiac cycle**.

It is important to remember that:

Cardiac auscultation can be used to evaluate:

- Rate and rhythm.
- Valve functioning (e.g. stenosis, regurgitation/ insufficiency).

- Anatomical defects (e.g. atrial septal defects, ventricular septal defect (VSD), hypertrophy).

It is vital that cardiac auscultation is carried out in conjunction with other clinical observations of the patient, such as:

- Pulse rate
- Blood pressure
- Respiratory rate

Accurate visual assessment of the patient should also be undertaken in order to make a sound clinical judgement on their condition.

Prior knowledge

Before attempting cardiac auscultation, make sure you are familiar with:

1 The anatomy and physiology of the cardiovascular and respiratory systems.
2 The electroconductive system in the heart.
3 The anatomical landmarks of the thorax and the correct terminology of anatomical positions, e.g. lateral, medial, inferior.
4 Normal heart sounds, particularly the first and second heart sounds.
5 Pathophysiology of common cardiovascular diseases (myocardial infarction, heart failure, atrial fibrillation, hypertension, shock, atherosclerosis, thrombosis/embolism, anaemia).

Background

Normal heart sounds are produced by the brief turbulence of blood flow occurring just as a valve closes. The sound made by the valves will be affected by the flow of the blood through the heart, for example during exercise, when the blood flows faster, the heart sounds will be more intense. Conversely when the rate of blood flow is slower, the heart sounds will be decreased and become quieter, e.g. in shock.

The heartbeat has two sounds – Lubb-Dubb. The first sound, Lubb (S1), is a prolonged low-pitched sound and is heard as the **atrioventricular valves** (i.e. the valves lying between the atria and the ventricles) close just prior to ventricular systole. It is best heard at the apex of the heart. These valves are also known as the mitral (on the right side of the heart) and tricuspid (on the left side of the heart) valves. The second heart sound, Dubb (S2), is briefer and higher pitched and is the sound of both **semi-lunar valves** closing just prior to diastole. It can be best heard over the aortic area (see **Figure 6.43**). These valves are also known as the aortic and pulmonary valves (Walsh 2002).

It is useful to be able to visualize in your mind the position of the heart and lungs within the chest cavity.

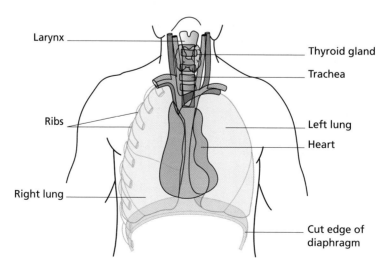

Larynx — Thyroid gland — Trachea

Ribs — Left lung — Heart

Right lung

Cut edge of diaphragm

Figure 6.43 Heart and lungs within the chest cavity.

A text on surface anatomy will help you do this (e.g. Lumley 2002).

Abnormal heart sounds

Certain abnormal heart sounds known as murmurs are often found on routine physical examination and can be described as a swishing sound caused by turbulent or abnormal blood flow across the heart valves. Murmurs can be heard in the absence of any medical or cardiac conditions when caused by increased cardiac output, e.g. during fever or pregnancy, or by the size of the heart, e.g. women and children have smaller hearts than men. These are known as benign flow murmurs (other names you might hear are innocent murmurs or functional murmurs). These findings should be reported to a senior colleague and must be analysed for their significance by taking a holistic view of the patient's condition.

Heart murmurs are soft sounds made as the blood flows through damaged or leaking heart valves (if not benign). They can be heard at different points in the cardiac cycle in relation to the normal S1 and S2 sounds, and more loudly in different areas over the heart depending on which valve is affected as the blood flows through the heart (Davey 2006). You will find a list of useful websites at the end of this section where you can listen to all the different heart sounds. In order to differentiate between the heart sounds, it is necessary to listen at various positions on the chest wall.

The third heart sound (S3) is heard immediately after S2 and is best heard at the apex of the heart when the patient is in the **left decubitus position**. It is a normal finding in children and young adults, but in adults over the age of 40 it is an abnormal (**pathological**) finding and is due to inefficient ventricular function. It can be an early indicator of heart failure or conditions such as mitral regurgitation or aortic regurgitation. In such adults it is known as a 'ventricular gallop'. It can also be heard when patients have an increased cardiac output in the absence of heart disease such as in hyperthyroidism, anaemia, and pregnancy. When the primary condition is corrected, the S3 gallop disappears.

The fourth heart sound (S4) is best heard over the tricuspid and mitral valve areas and comes immediately before S1. It may be present in healthy infants and children. In adults the S4 is produced with decreased compliance of the ventricle and may indicate myocardial infarction or shock.

Murmurs are graded according to the quality of the sound heard; Grade 1 is the softest-sounding murmur and Grade 6 is the loudest. A murmur graded 4, 5, or 6 is so loud you can actually feel a rumbling from it under the skin, often described as a 'cat purring'. If you feel this with your hand on the patient's chest over the pulmonary and aortic areas, this is known as a 'thrill' (Davey 2006).

It is not necessary for the nurse to be able to name murmurs or diagnose their presence. However, it is useful to have an insight into the common causes of heart murmurs in order to be able to understand presenting signs and link these to the condition of the patient you are caring for (see **Box 6.9**).

It is essential to have a good quality stethoscope with a bell and diaphragm (see **Figure 6.44**). The bell is sensitive to low-pitched sounds and the diaphragm is sensitive to high-pitched sounds. It must also have snug-fitting earplugs placed in the ear correctly, i.e. fitting positioned towards your nose; if they feel uncomfortable take them out and put them in with the earplugs facing forward. Ideally, the tubing should be no longer than 38 cm long with an internal diameter of 0.3 mm. You should be confident and competent in its use (Bickley and Szilagyi 2005) (see **Box 6.10**).

Box 6.9 Causes of heart murmurs

Heart valve disease is the most common cause of a heart murmur:

- Valve stenosis – a narrow, tight, stiff valve, limiting forward flow of blood.
- Valve regurgitation – a valve that does not close completely, allowing backward flow (a 'leaky' valve).
- The abnormal changes to the valve cause the abnormal heart sound (murmur).

Other causes of heart murmurs include:

- Hypertrophic cardiomyopathy.
- Septal defect.
- Functional causes – increased blood flow across the valve related to other medical conditions without heart disease, such as anaemia or hyperthyroidism.
- Innocent murmurs – those without any medical or heart condition. Two common examples include childhood murmurs and pregnancy.

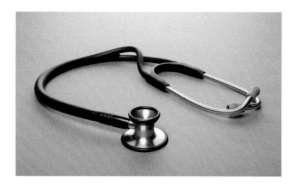

Figure 6.44 Stethoscope. Daniel Loiselle/istock.com.

Box 6.10 How to use a stethoscope

- Hold the diaphragm *firmly* in the correct anatomical position against the patient's skin. If the correct pressure has been applied you will see a slight ring mark on the patient's chest when you lift off the stethoscope.
- Hold the bell *lightly* in the correct anatomical position against the patient's skin. Holding the bell too firmly causes the skin to act as a diaphragm, thus obliterating the low-pitched sounds.
- Hair on the patient's chest may cause friction on the end and thus mimic abnormal breath sounds such as crackles (Beverage *et al*. 2005). You can minimize this problem by lightly wetting the hair before auscultating.
- Heart sounds and breath sounds are easy to hear in a quiet environment; closing your eyes will help you focus on what you are hearing. Concentrate your focus on the characteristics of one sound at a time.
- Always expose the chest area before auscultation. Never listen through clothing or try to undertake the procedure with the patient still dressed, as this will interfere with the quality of the sounds. You cannot carry out an effective examination through the 'buttonhole' window of a shirt or blouse or by 'creeping' between clothing.
- Warm the stethoscope in your hand first.

The stethoscope should be cleaned as per local policy; research suggests that cleaning once per day at the start of your shift using 66% ethyl alcohol is an effective method (Saloojee and Steenhoff 2001, Kennedy *et al*. 2003, Ramesh *et al*. 2004). However, some hospital policies recommend wiping the stethoscope before and after each patient and others recommend cleaning before and after each shift; disposable covers for stethoscopes can now also be purchased and used as single patient use items. It is therefore essential that you follow the policy of your employing authority. A suitable method is to wipe the stethoscope with an approved alcohol wipe (i.e. at least 66% ethyl alcohol concentration), starting at the earpieces (which helps prevent the spread of ear infections among staff). Clean around them and proceed down the tubing, finishing by wiping the bell and the diaphragm. Take the diaphragm apart to remove dust, lint, or debris and clean it well before reassembling it (Saloojee and Steenhoff 2000, Kennedy *et al*. 2003, Ramesh *et al*. 2004).

Patient's position for cardiac auscultation

It is important to ensure that the patient is sitting comfortably at 30–45° (see **Figure 6.45**), well supported by pillows and with clothing removed to allow visualization of the chest wall. At this point you can visually assess the chest for scarring from previous surgery, rashes, and other signs of disease, e.g. the blisters of shingles. You can also observe the rise and fall of the chest as the patient breathes. It may be possible to see on some slim-build or thin patients the beating of the heart at or medial to the left midclavicular line in the fifth or possibly fourth intercostal space. This is the pulsation of the left ventricle during contraction as it touches the chest wall. It is not visible in all patients and cannot be seen at all when the patient is supine (lying down) (Bickley and Szilagyi 2005).

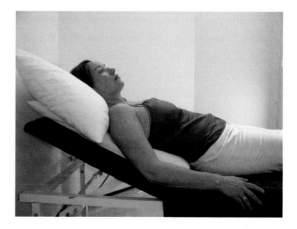

Figure 6.45 A patient lying at 35–40° awaiting cardiac auscultation. Clothing should be removed to allow visualization of the chest wall before starting the procedure.

Context

 When to use cardiac auscultation

Nurses typically use this skill to assess the rate and rhythm of the heart when the peripheral pulse is weak or irregular, or both, by listening to and counting the rate of the apical pulse, sometimes known as the **apex beat** or the point of maximum impulse (PMI) (Davey 2006). In addition to measuring the apical pulse, cardiac auscultation is used by doctors and other suitably qualified practitioners to diagnose and monitor irregularities of the cardiac function such as heart murmurs, and this should be undertaken as part of a full cardiac examination. It is an advanced clinical skill that needs to be practised regularly in order to maintain competence in identifying changes from the normal heart sounds and make clinically sound decisions about the patient's condition (March *et al.* 2005). The nurse is not expected to make diagnoses but should be able to recognize normal heart sounds and inform a senior colleague if abnormal heart sounds are heard.

Measuring a patient's apical pulse is an additional assessment of cardiac function to be used in conjunction with other clinical observations, e.g. temperature, pulse rate, respiratory rate, and blood pressure. It is particularly useful to use when the peripheral pulse is found to be weak, irregular, or both, indicating there is underlying pathology, e.g. atrial fibrillation. Auscultation of the apex beat is the normal method used to obtain the heart rate of infants and children.

 When not to use cardiac auscultation

- If the patient is collapsed and in need of cardiopulmonary resuscitation and the priority of care is airway and breathing.
- It should not be undertaken as the only assessment of the patient's condition but should be used to support any other abnormal baseline observations.

Additional interventions

Alternative interventions may be necessary if, for example, a rapid and/or irregular heart rate is palpated at the radial pulse and confirmed with cardiac auscultation of the apical beat, leading you to suspect the presence of a pulse deficit (when the radial pulse is less than the apical pulse due to an insufficient cardiac output). This can be confirmed by measuring an apical–radial pulse, which requires two nurses simultaneously to measure the radial pulse by palpation and the apical pulse by auscultation and compare the difference. (See later section on measurement of apical–radial pulse.)

Other investigations may be instigated such as an electrocardiograph (ECG) to record the electrical activity of the heart, or an echocardiogram to give accurate pictures of the heart muscle, chambers, and structures such as the valves, and the efficiency of the function of the heart.

Potential problems

The patient's heart rate may be too fast or too irregular to count accurately and this should be reported to a senior colleague.

Indications for assistance

If you are unable to locate the apical pulse and have tried alternative manoeuvres to locate it, seek the assistance of a senior colleague (see Special considerations box).

Interpreting findings

When considering your findings from auscultating the apical beat, ask yourself these questions:

- Am I confident that I was listening in the correct position on the chest for the age of the patient?
- Could I clearly hear the heart rate and rhythm?
- Have I taken into consideration the age of the patient and therefore the normal heart rate?
- Have I taken into account how the patient is presenting (see Section 6.1 on visual assessment of the cardiac patient)?
- What is the significance of the heart rate and rhythm (see Section 6.2 on pulse rate)?
- Did I hear two heart sounds (Lubb-Dubb) and were they clear?
- Were there any other sounds?
- Where were these heard loudest and clearest?

Special considerations

The position of the apical pulse will vary slightly according to the age/condition of the patient, for example:

- For adults, usually found at fourth to sixth intercostal space left midclavicular line.

- Elderly patients in heart failure may have an enlarged left ventricle. In this case the apical pulse will be located more laterally of the midclavicular line and can be felt and heard more easily by asking the patient to roll onto their left side (left lateral decubitus position).

- When examining a woman with large breasts it is often necessary to move the breast gently upward or laterally. It is acceptable to ask her to do this herself if she is physically able.

- In patients who are obese, have a very muscular chest wall, or have an increased anterior–posterior diameter of the chest (e.g. pigeon chest or barrel chest), it may be impossible to palpate the apical beat. Some apical impulses 'hide' behind the ribcage, despite positioning (Bickley and Szilagyi 2005).

- The apex beat may also be displaced by other conditions such as pleural or pulmonary disease, e.g. chronic obstructive pulmonary disease can lead to cor pulmonale and cardiomegaly (an enlarged heart). A pneumothorax may also lead to displacement of the apex beat.

- Rarely a patient may have a condition known as **dextrocardia** where the heart is situated on the right side. An apical pulse would then be heard in the same position on the right chest wall (Bickley and Szilagyi 2005).

Procedure: auscultating the apical pulse

Preparation

As with all patient encounters, always follow professional guidelines and recognize limitations (NMC 2008).

Prepare yourself
Wash your hands and put on any other equipment such as gloves and apron as necessary, i.e. follow universal precautions (Ayliffe *et al.* 2000).

Prepare the patient

- Ensure privacy by pulling the curtains around the patient's bed.
- Ensure that the patient is comfortable and happy with the procedure; assist them into a comfortable position between 30 and 45°, supported by pillows.
- Expose the chest by removing clothing; it is acceptable to unbutton pyjama tops, shirts, and blouses.

Prepare the equipment
Gather together all the necessary equipment:

- Stethoscope with a diaphragm and bell.
- A watch with a second hand.
- The observation chart available.
- A black ink pen.
- Clean the stethoscope (as described in the Background section) with alcohol wipes.

Step-by-step guide to auscultating the apical pulse

Step	Rationale
1 **Introduce yourself, confirm the patient's identity, explain the procedure, and obtain consent.**	To identify the patient correctly and gain informed consent. If the patient is unconscious, consent can be sought from next of kin to undertake the examination if they are present. Explain what you are about to do in order to allay fears or anxieties (DH 2001a, 2001b).
2 **Inspect anterior chest wall.** **Ensure the patient is recumbent at 30–45°.**	Close inspection of anterior chest wall may reveal the location of the apical pulse (seen as a visible pulsation in the precordial area of the chest) and the position of the beat will give an indication of the size of the heart (Bickley and Szilagyi 2005). Scars may reveal evidence of previous thoracic/cardiac surgery. In slim patients with a cardiac pacing device this can sometimes be seen. This is the best position for auscultating the heart.
3 **Locate the apical pulse, which is found on the midclavicular line, fifth intercostal space.**	Aids correct positioning of the stethoscope over the apex of the heart. This is the area to clearly hear the first heart sound, Lubb (S1), of the mitral and tricuspid valves closing, and the second heart sound, Dubb (S2), as the aortic and pulmonary valves snap shut.
4 **Place your warm stethoscope with the diaphragm on the skin of the chest wall over the apex.**	Ensures patient comfort. The diaphragm is most useful for picking up high-pitched sounds, e.g. S1, S2.
5 **Count the beats heard over 1 minute. Begin with zero, then one, two, three, etc. This is the rate of the heartbeat.**	Counting for a full minute ensures an accurate rate. Zero begins the time interval and should be included to give an accurate count.
6 **Note the rhythm of the heartbeat. Rhythms should be recorded as regular or irregular, and irregular heart rhythms should be further classified as irregularly irregular or regularly irregular.**	This will give a clear indication of the underlying cause of the abnormality.
7 **Discuss the findings with the patient.**	This keeps the patient informed of their condition and will help to alleviate anxiety and allow the patient to be a partner in their care.
8 **Record findings on the patient's notes.**	Communicates the findings to other members of the health care team. Supports legal requirements for recording care given to patients (NMC 2008).

Following the procedure

- Ensure that you act immediately if you believe the patient's condition is unstable or an emergency. Instigate any local resuscitation procedures, or, if not life-threatening, report your findings to the appropriate clinician.
- Wash your hands and clean the stethoscope as per hospital policy.
- If you suspect the patient has a pulse deficit, you should carry out an assessment of the apical–radial pulse (see next section).

Procedure: measurement of apical–radial pulse

Before seeking assistance in order to undertake the measurement of the apical–radial pulse:

- Assure yourself that the patient is stable; if they are collapsed call for immediate help.
- Have you correctly identified and palpated the radial pulse and recorded your findings?
- Have you checked other pulses, e.g. brachial and carotid, to confirm your suspicions?

Table 6.11 Interpreting findings

Finding	Interpretation
Pulse rate above 110 bpm	Tachycardia. Some possible causes are: Fever Anxiety Pain Hypotension Myocardial infarction Heart failure Ischaemic heart disease Sick sinus syndrome Respiratory failure Drugs (nicotine, caffeine, cocaine, adrenaline) Hyperthyroidisms Anaemia
S3 ventricular gallop	Could be: Normal in children and young adults Normal in last trimester of pregnancy Heart failure (ventricular hypertrophy) Acute myocardial infarction Associated with pulmonary oedema Mitral/tricuspid regurgitation Anaemia Hyperthyroidism (Kusumoto 2004)
S4 atrial gallop	Could be: Hypertension Pulmonic stenosis Coronary artery disease Aortic stenosis (Kusumoto 2004)
Pulse deficit	Insufficient cardiac output generated to produce a peripheral pulse. Could be due to: Atrial fibrillation Dissecting aortic aneurysm

Step-by-step guide to measuring the apical–radial pulse

Step	Rationale
1 Find an assistant.	This technique requires two nurses to undertake the procedure.
2 Check and confirm the patient's medical diagnosis by checking the medical and nursing notes. The patient may be able to tell you themselves.	It is important to know if this is a recognized symptom for the patient or a new symptom signifying a change in their condition.
3 Ensure the patient is sitting comfortably at 30–45°, well supported by pillows with clothing removed to allow visualization of the chest wall.	This is the best position to locate the apex beat and you can visually assess the chest for scarring, rashes, signs of disease, etc.
4 **First nurse:** Locate the apical impulse in the left fifth intercostal space on the midclavicular line.	This is the best position to hear the apical beat.
5 Warm the end piece of the stethoscope using your hands and place it at the located site on the patient's chest wall.	Ensures patient comfort as a cold stethoscope is uncomfortable and can startle the patient.
6 Signal the second nurse that you are ready to start counting.	It is essential that you begin and end counting at the same time.
7 **Second nurse:** Locate the patient's radial pulse as per Section 6.2. Signal the first nurse that you are ready and begin counting the heart rate simultaneously for 1 minute. Start with zero, then one, two, three, etc. Hold a watch with a second hand in view of both nurses.	This is the recommended method of taking the radial pulse. Simultaneous measurement of radial and apical pulses will ensure that if present the pulse deficit will be accurately obtained. Zero begins the time interval and should be included to get an accurate count. Both nurses can ensure the count is for a full minute.
8 Compare the findings.	See interpreting findings box.
9 Wash your hands.	Decreases the transmission of microorganisms and minimizes the risk of health care-associated infection.
10 Record the results.	Communicates the findings to other members of the health care team. Supports legal requirements for recording care given to patients.

- Is the patient on cardiac monitoring? Does the heart rate displayed on the monitor concur with the measurement you palpated?
- Carrying out an ECG will provide a visual record of the condition of the patient's heart.

Preparation

Explain to the patient that you are going to find a colleague to help you check their apical–radial pulse rate. You will need to explain to the patient what this is and what it means. For example, explain that their pulse rate is fast and/or irregular and you want to listen simultaneously to the heart while feeling the pulse at their wrist to ensure that you have an accurate record of the rate and rhythm of their heartbeat.

Ensure that the patient is comfortable, warm, and covered up; explain that you will be back as soon as you have found a colleague to assist you.

Ensure the second nurse understands their role and explain that you will signal to them when to begin counting the radial pulse as you auscultate the apex beat.

If you cannot find a colleague to assist, it is acceptable to count the radial pulse for 1 minute and note it, and then count the apical pulse for 1 minute and compare the difference. This is not as accurate as using two people but will suffice if no help is available to get a baseline observation. The procedure should be repeated with two nurses as soon as time allows.

Whichever method is used, if the radial pulse is higher than the apical then an error in technique has occurred and the apical–radial pulse should be reassessed.

> ### Interpreting findings
>
> - When interpreting your findings, assure yourself that the procedure was carried out correctly.
> - Work out the pulse deficit, expressed as heart rate (apical pulse) minus pulse rate (radial pulse) per minute.
> - In normal heart rates and rhythms there should be no difference between the peripheral pulse and heart rate.
> - If the apical pulse rate is higher than the radial pulse, this is a pulse deficit and a senior colleague should be informed.

> ### Recognizing patient deterioration
>
> Act appropriately (e.g. ask for assistance) depending on the following:
>
> - Were there audible heart sounds?
> - Did you clearly hear S1 and S2?
> - Were there added sounds?
> - Was the patient conscious?
> - Was the heart rate too fast to count?
> - Is the patient feeling and/or looking unwell?

Reflection and evaluation

When your observation of the patient is over, think about the following questions:

- Did you hear normal heart sounds S1 (Lubb) and S2 (Dubb)?
- Which did you hear the loudest? Were you able to hear the difference in the sounds?
- Were there any additional sounds heard?
- How did you feel? Did you think you made an accurate estimation and assessment of the patient's condition?
- Did you act on the information you gained appropriately?
- Consider how a fast, irregular heart rate would affect the patient. How would they feel, what signs would you expect to see when you looked at them, and what would their cognitive function be?

Further learning opportunities

Take every opportunity you can to listen to the heart sounds of real patients under the supervision of an experienced clinician, who can offer guidance and an explanation of what you hear. This way you will be able to recognize abnormal sounds with more certainty. Listen to auscultation sites on the Internet.

Reminders

- Assessment of heart sounds should *always* be correlated with the patient's clinical condition.

- Heart auscultation is only one part of your assessment of the patient.
- It can be difficult to hear the apical pulse in a busy, noisy ward area. Make sure you have a wellfitting, good quality stethoscope, and try closing your eyes before starting to count to focus your hearing on the sounds.

 Patient scenarios

1 You are taking the radial pulse of a patient and it measures 66 beats per minute, but the patient is complaining of a feeling of palpitations in his chest and feeling light-headed. What could this mean and what do you do?

2 One of your COPD patients has a marked anterior posterior deformity of his chest. When palpating his radial pulse you discover he has a tachycardia of 120 beats per minute, which is irregular. What will you take into consideration when listening for an apex beat?

Website

 http://www.oxfordtextbooks.co.uk/orc/ endacott

You may find it helpful to work through our short online quiz and additional scenarios intended to help you to develop and apply the skills in this chapter.

References

Ayliffe GAJ, Fraise AP, Geddes AM, and Mitchell K (2000). *Control of hospital infection. A practical handbook*, 4th edition. Arnold, London.

Beverage D, Mayer BH, Schaeffer L, and Thompson G (2005). *Assessment made incredibly easy*, 3rd edition. Lippencott Williams and Wilkins, Philadelphia.

Bickley LS and Szilagyi P (2005). *Bates' guide to physical examination and history taking*, 9th edition. Lippincott Williams and Wilkins, Philadelphia.

Davey P (2006). *Medicine at a glance*, 2nd edition. Bailliere Tindall, Oxford.

Department of Health (2001a). *Reference guide to consent for examination or treatment*. The Stationery Office, London.

Department of Health (2001b). *12 points on consent: the law in England*. DH, London.

Kennedy KJ, Dreimanis DE, Beckingham WD, and Bowden FJ (2003). *Staphylococcus aureus* and stethoscopes. *MJA*, **178**(9), 468.

Kusumoto, FM (2004). *Cardiovascular pathopysiology*. Hayes Barton Press, Oxford.

Lumley SP (2002). *Surface anatomy – the anatomical basis of clinical examination*, 3rd edition. Churchill Livingstone, Oxford.

March SK, Bedynek JL, and Chizner MA (2005). Teaching cardiac auscultation: effectiveness of a patient-centred teaching conference on improving cardiac auscultatory skills. *Mayo Clinic Proceedings*, **80**(11), 1443–8.

Nursing and Midwifery Council (2002). *The scope of professional practice*. NMC, London.

Nursing and Midwifery Council (2008). *Standards for medicine management*. NMC, London.

Ramesh CP, Chayya CV, Poonam S, Jairshree RK (2004) A prospective, randomised, double-blind study of comparative efficacy of immediate versus daily cleaning of stethoscope using 66% ethyl alcohol. *Indian Journal of Medical Science*, **58**(10),

Saloojee H and Steenhoff A (2001). The health professional's role in preventing nosocomial infections. *Postgraduate Medical Journal*, **77**, 16–19.

Walsh M (2002). *Watson's clinical nursing and related sciences*, 6th edition. Bailliere Tindal, London.

Useful further reading and websites

Excellent site by the University of Belfast demonstrating cardiac examination: **http://www.qub.ac.uk/ cskills/praecordium.htm**

Comprehensive physical examination and clinical education site for medical students and other health care professionals: **http://www.med.ucla.edu/ wilkes/intro.html**

Exciting science site: **http://www.blobs.org/science/ article.php?article=48fun**

Useful chapter on cardiac examination: **http://www.ncbi.nlm.nih.gov/books/bv.fcgi? indexed=google&rid=cardio.chapter.10**

 Answers to patient scenarios

1 The patient could be in atrial fibrillation and the cardiac output could be insufficient to register a radial pulse. It is necessary to palpate the apical pulse and

listen to the beat. Ask a colleague to assist you and measure and record the apical–radial pulse, noting any pulse deficit and informing a senior colleague of your findings.

2   The anterior posterior diameter of the chest can be increased in patients with long-standing COPD. It is essential to locate the apical pulse accurately; this can be done by asking the patient to lean over onto his left side. A deviated apical pulse can indicate ventricular hypertrophy of heart failure. It can also indicate **pleural effusion** or a pneumothorax.

6.15 **Anaphylaxis**

This is an advanced skill. You *must* check whether you can assist with or undertake this skill, in line with local policy.

Definition

The term anaphylaxis was coined in 1902 by a French scientist, Charles Richet (Dreskin 2005, Moneret-Vautrin *et al.* 2005). It comes from the Greek and means 'against protection', i.e. the opposite of prophylaxis.

Not all people present with the same symptoms, so it has been difficult to agree a universally accepted definition. Anaphylaxis was defined in 2001 by the European Association for Allergy and Clinical Immunology (EAACI) as 'a severe life threatening generalised or systemic hypersensitivity reaction' (EAACI 2001) and this is the definition used in the European Resuscitation Guidelines 2005 (Soar *et al.* 2005). The term anaphylactoid should not be used (EAACI 2001) but rather non-allergic anaphylaxis.

It is important to remember that:

- Median time to cardiac arrest for food-related reactions is 30 minutes (Pumphrey 2000).
- Median time to cardiac arrest for iatrogenic-related reactions is 5 minutes (Pumphrey 2000).
- More than 50% of people who die from anaphylaxis do so within the first 60 minutes (Sadana *et al.* 2000).
- Delay in adrenaline administration is likely to result in a poor outcome (Jowett 2000).

Prior knowledge

Make sure you are familiar with:

1   Cardiovascular anatomy and physiology.
2   Respiratory anatomy and physiology.
3   Basic immunology and allergy reaction.
4   Cardiopulmonary resuscitation.
5   Basic pharmacology.

Background

When a person is first exposed to an **allergen**, for example peanuts, the body produces a specific immuno-globulin E (IgE) antibody that attaches to mast cells and basophils. Mast cells are predominantly found in tissues open to the environment, e.g. intestinal and respiratory (Arshad 2002). The IgE antibody is specific to that allergen and on subsequent exposure to the allergen the hyper-sensitive reaction is triggered; the allergen and IgE anti-body fit together in the manner of a lock and key (Hendry and Farley 2001). This results in the mast cells and basophils breaking down (degranulation) and releasing a number of mediators, among them histamine, tryptase, and heparin. These mediators cause an increased vascular permeability, bronchoconstriction, and vasodilatation, which affects all body systems (**Figure 6.46**) and gives rise to the signs and symptoms (**Box 6.11**) associated with anaphylaxis (Arshad 2002, Finney and Ruston 2007). Allergic anaphylaxis resulting from an allergic reaction may or may not be IgE mediated. Anaphylaxis may also arise from a non-allergic reaction. The mechanism is different; however, since the treatment is the same it is not necessary to distinguish the mechanism prior to

Box 6.11 Signs and symptoms of anaphylaxis

- Skin/face – flushing, pruritis, urticaria, angioedema, and tingling lips.
- Respiratory system – sneezing, laryngeal oedema, and bronchospasm.
- Cardiovascular system – hypotension, tachycardia, and arrhythmias.
- Gastrointestinal tract – nausea, vomiting, cramps, and diarrhoea.
- Neurological system – anxiety, dizziness, and loss of consciousness.

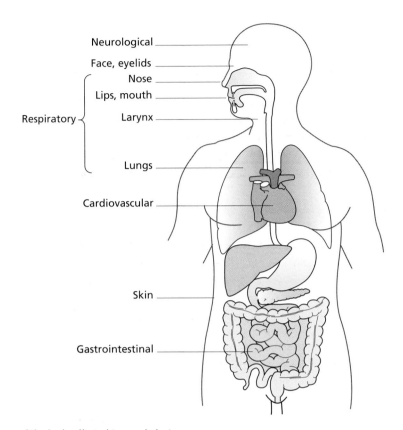

Figure 6.46 Organs of the body affected in anaphylaxis.

treatment. Follow-up care and investigations should help establish the type of reaction, which will be useful in aftercare and the avoidance of triggers.

Incidence and mortality

There has been a significant increase in allergies, particularly in the Western world, over the last few decades (Kay 2000, Gupta *et al*. 2007). Although admissions for anaphylaxis remain low (many patients are seen and then discharged from the emergency department), there has been a sevenfold increase from 5 per million in 1990/91 to 36 per million in 2003/04 (Gupta *et al*. 2007). Mortality figures vary as some deaths may be recorded as asthma rather than anaphylaxis. In the UK, Pumphrey (2003) identified 214 deaths between 1992 and 2001 as resulting from anaphylaxis. Asthmatic type reactions were most common in food allergies, and cardiovascular collapse (shock) in sting and drug reactions (Pumphrey 2000).

There are multiple triggers/causes for a reaction – in theory almost any food protein may provoke a reaction (Sampson 2000). The most common foods associated with reactions in Westernized countries are shown in **Box 6.12** and **Figure 6.47**, together with other triggers.

The management of life-threatening anaphylaxis relies upon swift recognition and early treatment. Anaphylaxis may be both over- and undertreated and there persists a lack of familiarity with the most appropriate treatment (Pumphrey 2000, Gompels *et al*. 2002, Johnston *et al*. 2003).

Medical and nursing staff must be alert to the early signs of anaphylaxis, make a rapid assessment of the patient, and be knowledgeable about the appropriate actions. They should call for help if necessary and institute administration of adrenaline and supportive airway measures without delay.

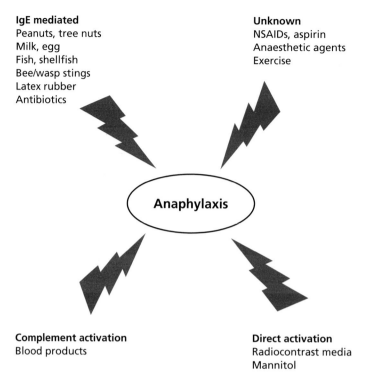

IgE mediated
Peanuts, tree nuts
Milk, egg
Fish, shellfish
Bee/wasp stings
Latex rubber
Antibiotics

Unknown
NSAIDs, aspirin
Anaesthetic agents
Exercise

Anaphylaxis

Complement activation
Blood products

Direct activation
Radiocontrast media
Mannitol

Figure 6.47 Some causes and mechanisms of action for anaphylaxis. With thanks to the Resuscitation Council (UK).

Box 6.12 Triggers of anaphylaxis

- Food – peanuts, tree nuts (walnuts, pecans etc.), shellfish, fish, milk, soy, wheat, eggs.
- Stinging insects (Hymenoptera order of insects) – bees, wasps, yellow jackets, hornets, ants (including the fire ant).
- Latex – car tyres, rubber bands, elastic, carpet backing, hospital and dental equipment, gloves, balloons, condoms.
- Medications – penicillin, sulfa antibiotics, allopurinol, muscle relaxants, vaccines, radiocontrast media, antihypertensives, insulin, blood products, NSAIDS, aspirin.
- Exercise and unknown causes.

Context

Some patients coming into hospital may already know they are allergic to some substance and thus be able to alert the health care team to the fact, but all other patients are still potential victims. In the UK the incidence of blood transfusion causing allergic reactions is 1 in 3293, and of severe anaphylactic reactions is 1 in 57 000 (Donaldson 2003). Nurses need to be able to recognize the signs and distinguish between other similarly presenting conditions such as episodes of vasovagal syncope and panic attacks (Box 6.13).

Box 6.13 Differential diagnoses

- **Anaphylaxis** – flushing, pruritis, urticaria, *angioedema*, sneezing, laryngeal oedema, bronchospasm, stridor, wheeze, *hypotension*, *tachycardia*, arrhythmias, nausea, vomiting, cramps, diarrhoea, anxiety, *dizziness, loss of consciousness, cardiac arrest.*
- **Vasovagal episode** – *dizziness, loss of consciousness*, bradycardia, *hypotension*.
- **Panic attack** – hyperventilation, **erythematous** rash, *tachycardia*, pallor, wheeze.

Special considerations

School nurses involved in vaccination programmes must be familiar with emergency procedures and any equipment and drugs available where they are working. Community and school nurses need to ascertain what the local policy is with regard to their being able to administer adrenaline. Most hospitals and health providers will have a patient group directive (PGD) covering this eventuality. School nurses should check their local policy with regard to their role in educating and supporting school staff in the care of pupils with a known hypersensitivity and the use of adrenaline auto-injectors.

People known to be at risk of anaphylaxis should wear a medic alert bracelet or necklace. Hospitals and care homes should have an easily recognized system for identifying patients with known allergies, for example red identity bands.

Procedure

Preparation

Preparation for medical emergencies is the key to successful and efficient treatment. Nurses caring for patients in hospital or the community must be ready to deal with emergencies whenever they arise. Staff should be familiar with emergency procedures, the equipment available, and how to raise additional assistance, i.e. the medical emergency team. Nursing staff who may be required to administer adrenaline should be familiar with the policy and contents of the PGD. Annual refresher sessions in the management of anaphylaxis are recommended for staff working in areas or with patients/clients most at risk, e.g. occupational health, practice and school nurses, X-ray staff, and chemotherapy department.

Step-by-step guide to treating anaphylaxis

Note: extended training will be required to institute all the treatments as listed, for example giving IM adrenaline or gaining IV access. However, knowing the correct procedure will mean the nurse will be ready to assist with greater effectiveness.

Step

Rationale

Step	Rationale
1 **Rapid ABCDE assessment of patient.**	To establish the patient's condition and gain an idea of what is wrong with the patient.
2 **Call for help.**	To ensure appropriate assistance comes quickly, including anaesthetic support.
3 **Give high-flow (15 litres) oxygen with a reservoir bag.**	To maximize oxygen delivery to tissues while patient is compromised.
4 **Put the patient in a semi-supine position. Or lie the patient flat and in recovery position if unconscious.**	If the patient has breathing difficulties this may be the most comfortable position. As blood pressure is compromised, lying the patient down will reduce cerebral hypoxia. Putting the patient in the recovery position will protect the airway.
5 **Give adrenaline IM 500 micrograms i.e. half a ml of 1:1000. (Caution: this is the adult dose. Dose differs for infants and children.)**	Adrenaline counteracts the vasodilatation associated with anaphylaxis and helps to maintain the blood pressure. IM is the route of choice.

continued overleaf

6	Gain (early) IV access.	Patient will need intravenous fluids to maintain blood pressure. It is important to gain access early as it may be very difficult later.
7	Record observations of vital signs continuously during the acute episode.	To ensure signs of either deterioration or improvement are noted, and if deterioration, that further action is taken (e.g. supported ventilations, further doses of adrenaline).
8	Give chlorphenamine and hydrocortisone IM or slow IV (see Figure 6.48). NB IV adrenaline is not a first line treatment.	Chlorphenamine is an antihistamine and steroids will help protect against late sequelae.
9	Continuously review ABCDE assessment.	To ensure improvement/deterioration in the patient's condition is known at all times so appropriate action can be instituted.

If the condition is unresponsive to IM adrenaline, titrated IV boluses may be required but only under experienced medical supervision with the patient on a cardiac monitor.

NB IV adrenaline is hazardous and is not a first line treatment (see **Figure 6.48** for recommendations).

Following the procedure

In the immediate post-event phase, patients need monitoring in a high dependency unit or equivalent. Second phase reactions can arise and patients may need admission for up to 24 hours (Nolan *et al.* 2006).

Bloods for serum tryptase levels will help confirm the diagnosis of anaphylaxis (this blood test can also be used to confirm diagnosis post-mortem). Tryptase levels are raised for 3 hours after an event; therefore ensure samples are taken within this time window (Fisher 2003).

Above all, someone experiencing an anaphylactic reaction needs reassurance and comfort following this frightening (and generally unexpected) event. Patients who experience an anaphylactic reaction also need to be fully investigated and in the longer term referred to an immunologist for advice on how to prevent or reduce recurrent episodes.

Additional information

Nursing staff in and out of hospital (e.g. school nurses) may be covered by a PGD to administer IM adrenaline for anaphylaxis without waiting for a medical order. Always ensure you know what help is available to you in your place of work and how to call it.

Recognizing patient deterioration

Signs of deterioration of the patient include appearance or resurgence of:

- **A**irway – **stridor**, wheeze.
- **B**reathing – respiratory distress, tachypnoea.
- **C**irculatory – hypotension, tachycardia.
- **D**isability – reduced GCS.
- **E**xposure – angioedema, rash.
- Cardiac arrest!

Reflection and evaluation

Think about the following questions:

1 If a patient on your ward collapsed, how would you assess them to exclude anaphylaxis?
2 Are you or were you familiar with the location and function of the emergency trolley on your most recent clinical placement?
3 Are you familiar with the procedure for summoning emergency assistance to your clinical area?
4 Have you read the local anaphylaxis policy?
5 How would you guide a junior doctor unfamiliar with the management of anaphylaxis?

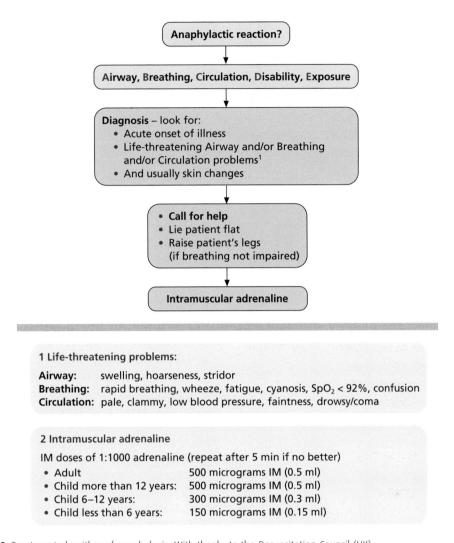

1 **Life-threatening problems:**

Airway: swelling, hoarseness, stridor
Breathing: rapid breathing, wheeze, fatigue, cyanosis, SpO$_2$ < 92%, confusion
Circulation: pale, clammy, low blood pressure, faintness, drowsy/coma

2 **Intramuscular adrenaline**

IM doses of 1:1000 adrenaline (repeat after 5 min if no better)
- Adult   500 micrograms IM (0.5 ml)
- Child more than 12 years: 500 micrograms IM (0.5 ml)
- Child 6–12 years: 300 micrograms IM (0.3 ml)
- Child less than 6 years: 150 micrograms IM (0.15 ml)

Figure 6.48 Treatment algorithm of anaphylaxis. With thanks to the Resuscitation Council (UK).

Further learning opportunities

Become familiar with:

- Anaphylaxis algorithm (RCUK)
- CPR (RCUK)
- Emergency equipment

A patient who has collapsed or is in the process of collapsing needs emergency assistance ASAP, ranging from summoning help to instituting CPR. It is worthwhile practising your ABCDE assessment and updating your CPR as often as possible to enable your contribution to become second nature in any emergency situation.

Reminders

Ensure familiarity with both local policies and current algorithms for management of anaphylaxis.

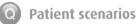 **Patient scenarios**

1   You are accompanying a patient to X-ray for an angiogram. Following a bolus injection of contrast the patient complains of feeling strange, they start to cough, and their breathing becomes wheezy. What do you do?

2 A patient is being sedated with midazolam for elective synchronized cardioversion. Vital signs are stable but a rash is noted over the upper body. You perform an ABCDE assessment and identify the following:

   ● A – patent.
   ● B – normal quiet respiration.
   ● C – pulse rate 110 fast AF BP 110/70.
   ● D – drowsy.
   ● E – a patchy rash.
     What do you do?

3 A 25-year-old woman visiting her husband in hospital experiences difficulty in breathing 10 minutes after eating some nuts. You perform an ABCDE assessment and find the following:

   ● A – patent.
   ● B – some inspiratory stridor but no wheeze, SpO_2 98%.
   ● C – pulse rate 90 BP 140/80.
   ● D – alert and slightly anxious.
   ● E – no erythema observed.
     How do you manage this situation?

Website

  http://www.oxfordtextbooks.co.uk/orc/ endacott

You may find it helpful to work through our short online quiz and additional scenarios intended to help you to develop and apply the skills in this chapter.

References

Arshad SH (2002). *Allergy: an illustrated colour text*. Churchill Livingstone, Edinburgh.

Donaldson L (2003). A precious gift: better blood transfusion. In L Donaldson. *Annual Report of the Chief Medical Officer 2003*, pp. 26–35. Department of Health, London.

Dreskin S (2005). Anaphylaxis *eMedicine Specialties* [online] **http://www.emedicine.com/ specialties.htm** accessed 29/08/08, article last updated 07/10/05.

EAACI (2001). A revised nomenclature for allergy: an EAACI position statement from the EAACI nomenclature task force. *Allergy*, **56**(9), 813–24.

Finney A and Ruston C (2007). Recognition and management of patients with anaphylaxis. *Nursing Standard*, **21**(37), 50–7.

Fisher M (2003). Anaphylaxis. In AD Bersten, N Soni, and TE Oh, eds. *Oh's intensive care manual*, pp 617–20. Butterworth Heinemann, London.

Gompels L, Bethune C, Johnston S, and Gompels M (2002). Proposed use of adrenaline (epinephrine) in anaphylaxis and related conditions: a study of senior house officers starting accident and emergency posts. *Postgraduate Medical Journal*, **78**, 416–18.

Gupta R, Sheikh A, Strachan D, and Anderson H (2007). Time trends in allergic disorders. *Thorax*, **62**, 91–6.

Hendry C and Farley A (2001). Understanding allergies and their treatment. *Nursing Standard*, **15**(35), 47–54.

Johnston S, Unsworth J, and Gompels M (2003). Lesson of the week: adrenaline given outside the context of life threatening allergic reactions. *BMJ*, **326**, 589–90.

Jowett N (2000). Letter: speed of treatment affects outcome in anaphylaxis. *BMJ*, **321**, 571.

Kay AB (2000). Allergy and allergic diseases: with a view to the future. *British Medical Bulletin*, 56(4), 843–64.

Moneret-Vautrin D, Morisset M, Flabbee J, Beaudouin E, and Kanny G (2005). Epidemiology of life-threatening and lethal anaphylaxis: a review. *Allergy*, **60**(4), 443–51.

Nolan J, Soar J, Lockey A *et al.*, eds (2006). *Advanced life support*, 5th edition. Resuscitation Council (UK), London: 130–3.

Pumphrey (2000). Lessons for management of anaphylaxis from a study of fatal reactions. *Clinical and Experimental Allergy*, **30**(8), 1144–50.

Pumphrey (2003). *Anaphylaxis No. 257 eBooks*. Novartis Foundation Symposium [buy online] **http://www.ebookmall.com/ebooks-authors/ novartis-foundation-symposium-ebooks.htm** accessed 29/08/08.

Sadana A, O'Donnell C, Hunt M, and Gavalas M (2000). Letter: managing acute anaphylaxis. *BMJ*, **320**, 937.

Sampson H (2000). Food anaphylaxis. *British Medical Bulletin*, **56**, 925–35.

Soar J, Deakin CD, Nolan JP *et al.* (2005). European Resuscitation Council Guidelines for Resuscitation 2005. Section 7 Cardiac arrest in special circumstances. Subsection 7g. *Anaphylaxis Resuscitation*, **67**(Suppl 1), S151.

Useful further reading and websites

The Anaphylaxis Campaign:
 http://www.anaphylaxis.org.uk
Asthma and allergy information and research:
 **http://www.users.globalnet.co.uk/~aair/
 anaphylaxis.htm**
Resuscitation Council UK: **http://www.resus.org.uk**
Epipen information: **http://www.epipen.com/
 causes_main.aspx**
Jevon P and Dimond B (2004). *Anaphylaxis: a practical
 guide*, eds J North, D Bowden, and J Singh Poona.
 Butterworth-Heinemann, Edinburgh.

 Answers to patient scenarios

1 A rapid ABCDE assessment. Depending on the findings, you may need to do the following:
  - Call emergency medical assistance.
  - Give high flow oxygen via a mask with reservoir bag.
  - Give 500 micrograms of adrenaline IM (0.5 ml of adrenaline 1:1000). Note the time.
  - Lie patient flat (semi-supine if breathing difficulties necessitate).
  - Remove IV cannula used for contrast administration.
  - Site a new IV and give 500 ml normal saline.
  - Monitor breathing, pulse, and blood pressure continuously.
  - Support and reassure patient, giving explanations.
  - Give slow injection IV of chlorphenamine 10 mg and 200 mg of hydrocortisone.

(Depending on the response, patient may need transfer to a high dependency area for observation, with bloods taken and detailed notes made in patient records.)

2 Administer oxygen and continue with cardioversion – the flushing is likely to be due to anxiety, no other systemic signs.

3 Life-threatening anaphylaxis is not present. Consider inhalation of foreign body. Escort to Emergency Department for full assessment.

7 Respiratory system

Skills

7.1 **Visual respiratory assessment**

Introduction

Initial assessment of all patients should incorporate a visual respiratory assessment to include: observation of the patient's respiratory rate, depth, and pattern, temperature, assessment of the peripheries, and observation of level of consciousness.

It is important to remember that:

- Rapid visual respiratory assessment is required to ensure appropriate and prompt intervention.
- If abnormal results are obtained, advice from a senior practitioner or doctor should be sought.

Prior knowledge

Before undertaking a visual respiratory assessment, make sure you are familiar with:

1 Respiratory and cardiovascular anatomy.
2 Physiology of respiration.
3 Pathophysiology of common respiratory diseases.

Background

In order to understand visual respiratory assessment, it is essential to have knowledge of the anatomy and physiology of the respiratory system. Where possible, you should have some background knowledge of the patient's previous medical history. Healthy breathing is quiet and uses minimal effort, while an increase in the work of breathing will result in a rise in respiratory rate, noisy breathing, and increased use of accessory muscles (which can be observed in the chest and also the neck).

Observation is a skilled process, requiring practice. It allows the nurse to assess characteristics of underlying health and illness. This section explains key features of visual assessment in respiratory patients and examines the relevance of observations of the individual patient in the context of their illness (see **Table 7.1**). In general terms, it should include the following (Francis 2006):

- **Respiration rate and pattern**, which will allow you to assess whether a patient is having to breathe faster than normal to compensate for a lack of oxygen, or slower or more irregularly than normal due to some underlying pathology. This is especially important as alterations in respiratory rates can be a crucial and early sign of patient deterioration.
- **Respiration depth**, which allows you to assess many things: shallow breathing, for example, may indicate pain or trauma, as the patient is unable to breathe deeply because it is painful.
- **Skin colour**, which allows you to assess whether a patient has sufficient oxygen circulating in their body. This is an essential observation in many acute illnesses (such as exacerbations of asthma, where the airways are constricted) and chronic illnesses (such as chronic obstructive pulmonary disease or COPD, where the airways are unable to function properly due to their deterioration). These conditions mean that there is insufficient oxyhaemoglobin in the skin or mucous membranes, so the skin appears pallid. An increase in deoxyhaemoglobin also causes a blue discoloration of the skin (cyanosis).
- Physical condition, which allows a general observation of important factors such as confusion, exhaustion, and use of accessory muscles. Emaciation indicates malnourishment, an important feature of lung cancer and other chronic lung diseases, requiring nutritional assessment and support.
- **Presence of cough**, which can indicate, for example, infection, tuberculosis, or heart failure, as well as being an early indicator of lung cancer.

- **Breath sounds**, for example wheezing indicates asthma.

Context

 ### When to use visual assessment

Visual assessment should be performed regularly and used whenever observation of a patient's vital signs is being undertaken, either in the hospital setting or in the patient's own home. It is important that if visual assessment reveals a problem or abnormality, it is dealt with immediately and brought to the attention of a senior nurse or doctor.

 ### When not to use visual assessment

You should always undertake a visual assessment of the patient. However, visual assessment does not provide accurate recordings, for example it is not possible to estimate the level of oxygen in the blood visually when a patient has been identified as being **cyanotic** (a bluish skin colour indicating a lack of oxygen). In these circumstances the use of pulse oximetry and arterial blood gas measurement are also required.

Alternative interventions

If you suspect the patient's condition has deteriorated, it is important to obtain accurate physiological readings in order to instigate appropriate patient management.

Interpreting readings

As with all patient assessment, it is important that you understand the findings of your visual assessment and take account of the patient's 'resting' condition when interpreting their respiratory rate. Respiratory rate should be 14–20 breaths per minute in the fit and healthy adult (Timby 1989). The following should therefore all be a prompt for an urgent review by a senior practitioner or doctor (Smith 2000):

- A recording of under eight (bradypnoeic) or above 30 (tachypnoeic) breaths per minute.

- Acute onset of dyspnoea (difficulty in breathing).

- Patient states that they cannot breathe.

Table 7.1 Interpreting visual assessment data

Observation (and how assessed)	Possible cause
Increased respiratory rate or tachypnoea (by counting the patient's breathing)	Infection Possible deterioration in condition Anxiety Pain
Lower respiratory rate or bradypnoea (by counting the patient's breathing)	Depression of the respiratory centre in the brain, caused by the use of opiate medication or a cerebrovascular event Hypothermia
Cyanosis (by observation of nail beds, skin colour, and assessment using pulse oximetry)	Insufficient oxygen to maintain acceptable saturation level Could be due to *acute shortness of breath*, e.g. in asthma, or *chronic shortness of breath*, as in COPD May also be a combination of acute and chronic cyanosis for some patients These factors will be assessed by arterial blood gas analysis
Confusion (by questioning and observation)	Severe respiratory distress
Orthopnoea (by observation of the patient's breathing pattern in different positions)	Prolonged hypoxia, or hypercapnia Left ventricular failure Asthma
Paroxysmal nocturnal dyspnoea (by observation at night)	Pulmonary oedema and left ventricular failure
Kussmaul breathing or air hunger (by observation of breathing patterns)	Ketoacidosis Renal failure
Cheyne–Stokes respiratory pattern (by observation of breathing patterns)	Left ventricular failure Cerebral injury End of life (Jevon and Ewens 2001)
Pain on inspiration (by observation)	Pneumothorax Infection
Cough (by observation)	Asthma Tuberculosis
Sputum (by observation)	White: asthma, COPD Yellow/green: infection Blood: lung tumour, pneumonia, pulmonary embolism, tuberculosis

Visual examples of both peripheral and central cyanosis can be found at **http://www.emedicine.com/med/topic3002.htm**.

Special considerations

- Elderly patients may have an increased resting respiration rate, especially if the patient is a past or current smoker.

- If undertaking a visual assessment in the patient's home, ascertain their level of activity immediately prior to the assessment (have they rushed down two flights of stairs to answer the door?)

The procedure

Preparation

Visual assessment should be an essential component of the nursing care of any patient, so, apart from an introduction to the patient, there is no other key preparation required prior to undertaking this skill.

Step-by-step guide to visual respiratory assessment

Step	Rationale
1 Introduce yourself, confirm the patient's identity, explain the procedure, and obtain consent.	To correctly identify the patient and gain informed consent.
Respiratory rate and pattern	
2 Count respiratory rate for a full 60 seconds.	To ensure that an accurate count is made, and to assess for irregularities in pattern and rate (Adam and Osborne 2005). Rate should be 14–20 breaths per minute in the fit and healthy adult (Timby 1989).
3 If possible, observe respiratory rate when the patient is at rest and while recording other vital signs. Possible causes of tachypnoea (fast respiratory rate) and bradypnoea (slow respiratory rate) along with other examples of respiratory observations can be found in Table 7.1 (Kenward *et al.* 2001).	This should ensure that they do not alter their breathing rate or pattern because they are aware that the nurse is observing them.
Respiratory depth	
4 Assess depth of respiration by observing the patient's chest movement, which should be equal and symmetrical, and the work of breathing (meaning how hard the patient needs to work to take breaths) (Jevon and Ewens 2001).	Respiratory depth is the volume of air that is moved in and out with each respiration. In fit, healthy people, the main respiratory muscles used in breathing are the diaphragm, sternomastoid, and intercostal muscles.
Sound of breath	
5 Noisy breathing is characterized by three different sounds: stridor, wheeze, and rattle. Listen for stridor (can be inspiratory or expiratory). This produces a high-pitched sound, usually on inspiration.	Caused by laryngeal or tracheal obstruction, such as foreign body or laryngeal oedema.

continued overleaf

6	Listen for wheeze. This produces a musical sound, which is more pronounced on expiration.	Produced when air passes through narrowed bronchi and bronchioles. A wheeze can be heard in asthma and COPD.
7	Listen for rattle. This produces a gurgling sound resulting from fluid in the upper airway (Jevon and Ewens 2001, Ahern and Philpot 2002, Bennett 2002).	Can be caused by pulmonary oedema or sputum retention.
8	Check for dyspnoea (difficulty in breathing). Three types are described: exertional dyspnoea (shortness of breath on exercise); orthopnoea (shortness of breath on lying down); paroxysmal nocturnal dyspnoea (sudden breathlessness that occurs at night when the patient is lying down).	Dyspnoea is a symptom of much underlying respiratory pathology.

Skin colour

| 9 | Assess skin colour. | Provides information about the efficiency and basic functioning of the respiratory system. If hypoxic (low in oxygen), the skin will appear pale as hypoxia causes vasoconstriction. The blue skin colouring known as cyanosis, which can be observed in nail beds, lips and mouths, tip of nose, and earlobes, is usually associated with hypoxia (Francis 2006). Cyanosis is an indication that there isn't enough oxygen to maintain the oxygen saturation level at above 80%; this is serious and should be reported immediately. |

Cough

10	Observe for a cough. Coughing is a reflex action that occurs when a deep inspiration is followed by an explosive expiration and is directed towards the removal of a foreign body, such as sputum.	It is a common respiratory symptom that can indicate certain conditions.
11	Note if patient has a strong, dry, or hoarse cough and how frequent it is.	A cough that is worse at night might be suggestive of asthma or heart failure (Jevon and Evans 2001).
12	Sputum produced should be assessed by colour, consistency, and quantity.	Consistent sputum production is most often related to inflammation or disease of the airways, such as asthma, COPD (Wilkins *et al*. 2005).

Physical condition (presence of any of the following must prompt review by a senior practitioner or doctor)

13	Assess physical condition, including increased use of accessory muscles.	Indicator of change in clinical condition. Can be indicator of respiratory failure.
14	Check for exhaustion, confusion, anxiety, or unresponsiveness.	Indicator of change in clinical condition. Can be indicator of respiratory failure.
15	Assessment of non-verbal expressions of pain related to breathing, particularly on either inspiration or expiration. Sit the patient upright and repeat the assessment.	Pain could indicate a pneumothorax or infection. Posture and position of the patient can improve symptoms of breathlessness. Breathing can improve if the patient sits upright, enabling improved lung expansion.

Reflection and evaluation

When you have completed the visual assessment, ask yourself the following questions:

1 How easy was it to complete a visual assessment? Were there any aspects that were more difficult?
2 Do you feel that your assessment was accurate?
3 Did your visual assessment lead you to take further action? If so, in the light of what you now know, were your actions appropriate? If not, what have you learnt and how could your care be improved next time?
4 Were you able to distinguish between respiratory problems, for example central and peripheral cyanosis or different types of dyspnoea?

Further learning opportunities

- When assessing vital signs with your next patient, observe their breathing pattern and look at the depth of each breath.
- Observe several patients and note whether they become more short of breath on lying down or at night.
- Use the *Reflection and evaluation* section to identify aspects of visual assessment where you need more experience.

Reminders

- The management of a patient's airway may take priority over a respiratory assessment in acute situations such as cardiac or respiratory arrest or if the airways are obstructed or blocked physically with an inhaled object. Students should be mindful of the need to assess a patient's airways at all times, including during visual assessment.
- Visual assessment can indicate important aspects of a patient's condition that require further investigation, nursing care, and treatment.
- Anything that appears untoward, such as a sudden change in the patient's respiratory rate, is probably important, or even life-threatening, for the patient. New treatments may need to be initiated.
- Even if nothing untoward is observed, trends such as respiratory rates slowly decreasing over several days from a fast peak can indicate that treatment is working and that the patient is improving.

 Patient scenarios

Consider what you should do in the following situations, then turn to the end of this skill to check your answers.

1 Patient A has been admitted to your ward and you are undertaking your first respiratory assessment. What six key elements will you assess?
2 Patient B has a respiratory rate of 30, has become suddenly short of breath, and states that they have difficulty in breathing. What action should you take next?
3 Patient C is found to be tachypnoeic on assessment. What might this indicate?

Website

 http://www.oxfordtextbooks.co.uk/orc/ endacott

You may find it helpful to work through our short online quiz and additional scenarios intended to help you to develop and apply the skills in this chapter.

References

Adam SK and Osborne S (2005). *Critical care nursing: science and practice*. Oxford Medical Publications, Oxford.

Ahern J and Philpot P (2002). Assessing acutely ill patients on general wards. *Nursing Standard*, **16**(47), 54–7.

Bennett C (2002). Respiratory care. In B Workman and C Bennett, eds. *Key nursing skills*, pp. 178–213. Whurr, London.

Francis C (2006). *Respiratory care: essential clinical skills for nurses*. Blackwell Publishing, Oxford.

Jevon P and Ewens B (2001). Assessment of a breathless patient. *Nursing Standard*, **15**(16), 48–53.

Kenward G, Castle N, and Hodgetts T (2001). Time to put the R back into TPR. *Nursing Times*, 97(40), 32–3.

Smith G (2000). *Acute life threatening events: recognition and treatment manual*. University of Portsmouth Open Learning publication, Portsmouth.

Timby B (1989). *Clinical nursing procedure*. JB Lippincott, Philadelphia.

Wilkins R, Sheldon R, and Krider S (2005). *Clinical assessment in respiratory care*, 5th edition. Elsevier Mosby, St Louis.

Useful further reading and websites

Bourke SJ (2007). *Lecture notes on respiratory medicine.* Blackwell Publishing, Oxford.

 Answers to patient scenarios

1 The six components of visual assessment are: respiration rate and pattern, respiration depth, skin colour, physical condition, presence of cough, sound of breath.

2 If these three elements are present then you should contact a senior practitioner or a doctor.

3 If a patient is tachypnoeic, this could indicate infection, pain, or anxiety.

7.2 Monitoring oxygen saturation using pulse oximetry

Definition

Pulse oximetry provides an immediate, non-invasive means of assessing **oxygen saturation** (the carriage of oxygen by haemoglobin (Hb) molecules). The amount of haemoglobin carrying oxygen (SaO_2) is expressed as a percentage of the total oxygencarrying capacity, for example SaO_2 98%. The pulse oximeter also calculates and displays heart rate.

It is important to remember that:

- The purpose of evaluating a person's oxygen status is to determine how much oxygen is reaching the cells of the body. Arterial oxygen saturation only provides part of this information and does not indicate the efficiency of gas exchange in the lungs or tissues.
- A pulse oximeter is easy to use and convenient; however, nursing and medical staff can have potentially dangerous gaps in their knowledge of oximetry (Howell 2002).
- Familiarizing yourself with the equipment before trying to use it will aid patient confidence.

Prior knowledge

Before using pulse oximetry to monitor oxygen saturation, make sure you are familiar with:

1 Respiratory and cardiovascular anatomy.
2 Physiology of respiration (in particular gas exchange).
3 Pathophysiology of common respiratory diseases.
4 Mechanisms of oxygen transport.
5 Factors influencing oxygen transport.
6 The *principles* of the oxyhaemoglobin dissociation curve.
7 The equipment you'll be using.

There are situations in which the recording of oxygen saturation with a pulse oximeter may give an inaccurate reading. Review of the areas above will help you recognize many of these situations (but not all, e.g. equipment-related problems).

Background

In order to understand why pulse oximetry is useful, it is helpful to consider oxygen transport as a four-stage journey (see **Table 7.2**); this will pinpoint the cause of inadequate tissue oxygenation. Oxygen is transported in the blood in two ways: dissolved in plasma (referred to as PaO_2 – partial pressure of arterial oxygen); and attached to haemoglobin (oxygen saturation). These two are inextricably linked: in order for oxygen to bind with haemoglobin, an adequate PaO_2 is required.

How does pulse oximetry work?

Readings are obtained using a two-sided probe, commonly placed over the fingertip (see **Figure 7.1**). Infrared light is passed through the fingertip and the rate of absorption varies according to the number of oxygen molecules linked to each haemoglobin molecule. The pulse oximeter translates this absorption of light into a percentage reading. This reading is commonly referred to as SaO_2, although as the reading is taken from peripheral capillaries, it is more accurately identified as SpO_2 (Jubran 2004).

The pulse oximeter also commonly displays a waveform or bar graph (see **Figure 7.2**); this reflects changes in blood flow through the capillary bed during systole and

Table 7.2 Potential problems at different stages of oxygen transport

Stage of oxygen transport	Potential problems	Some causes
VENTILATION 1 The movement of oxygen into the alveoli	Reduced airway diameter	■ Airway blockage (sputum plugs, aspirate, blood, foreign body) ■ Bronchoconstriction ■ Pulmonary oedema
	Lowered respiratory rate/depth	■ Pneumothorax ■ Reduced movement of diaphragm (paralysis; abdominal pain, surgery, or injury) ■ Inappropriate stimulation of central and peripheral chemoreceptors (change in blood pH/CO_2; damage or depression of medulla oblongata in brain)
	Inadequate available oxygen	■ Smoke inhalation ■ High altitude
2 Diffusion of oxygen across the alveolar capillary membrane	Reduced surface area in alveoli for gas exchange	■ Infection ■ Pulmonary oedema
	Reduced pulmonary circulation	■ Chest trauma ■ Pulmonary embolism
OXYGENATION 3 Transport of oxygen on the haemoglobin molecule (oxygen saturation – SaO_2)	Lowered plasma oxygen (PaO_2)	■ May be caused by any of the above
	Lowered haemoglobin levels	■ Anaemia
	Inability of Hb to transport O_2	■ Carbon monoxide poisoning
4 Movement of oxygen from the haemoglobin to the tissues	Reduced dissociation of O_2 from Hb at the tissues	■ Lowered body temperature ■ Reduced PaO_2 ■ Rise in blood pH (alkalosis)
	Increased diffusion distance	■ Tissue oedema
	Inadequate tissue blood supply	■ Local injury ■ Vascular disease

(adapted from Endacott 2002)

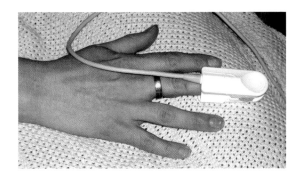

Figure 7.1 Pulse oximeter probe.

diastole. Pulse oximetry can be used to measure oxygen saturation at any place where a pulse is accessible. In practice, the most common site of application is the finger. The earlobe may be used as an alternative, or a probe can be taped to the bridge of the nose.

The pulse oximeter also displays the patient's pulse rate. However, as the pulse rate is recorded at the site of the probe, irregular rhythms such as atrial fibrillation may cause inaccuracies.

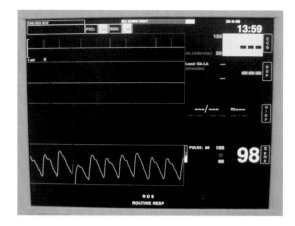

Figure 7.2 Pulse oximeter display.

Understanding pulse oximeter readings

Oxygen is carried in the blood attached to haemoglobin molecules. Oxygen saturation is a measure of how much oxygen the blood is carrying as a percentage of the maximum possible.

One haemoglobin molecule carries a maximum of four molecules of oxygen. If a haemoglobin molecule is carrying three molecules of oxygen, then it is carrying 3/4 or 75% of the maximum amount of oxygen it could carry.

One hundred haemoglobin molecules could together carry a maximum of 400 (100×4) oxygen molecules. If 100 haemoglobin molecules are carrying 360 oxygen molecules, they are carrying ($360/400$) $\times$ 100 = 90% of the maximum number of oxygen molecules. So together they are 90% saturated.

Context

 When to use pulse oximetry

Pulse oximetry is used when a patient is hypoxic or at risk of developing hypoxia, and during oxygen therapy to monitor its effect. Anaemia and jaundice have little or no effect on the function of the oximeter, although previous studies have found that skin pigmentation may give a falsely high (Bickler *et al.* 2005) or inaccurate (Feiner *et al.* 2007) reading when the patient is hypoxic. Pulse oximetry may also be used during exercise testing, when assessing an individual's fitness for flying, or to assess oxygenation during administration of drugs that may have a depressant effect on respiration (e.g. patient-controlled analgesia).

In primary care settings, pulse oximetry may be used as a single measurement to assess patients with chronic respiratory disease and those on long-term oxygen therapy.

When not to use pulse oximetry

A pulse oximeter will not work in the following situations:

- When a patient has **carbon monoxide poisoning**, the Hb carrying carbon monoxide (CO) will register as saturated, hence the patient will have a (false) oxygen saturation reading of close to 100%. This is because CO has a greater affinity for haemoglobin than oxygen and therefore binds with haemoglobin more readily. If haemoglobin is carrying CO, it cannot carry oxygen.

- If the patient is **peripherally vasoconstricted** (e.g. in severe hypotension or hypothermia, hypovolaemia, or peripheral vascular disease) the reading may be unreliable. Pulse oximetry is only considered reliable for individuals with a systolic blood pressure greater than 80 mmHg (Hinkelbein *et al.* 2005). Warm extremities are essential to obtain an accurate reading. It is common for elderly people with respiratory disease to have either poor circulation or cold extremities.

- Excess patient movement or a poorly fitting probe may cause too much light to reach the sensor, producing a distorted reading. Readings may not be considered reliable in a patient who is shivering excessively, convulsing, or having a rigor.

- The pulse oximeter can give inaccurate readings at **low levels of SaO$_2$**; previous studies have found inaccuracies below 82%, depending on the model of oximeter (Carter *et al.* 1998, Chiappini *et al.* 1998, Jubran 2004). In practice this is of limited significance; if the patient has an oxygen saturation level below 85%, it is likely that other interventions will be underway to increase their oxygenation. It is also likely that alternative steps to measure oxygenation, such as arterial blood gas analysis, will be taken.

- Interference from other electronic devices (e.g. diathermy in the operating theatre) may disrupt readings.
- Inflating a BP cuff above the level of the probe will disrupt readings.

There is conflicting evidence regarding the effect of nail polish on the accuracy of the pulse oximeter (Jubran 2004, Hinkelbein *et al.* 2007, Rodden *et al.* 2007). It is safest to remove dark nail polish. If the urgent need for monitoring precludes this, document the presence of nail polish on the observations chart.

Alternative interventions

There may be situations in which you suspect the patient may be hypoxic but you don't have access to a pulse oximeter. In such cases, use your visual assessment skills (see Section 7.1).

Interpreting pulse oximetry readings

- 100% Not achieved when breathing air; may be achieved using supplementary oxygen.

- 95–98% Normal saturation range.

- 90–94% Acceptable for patients with COPD (NICE 2004).

- <90% Indicates respiratory failure *but* may be normal for patient with chronic respiratory disease.

- 75% Inadequate but may be tolerated short term.

- <75% Inadequate – tissue hypoxia and arrhythmias can be expected.

NB readings below 85% cannot be deemed accurate, and since they may indicate serious pathology, alternative (and more accurate) means of assessment should be used (i.e. arterial blood gases).

The waveform/bar graph displayed on the oximeter indicates the adequacy of the signal (Figure 7.2), highlighting the need for nurses to be able to recognize an abnormal waveform/bar graph.

Potential problems

There are reports of cutaneous necrosis associated with continuous use of finger probes (Wille *et al.* 2000), hence the requirement to change probe position every 4 hours. A further potential problem is the time lag between the display and an actual event that may have caused oxygen saturation to fall. Other potential problems include failure of the nurse to acknowledge the limitations of the pulse oximeter (they don't provide all the information you need to make your assessment), and, as with any electrical device, the potential for the oximeter to develop a fault.

Indications for assistance

As with all patient assessment and monitoring, it is essential that you understand the readings (see Interpreting readings box). It is inappropriate to take a recording if you do not understand the significance of the reading and how to interpret it in the context of the overall condition of the patient.

Observations and monitoring

Pulse oximetry should always be considered an adjunct to visual assessment of the patient's respiratory function. The use of oximetry means that the patient is considered to be at risk of becoming hypoxic, so full vital signs should be recorded at regular intervals. Assessment of the patient's colour, accessory muscle use, respiratory rate, breath sounds, signs of chronic respiratory disease, and their position (e.g. orthopnoeic position) is also essential in the interpretation of oxygen saturation and may alert you to a reading that appears higher or lower than you would expect.

Procedure

Preparation

Prepare yourself
Ensure you understand how the equipment works, how to set alarms, and how to interpret readings. Wash your hands.

Step-by-step guide to pulse oximetry

Prepare the patient

The procedure should be fully explained to the patient (see box below).

Prepare the equipment

Select the probe most appropriate for the patient's age and condition (depending on availability). Clean the probe according to the manufacturer's instructions. Where possible run the oximeter from the mains.

> **Discussing the procedure with the patient and family**
>
> ■ Explain what is being measured and why.
>
> ■ Place the probe on your own finger to reassure the patient that it is not painful.
>
> ■ Assure the patient that their condition will not get worse if the probe drops off. However, remind them of the need to keep it on constantly.
>
> ■ Ask them to let a nurse know if it is uncomfortable, rather than removing it.
>
> ■ Explain and demonstrate the alarm sounds.
>
> ■ If possible/appropriate, turn off the constant audible pulse.

Step-by-step guide to using pulse oximetry to measure oxygen saturation

Step	Rationale
1 Introduce yourself, confirm the patient's identity, explain the procedure, and obtain consent.	To identify the patient correctly and gain informed consent.
2 Assess for factors that may alter the accuracy of the pulse oximeter reading (e.g. shivering, peripheral vasoconstriction).	Readings from the oximeter may be inadequate.
3 Clean the patient's skin; remove nail polish if worn.	Prior to applying the oximeter probe, the skin should be clean, dry, and warm. Nail polish can make readings less accurate.
4 Attach the probe according to the manufacturer's instructions. Plug the cable into the oximeter and switch on.	It may be necessary to transport the oximeter, so the battery should be kept fully charged.
5 Ensure the oximeter is displaying a normal waveform or bar graph and that the pulse displayed corresponds with the patient's pulse rate.	A shallow waveform indicates poor blood flow or poor reading of blood flow by the oximeter. If the pulse displayed does not correspond with the patient's pulse rate, the oxygen saturation measurements are likely to be inaccurate.

6	Set alarm limits.	Alarm limits should be agreed with senior clinical staff and set at a level that identifies a significant change in saturation. The patient's normal respiratory function should be taken into account when setting alarm limits; a patient with COPD may function with a saturation level below 90%.
7	Note the time and site the probe is placed at. Change the site at least every 4 hours.	The site used should be changed frequently to avoid discomfort from the pressure of the probe or the heat source. Time between changes of probe site should be individualized according to the skin condition and peripheral circulation.
8	If intermittent readings are to be taken, remove the probe between readings.	Reduce unnecessary patient discomfort.
9	If the pulse oximeter is to be used for continuous monitoring, ensure leads do not present a hazard.	Maintain a safe environment for patient and staff.
10	Document oxygen saturation, noting whether the patient is receiving oxygen therapy (with %) or air.	Provides a baseline measurement.

Following the procedure

Oximetry may be used for single measurements or for continuous monitoring. Regardless, respiratory observations should be continued. Be aware that there is a potential time lag between the onset of a hypoxic event and a drop in saturation. Identify the goals of management for the patient, for example administration of oxygen to maintain oxygen saturation at a particular level. If SaO_2 remains consistently at 100%, senior clinical staff may review oxygen administration. Ensure any abnormal measurement is reported to the clinical team.

After use, clean the probe (as per the manufacturer's instructions). Surface colonies of microorganisms may be transferred on the probe. Liquids that have dried on the probe may interfere with readings (Woodrow 1999). Store the equipment in accordance with the manufacturer's instructions and charge the battery if necessary.

Reflection and evaluation

When you have undertaken pulse oximetry with a patient, think about the following questions:

1 Did the oximeter give the reading you were expecting for that particular patient?
2 Were you able to answer the patient's questions?
3 Did your visual respiratory assessment of the patient alert you to any potential problems with using the pulse oximeter?
4 Were you able to interpret the reading, in the light of the patient's medical condition?

Further learning opportunities

At the next available opportunity, try out the probe on yourself.

- Does it make any difference to the comfort or saturation readings if the light source is placed over tissue or the nail bed?
- Do the readings change when you move your arms around?
- How long is it before the heat of the probe becomes uncomfortable?

Reminders

Don't forget to:

- Connect the oximeter to the mains.
- Discuss the alarm sounds with the patient.
- Record application of the probe in the patient's notes.

 Patient scenarios

Consider what you should do in the following situations, then turn to the end of this skill to check your answers.

1 Patient A has become tachypnoeic, with a rapid and shallow breathing pattern. His oxygen saturation readings have not changed. What might be the problem?
2 Patient B is disorientated and keeps removing the probe. What is the best way to manage this situation?
3 The oxygen-carrying capacity of the blood is determined by the oxygen saturation and haemoglobin level. Patient C has a haemoglobin level of 14 g/dl and patient D has a haemoglobin level of 12 g/dl. Both patients have oxygen saturation readings that fluctuate between 95 and 96%. Which patient is actually carrying the most oxygen in their blood?

Website

 http://www.oxfordtextbooks.co.uk/orc/ endacott

You may find it helpful to work through our short online quiz and additional scenarios intended to help you to develop and apply the skills in this chapter.

References

Bickler PE, Feiner JR, and Severinghaus JW (2005). Effects of skin pigmentation on pulse oximeter accuracy at low saturation. *Anesthesiology*, **102**(4), 715–19.

Carter BG, Carlin JB, Tibballs J, Mead H, Hochmann M, and Osborne A (1998). Accuracy of two pulse oximeters at low arterial hemoglobin-oxygen saturation. *Critical Care Medicine*, **26**(6), 1128–33.

Chiappini F, Fuso L, and Pistelli R (1998). Accuracy of a pulse oximeter in the measurement of the oxyhaemoglobin saturation. *European Respiratory Journal*, **11**(3), 716–19.

Endacott R (2002). Emergency care of the adult patient. In G Jones, R Endacott, and R Crouch, eds. *Emergency nursing care: principles and practice*, pp. 47–74. Greenwich Medical, London.

Feiner JR, Severinghaus JW, and Bickler PE (2007). Dark skin decreases the accuracy of pulse oximeters at low oxygen saturation: the effects of oximeter probe type and gender. *Anaesthesia and Analgesia*, **105**, S18–S23.

Hinkelbein J, Genzwuerker HV, and Fiedler F (2005). Detection of a systolic pressure threshold for reliable readings in pulse oximetry. *Resuscitation*, **64**, 315–19.

Hinkelbein J, Genzwuerker HV, Sogl R, and Fiedler F (2007). Effect of nail polish on oxygen saturation determined by pulse oximetry in critically ill patients. *Resuscitation*, **72**, 82–91.

Howell M (2002). Pulse oximetry: an audit of nursing and medical staff understanding. *British Journal of Nursing*, **11**, 91–7.

Jubran A (2004). Pulse oximetry. *Intensive Care Medicine*, **30**, 2017–20.

National Institute for Health and Clinical Excellence (2004). *Chronic obstructive pulmonary disease. Management of chronic obstructive pulmonary disease in adults in primary and secondary care. Clinical Guideline 12*. NICE, London.

Rodden AM, Spicer L, Diaz VA, and Stever TE (2007). Does fingernail polish affect pulse oximeter readings? *Intensive and Critical Care Nursing*, **23**, 51–5.

Wille J, Braams R, van Haren WH, and van der Werken C (2000). Pulse oximeter-induced digital injury: frequency rate and possible causative factors. *Critical Care Medicine*, **28**(10), 3555–7.

Woodrow P (1999). Pulse oximetry. *Nursing Standard*, **13**(42), 42–6.

Useful further reading and websites

Moore T (2007). Respiratory assessment in adults. *Nursing Standard*, **21**(49), 48–56.

More details regarding how the pulse oximeter detects oxygen saturation can be found at: **http://www. oximetry.org/pulseox/principles.htm**

Answers to patient scenarios

1 High carbon dioxide levels in the blood. The pulse oximeter measures the saturation of haemoglobin by oxygen but does not indicate carbon dioxide level.

2 Take single readings and remove the probe each time.

3 Patient C. Arterial oxygen saturation does not provide a picture of the overall efficiency of gas exchange in the lungs or the tissues, merely the transport of oxygen on the haemoglobin molecules.

7.3 Measuring peak expiratory flow rate (PEFR)

Definition

Peak flow meters measure the highest rate at which air can be expelled from the lungs through an open mouth. The value given is known as the peak expiratory flow rate (PEFR) and is a commonly used and simple test of lung function.

It is important to remember that:

The technique of performing PEFR is important to ensure an accurate measurement, as inadequate effort can lead to an overestimate of airway obstruction.

Prior knowledge

Before undertaking PEFR measurement, make sure you are familiar with:

- Respiratory anatomy.
- Physiology of respiration.
- The reasons for measuring lung function.

Background

PEFRs are essential measurements for patients with asthma and COPD. These conditions are characterized by constriction in the airways, which reduces oxygenation and can be life-threatening. PEFR measurements are important because they:

- Measure the extent of constriction in the patient's airways.
- Indicate the degree of reversibility that is achievable with bronchodilator and steroid medications.
- Provide important clinical indicators of deterioration in patients with asthma and COPD.
- Measure improvement following treatment in patients with COPD and asthma.

Patients with asthma and COPD should be encouraged to monitor their own peak flow measurements while at home and in hospital.

Asthma is a variable condition and a single 'normal' peak expiratory flow (PEF) reading does not exclude a diagnosis of asthma. Serial PEF readings should be taken over a 2- to 3-week period to confirm a diagnosis. A diurnal (morning and evening) variation of more than 20% of the best peak flow with a minimum change of at least 60 litres/minute, ideally for 3 days in a week over the 2-week period, is considered diagnostic (British Thoracic Society (BTS) and Scottish Intercollegiate Guidelines Network (SIGN) 2007).

When interpreting peak flow results in the context of illness it should be recognized that single peak flow readings are of limited use (Kendrick and Smith 1992). Instead serial peak flow recordings should be undertaken, as this provides information regarding the trend of the patient's large airway function and the effect of inhaled treatments such as bronchodilators (e.g. Salbutamol). For patients with asthma, the BTS and SIGN (2007) recommend taking measurements prior to inhaled medication twice daily in the morning and evening, and then 30 minutes after inhaled medication. When the patient is acutely unwell in hospital, PEFR will be measured more frequently and at least 6-hourly.

PEFR is dependent on age, gender, and height. Charts (see **Tables 7.3** and **7.4**) should be available with these ranges mapped out in your hospital, or can be downloaded from the Clement Clarke website address given in the footnotes of Table 7.4, and these give the predicted 'best' values for men and women based on age and height. For example, a 35-year-old man, 175 cm tall, might achieve 635 litres/minute, while a woman of the same age, 160 cm tall, would only achieve 424 litres/minute. In COPD, the PEFR will be consistently

Table 7.3 Normal values for PEF in men (in litres/minute)

Height (cm)	20 years	30 years	35 years	40 years	50 years	60 years	70 years	80 years
190	600	660	670	660	640	590	540	500
175	570	630	635	630	610	570	520	470
160	540	590	600	598	570	530	490	440

Table 7.4 Normal values for PEF in women (in litres/minute)

Height (cm)	20 years	30 years	35 years	40 years	50 years	60 years	70 years	80 years
183	450	465	462	458	440	410	380	350
160	410	425	424	420	400	375	350	320

All Table 7.3 and 7.4 values are from Clement Clarke, **http://www.clement-clarke.com**. Select 'Product Information' and click on 'Peak Flow'.

less than in healthy adults and will worsen during acute exacerbations.

How to use a peak flow meter

The timing and frequency of peak flow recordings should be explained to the patient. Peak flow meters are for single patient use only unless an antibacterial filter is used. It is helpful to demonstrate the technique first to the patient.

Context

 When to measure PEFR

PEFR is used to:

- Diagnose and monitor asthma, as part of a personal asthma management plan.
- Assess the severity of an asthma attack or an exacerbation of COPD.
- Monitor response to medication/therapy in asthma and COPD.

 When not to measure PEFR

Peak flow measurement should not be undertaken if the patient is unable to perform the procedure, for example if they are semi-conscious.

Alternative interventions

Spirometry, another non-invasive method, is a breathing test that detects airway obstruction by measuring forced expiratory volume in one second and forced vital capacity. This test is performed by a variety of experienced personnel such as respiratory nurse specialists, specialist nurse practitioners, and lung function technicians. It is a more useful test in the diagnosis of COPD than PEFR, but is not routinely available in a ward setting.

Pulse oximetry is a common non-invasive assessment that is used in ward settings as a crude measure of a patient's peripheral oxygen saturation (the concentration of oxygen circulating in the body); this is covered in more depth in Section 7.2.

Interpreting readings

In patients with asthma, PEFR readings will usually vary over time and in response to medication. Patient with COPD, on the other hand, will have a relatively fixed, if low, PEFR reading.

PEFR readings can give an indication of the level of severity of an asthmatic attack. For example, a PEFR reading less than one-third of their best is described as life-threatening asthma (BTS/SIGN 2007).

If a patient demonstrates a PEFR that shows significant diurnal variation over at least a month, they should be reviewed by an asthma specialist.

Procedure

Preparation

Prepare yourself
Ensure you understand how the equipment works and how to interpret readings. Establish the patient's usual/best peak flow. Patients with long-standing conditions will usually know this, or it will be recorded in their notes or charts from previous admissions. Predicted values for normal patients can be found in Tables 7.3 and 7.4.

Prepare the patient
The procedure should be fully explained and demonstrated to the patient.

Prepare the equipment
Ensure all equipment is available and functions correctly.

Step-by-step guide to measuring PEFR

	Step	Rationale
1	Introduce yourself, confirm the patient's identity, explain the procedure, and obtain consent.	To identify the patient correctly and gain informed consent.
2	Patient should stand or sit. If this is not possible, the most upright position possible should be achieved.	To ensure best lung expansion and consistency of readings.
3	Patient to hold peak flow meter horizontally (with fingers well away from the gauge marker) and ensure that gauge marker is at the bottom of the scale.	To ensure accuracy and that fingers do not interfere with the readings.
4	Patient should breathe in deeply and place lips and teeth around mouthpiece, forming a tight seal.	To ensure accuracy.
5	The patient should breathe out deeply as quickly and hard as possible.	To take the reading.
6	Read the position that the marker arrow has now reached and record this result.	To record the reading.
7	Repeat steps 1–5 twice more. The three readings should be within a 20 litre/minute range; if not the procedure should be repeated up to five times (Booker 2007).	To ensure that the correct technique is used and that the results are reliable.
8	Record the highest peak flow reading.	To provide an accurate record of assessment.

Following the procedure

Make sure the patient is comfortable. If the patient is learning to record their own PEFR, note any learning needed in the patient record.

Recognizing patient deterioration

PEFR is a very useful recording that can indicate a change or deterioration in the condition of a patient in the home, in the acute hospital setting, and in the GP practice. A sudden and consistent drop in peak flow rate with an increase in wheeze or shortness of breath should alert the nurse to request an urgent review by a senior practitioner or doctor.

Reflection and evaluation

When you have taken a peak flow reading, think about the following questions:

1 Did the patient understand what was required?
2 Were they able to perform the test correctly?
3 Did you understand the significance of the results?
4 Did you record them accurately? Were you clear about when to alert senior colleagues to the test results?

Further learning opportunities

- Try using a peak flow meter yourself and record the readings on the peak flow chart.
- When patients are admitted, look at their diagnosis. If the patient has asthma, does their peak flow vary in line with diurnal variations (morning and evening) or in response to treatment? If the patient has COPD, is the PEFR variable or fixed even in response to treatment (in COPD expect very small variations)?
- Patient UK has a number of useful information sheets on PEF measurements and asthma at **http://www.patient.co.uk/** (search for peak flow measurement).
- The Mini-Wright peak flow meter site has charts for normal adult and children's PEF values, pictures of these common peak flow meters, and explanations of related issues at **http://www.peakflow.com/ top_nav/normal_values/index.html**. You can get personalized predicted normal values at **http://www.peakflow.com/top_nav/ normal_values/PEFNorms.html**.

Reminders

- A single peak flow recording is of little use.
- Asthmatic patients are likely to have variation in their peak flow recording because their illness has some element of reversibility.
- COPD patients are likely to have low, fixed peak flow recording because their illness has very little reversibility.

Patient scenarios

Consider what you should do in the following situations, then turn to the end of this skill to check your answers.

1 Patient A has been admitted with an asthma attack. You have been asked to monitor their PEFR – how often should this be undertaken?
2 Patient B has been diagnosed with asthma. How might this be confirmed using a PEF meter?
3 Patient C suffers from asthma and has a best PEFR of 450. They have arrived in the GP surgery short of breath and wheezy, with little relief being gained from their bronchodilators. Their PEFR is now 100. What does this indicate?

Website

 http://www.oxfordtextbooks.co.uk/orc/ endacott

You may find it helpful to work through our short online quiz and additional scenarios intended to help you to develop and apply the skills in this chapter.

References

Booker R (2007). Peak expiratory flow measurement. *Nursing Standard*, **21**(39), 42–3.

British Thoracic Society and Scottish Intercollegiate Guidelines Network (2007). *British guideline on the management of asthma, A national clinical guideline* [online] http://www.brit-thoracic.org.uk/ Guidelinessince%201997_asthma_html accessed 24/10/07.

Kendrick AH and Smith EC (1992). Respiratory measurements 2: interpreting simple measurements of lung function. *Professional Nurse*, **7**(11), 748–54.

Useful further reading and websites

Bourke SJ (2007). *Lecture notes on respiratory medicine.* Blackwell Publishing Ltd, Oxford.

 Answers to patient scenarios

1 PEF recordings should be taken at least 6-hourly when in hospital. They should be recorded prior to inhaled medication and 30 minutes after inhaled medication.

2 PEF readings should be taken over a 2- to 3-week period to confirm diagnosis. A diurnal variation of more than 20% of the best peak flow for at least 3 days in a week is considered diagnostic.

3 PEF readings give an indication of the level of severity of an asthmatic attack. A peak flow reading of 100 is less than one-third of their best and therefore described as life-threatening asthma.

7.4 **Non-invasive respiratory support and oxygen therapy**

Definition

Non-invasive respiratory support augments lung function and lessens the work of breathing without requiring an (invasive) endotracheal tube. Airway adjuncts are used to maintain a patent airway through provision of a passage for airflow by separating the pharyngeal wall from the tongue (Jevon 2002). The two most commonly used are oropharyngeal (Guedel) and nasopharyngeal airways.

Two other techniques are used for patients who require additional respiratory support: BiPAP (bi-level positive airway pressure, sometimes referred to as non-invasive ventilation) and CPAP (continuous positive airway pressure).

It is important to remember that:

- Oxygen is a prescription-only medication and therefore should be prescribed for a specific patient (Jamieson *et al.* 2002). Patients should be made aware of this and asked not to alter the settings themselves as this may be dangerous.

- The effectiveness of oxygen therapy should always be monitored; pulse oximetry will confirm an adequate oxygen flow rate but will not exclude hypercapnia (raised carbon dioxide level). In order to do this, arterial blood gas measurements are required.

- An oropharyngeal airway should only be used if the patient is unconscious as it can cause vomiting and **laryngospasm.**

- CPAP delivers one pressure setting and requires a patient to be able to breathe in. BiPAP delivers two settings and has the provision of an underlying back-up rate that will cut in if the patient fails to breathe.

Prior knowledge

Before using respiratory support or oxygen therapy, make sure you are familiar with:

1 Respiratory anatomy.

2 Respiratory physiology (gas exchange).

3 Knowledge of the normal doses, side effects, precautions, and contraindications of oxygen.

4 Understand which patients may benefit from oxygen and which patients require controlled oxygen to be administered.

5 Basic understanding of airway management.

Background

In order to understand the use of oxygen therapy it is necessary to understand the major function of the respiratory system, which is the delivery of oxygen to and elimination of carbon dioxide from the cells via the blood. When this function is not performed, this will result in respiratory failure. Oxygen delivery may then be required.

Oxygen is a colourless, odourless, tasteless, transparent gas that is slightly heavier than air. Oxygen is essential for functioning and survival of the cells of the body. Breathing and respiration together in normal, fit, healthy people ensure that the correct concentration of oxygen is maintained within the tissues.

In healthy people, oxygen concentration is maintained at 12–14 kPa (90–105 mmHg) in arterial blood (Guyton and Hall 2000); however, it can be impaired in many conditions (see Table 7.2). Obviously, prolonged shortage of oxygen is a serious condition and can cause brain and organ damage and ultimately death. If you suspect that a patient's condition is deteriorating rapidly, act quickly and summon senior colleagues. Use the emergency call bell if necessary and be prepared to initiate basic life support procedures.

Oxygen therapy in respiratory care is used to correct:

- Type I respiratory failure (**hypoxaemia**, when a patient is low in oxygen).
- Type II respiratory failure (hypoxaemia, when a patient is low in oxygen, and hypercapnia, when there is a raised carbon dioxide level).
- Palliative relief of shortness of breath (Esmond 2001).

In emergency situations, such as acute severe asthma or pneumonia with no evidence of raised carbon dioxide, high flow oxygen should be delivered in a sufficient amount to correct the hypoxaemia. This amount will vary for different patients, with some requiring 60–100%. Monitoring of patients receiving high flow oxygen should include oxygen saturation monitoring via a pulse oximeter and an arterial blood gas measurement. Once hypercapnia has been excluded, repeated arterial blood gas measurements are not required (Francis 2006).

In acute respiratory emergencies where there is a risk of ventilatory failure (type II respiratory failure), controlled oxygen is administered at 24–28%. In patients with type II respiratory failure, the rise in carbon dioxide within their bloodstream suppresses inspiration. When additional oxygen is administered there is an increase in the oxygen concentration in the patient's blood, which may cause a reduction in the rate and depth of breathing. It is essential that arterial blood gas analysis is undertaken on a regular basis for these patients (Bateman and Leech 1998). Arterial blood gas sampling and analysis are skills that can be undertaken by doctors, nurses, and other health care professionals depending on local organizational guidelines (Dodds and Williamson 2007), but this is not something that a student nurse should ever undertake.

There are a number of precautions to be taken when using oxygen cylinders in hospital, community settings, or the patient's home (see **Box 7.1**).

Oxygen may be given to patients via cylinders through masks that fit over the nose and mouth or via nasal cannulae that sit in the nostrils. In hospital settings, oxygen is

Box 7.1 Precautions to be taken with oxygen cylinders (BOC Medical 2006)

- Cylinders should be stored under cover (preferably inside), kept dry and clean, and not subjected to extremes of heat or cold.
- Cylinders should be stored separately from industrial and other non-medical cylinders.
- Full cylinders should be stored separately from empty cylinders.
- Cylinders should be used in strict rotation so that those with the earliest filling dates are used first.
- Cylinders should be stored separately from other medical cylinders.
- Smoking and naked lights must not be allowed within the vicinity of cylinders or pipeline outlets. Warning notices must be posted clearly.
- F size cylinders and larger should be stored vertically. E size cylinders and smaller should be stored horizontally.
- Cylinders should be handled and used with care.

piped into wards and departments and accessed via a tap located in the wall behind bed or trolley spaces.

If oxygen alone is not successful or not likely to be successful, non-invasive ventilation (NIV) may be considered. Treatment decisions for the use of oxygen therapy and NIV are usually made by doctors, but the nurse's role is crucial in reporting signs of distress and deterioration in a patient's condition, setting up equipment, and monitoring progress and treatment (see Section 7.1, *Visual respiratory assessment*).

Oxygen delivery devices

There are several types of delivery device for oxygen delivery:

- Fixed performance.
- Variable flow (Francis 2006).
- Non-rebreathe masks.
- Humidification.

Selection of an oxygen delivery device is based on several factors (Vines *et al.* 2000, Jevon and Ewens 2001, Bennett 2003). These include:

- Type of respiratory failure.
- Rate and depth of patient's inspiration and expiration.

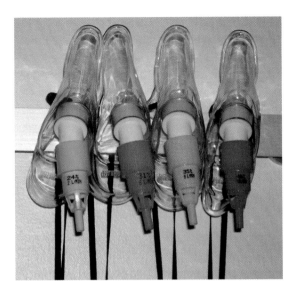

Figure 7.3 Venturi masks.

- Amount of oxygen prescribed.
- Length of oxygen therapy required.
- Requirement for humidification.
- Patient tolerance and preference.

All oxygen delivery systems consist of an oxygen source – a cylinder, a concentrator, or a liquid oxygen system. When a fixed amount of oxygen is delivered to a patient with the use of a Venturi adaptor, this is a fixed performance system. The Venturi principle allows for the mixing of oxygen with air, as air is drawn into the system through holes in the adaptor. The Venturi adaptor will have an indicator on it showing the flow rate of oxygen required (see **Figure 7.3**). For example, delivering a 24% concentration by the Venturi principle using a mask made by Respironics requires a flow rate of 3 litres/minute. It is important to check each Venturi mask prior to administering oxygen, as some company products require different flow rates. Patients will continue to receive a concentration of oxygen therapy not reliant on their rate or depth of breathing.

Variable performance devices include nasal cannulae and a basic oxygen mask, which does not include a Venturi adaptor. With these devices it is difficult to ensure that an accurate percentage of oxygen is delivered. Nasal cannulae are particularly useful for patients who may be claustrophobic with a mask or who need to have oxygen continuously and want to be able to eat and drink while receiving it.

Non-rebreathe masks provide high concentrations of oxygen (up to 95%) at a flow rate of 12 litres/minute. This is only suitable for short-term therapy (Vines *et al.* 2000). The reservoir should be able to expand freely and should not be kinked or restricted in any way.

The use of humidification systems will reduce some of the complications associated with oxygen therapy. They should be used when a high flow rate (greater than 4 litres/minute) is required (Bateman and Leech 1998), where a patient has thick secretions and has difficulty expectorating, and when oxygen is likely to be required for longer than 4 hours. It is important to use them to prevent blocking of tracheostomy tubes (see Section 7.5) and respiratory tract mucosal drying.

Modes of non-invasive ventilator (NIV) support

NIV provides ventilatory support through the patient's upper airway using a mask or similar device (British Thoracic Society Standards of Care Committee 2002). While CPAP delivers one pressure setting and requires a patient to be able to breathe in, BiPAP delivers two settings and includes patient-triggered inspiratory support spontaneous mode with provision of an underlying back-up rate spontaneous timed mode that will cut in if the patient fails to breathe, as well as a timed mode that can deliver all breaths. The two settings are:

IPAP (inspiratory positive airways pressure)
- Increases tidal volume.
- Reduces hypercapnia.
- Reduces the work of breathing.

EPAP (expiratory positive airways pressure)
- Increases lung volume.
- Improves oxygenation.
- Maintains an open airway.
- Reduces the work of breathing.

BiPAP also compensates for leaks in the system, such as ill-fitting masks or an inadequate mouth seal, but this compensation is not unlimited, so these problems should be quickly corrected (Elliott 1997).

The patient will need to wear a tight-fitting mask attached to a portable ventilator via wide smooth bore tubing (see **Figure 7.4**).

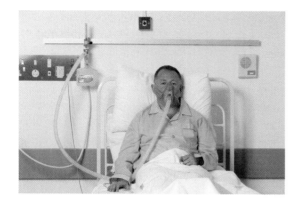

Figure 7.4 Non-invasive ventilation mask.

CPAP works by increasing airway pressure and therefore improves ventilation to the collapsed areas of the lung. Oxygenation is improved by the positive pressure generated by CPAP, which prevents the alveoli from collapsing at the end of expiration (Cull and Inwood 1999). CPAP will increase lung volume in order for gaseous exchange to take place; this will enable the work of breathing and the amount of oxygen required to be reduced (Oh 1997).

Patients with **obstructive sleep apnoea** (obstruction to, and stopping of, the respiratory airflow for periods of 10 seconds or longer during sleep) use CPAP machines. The use of CPAP prevents occlusion and apnoeic periods as it can be set to a constant pressure to keep the airways open when the patient is asleep (Phillipps 2005).

Context

When to use oxygen

Additional oxygen will be required when the PaO_2 has fallen to 8 kPa (60 mmHg) or less (Oh 1997).

When not to use oxygen

In patients who always retain carbon dioxide and are usually hypercapnic due to COPD, oxygen should be used carefully. It should be used at 24–28% with settings carefully controlled, close monitoring of saturations and blood gases, and with the patient in an area of the ward where they can be closely observed by nursing staff at all times.

If a patient persists with smoking this should be discouraged, as there is limited benefit for patients who continue to smoke. As oxygen supports combustion, no smoking should be allowed in the vicinity of oxygen (piped or delivered via cylinder).

When to use airway adjuncts

An oropharyngeal (Guedel) airway can be used when there is obstruction of the upper airway due to backward displacement of the tongue (Jevon 2006). The curved body of the airway is designed to fit over the back of the tongue. It is commonly used in the initial stages of resuscitation and during anaesthesia. Oxygen administration will be required if the patient is unconscious or not breathing (see Section 6.9, *Cardiopulmonary resuscitation*).

A nasopharyngeal airway is used when an airway is at risk of being compromised. It can be used in a patient who is semi-conscious or conscious and is sometimes used in the post-resuscitation phase (Jevon 2006) and when removal of secretions from the chest is required. It can be life-saving in a patient with a clenched jaw or maxillofacial injuries. Oxygen administration will be required if the patient is unconscious or not breathing.

When not to use airway adjuncts

A nasopharyngeal airway is contraindicated in patients with a fractured base of skull.

When to use BiPAP

BiPAP has been shown to be an effective treatment for acute hypercapnic (raised carbon dioxide) respiratory failure, which is a feature in many patients with COPD. It can also be used for patients with neuromuscular disease and chest wall deformities, who may have chronic respiratory failure due to poor arterial blood supply or altered lung mechanics (Phillipps 2005).

When not to use NIV (CPAP or BiPAP)

NIV should not be used as a substitute for intubation and invasive ventilation. See **Box 7.2** for contraindications to NIV.

Box 7.2 Contraindications to NIV

- Recent facial or upper airway surgery.
- Inability to protect the airway.
- Copious respiratory secretions.
- Vomiting.
- Life-threatening hypoxaemia (low level of oxygen in the blood).
- Several comorbidities.
- Confusion/agitation.
- Pneumothorax (unless an intercostal drain has been inserted).
- Asthma.
- Severe respiratory acidosis (British Thoracic Society Standards of Care Committee 2002).
- Unconscious patient.

 ## When to use CPAP

CPAP is used when a patient is hypoxic but not hypercapnic; it is a treatment most appropriate for patients having problems with oxygenation and not ventilation (Brigg 1999, Place 1997). Conditions where CPAP may be considered include pneumonia, pulmonary oedema, and interstitial lung disease.

 ## When not to use CPAP

CPAP should not be used in patients with COPD as it has the potential to increase hyperinflation and hypercapnia in these patients (Brochard 1996). CPAP should not be used in patients who are vomiting, as this may lead to aspiration of stomach contents.

Procedure

Preparation

Prepare yourself
Ensure that you have undertaken the procedure before and are aware of the correct procedure. You should understand the reasons for commencing oxygen therapy, have the oxygen dose prescribed, and understand the need for appropriate monitoring.

If inserting an airway, you should be released from other responsibilities while doing this and caring for the patient. This may take place in an emergency situation such as a cardiac or respiratory arrest.

Similarly, if you are helping to establish a patient on NIV/CPAP, you need to give this your undivided attention, as this will contribute to the compliance of the patient with using the NIV/CPAP. All non-invasive ventilation is given under medical supervision and should not be initiated by nurses unless they are specialists in the field. It is not a task that a student nurse would initiate or manage, but will be encountered in settings including respiratory wards, emergency departments and medical admissions units, theatres, and recovery and intensive care units.

Prepare the patient
Explain the procedure to the patient and their relatives, and explain why they require this treatment. Show them the equipment in order to reduce anxiety and aid compliance.

Prepare the equipment/environment
The environment should be conducive to the patient receiving treatment. The equipment should be made available at the patient's bedside. Safety principles regarding the use of oxygen should be adhered to whether the patient is receiving oxygen therapy in a hospital, community setting, or their own home (see Box 7.1). If an airway is being inserted, privacy should be maintained.

See Figure 6.29 in the previous chapter, which shows how to select an oropharyngeal airway of the correct size.

Step-by-step guide to commencing oxygen therapy

Step		Rationale
1	Introduce yourself, confirm the patient's identity, explain the procedure, and obtain consent.	To identify the patient correctly and gain informed consent.
2	Ensure that the oxygen therapy has been prescribed, with flow rate, method of delivery, duration, and monitoring clearly stated.	Oxygen is a drug and must be prescribed; however, local policy may enable oxygen to be administered against a patient group direction or local guidelines, particularly in an emergency situation.
3	Assess the patient and, using the prescription, select the most appropriate delivery device.	To establish patient and clinical preference and to ensure compliance with oxygen therapy.
4	Set the prescribed flow rate/oxygen concentration according to the prescription and device instructions.	To ensure correct flow rate according to the individual delivery device.
5	Administer oxygen and assess the effectiveness of treatment using oxygen saturation recording/ arterial blood gas monitoring.	To monitor any change or deterioration in condition.

Step-by-step guide to insertion of an oropharyngeal airway

Step		Rationale
1	Introduce yourself, confirm the patient's identity, explain the procedure, and obtain consent.	To identify the patient correctly and gain informed consent.
2	Apply gloves.	To protect hands from body fluids.
3	Clear the patient's airway using suction.	To ensure a clear passage for the airway and prevent contents of mouth being pushed into lungs.
4	Select an airway with a length equal to the vertical distance between the patient's incisors and angle of the jaw – see Figure 6.29 (UK Resuscitation Council 2006).	If too small a Guedel airway is used then it may occlude the patient's airway by pushing the tongue back. If too big an airway is used it may occlude the patient's airway by displacing the epiglottis and cause damage to the laryngeal structures (Jevon 2002).
5	Insert the airway in the inverted position. As it passes over the soft palate, rotate the airway through 180°.	The curved part will depress the tongue and prevent it from being pushed back.
6	Check position of the airway. The flattened, reinforced section should be positioned between the patient's teeth or gums (Resuscitation Council (UK) 2000). Continue to monitor patency and position of airway.	To ensure that potential blockages such as vomit, secretions, and blood are noticed and removed. The reinforced section stops the patient biting through the airway.

Step-by-step guide to insertion of a nasopharyngeal airway

Step		Rationale
1	Introduce yourself, confirm the patient's identity, explain the procedure, and obtain consent.	To identify the patient correctly and gain informed consent.
2	Apply gloves.	To protect against bodily secretions.
3	Select an appropriate-sized airway. Sizes 6 or 7 are suitable for male and female adults.	Too short an airway will be ineffective; too long an airway may enter the oesophagus, causing distension.
4	Assess the right nostril; lubricate the airway using water-soluble jelly.	To aid the passage of the airway and reduce discomfort (the right nostril is commonly used so that the distal opening is at the correct angle).
5	Advance the airway up into nostril bevel. Pass it vertically along the floor of the nose, into the posterior pharynx (Resuscitation Council (UK) 2000). Once the flange of airway is at the level of the nostril, secure with tape and place a safety pin through the flange (Jevon 2006).	The safety pin will help prevent inhalation of the airway.

Step-by-step guide to commencing patient on NIV

Step		Rationale
1	Introduce yourself, confirm the patient's identity, explain the procedure, and obtain consent.	To identify the patient correctly and gain informed consent.
2	Prepare equipment at the bedside; set up CPAP circuit or NIV machine.	So equipment is ready for procedure.
3	Using a measuring gauge to select the mask size, assess suitability for nasal or full face mask.	In order to obtain the correct mask type and size.
4	Ensure patient is in a comfortable position, sitting up in bed.	To ensure comfort and help lung expansion.
5	Explain to the patient how the mask is going to be applied. Encourage them to hold the mask themselves and feel the amount of pressure being delivered.	To relieve anxiety and give control to the patient, thus promoting compliance.
6	Once the patient is comfortable with the mask, apply the head straps.	To hold the mask in place and for patient comfort.

continued overleaf

7	Adjust the mask and head straps to ensure that no leaks are present.	A tight seal is required in order to ensure that the system functions properly.
8	Explain how long they are likely to have the mask in place before stopping for a break. Ensure the nurse call button is placed within close reach.	To inform the patient of the plan of care, reduce anxiety, and aid compliance.
9	Ensure that the mask is not too tight. Assess facial skin integrity regularly, particularly over nasal bridge, and apply protective dressing if required.	To alleviate pressure and prevent skin breakdown.
10	Reassure the patient and monitor respiratory rate, pulse oximetry, blood pressure, pulse, and temperature.	To ensure compliance and identify change in condition and benefits of treatment.

Recognizing patient deterioration

Before any patient is commenced on NIV or CPAP there should be a clear medical plan for if the patient deteriorates. Deterioration may be indicated by worsening pulse oximetry or arterial blood gas analysis, worsening cyanosis, worsening confusion and drowsiness, or inability to tolerate the mask or machine settings. These signs must be monitored accurately and reported promptly as they can indicate an approaching emergency situation. Deteriorating patients are likely to require intubation and urgent transfer to the intensive care department, or a decision to stop the NIV or CPAP treatment if such measures are not appropriate.

Reflection and evaluation

1 When you next look after a patient who has oxygen in place, think about the delivery device. Is it the most appropriate for the patient's condition?
2 When you have set a patient up on NIV, ask them how it feels – can you make the mask more comfortable?

Further learning opportunities

- Try putting an oxygen mask and nasal cannulae on. Do they feel comfortable?
- Try using humidified oxygen. Is it noisy?
- Often the use of an oropharyngeal airway takes place in an emergency situation; it is therefore useful to practise the insertion technique regularly using a model.

- Practise setting up NIV and put it on yourself. Are you able to keep it on for more than a minute – how does it feel?

Reminders

- Oxygen is a drug and should always be prescribed.
- Ensure you always have the correct oxygen delivery device according to the prescription.
- Always measure an airway prior to insertion.
- Allow time when commencing a patient on NIV in order to improve compliance.

Patient scenarios

Consider what you should do in the following situations, then turn to the end of this skill to check your answers.

1 Patient A has been admitted to the ward and has been prescribed oxygen therapy. They have been given a mask with a 24% Venturi but they suffer from claustrophobia. What alternative device would you obtain for the patient?
2 Patient B has pneumonia, is semi-conscious, and is having great difficulty coughing and clearing any secretions from their chest. Which airway might be suggested as an aid for this patient?
3 Patient C has been admitted in type II respiratory failure and requires assisted ventilation; will they need to have CPAP or NIV?

Website

 http://www.oxfordtextbooks.co.uk/orc/ endacott

You may find it helpful to work through our short online quiz and additional scenarios intended to help you to develop and apply the skills in this chapter.

References

Bateman NT and Leech RM (1998). ABC of oxygen: acute oxygen therapy. *British Medical Journal*, **317**, 798–801.

Bennett C (2003). Nursing the breathless patient. *Nursing Standard*, **17**(17), 45–51.

BOC Medical (2006). *Medical Gas Data Sheet. Medical oxygen (compressed gas)*. BOC Medical, Manchester.

Brigg C (1999). The benefits of non-invasive ventilation and CPAP therapy. *British Journal of Nursing*, **8**(20), 1355–61.

British Thoracic Society Standards of Care Committee (2002). Non-invasive ventilation in acute respiratory failure. *Thorax*, **57**, 192–211.

Brochard L (1996). Non-invasive ventilation in acute respiratory failure. *Respiratory Care*, **41**(5), 456–65.

Cull C and Inwood H (1999). Weaning patients from mechanical ventilation. *Professional Nurse*, **14**(8), 535–8.

Dodds S and Williamson GR (2007). Nurse-led arterial blood gas sampling for patients requiring long term oxygen therapy. *Nursing Times Respiratory Supplement*, **103**(44) [online] **http://www. nursingtimes.net/nursingtimes/pages/ DevelopmentNurseLedarterialbloodgassamplingfor patients** accessed 09/07/2007.

Elliott MW (1997). Non-invasive ventilation in COPD. *British Journal of Hospital Medicine*, **57**(3), 83–6.

Esmond G (2001). *Respiratory nursing*. Baillere Tindall, Edinburgh.

Francis C (2006). *Respiratory care*. Blackwell Publishing, Oxford.

Guyton A and Hall J (2000). *Textbook of medical physiology*, 10th edition. WB Saunders, Philadelphia.

Jamieson EM, McCall JM, and Whyte LA (2002). *Clinical nursing practices*. Churchill Livingstone, Edinburgh.

Jevon P (2002). *Advanced cardiac life support*. Butterworth Heinemann, Oxford.

Jevon P and Ewens B (2001). Assessment of a breathless patient. *Nursing Standard*, **15**(16), 48–53.

Oh TE (1997). *Intensive care manual*. Butterworths, Sydney.

Phillipps T (2005). Home non-invasive ventilation: a brief guide for primary care staff. *Nursing Times*, **101**(57), 35–8.

Place B (1997). Care is critical. Using airway pressure. *Nursing Times*, **93**(31), 42–4.

Resuscitation Council (UK) (2000). *Advanced life support provider manual*. Resuscitation Council (UK), London.

UK Resuscitation Council (2006). *Immediate life support*, 2nd edition. UK Resuscitation Council, London.

Vines DL, Shelledy DC, and Peters J (2000). Current respiratory care. Part 1: oxygen therapy, oximetry, bronchial hygiene – among many devices and methods, how to choose those that meet therapeutic goals. *Journal of Critical Illness*, **15**(9): 507–15.

Woodward P (2003). Using non-invasive ventilation in acute wards. Part 7. *Nursing Standard*, **18**(1): 39–44.

Useful further reading and websites

PatientPlus has some more technical material on oxygen therapy at: **http://www.patient.co.uk/** (search for oxygen therapy).

 Answers to patient scenarios

1 Patient A may benefit from nasal cannulae, which would also enable them to eat and drink while continuing to receive oxygen.

2 Patient B would benefit from the use of a nasopharyngeal airway, which would enable suctioning of the secretions from the chest.

3 Patient C has been admitted in type II respiratory failure, which means that they will also have a raised carbon dioxide level. They will require NIV as this is a ventilatory problem and not an oxygenation one.

7.5 Tracheostomy management

Definition

A tracheostomy is an opening in the front (anterior) wall of the trachea below the cricoid cartilage and between the second and third tracheal cartilage rings, which may be formed surgically (in an operating theatre) or **percutaneously** (through the skin using a needle and dilators in an intensive care unit). A tracheostomy tube is then inserted through the opening – the tube may or may not have an inflatable cuff to create an air seal in the trachea above the internal opening of the tracheostomy tube.

Tracheostomy management includes the following skills:

- Care of inner tubes.
- Changing a tracheostomy dressing.
- Removing the tracheostomy tube.

It is important to remember that:

- A patient with a tracheostomy tube will require skilled nursing assessment, monitoring, and care, due to the potential for complications.
- The patient is dependent on the tube being kept clean and patent in order to be able to breathe.
- The patient may not be able to communicate verbally – ensure that there is a call bell within reach and that you provide some alternative means of communication (pen and paper, spelling/symbols chart).
- Spare tubes (the same size, a half-size (if available), and a size smaller), a spare inner tube, and tracheal dilators must be kept with the patient, in case the tube becomes blocked or accidentally displaced.

Prior knowledge

Before undertaking care of a patient with a tracheostomy tube, make sure you are familiar with:

1 Anatomy and physiology of the upper airway.
2 Reasons that a patient may need a tracheostomy.
3 Signs of airway obstruction and respiratory distress.
4 Emergency equipment, including how tracheal dilators work.
5 The different types of tracheostomy tubes used in your health care setting.
6 Resources available within your Trust, such as a head and neck nurse specialist, speech and language therapists, or staff in the intensive care unit.
7 Local policy on management of patients with tracheostomy tubes.

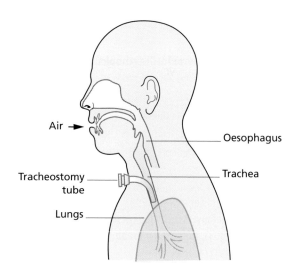

Figure 7.5 A tracheostomy tube *in situ*.

Background

Insertion of a tracheostomy tube may be necessary following complicated head and neck surgery, or as an aid to weaning patients from a ventilator in an intensive care unit. A tracheostomy provides a secure airway for the patient and allows secretions to be cleared from the patient's chest (see Section 7.6). **Figure 7.5** shows a tracheostomy tube *in situ*.

Principles of tracheostomy tube design

One of the key nursing objectives when caring for patients with tracheostomy tubes is to ensure that the tube is kept patent and does not become occluded with secretions. Most tracheostomy tubes will accommodate a removable inner tube – this should be inserted when the tracheostomy is inserted, to prevent the build-up of secretions on the inner wall of the tube. It is important to remember that inserting an inner tube into a tracheostomy tube will reduce the inner diameter of the tracheostomy tube.

Types of tracheostomy tubes

There are many different types of tracheostomy tube available in different sizes, so it is advisable to familiarize yourself with the tracheostomy tubes used in your health care setting. Tracheostomy tubes are commonly manufactured from:

- Polyvinyl chloride (PVC).
- Silicone.
- Silver.

(Serra 2000)

The first two are most commonly used; they are disposable but can be fitted with a removable inner tube that can be cleaned. Silver tubes are expensive, but can be re-sterilized (Russell 2005).

The size of the tracheostomy tube (e.g. 8.0, 7.5) refers to the internal diameter of the tube in mm – a size 8.0 tracheostomy tube has an 8 mm internal diameter.

Cuffed tubes

Cuffed tracheostomy tubes have an inflatable cuff that is situated above the internal opening of the tube (see **Figure 7.6**). This type of tube will be needed if a patient requires artificial ventilation or is at risk of aspiration. Once inflated, the cuff creates an air seal within the trachea – this prevents air from escaping during ventilation. The cuff also provides anchorage for the tube in the trachea and minimizes the risk of aspirating saliva or gastric contents. Cuffed tubes have a pilot tube and cuff through which air is introduced to inflate the internal cuff.

Ideally, the internal cuff should be what is termed a high volume, low pressure cuff – these enable an air seal to be created while exerting the least possible pressure

on the tracheal mucosa. Excessive pressure on the tracheal mucosa can cause injury and necrosis (Serra 2000). The pressure within the cuff should be kept at between 20 mmHg (Pritchard 1994) and 25 mmHg (Guyton *et al*. 1991). There are pressure gauges available to measure this; check that these are available on your ward.

If the cuff is inflated, the patient will not be able to talk, since air will not pass through their vocal cords on expiration.

Uncuffed tubes

This type of tube may be used for patients who can breathe for themselves and who have been assessed as safe to swallow, since uncuffed tubes offer no protection against aspiration.

Fenestrated tubes

These tubes have single or multiple holes (fenestrations) in the outer tube on its uppermost side and matching removable fenestrated inner tubes (as well as non-fenestrated inner tubes). With the cuff deflated, these fenestrations allow more air to pass through the upper airway compared with non-fenestrated tubes (see **Figure 7.7**). This can make expiration easier if the tracheostomy tube is capped or a speaking valve is used, particularly if the tracheostomy tube is relatively large for the diameter of the patient's trachea.

It is important to remember that if your patient has a fenestrated tracheostomy tube, the nonfenestrated inner

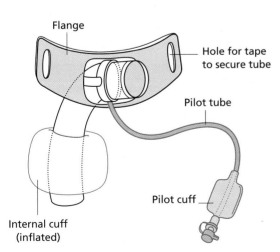

Figure 7.6 A cuffed tracheostomy tube, showing the internal cuff inflated around the tube.

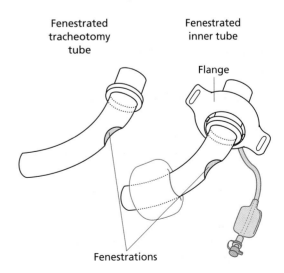

Figure 7.7 Fenestrated tracheostomy tube with fenestrated inner tube.

tube is inserted for suctioning. This is because the suction catheter could pass through the fenestrations and cause trauma to the posterior tracheal wall (Billau 2004).

It is also important to remember that a fenestrated tracheostomy tube may have a larger outer diameter than the same (internal) size non-fenestrated tube. This means that a size 8.0 non-fenestrated tube may not be able to be exchanged for a size 8.0 fenestrated tube, as the latter may not fit through the opening in the patient's neck. This is because the size of the fenestrated tube refers to the diameter of the removable inner tube, rather than the outer tube.

Adjustable flange tubes

These are used for patients in whom a standard tube does not fit through the neck and into the trachea. These tubes are longer than standard tracheostomy tubes and have an adjustable flange that enables the functional length of the tube to be varied to fit the patient.

Humidification

The nose and upper airway warm and moisten inhaled air. If a patient has a tracheostomy, these structures are bypassed. Therefore, the air/gases a patient with a tracheostomy breathes in have to be humidified by other means. This is very important as secretions need to be kept humidified in order to prevent them becoming dry and sticky, and potentially blocking the tracheostomy tube.

This will usually be achieved by using a 'wet' humidification system such as a Fisher Paykel system (a reservoir of water is heated that warms and moistens gases as they pass over the water surface) or a filter that traps heat and moisture from exhaled gases and then warms and moistens the next inhaled breath. Practice can vary; check your employer's policy regarding tracheostomy humidification. It is also important to monitor the type of secretions obtained when the patient is suctioned for signs of adequate humidification (are they loose, easy to clear?).

Removal of tracheostomy tubes

The tracheostomy tube can be removed once the patient has been assessed by the multidisciplinary team as being safe to breathe and clear secretions without it. Indications may include the ability to clear secretions out of the tra-

Box 7.3 Potential complications following a tracheostomy

- Bleeding.
- Infection.
- Tube misplacement.
- Tube displacement.
- Blockage of the tube.
- Tracheal stenosis.

cheostomy tube independently and the ability to breathe for long periods with a speaking valve in place.

A tracheostomy provides a secure airway for the patient. It can enable secretions to be cleared by suctioning and, with the cuff inflated, can minimize – though not completely prevent – the risk of the patient aspirating saliva or gastric contents (Hales 2004). There are, however, some potential complications that may occur following a tracheostomy, which are listed in **Box 7.3**.

Sometimes, a mini-tracheostomy (or cricothyroidotomy) may be inserted through the cricothyroid membrane. It is a thin tube and does not have a cuff. It is usually inserted to assist the patient to clear secretions, but may be inserted in emergency situations if the patient has severe or complete airway obstruction (Joynt 2003). Because it is a very thin tube, only small suction catheters can be passed through it (size 10Fg). Some secretions can be cleared via the catheter (although this may be difficult if secretions are thick) but some will be cleared via the upper airway by the patient's own cough, as a cough reflex will be initiated by passing through the suction catheter.

Speaking valves

As described earlier, if the tracheostomy tube cuff is inflated, air will not pass through the patient's vocal cords and they will be unable to speak. This can be a source of frustration for both the patient and those caring for them. Once a patient has been assessed as being safe to try deflating the cuff, the use of a speaking valve can be considered.

A speaking valve can be used with both fenestrated and non-fenestrated tracheostomy tubes. The key point to remember is that the cuff *must* be deflated, as if the cuff is not deflated with the speaking valve in place, the patient will be unable to breathe out. Speaking valves work using a one-way valve that allows air in during inspiration but closes during expiration, thus forcing air to escape through the patient's vocal cords and upper airway.

Some tracheostomy tubes have an integral port to aspirate secretions from above the cuff. If present, the port should be aspirated using a 10 ml syringe to remove any pooled secretions before deflating the cuff, in order to prevent these being aspirated by the patient. If there is no port on the tracheostomy, a second person should be present to perform tracheal suction as you deflate the cuff, in case secretions are pooled above the cuff. Prepare the patient before performing suction (see Section 7.6) and advise them that their voice may sound different with a speaking valve in place.

A patient with a non-fenestrated tube may experience some difficulties in breathing out with a speaking valve in place, particularly if the tracheal tube is proportionally large in relation to the diameter of their trachea. This is because they can only breathe out through the space between the tracheostomy tube and their trachea. Assess the patient closely for signs of respiratory distress and remove the speaking valve if these develop. Assistance from an experienced member of staff should also be obtained.

Context

 ### When to use tracheostomy tubes

Patients may have had a tracheostomy tube inserted for a number of reasons. These may include:

- A lengthy period of artificial ventilation, usually in an intensive care unit. Patients will generally tolerate a tracheostomy tube much better than an endotracheal tube (see Section 7.9). This enables sedation to be reduced or stopped and allows weaning off ventilatory support.
- Following head and neck surgery, such as neck dissection.
- Upper airway obstruction due to infection (such as epiglottitis) or a tumour.
- Impaired swallowing ability with an associated risk of aspiration (Price 2004).
- Vocal cord paralysis (Serra 2000).

Potential problems

Some potential complications following a tracheostomy are listed in Box 7.3. Two problems that will require immediate attention and medical assistance are:

- Displaced tubes
- Blocked tubes

As the stoma may close slightly when either of these problems arises, a smaller tube may have to be inserted instead of one the same size.

Displaced tubes

A tracheostomy tube can become displaced by falling completely out of the stoma, or displacing from the trachea into the soft tissues. In the latter situation, it may not be visually obvious that the tube is displaced, except for signs of respiratory distress. Summon appropriate assistance immediately, in order that a new (or, in an emergency, the old tube) can be inserted. A smaller-sized tracheostomy tube may be needed. The tracheostomy stoma can be kept open using tracheal dilators. These are inserted 'sideways-on' (horizontally) and separate the tracheal rings when the handles are squeezed together.

Blocked tubes

This is usually caused by a large plug or crust of sputum (Serra 2000), which is why good humidification and cleaning of the inner tube are so important. If attempts to clear the blockage by tracheal suction or changing the inner tube fail, the tracheostomy tube will need to be removed and the stoma held open using tracheal dilators. Summon appropriate assistance immediately.

Procedure

Preparation

Prepare yourself

If you have not undertaken the procedure before, make sure you have appropriate supervision available. Ensure you understand the reasons for the procedure. If undertaking a tracheostomy dressing, ensure you have assistance from a second practitioner: one person should hold the tube while the other changes the dressing.

Prepare the patient

Explain the procedure to the patient and their relatives, and explain why it needs to be undertaken. Show them the equipment in order to reduce anxiety and aid compliance.

Prepare the equipment/environment

The environment should be conducive to the patient receiving treatment. The equipment should be made available at the patient's bedside. Ensure patient privacy is maintained.

Step-by-step guide to caring for inner tubes

Step	Rationale
1 Introduce yourself, confirm the patient's identity, explain the procedure, and obtain consent.	To identify the patient correctly and gain informed consent.
2 Check the patient's secretions at least 4-hourly initially after insertion.	The frequency of cleaning the inner tube should be determined by the nature and quantity of the patient's secretions. Checking at 4-hourly intervals will help determine the frequency of subsequent inner tube changes.
3 Remove the inner tube and replace it with a second spare tube.	To allow cleaning of the tube that was *in situ* and to maintain airway patency during tube cleaning.
4 Clean the tube with warm, running tap water and a brush (Russell 2005). Some hospitals advocate using sterile 0.9% saline, so check local policy (St. James's Hospital 2000, Trundle and Brooks 2004).	This allows the build-up of sputum and microorganisms to be removed.
5 Leave the newly cleaned tube in a clean place, or dry container with a lid if available, near the patient.	Spare tubes should be near at hand in case ones *in situ* fall out, and for when cleaning is required again.
6 Re-tie the tracheostomy tapes, or reapply the purpose-made Velcro straps, through the flanges (see Figure 7.6).	To ensure that the tube remains *in situ*.

Step-by-step guide to changing a tracheostomy dressing

Step		Rationale
1	Introduce yourself, confirm the patient's identity, explain the procedure, and obtain consent.	To identify the patient correctly and gain informed consent.
2	Assess the volume of secretions escaping from the wound, and assess the patency and appearance of the dressing.	A tracheostomy is a surgical wound so should be kept clean and dry to reduce the risk of infection at the site. The frequency of dressing changes should be determined by the volume of secretions escaping from around the tracheostomy tube, rather than being performed as a 'ritualized activity' simply because it is 'due' to be done.
3	Clean the stoma site with 0.9% saline (Blunt 2001) using aseptic technique and apply a purpose-made tracheostomy dressing.	Aseptic technique is usually required to change dressings, although there is some debate as to whether this should be by an aseptic or clean technique (Serra 2000). Check your local policy on this. The tracheostomy dressing should be thin, so as not to displace the tube (Russell 2005), and absorbent, to keep the skin around the stoma dry; purpose-made dressings are best for this.
4	Assess whether it is necessary to lift the flange of the tracheostomy tube in order to clean the skin around the stoma and replace the dressing.	This will be necessary if the stoma is dirty or inflamed to ensure thorough cleaning. If so, a second person may be needed to hold the tracheostomy tube while you loosen or remove the securing tapes and clean and redress the stoma site, to avoid displacing the tube.
5	If necessary, re-tie the tracheostomy tapes, or reapply the purpose-made Velcro straps, through the flanges (see Figure 7.6).	To ensure that the tube remains *in situ*.

Step-by-step guide to tracheostomy tube removal

Step		Rationale
1	Introduce yourself, confirm the patient's identity, explain the procedure, and obtain consent.	To identify the patient correctly and gain informed consent.
2	Remove the dressing and untie the tapes.	To allow smooth removal of the tube.
3	Check if the tracheostomy tube is still inflated; if so deflate the cuff fully via the port using a 10 ml syringe.	To allow smooth removal of the tube.

continued overleaf

4	Ask the patient to take a deep breath and pull the tube out in a quick, smooth motion. Cover the stoma immediately with an airtight dressing.	To avoid triggering a cough during tube removal. The dressing will prevent air entering and escaping via the stoma.
5	The patient should be advised to support the dressing when they speak and particularly when they cough.	To prevent the dressing being displaced by pressure of exhaled air. The dressing will need to be changed as required.
6	Inform the patient that the stoma will usually close relatively quickly and without the need for surgical intervention (Russell 2005), particularly with a **percutaneous** tracheostomy.	To ensure the patient is fully informed and to reduce anxiety.
7	Observe the patient for signs of respiratory distress.	In case they are not able to breathe well on their own immediately after the tracheostomy removal.

Following the procedure

Document your actions according to local policy in order to enable continuity of care and provide a written record of the patient's tracheostomy.

Reflection and evaluation

When you have cared for a patient with a tracheostomy, think about the following questions:

1 Why did the patient need a tracheostomy?
2 Were there any communication issues with the patient, and if so how did you manage this?
3 Was appropriate equipment at the bedside (spare tracheostomy tubes of the same size and one size smaller; tracheal dilators)?

Further learning opportunities

Observe the insertion of a tracheostomy in order to understand what happens and what the patient experiences. Try to get involved in cleaning, changing dressings, and removal of the tubes.

Reminders

Don't forget to:

● Always deflate a tracheostomy tube cuff before attaching a speaking valve.

● Remember that patients may have difficulty with communication and experience frustration.
● Ensure that spare tracheostomy tubes and tracheal dilators are at the patient's bedside.
● Ensure that humidification is used and is adequate for the patient.

Patient scenarios

Consider what you should do in the following situations, then turn to the end of this skill to check your answers.

1 Patient A has a size 8.0 tracheostomy tube in place. What size tubes should be available at the bedside?
2 The same patient has been assessed as being ready to try a speaking valve. What should you do before attaching the speaking valve?
3 The same patient has had the speaking valve removed. A few hours later they appear to be struggling to breathe. What should you do?

Website

 http://www.oxfordtextbooks.co.uk/orc/ endacott

You may find it helpful to work through our short online quiz and additional scenarios intended to help you to develop and apply the skills in this chapter.

References

Billau C (2004). Suctioning. In C Russell and B Matta, eds. *Tracheostomy: a multi-professional handbook*, pp. 157–71. Cambridge University Press, Cambridge.

Blunt J (2001). Wound cleansing: ritualistic or research-based practice? *Nursing Standard*, **16**(1), 33–6.

Guyton D, Banner MJ, and Kirby (1991). High-volume, low pressure cuffs: are they always low pressure? *Chest*, **100**, 1076–81.

Hales P (2004). Swallowing. In C Russell and B Matta, eds. *Tracheostomy: a multi-professional handbook*, pp. 187–210. Cambridge University Press, Cambridge.

Joynt GM (2003). Airway management and acute upper airway obstruction. In AD Bersten, N Soni, and TE Oh, eds. *Oh's intensive care manual*, 5th edition, pp. 283–96. Butterworth Heinemann, London.

Price T (2004). Surgical tracheostomy. In C Russell and B Matta, eds. *Tracheostomy: a multi-professional handbook*, pp. 35–58. Cambridge University Press, Cambridge.

Pritchard A (1994). Tracheostomy. *Care of the Critically Ill*, **10**(2), 66–8.

Russell C (2005). Providing the nurse with a guide to tracheostomy care and management. *British Journal of Nursing*, **14**(8), 428–33.

Serra A (2000). Tracheostomy care. *Nursing Standard*, **14**(42), 45–52.

St. James's Hospital/Royal Victoria Eye and Ear Hospital (2000). *Tracheostomy care guidelines* [online] **http://www.stjames.i.e/PatientsVisitors/ Departments/Otolaryngology/ TracheostomyCareGuidelines/PrintableVersion/ file,7385,en.PDF** accessed 01/05/07.

Trundle C and Brooks R (2004). Infection control issues in the care of a patient with a tracheostomy. In C Russell and B Matta, eds. *Tracheostomy: a multi-professional handbook*, pp. 345–59. Cambridge University Press, Cambridge.

(A) Answers to patient scenarios

1 Size 8.0, 7.5, and 7.0. If the tracheostomy tube is displaced, it may be necessary to re-intubate with a smaller tube.

2 Explain what you are going to do; clear secretions from above the cuff if possible; deflate the cuff; perform suction.

3 Summon appropriate assistance immediately and check that the tube is patent – try suctioning/changing the inner tube. You may need to be prepared to assist with removing the tracheostomy tube.

7.6 **Oropharyngeal, tracheal, and endotracheal suctioning** (A)

This is an advanced skill. You *must* check whether you can assist with or undertake this skill, in line with local policy.

Definition

Oropharyngeal, tracheal, and endotracheal suction are methods of clearing secretions by the application of negative pressure via either a yankauer sucker (oropharyngeal) or an appropriately sized tracheal suction catheter (tracheal/endotracheal). This procedure may be required in an emergency situation or as part of a patient's planned care.

It is important to remember that:

- The purpose of performing oral suction is to maintain oral hygiene and comfort for the patient or to remove blood and vomit in an emergency situation.
- The purpose of tracheal/endotracheal suction is to remove pulmonary secretions in patients who are unable to cough and clear their own secretions effectively. The patient may be fully conscious or have an impaired conscious level.
- Secretions are cleared from these patients' airways in order to maintain airway patency, to prevent atelectasis secondary to blockage of smaller airways (Royal Free Hampstead NHS Trust 1999), and to ensure that adequate gas exchange (particularly oxygenation) occurs.

Prior knowledge

Before undertaking suction, make sure that you are familiar with:

1 Respiratory anatomy and physiology.

2 Cardiovascular physiology.

3 The reasons that patients may require an artificial airway (e.g. a patient may need a tracheostomy if they have been intubated for a long time and may arrive in the ward with it still *in situ*. They may require an endotracheal tube after an emergency situation such as a cardiac arrest, or during surgery).

4 Causes for an impaired conscious level/cough.

5 Oral anatomy.

6 Your employer's infection control policy with regard to tracheal suction.

Background

Patients will require suction to be performed for a number of reasons:

- Oropharyngeal suction may be required for a patient who has undergone head and neck surgery, or whose conscious level is impaired and/or has an absent or impaired swallow reflex. Care should be taken to avoid trauma to the oral mucosa, particularly in patients with clotting disorders.
- Tracheal suction may be indicated in patients who are unable to clear their secretions themselves and will be required in those patients who need an artificial, secure airway (tracheostomy, endotracheal tube). An artificial airway may be needed after surgery or in order to provide mechanical ventilation, for example in an intensive care unit.

The purpose of performing suction is to clear vomit, blood, or secretions from the oropharynx or trachea in patients who are unable to do so independently, due either to their underlying illness, following surgery, or because of an impaired conscious level. Lower airway secretions that are not cleared may provide a medium for bacterial growth (Woodrow 2000). Suction may be performed using a yankauer sucker to clear oral secretions from the mouth and oropharynx, or by passing a suction catheter into the upper airway in order to clear tracheal secretions (see **Figure 7.8**).

Suctioning has been identified by patients as causing anxiety and discomfort (Puntillo 1990). It may be useful to liaise with other health care professionals, such as your ward physiotherapist, for help and advice regarding suctioning.

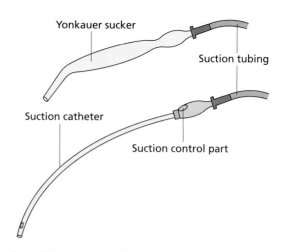

Figure 7.8 Yankauer sucker and suction catheter.

Tracheal suction can be performed via a variety of routes:

- Orally, using an oropharyngeal airway (unlikely to be tolerated by a conscious patient).
- Nasally, using a nasopharyngeal airway (contraindicated if the patient has clotting abnormalities or a fractured base of skull).
- Via a mini-tracheostomy tube.
- Via a tracheostomy tube.
- Via an endotracheal tube.

When suction is performed, an assessment should be made of the type of secretions obtained and any changes noted. Secretions may be:

- Copious
- Minimal
- Mucopurulent (green or yellow) if infection is present
- Frothy (possibly seen if the patient has pulmonary oedema)
- Bloodstained (possibly from trauma to the tracheal mucosa)
- Thick
- Watery

A sputum sample may be requested for microbiological investigation. A sputum trap should be used to collect a sputum sample; if you are unsure how to add this to a suction circuit, seek further advice/assistance from senior colleagues.

While tracheal/endotracheal suctioning may be a necessary procedure, it can be associated with some potentially harmful effects. These may include:

- Hypoxaemia (Bersten *et al.* 2003), as oxygen as well as secretions may be removed from the lungs when suctioning (Woodrow 2000).
- Vasovagal response causing arrhythmias and hypotension (Wainright and Gould 1996, Bersten *et al.* 2003).
- Mucosal trauma (Moore 2003). Suction should only be applied when withdrawing the catheter, *never* when inserting it.
- Cross-infection (Woodrow 2000, Moore 2003).

Suction procedures should therefore be as brief as possible, lasting approximately 15 seconds (Woodrow 2000). The instilling of 0.9% saline via a tracheostomy or endotracheal tube prior to suctioning is sometimes performed; however, there is little evidence to support this practice and it could potentially cause harm (Akgul and Akyolcu 2002, Ridling *et al.* 2003).

Choosing the right sized suction catheter

The suction catheter diameter should be half the diameter (or less) of the tracheal tube. This prevents occlusion of the airway and avoids the generation of large negative intra-thoracic pressures (Bersten *et al.* 2003). A method of calculating the correct size of suction catheter is shown in **Box 7.4**.

Setting the correct pressure

The negative pressure set on the suction machine needs to be sufficiently high to clear secretions while avoiding

---

Box 7.4 Sizing a suction catheter (Fg – French gauge)

$$\frac{\text{Diameter of tracheal tube (mm)} \times 3}{2}$$

Example:
For a size 8 tracheostomy:

$$8 \times 3 = 24$$

$$24/2 = 12 \text{ (Fg) suction catheter.}$$

---

trauma to the bronchial mucosa. Ashurst (1997) recommends a setting of 120 mmHg (16 kPa). In practice, it is sometimes necessary to apply higher levels of negative pressure to clear thick, tenacious secretions; this should be done cautiously, and advice should be sought regarding therapies to help loosen secretions, such as ensuring adequate patient hydration (Akgul and Akyolcu 2002), mucolytic agents, and sufficient airway humidity (Blackwood 1999).

Context

 ### When to perform suction and in whom

Potential indications for tracheal or endotracheal suctioning (Woodrow 2000) include:

- Raised respiratory rate.
- Inability to clear secretions effectively.
- Reduced air entry on auscultation.
- Audible secretions.
- Spontaneous but ineffective cough.
- Reduced oxygen saturation levels.

However, the need for suction should be assessed on an individual basis rather than as a 'ritualized' activity, meaning that patients should only receive suctioning when they need it, not because a certain length of time has elapsed since it was last performed (Royal Free Hampstead NHS Trust 1999, St. James's Hospital/Royal Victoria Eye and Ear Hospital 2000, Moore 2003, Redditch and Bromsgrove PCT 2004).

 ### When not to perform suction

Oral suctioning can cause trauma if the oral mucosa is damaged; it should also be undertaken with extreme caution in patients with clotting disorders. Suction should never be applied during insertion of the suction catheter.

Alternative interventions

A fine gauge suction catheter is preferable to a yankauer sucker for oral suction in patients with damaged oral mucosa. In patients who are fully awake, suction is less likely to be tolerated. With assistance or advice from a physiotherapist, encourage the patient to clear their airways by coughing if possible. Appropriate positioning of the patient is essential.

Indications for assistance

Seek assistance from a more senior colleague if you experience any difficulty at any stage of the procedure.

Procedure

Preparation

Prepare yourself

Ensure that you understand how the equipment works, how to assemble it, and the reason you need to perform suction. Wash your hands.

Prepare the patient

The procedure should be fully explained to the patient (see Discussing the procedure box).

Prepare the equipment

Assemble the correctly sized catheter, gloves (sterile or non-sterile depending on your employer's infection control policy), and other equipment. Ensure that the suction machine works.

Discussing the procedure with the patient and family

- Explain what you are going to do and why it is necessary/important.

- Explain that the procedure is likely to be uncomfortable, but will be brief.

- Explain that the procedure may need to be done more than once.

- Depending on the conscious level of the patient, explain that the patient may cough for a short while after the procedure.

Step-by-step guide to performing tracheal suction

Step	Rationale
1 Introduce yourself, confirm the patient's identity, explain the procedure, and obtain consent.	To identify the patient correctly and gain informed consent.
2 Assess the patient to ensure that suction is necessary (including the effectiveness of their cough).	To reduce potential complications from endotracheal suction and avoid unnecessary interventions.
3 Assist the patient into an upright position (if possible).	To allow optimum lung expansion and effective cough.
4 Apply an oxygen saturation (SpO_2) probe.	To enable evaluation of patient's oxygenation prior to and following the suction procedure (see Section 7.2).
5 Wash hands.	To reduce the risk of cross-infection.
6 Put on disposable apron and protective visor/eye wear, according to local policy.	To reduce risk of cross-infection and to protect yourself from droplets/sputum contamination.
7 Connect suction catheter to suction tubing and turn suction machine on.	To allow suction to begin.

8	Use sterile/clean non-sterile glove* on the hand manipulating the catheter and clean non-sterile glove on other hand.	To reduce risk of cross-infection to the patient and to yourself.
9	Withdraw suction catheter from sleeve with clean gloved hand and grasp catheter with sterile/clean non-sterile gloved* hand away from catheter tip.	To reduce risk of cross-infection.
10	Advance catheter gently until a cough is stimulated or resistance is felt. *Do not apply suction during catheter insertion.*	To minimize risk of mucosal trauma.
11	When a cough is initiated or resistance is felt, withdraw the catheter approximately 1 cm and apply suction by occluding suction control port on catheter with thumb. Withdraw gently. *Procedure should last no more than 15 seconds.*	To reduce potential complications from suctioning.
12	Dispose of suction catheter and gloves in clinical waste disposal bin.	To reduce risk of cross-infection and ensure clinical waste is correctly disposed of.
13	Rinse suction tubing with sterile/non-sterile* water.	To ensure sputum is removed from suction tubing.
14	Clear patient's oral secretions if required.	To maintain patient comfort.
15	Dry the container used for rinsing and wash hands.	To reduce risk of cross-infection to the patient and to yourself.
16	Repeat procedure if required, having checked the patient's SpO$_2$. Seek assistance from a more experienced colleague. Allow the patient to rest/recover between each suction procedure.	If the patient has a sustained lower SpO$_2$ compared to before the procedure, they may require oxygen for a period of time.

*Refer to your local infection control policy.

Following the procedure

Ensure the patient is comfortable and has everything they require within reach. Document any problems with the procedure in the patient records, noting the amount, colour, and consistency of the secretions.

Reflection and evaluation

After you have performed tracheal suction on a patient, think about the following questions:

1 What made you decide that the patient required suction?

2 Did you explain the procedure so that the patient understood what was going to happen?

3 Was there an improvement in the patient's respiratory condition after the procedure had been performed?

4 Did you observe and record the volume, colour, and consistency of the patient's secretions?

Further learning opportunities

Suctioning is a delicate art, and requires practice and patience to perfect. Watch how experienced staff do it. Note what they do well or badly. Ask to have practice, under supervision, when it is appropriate to do so. It may be possible to organize a practice placement with your employer's intensive care unit or head and neck surgical ward to gain further experience.

Reminders

Don't forget to:

- Use the correct size of suction catheter.
- Explain the procedure to the patient.
- Only apply suction when withdrawing the catheter.

 Patient scenarios

Consider what you should do in the following situations, then turn to the end of this skill to check your answers.

1 For what reasons might a patient require tracheal suctioning?

2 You are caring for a patient with a tracheostomy. You notice when undertaking suction that his secretions are very thick and difficult to clear. What interventions/therapies might you consider to alleviate this?

3 You are asked by a junior student what complications might occur when you perform a suction procedure. What will you include in your response?

Website

 http://www.oxfordtextbooks.co.uk/orc/ endacott

You may find it helpful to work through our short online quiz and additional scenarios intended to help you to develop and apply the skills in this chapter.

References

Akgul S and Akyolcu N (2002). Effects of normal saline on endotracheal suctioning. *Journal of Clinical Nursing*, **11**(6), 826–30.

Ashurst S (1997). Nursing care of the mechanically ventilated patient in ITU. *British Journal of Nursing*, **6**(8), 447–54.

Bersten AD, Soni N, and Oh TE, eds (2003). *Oh's intensive care manual*, 5th edition. Butterworth Heinemann, London.

Blackwood B (1999). Normal saline instillation with endotracheal suction: primum non nocere (first do no harm). *Journal of Advanced Nursing*, **29**(4), 928–34.

Moore T (2003). Suctioning techniques for the removal of respiratory secretions. *Nursing Standard*, **18**(9), 47–53.

Puntillo KA (1990). Pain experiences of intensive care unit patients. *Heart and Lung*, **19**(5), 526–33.

Redditch and Bromsgrove Primary Care Trust (2004). *Suction guidelines for adult patients in a community setting* [online] **http://www. worcestershirehealth.nhs.uk/RBPCT_Library/ lesleyway/suction%20guidelines%202004.doc** accessed 01/05/07.

Ridling DA, Martin LD, and Bratton SL (2003). Endotracheal suctioning with or without instillation of isotonic sodium chloride in critically ill children. *American Journal of Critical Care*, **12**, 212–19.

Royal Free Hampstead NHS Trust (1999). *Guidelines for tracheal suction* [online] **http://www. bahnon.org.uk/Professional Guidelines/ TrachealSuction.doc** accessed 01/05/07.

St. James's Hospital/Royal Victoria Eye and Ear Hospital (2000). *Tracheostomy care guidelines* [online] **http://www.stjames.ie/PatientsVisitors/ Departments/Otolaryngology/ TracheostomyCareGuidelines/PrintableVersion/ file,7385en.PDF** accessed 01/05/07.

Wainright S and Gould D (1996). Endo-tracheal suctioning: an example of the problems of relevance and rigour in clinical research. *Journal of Clinical Nursing*, **5**(6), 389–98.

Woodrow P (2000). *Perspectives in intensive care nursing*. Routledge, London and New York.

 Answers to patient scenarios

1 Patients with an artificial airway or those with an ineffective cough.

2 Adequate humidification, patient hydration, or mucolytic agents.

3 Your answer should include: hypoxia, cardiac arrhythmias, hypotension, mucosal trauma, and cross-infection.

7.7 **Lung auscultation**

This is an advanced skill. You *must* check whether you can assist with or undertake this skill, in line with local policy.

Definition

Lung **auscultation** is a simple, non-invasive way of listening to the sounds produced within the lungs. Identification and interpretation of the characteristic sounds produced following pathological changes within the lungs forms a key component of the assessment of a patient's respiratory function (Gross *et al.* 2000).

It is important to remember that:

- Auscultation is a simple, cost-effective way of assessing a patient's respiratory function; however, the interpretation of sound is subjective and this is compounded by the lack of formal recognized **nomenclature** (terminology) to describe lung sounds.
- Reliability from one therapist to the next is only average; however, improvements in reliability can be achieved following education sessions on standardized nomenclature, technique, and interpretation (Brooks and Thomas 1995).
- Regardless of the reliability of auscultation, it should only be undertaken as part of a full respiratory assessment.

Prior knowledge

Before undertaking lung auscultation, make sure you are familiar with:

1 Respiratory and cardiovascular anatomy.
2 Physiology of respiration.
3 Surface anatomy of the lungs.
4 The stethoscope and limitations of use.
5 Definitions of terms to describe auscultation findings.
6 Pathophysiology of common respiratory diseases and their clinical presentation.

The skill of auscultation is part of the respiratory assessment and therefore needs to be treated as such. Review of the areas above will enable you to look at the patient with an idea of what auscultation findings you might expect.

Background

Auscultation is the technical term for listening to the internal sounds of the body, usually using a stethoscope.

Auscultation is normally performed for the purposes of examining the circulatory system, respiratory system, and gastrointestinal system.

The reliability of auscultation has been questioned. Brooks and Thomas (1995) looked at the reliability of physical therapists in recognizing auscultation findings from a tape rather than *in vivo* lung sounds. They concluded that there was only fair inter-rater reliability amongst physical therapists when auscultating lung sounds. This was also demonstrated by earlier studies (Pasterkamp *et al.* 1987, Aweida and Kelsey 1990, Brooks *et al.* 1993). Despite this, auscultation remains an important component of respiratory assessment.

In order to understand the skill of auscultation and why it is useful, we first need to understand how the stethoscope works. The development of the stethoscope was carried out in 1816 by a French physician called Laennec (Mangione and Nieman 1999). Since then the stethoscope has developed from the original rolled up paper to wood and now the expensive pieces of equipment we use today. They do, however, remain very simple instruments used simply to conduct the sound between the body surface and the ears (Pasterkamp *et al.* 1997). **Figure 7.9** shows the hollow tube that connects the diaphragm and bell to the earpieces. High frequency sound is transmitted more effectively using the diaphragm and lower frequency sound via the bell.

Breath sounds are essentially generated by the movement of the air through mainly the larger airways, producing various sounds in accordance with the patient's clinical presentation. Despite the wealth of articles

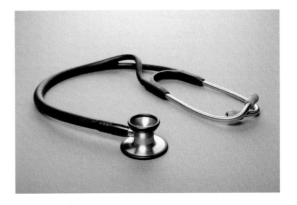

Figure 7.9 Stethoscope. Daniel Loiselle/istockphoto.com

dedicated to this topic, there is still no formal defined nomenclature for the most common breath sounds that are heard (Pasterkamp *et al.* 1987, Wilkins *et al.* 1990, Gross *et al.* 2000, Mangione and Duffy 2003). The main reason is that oral or written description of what one hears with a stethoscope requires an ability to describe one sensory experience by analogy to others. Despite being easier than cardiac auscultation, pulmonary auscultation remains hampered by a descriptive and confusing terminology (Mangione and Nieman 1999).

The most common breath sounds are described in the following sections using the classification that the authors have both used over the course of their careers.

Breath sounds can be classified into two main categories: normal or abnormal. They originate in the large airways where air velocity and turbulence caused by secretions, for example, induce vibrations in the airway walls. Examples of breath sounds are available at **http://www.rale.ca/repository.htm**.

Normal breath sounds

Normal breath sounds are a variety of high, medium, and low-pitch frequencies that originate in the large airways. Normal lung tissue attenuates the higher frequency sounds, resulting in softer, lower-pitched sounds audible in the periphery during inspiration and briefly during expiration (Webber and Pryor 1993).

Abnormal breath sounds

Crackles

Crackles are discontinuous, explosive, 'popping' sounds that originate within the airways. They are heard when an obstructed airway suddenly opens and the pressures on either side of the obstruction suddenly equilibrate, resulting in transient, distinct vibrations in the airway wall. The airway obstruction can be caused by either accumulation of secretions within the airway lumen or airway collapse due to pressure from inflammation or oedema in the surrounding pulmonary tissue.

Crackles can be heard during inspiration when intrathoracic negative pressure results in opening of the airways or on expiration when thoracic positive pressure forces collapsed or blocked airways open. Crackles are heard more commonly during inspiration than expiration.

They are significant as they imply either accumulation of fluid secretions or exudate within airways, or inflammation and oedema in the pulmonary tissue.

Wheeze

Wheezes are continuous musical tones that are most commonly heard at end inspiration or early expiration. They result as a collapsed airway gradually opens during inspiration or gradually starts to close during expiration. As the airway diameter becomes smaller, the air flow increases, resulting in harmonic vibration of the airway wall and thus the musical tonal quality.

Wheezes can be classified as either high-pitched or low-pitched wheezes. High-pitched normally infers that bronchospasm is the cause and low-pitched wheeze normally means that sputum is the cause. Wheezes may be monophonic (a single pitch heard over an isolated area) or polyphonic (multiple pitches heard over a variable area of the lung).

Wheezes are significant as they imply decreased airway lumen diameter. This may be due to thickening of reactive airway walls, or collapse of airways due to pressure from surrounding pulmonary disease or the presence of secretions in the airways.

Bronchial breath sounds

Bronchial breath sounds are loud, harsh, high-pitched sounds with a short pause between inspiration and expiration and a distinctive, hollow expiratory sound. Normal bronchial breath sounds can be heard by placing the stethoscope over the trachea.

Bronchial breath sounds occur over consolidated lung tissue where there is no active ventilation occurring secondary to the infective process of pneumonia. The sounds that are heard therefore occur due to normal breath sounds being transmitted through the consolidated tissue. Bronchial breath sounds can also be heard over the upper level of a pleural effusion, as the surface level of the liquid augments sound transmission, and over an area of lung collapse with a patent bronchus.

Pleural rub

Pleural rub is a sound that is similar to creaking leather or the sound of walking in snow, and is caused primarily by inflammation between the parietal and visceral pleural membranes.

Table 7.5 Frequently heard breath sounds with corresponding clinical features

	Diagnosis	Percussion note	Palpation
Fine crackles	Interstitial lung disease	Normal	Normal
Course crackles	1 Secretions in larger airways (chest infection)	Normal	Palpable secretions
	2 Possible sublobar collapse (atelectasis)	Slightly dull	Decreased expansion at affected zone
Low-pitched wheeze	Secretions in smaller airway (chest infection)	Normal	Palpable secretions
High-pitched wheeze	Bronchospasm (asthma)	Normal	Normal
Bronchial breathing	1 Consolidation (pneumonia)	Dull	Decreased expansion over affected zone
	2 Pleural effusion	Stony dull	
	3 Collapse with a patent bronchus	Dull	
Pleural rub	Pleural inflammation, infection, or neoplasm	Normal	Normal
Stridor	Laryngeal obstruction (foreign body, swelling, or tumour)	Normal	Normal
Absent	1 Pneumothorax	Hyper-resonant	All would have decreased expansion over affected side
	2 Pleural effusion	Stony dull	
	3 Lobar collapse		
	4 Obese patients		
	5 Poor position	Dull	
	6 Pain		

Stridor

Stridor is a harsh, high-pitched sound audible from the end of the bed on inspiration. It indicates laryngeal/tracheal obstruction that is a potential life-threatening emergency.

Table 7.5 shows common breath sounds with corresponding clinical features.

As Table 7.5 demonstrates, there are several possibilities for the cause of certain breath sound findings on auscultation, so this is a skill that must be used as part of a full respiratory assessment. For example, if a patient presents following chest trauma with rib fractures and begins to become tachycardic and hypotensive, as well as having absent breath sounds unilaterally and decreased expansion, you might expect them to have a pneumothorax.

How can I be sure where I am listening?

It is very difficult to be entirely accurate as to which lobe you are listening to when you are assessing a patient. It is therefore much easier to divide up the thorax into zones marked by easily found bony landmarks (see Table 7.6).

This is shown in **Figure 7.10**.

Context

 When to use auscultation

Auscultation is a tool that is used as part of a respiratory assessment that would incorporate everything from the patient's history to arterial blood gases and chest X-rays.

Table 7.6 Division of the thorax

Upper zone	2 cm above medial third of clavicle to axilla
Mid zone	Axilla to xiphisternum
Lower zone	Xiphisternum to diaphragm (sixth rib anteriorly, tenth rib posteriorly)

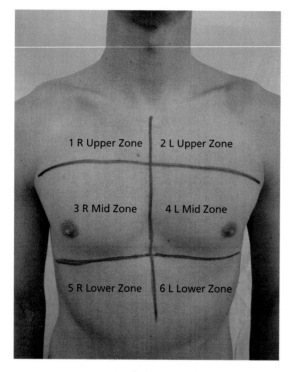

Figure 7.10 Division of the thorax used to guide stethoscope placement.

It can therefore be used on any patient in any clinical setting.

It is a useful tool to assess a patient quickly and at the bedside if they demonstrate any deterioration in respiratory function such as an increase in respiratory rate or work of breathing, or a decrease in oxygen saturations.

Alternative interventions

Interpretation of the clinical significance of auscultation findings can be facilitated by the addition of simple techniques that can be carried out during and after lung auscultation.

- **Vocal resonance** is the sound of speech transmitted through the chest wall to the stethoscope. Normal lung tissue attenuates high-frequency sounds, allowing lower frequencies to dominate and resulting in a low-pitched mumble. Consolidated lung tissue transmits higher frequencies better, resulting in normal speech being heard. This is normally assessed by asking the patient to repeatedly say '99' (Webber and Pryor 1993).
- **Percussion** is the technique of tapping the chest wall (using the middle finger of the right hand to tap the middle finger of the left, which is resting on the chest wall) to assess the resonance generated when the chest wall vibrates over the underlying tissue. Normal resonance is generated over aerated lung tissue (Webber and Pryor 1993) (see **Figure 7.11**).
- Palpation of the thoracic cage with the hands allows accurate assessment of chest expansion, equality of movement, and any additional palpable vibrations potentially resulting from secretions within the chest.

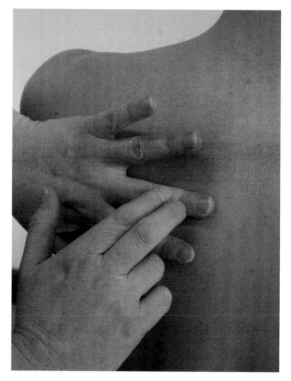

Figure 7.11 Percussion technique for assessment of chest wall resonance.

Interpreting findings

Auscultation findings cannot be interpreted independently and will need to be interpreted alongside a good patient history and all the other components of the respiratory assessment. Auscultation is also a skill that needs practice over a significant period of time, and is best learnt alongside an experienced practitioner who will be able to give feedback about the breath sounds that are being listened to.

Special considerations

- **Body size**: size can influence respiratory sound. There is a distinct quality of sounds produced that Pasterkamp *et al.* (1997) attribute to the acoustic transmission through thinner chest walls and smaller lungs. Auscultation can be very difficult to carry out accurately in the obese population due to the larger distance the sound has to travel from the lung to the skin surface.

- **Body position** can significantly hinder interpretation of lung sounds. Ideally the patient should be seated with legs down to avoid compression of the lower zones (see **Figure 7.12**). Modification may be required in critically ill ventilated patients who are unable to move, rendering posterior chest wall assessment difficult.

- Patients who have had surgery that has meant large **dressings over the chest wall**, for example following some thoracic surgery and some plastics procedures such as reconstructive breast surgery and burns victims.

- **Ventilated patients**: auscultation sounds can be markedly altered by the transmission of sounds produced by mechanical ventilators (Lichtenstein *et al.* 2004).

- If undertaking the skill in the patient's home or on a busy ward, remember that **environmental noise** can hinder the procedure.

- Consider asking the patient to cough prior to assessment if **secretions** are audible within the upper respiratory tract.

- Chest drains, humidification systems, and water in breathing circuits can transmit **additional sounds**, making interpretation difficult.

- **Elderly patients** frequently present with multiple pathology, which may result in multiple sounds being heard that may be difficult to interpret. For example, left ventricular failure with underlying infection.

- In all of the above patients, we would need to rely on other components of the respiratory assessment to be able to treat them accurately.

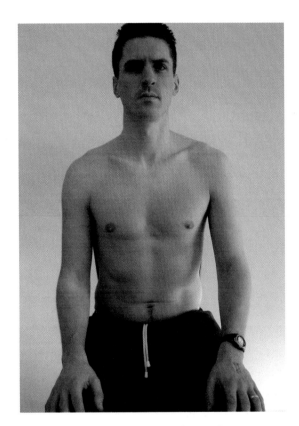

Figure 7.12 Optimal body position for auscultation.

Procedure

Preparation

Prepare yourself

Ensure you understand how the stethoscope works and how you interpret the findings. Wash your hands.

Prepare the patient

The procedure should be fully explained to the patient (see Discussing the procedure box). The patient should be suitably undressed and in an appropriate position to enable a complete assessment (see Special considerations box and Figure 7.12). Ensure that the patient's dignity is maintained at all times.

Prepare the equipment/environment

Clean the stethoscope according to the manufacturer's instructions, ensuring the diaphragm is dry prior to contact with the patient's skin. Where possible, try to assess in a quiet environment to make assessment easier.

Discussing the procedure with the patient and family

- Explain what is being assessed and why.

- Explain that you will warm the end of the stethoscope that will be in contact with the patient's skin.

- Give clear instructions to the patient as to what is required during the assessment and demonstrate if necessary.

- Make sure the patient knows to let the nurse know if the position or the assessment is uncomfortable.

Step-by-step guide to lung auscultation

Step	Rationale
1 Introduce yourself, confirm the patient's identity, explain the procedure, and obtain consent.	To identify the patient correctly and gain informed consent.
2 Pull the curtains around the bed space.	To maintain privacy.
3 Undertake a full respiratory assessment.	Lung auscultation should not be interpreted independently and should form part of a complete respiratory assessment.
4 Place earpieces facing forwards into the ears.	To enable transmission of sound into the ears.
5 Tap diaphragm with finger and listen for sound. If no sound heard, twist tubing to ensure correct alignment with diaphragm.	To test the stethoscope and ensure alignment of the stethoscope tubing with the diaphragm.
6 Expose the patient's skin, ensuring patient dignity is maintained at all times.	To prevent transmission of extraneous sounds (e.g. nightwear).
7 Place diaphragm of stethoscope flat against chest wall. (NB body hair can interfere with contact of diaphragm with the skin, resulting in the transmission of sounds similar to crackles).	To ensure maximum contact with the skin.
8 Ask patient to breath in and out slowly through the mouth.	To prevent turbulence from the nose transmitting extraneous sounds.
9 Listen for normal, abnormal, reduced, or absent breath sounds and any added sounds.	To assess for pathological lung sounds produced within the chest.

10 Move stethoscope across the chest wall (see Figure 7.12 and Table 7.6), comparing alternate sides of the chest anteriorly and posteriorly.

To facilitate assessment of the whole chest and all lung fields.

11 After completion of assessment, remove stethoscope and assist patient with nightwear and repositioning as required.

To maintain patient dignity and comfort.

Following the procedure

Clean the stethoscope according to the manufacturer's instructions, as surface colonies of microorganisms may be transferred on the stethoscope. Document the findings of your assessment.

Reflection and evaluation

When you have completed the respiratory assessment including auscultation, think about the following questions:

1 Could you hear breath sounds everywhere?
2 Were they normal, abnormal, or reduced?
3 Were there any added sounds?
4 Were the auscultation findings consistent with what you anticipated?
5 Were you able to interpret the lung sounds in light of the patient's medical condition?
6 Were you able to answer the patient's questions?
7 Is there anything that you would do differently next time?
8 Would it have been beneficial to have used a double-ended teaching stethoscope?

Further learning opportunities

At the next available opportunity, try and use the stethoscope on yourself or colleagues.

- Does it make a difference to the sound heard if the stethoscope tubing comes into contact with your colleague's arm, clothes, or bedding?
- Does it make a difference if your colleague talks to you during the assessment?
- Ask your colleague to breathe in and out through their mouth and then through their nose. Does this make a difference and why?

Reminders

Don't forget to:

- Clean the stethoscope before and after your assessment.
- Ensure the patient is well positioned and dignity is maintained at all times.
- Tap the diaphragm to ensure correct alignment prior to assessment.

Ⓠ Patient scenarios

Consider what you should do in the following situations, then turn to the end of this skill to check your answers.

1 Patient A has become pyrexial 2 days post-laparotomy with slightly increased work of breathing. What would you expect to hear on auscultation and what could be the cause?
2 Patient B has fractured three ribs falling off a horse. They are now in a slumped position in bed and have absent breath sounds in both lower zones. What are the possible causes?
3 Patient C is mechanically ventilated. Your assessment has shown stable respiratory rate, oxygen saturations, and arterial blood gases, and a clear chest X-ray. On auscultation you hear continuous added sounds on inspiration and expiration that you were not expecting. What might be the cause?

Website

 http://www.oxfordtextbooks.co.uk/orc/ endacott

You may find it helpful to work through our short online quiz and additional scenarios intended to help you to develop and apply the skills in this chapter.

References

Aweida D and Kelsey CJ (1990). Accuracy and reliability of physical therapists in auscultating tape recorded lung sounds. *Physiotherapy Canada*, **42**, 279–82.

Brooks D and Thomas J (1995). Interrater reliability of auscultation of breath sounds among physical therapists. *Physical Therapy*, **75**(12), 1082–8.

Brooks D, Wilson L, and Kelsey CK (1993). Accuracy and reliability of 'specialized' physical therapists in auscultating tape recorded lung sounds. *Physiotherapy Canada*, **45**, 21–4.

Gross V, Dittmar A, Penzel T, Schuttler F, and von Wichert P (2000). The relationship between normal lung sounds, age, and gender. *American Journal of Respiratory Critical Care Medicine*, **162**, 905–9.

Lichtenstein D, Goldstein I, Mourgeon MD, Cluzel P, Grenier P, and Rouby JJ (2004). Comparative diagnostic performances of auscultation, chest radiography, and lung ultrasonography in acute respiratory distress syndrome. *Anesthesiology*, **100**, 9–15.

Mangione S and Duffy D (2003). The teaching of chest auscultation during primary care training: has anything changed in the 1990s? *Chest*, **124**, 1430–6.

Mangione S and Nieman LZ (1999). Pulmonary auscultatory skills during training in internal medicine and family practice. *American Journal of Respiratory Critical Care Medicine*, **159**, 1119–24.

Pasterkamp H, Kraman SS, and Wodicka GR (1997). Respiratory sounds. Advances beyond the stethoscope. *American Journal of Respiratory Critical Care Medicine*, **156**, 974–87.

Pasterkamp H, Montgomery M, and Wiebicke W (1987). Nomenclature used by health care professionals to describe breath sounds in asthma. *Chest*, **92**, 346–52.

Webber BA and Pryor JA (1993). *Physiotherapy for respiratory and cardiac problems*. Churchill Livingstone, London.

Wilkins RL, Dexter JR, Murphy RL, DelBono EA, and Delbono JR (1990). Lung sound nomenclature survey. *Chest*, **98**, 886–9.

Useful further reading and websites

Hoevers J and Loudon RG (1990). Measuring crackles. *Chest*, **98**, 1240–3.

Moore KL (1992). *Clinically oriented anatomy*. Williams and Wilkins, London.

Examples of breath sounds are available at: **http://www.rale.ca/repository.htm** and at: **http://www.cvmbs.colostate.edu/clinsci/callan/breath_sounds.htm**

 Answers to patient scenarios

1 You would expect to hear course crackles throughout chest likely to be caused by a post-operative chest infection.

2 The possible causes could be:
   a) Pain secondary to the trauma causing reduced tidal volumes and subsequent absent breath sounds in lower zones. Assess patient's pain score as part of the assessment.
   b) Poor position can result in compression of the lower zones, resulting in absent breath sounds. Always attempt to have patient in optimal position before assessment.

3 The most likely cause for the unexpected breath sounds is transmission from the mechanical ventilator.

7.8 Intrapleural drainage

This is an advanced skill. You *must* check whether you can assist with or undertake this skill, in line with local policy.

Definition

Intrapleural or 'chest' drainage is the insertion of a drain for the purpose of removing fluids or air (or both) from the pleural space.

It is important to remember that:

● A chest drain may be inserted for a number of reasons.
● A patient with a chest drain will require skilled nursing assessment, monitoring, and care, due to the potential for serious complications.
● Insertion of a chest drain is likely to be frightening and painful for the patient, and an indwelling chest drain tube may cause further pain or discomfort.

- Chest drain clamps should be available (kept with the patient) in the event of accidental disconnection.
- As a general rule, chest drains should not be left clamped, as a tension pneumothorax may develop. A bubbling chest drain should never be clamped (Laws *et al.* 2003).

Prior knowledge

Before undertaking the care of a patient with a chest drain, make sure you are familiar with:

1 Respiratory anatomy and physiology, with particular regard to the pleura.
2 Cardiovascular physiology, with regard to the pulmonary vasculature and the matching of lung perfusion to ventilation.
3 Reasons that patients may require a chest drain.
4 The different types of chest drains and bottles used in your Trust.
5 Your employer's policy on management of chest drains.
6 The signs of respiratory distress, tension pneumothorax, and circulatory failure.

Background

There are two pleural membranes: the visceral pleura covers the external surface of both lungs and the parietal pleura lines the thoracic cavity (see **Figure 7.13**). The pleural space is normally a potential space, containing a very small volume of fluid regulated by the pleura. The

pressure within the space is negative, which holds the membranes together, thereby holding the lungs to the chest wall so they expand and recoil during inspiration and expiration (Tortora and Anagnostakos 1990, Allibone 2003). These features mean:

- The pleura are able to slide over each other as the lungs expand and contract during inspiration and expiration.
- The lungs are held to the chest wall, which means the lung expands during inspiration and recoils during expiration (expiration is a passive process, aided by the elasticity of the ribcage and lung tissue).

Fluid or air may fill the pleural space as a result of disease processes or trauma. If air or excess fluid enters the pleural space, negative pressure will be lost, which may cause partial or complete lung collapse (Bourke and Brewis 1998). The patient may well show signs of respiratory distress, such as breathlessness and a raised respiratory rate.

Pneumothorax

Air may enter the pleural space for a number of reasons. Pneumothoraces can be classified as follows (Allibone 2003):

- **Spontaneous**: usually occurring in young, thin men as a consequence of ruptured apical blebs or bullae (Bourke and Brewis 1998). It may also occur in patients with underlying respiratory disease such as asthma or COPD.
- **Traumatic**: as a consequence of internal chest injuries such as fractured ribs or penetrating injuries, or from oesophageal or tracheal rupture (Bourke and Brewis 1998).
- **Iatrogenic**: as a consequence of central line insertion, positive pressure ventilation with high airway pressures, or surgery.
- **Tension**: this is a medical emergency and requires prompt intervention by the insertion of a 12 or 14 Fg IV cannula into the second intercostal space, midclavicular line on the affected side, or chest drain (Clarke 2003), as it may be life-threatening. It occurs if the opening into the pleural space acts as a one-way valve, trapping air in the pleural space, so the volume of trapped air will increase with each breath.

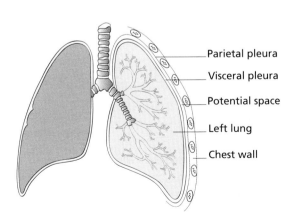

Figure 7.13 Anatomy of the lung showing the pleura.

Parietal pleura
Visceral pleura
Potential space
Left lung
Chest wall

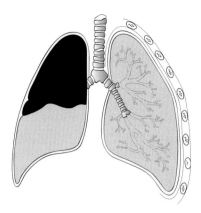

Figure 7.14 Right tension pneumothorax.

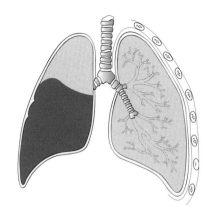

Figure 7.15 Right pleural effusion.

There is a consequent increase in pressure in the pleural space, which causes the lung to collapse on the affected side. This can cause the mediastinum and trachea to shift away from the affected side. Venous return to the heart is impaired and the cardiac chambers may also be compressed, leading to reduced cardiac output and low blood pressure (see **Figure 7.14**).

If a stethoscope were used to listen to the patient's chest, there would be no breath sounds on the affected side. If the chest were percussed, the affected side would sound hyper-resonant (see Section 7.7).

Haemothorax

Blood may enter the pleural space as a consequence of chest trauma, such as fractured ribs following a fall (if the patient is on anticoagulant therapy they will be at increased risk) or penetrating chest injuries. If blood loss into the pleural space is large, the patient may well show signs of shock.

Pleural effusion

As discussed previously, the pleura normally regulate the volume of fluid in the pleural space by balancing fluid filtration by the parietal pleura and fluid absorption by the visceral pleura (Bourke and Brewis 1998). Excess fluid may accumulate in conditions such as:

● Left ventricular failure or renal failure (increased filtration due to increased capillary pressure).

● Low albumin levels (increased filtration due to low plasma oncotic pressure).
● Disease of the pleura (increased filtration due to increased 'leakage' from capillaries).
● Disease of the lymphatic system (reduced absorption due to lymphatic obstruction by a tumour).
● Pneumonia (due to inflammation of the pleura).

Pleural effusions may also be classified as transudates or exudates. Transudates have low protein content (Bourke and Brewis 1998) and are often caused by problems outside of the lungs, such as heart or kidney failure. Exudates have high protein content and are often caused by disease of the pleura, such as primary (mesothelioma) or secondary (lung or breast) malignancy (Bourke and Brewis 1998) (see **Figure 7.15**).

If a stethoscope were used to listen to the patient's chest, the breath sounds would be muffled on the affected side. If the chest were percussed, it would sound stony dull (see Section 7.7).

Empyema

Empyema, or pus in the pleural cavity, occurs when a pleural effusion becomes infected with bacteria and is particularly associated with aspiration pneumonia (Bourke and Brewis 1998, Gomersall 2003). Although this can often be treated straightforwardly with a chest drain, some patients with an empyema may need surgery. This may be open (making a surgical incision in the patient's chest such as a thoracotomy) or using a scope (a small hole is made to enable a scope to be introduced into the patient's chest) (Gomersall 2003).

Chylothorax

The presence of chyle (digested fat) in the pleural space may be caused by damage to the thoracic duct following thoracic surgery or chest trauma, incorrect placement of a parenteral feeding catheter, or malignancy of the thoracic duct (Bourke and Brewis 1998). Chyle is milky in appearance.

How does a chest drain work?

A chest drain should allow fluid or air to escape from the pleural cavity and not re-enter it. This can be achieved with:

- An underwater seal chest drain bottle (see **Figure 7.16**). The chest drain tubing is connected to a tube incorporated with the chest drain bottle (which is filled to a marked priming line with sterile water). The end of the tube in the chest drain bottle sits approximately 2 cm under the water (Allibone 2003). This means that air can escape or 'bubble' out, but not re-enter the chest drain tube. Fluid will drain by gravity; therefore the bottle must be kept below the level of the patient's chest.
- A flutter valve system: this is used with a bag, rather than a bottle, for drainage of air. Fluid will tend to block the valve (Laws *et al.* 2003), so this system should not be used for draining effusions, empyemas, or haemothoraces. This system can allow greater mobility for patients.
- A drainage bag may be used for patients with pleural effusions. Fluid will drain by gravity and, again, the bag should be kept below the level of the patient's chest.
- The drain tubing should be secured to the patient's skin by a suture and a closure suture sited (purse-string sutures are not recommended; Laws *et al.* 2003).

Context

 ## When to use chest drainage

Patients may require the insertion of a chest drain for a number of reasons. This may be in an acute situation, for example in a trauma patient with a haemothorax, or may be associated with more chronic conditions, such as effusions or empyema (see **Table 7.7** for an explanation of these terms).

The urgency for chest drain insertion may depend on the degree of respiratory or circulatory failure. Some patients have chest drains inserted into the mediastinum and pericardium following cardiac surgery – these are not dealt with specifically in this section.

The size of the chest drain tube inserted may depend on the underlying cause and the preference of the person performing the procedure. In general, small drains are more comfortable for patients and may be used to drain pneumothoraces, effusions, and empyemas. Large bore chest drains are recommended for draining acute haemothoraces (Laws *et al.* 2003).

The underlying cause may also determine where the chest drain is sited. The most common site for chest drain insertion is the midaxillary line at the fourth, fifth, or sixth

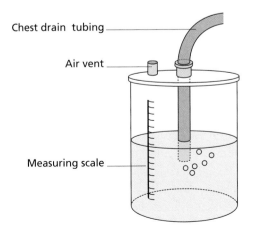

Figure 7.16 A chest drain bottle.

Table 7.7 Some terms and definitions for air or fluid in the pleural space

Term	Definition
Pneumothorax	Air in the pleural space.
Haemothorax	Blood in the pleural space.
Pleural effusion	Fluid in the pleural space.
Empyema	Pus in the pleural space.
Chylothorax	Digested fat from the lymphatic system in the pleural space.

intercostal space, to minimize risk to underlying structures such as the internal mammary artery and to avoid damaging muscle or breast tissue (Bourke and Brewis 1998, Laws *et al.* 2003). The insertion site may also depend on where the underlying problem is sited. Apical pneumothoraces may need a drain in the second intercostal space in the midclavicular line, while a loculated pleural effusion may require ultrasound guidance to site the drain where the collection is (Laws *et al.* 2003). The tip of the chest drain tube should be aimed towards the apex of the lung for a pneumothorax (because air rises) and towards the base of the lung for fluid (Laws *et al.* 2003).

Potential problems

There are several potential problems associated with chest drain insertion and management, so this is where your nursing assessment skills are very important!

1. Pain

This can be a problem both during the insertion of the chest drain and afterwards, while the drain is in place. Premedication should be given prior to the chest drain being inserted, together with a local anaesthetic (Laws *et al.* 2003). Following the procedure, ensure that the patient's pain is assessed regularly (using a pain assessment tool) and that analgesia is given as required. If analgesia is inadequate, inform the medical team and ask them to review the patient's medication. The pain may be so severe that some patients may require opiates to control it.

2. Lack of drainage

This could be due to kinked tubing causing a blockage, or may occur if the underwater seal chest drain bottle becomes full of fluid, as there is increased pressure to overcome before fluid can drain (Compeau and Johnston 1999). Check the tubing and correct any kinks, and change the bottle if it is becoming full (possibly before it reaches the maximum mark). It is also important to remember that lack of drainage could be due to resolution of the underlying problem.

3. Accidental disconnection

If this happens, the chest tube should be clamped immediately, to prevent air from re-entering the pleural space

(Allibone 2003). The drain and bottle should be reconnected as soon as possible using a new sterile system. A chest X-ray may be required, so a member of the medical team must be informed. There does not seem to be definitive advice regarding the taping of connections to prevent the tubing coming apart (Allibone 2003) – one concern is that any disconnection might be hidden by tape (Avery 2000).

4. The chest drain bottle falls over

Stand the bottle upright again and make sure that the end of the bottle tube is under the water/fluid level. This may mean that the chest tube has to be briefly clamped and the bottle tipped to reposition drained fluid correctly.

5. The chest drain falls out

The wound should be sealed using a closure suture if present (purse-string sutures are not recommended, see Laws *et al.* 2003) or an air-occlusive dressing. Medical staff must be informed and the patient's vital signs (pulse, respiration rate, blood pressure) should be checked and monitored.

6. Subcutaneous or 'surgical' emphysema

Air may enter the subcutaneous tissue if the drainage holes of the chest drain move out of the pleural space, or if the tube becomes blocked (Avery 2000) or is clamped (Laws *et al.* 2003). This can be very uncomfortable or distressing for the patient. If this happens, the chest drain should be unclamped and the tube unblocked or a new tube re-sited.

7. Other problems

Other problems that may occur during chest drainage include:

- Perforation of the heart, liver, lung, aorta, stomach (Allibone 2003), or pulmonary artery. The risk of this occurring is reduced if blunt dissection is used to make an opening in the chest wall for the chest drain, rather than using the trocar found with larger chest drain tubes (Compeau and Johnston 1999).
- Infection may occur at the insertion site or within the pleural space.

Special considerations

- Occasionally, patients who have had large pleural effusions drained have developed what is called 're-expansion' pulmonary oedema (Laws *et al.* 2003). For this reason, it is suggested that no more than 1.5 litres be drained at any one time, or that drainage should be slowed to 500 ml/hour (Laws *et al.* 2003).

- Sometimes, suction may be applied to the chest drain bottle in order to assist lung re-expansion in cases where a pneumothorax has not resolved. This will require a low-pressure suction unit, with lower pressures than the high-pressure suction units used for oral suction, which are normally found on the wall behind the bed in hospital wards. The medical team will determine the level of suction required. If the air leak is large, this may require the changing of the chest drain bottle to an appropriate type designed for this purpose – this type of chest drain may require a high-pressure suction unit. If you are unsure, seek advice from senior colleagues. If suction is applied to the chest drain bottle, *the suction unit should not be switched off without first disconnecting the attached suction tubing.* If this is not done, there will be nowhere for air draining from the pleural cavity to escape to (the chest drain bottle is normally vented to atmosphere, commonly where the suction tubing attaches to the bottle). This could lead to a tension pneumothorax developing.

- As a general rule, chest drains should not be clamped, unless directed to do so by the patient's medical team (chest drains are sometimes clamped for a period of time prior to their removal). This is because of the risk of a tension pneumothorax developing. If the drain is clamped, the patient should be closely monitored and should not leave the ward. If the patient becomes breathless or develops subcutaneous emphysema, the clamp should be removed and the medical team informed (Laws *et al.* 2003).

- There is no need to clamp a chest drain if the patient is mobilizing or needs to attend the X-ray department, but you should ensure that the patient understands that the chest drain bottle needs to be kept upright and below the level of their chest.

Observations and monitoring

After a chest drain has been sited, the patient should be carefully monitored, with close observation of their respiratory status including respiratory rate, oxygen saturation, oxygen requirements (if receiving supplementary oxygen), effort of breathing, and breath sounds.

The chest drain and tubing should also be observed for the following:

- 'Swinging': fluid in the tubing of the chest drain should move up and down with the patient's respiration. This reflects changes in intra-thoracic pressure. As the patient breathes in (generating negative intra-thoracic pressure), fluid is drawn up the tubing. As the patient breathes out (intra-thoracic pressure returns to atmospheric pressure), fluid drops down the tubing. If this movement is not seen, the tubing may be kinked or blocked, or the underlying problem has resolved.

- 'Bubbling': this shows that air is draining from the pleural space. It may be visible all the time, or when the patient coughs (you may need to ask them to cough). Again, if the bubbling stops, it may mean that the tubing is kinked, that the tube is displaced, or that the pneumothorax has resolved.

- Drainage volumes should be recorded as often as the patient's condition demands (a patient who has had surgery may require more frequent observations than a patient having a pleural effusion drained). Senior colleagues and medical staff should be informed if the volume suddenly increases or hourly volumes are high (more than 100 ml/hour; Nelson and Tully 1998). Don't forget to check the patient's vital signs for evidence of shock.

- The tubing should be secured to prevent it falling out (Laws *et al.* 2003). This includes the use of sutures around the tubing to secure it to the patient's skin at the insertion site, plus additional taping around the tube, again to secure it to the skin.

- The dressing should be checked and changed according to your Trust's infection control/tissue viability/ward's policies. There appears to be little evidence to support one particular type of dressing (Godden and Hiley 1998, Laws *et al.* 2003).

Procedure

Assisting with chest drain insertion

Your role in the procedures for chest drain insertion may involve assisting a member of the medical team or a senior colleague and helping prepare the patient physically (such as positioning or checking/administering medication) and emotionally (providing explanations or support).

Chest drain removal

Your role in chest drain removal may involve assisting a senior colleague to prepare the patient or removing the drain, which will require two people. The patient may be asked to perform one of the following just prior to chest drain removal, depending on your employer's practice/guidelines:

- A Valsalva manoeuvre (holding the breath while trying to breathe out against a closed glottis) (McMahon-Parkes 1997, Laws *et al.* 2003).
- Expiration (Laws *et al.* 2003).
- Take a deep breath and hold their breath (Mallett and Dougherty 2000).

One person should remove the drain with a brisk, firm movement and the second person should tie the closure suture (Laws *et al.* 2003) or apply an occlusive dressing over the site (Allibone 2003).

Preparation

Prepare yourself

Ensure you understand what the procedure involves and what you may need to monitor during and after it. Check that you know what equipment is required and that you understand how it works.

Prepare the patient

The procedure should be fully explained to the patient (see Discussing the procedure box).

Prepare the equipment

For chest drain insertion, you may be asked to prepare a selection of chest drain tubes, sutures, dressings, cleaning solutions, or chest drain bottles.

For chest drain removal, you are likely to require dressings, clamps, stitch-cutters, and an appropriate disposal container for the chest drain bottle.

Discussing the procedure with the patient and family

- Explain what you are going to do and why it is necessary/important.

- Explain that the procedure is likely to be uncomfortable, but will be brief.

Step-by-step guide to assisting with chest drain insertion

Step	Rationale
1 Introduce yourself, confirm the patient's identity, explain the procedure, and obtain consent.	To identify the patient correctly and gain informed consent.
2 Ensure the patient receives prescribed analgesia prior to the procedure.	To ensure the patient does not experience unnecessary pain/discomfort.
3 Explain that you will be monitoring them closely afterwards for a period of time and that this is normal practice. Explain that they will need a chest X-ray after the procedure.	To reassure the patient and make sure that they are fully informed.

4	Assist with the procedure as required. It will be carried out by a doctor. Afterwards, dress the site with an appropriate dressing.	To make sure the procedure goes smoothly and is as pain-free as possible. To keep the site clean and dry and to prevent air leakage.
5	Ensure that the patient is comfortable and that they have a pain assessment at an appropriate time and receive prescribed analgesia if needed.	To ensure good pain relief is achieved.
6	Wash your hands.	To prevent cross-infection.

Step-by-step guide to chest drain removal

Step		Rationale
1	Introduce yourself, confirm the patient's identity, explain the procedure, and obtain consent.	To identify the patient correctly and gain informed consent.
2	Ensure the patient receives prescribed analgesia prior to the procedure.	To ensure the patient does not experience unnecessary pain/discomfort.
3	Assess the patient, ensuring that there has been no sudden drainage/recommencing of bubbling via the chest drain.	To ensure patient safety.
4	Assist the patient into an upright position in bed.	Allows for better lung expansion and makes it easier for the patient to perform the chosen manoeuvre prior to chest drain removal.
5	Explain what you are going to do and what you wish the patient to do.	To ensure the patient understands what will happen.
6	Wash hands.	To reduce the risk of cross-infection for you and the patient.
7	Put on disposable apron and gloves.	To reduce the risk of cross-infection for you and the patient.
8	Remove the dressing from around the drain site and dispose of in clinical waste bag.	To reduce the risk of cross-infection for you and the patient.
9	Cut and remove the suture securing the tubing to the patient's skin, leaving the closure suture (if present) in place. Ensure that any sharps are disposed of correctly.	To ensure that the chest drain can be removed and the wound sealed afterwards. To prevent injury to you or the patient.

continued overleaf

10	Remind the patient what it is you want them to do.	To ensure the procedure happens correctly.
11	In a coordinated manner: The person removing the chest drain should ask the patient to perform the required manoeuvre and remove the chest drain with a brisk, smooth movement (Laws *et al.* 2003). The person managing the closing suture/dressing should pull/apply as the chest drain is removed.	To ensure that the chest drain is removed quickly and the wound is sealed.
12	Remind the patient that they should stop performing the manoeuvre and should breathe normally.	To promote patient comfort.
13	If required, a dressing should be applied to the wound site, according to local policy.	To promote wound healing.
14	The chest drain tubing and bottle should be disposed of in an appropriate container.	To prevent leakage of fluid and cross-infection.
15	Ensure that the patient is comfortable. See that they have a further pain assessment at an appropriate time and receive prescribed analgesia if needed.	To ensure good pain relief is achieved.
16	Explain that you will be monitoring them closely for a period of time and that this is normal practice. Explain that they will need a chest X-ray after the procedure.	To make sure the patient is fully aware of what will happen.
17	Wash your hands.	To prevent cross-infection.

Following the procedure

The patient's vital signs should be checked initially and then at regular intervals so that any deterioration in their respiratory or cardiovascular function can be detected and treated promptly. It is possible that the presenting problem may reoccur (or a new problem develop, such as bleeding). Any changes or deterioration should be reported to the medical team.

Reflection and evaluation

When you have cared for a patient with a chest drain, or helped to remove one, think about the following questions:

1 Why did the patient need a chest drain?
2 Did you observe any changes in the patient's respiratory observations after the drain was inserted compared to before?
3 Were you able to observe 'swinging' or 'bubbling' in the chest bottle and tubing?

Further learning opportunities

Try to get involved in chest drain insertion and removal. Assist a qualified nurse and gain confidence and skills in that way. Then try to get involved with minimal supervision.

Reminders

Don't forget:

- Never clamp a bubbling chest drain.
- To assess a patient's vital signs when the chest drain is removed.
- To ensure that the drain is kept below the level of the patient's chest.

 Patient scenarios

Consider what you should do in the following situations, then turn to the end of this skill to check your answers.

1 Patient A has been admitted with shortness of breath. You learn that when their chest is auscultated, their breath sounds are muffled, and when percussed, the sound is stony dull. What may be the problem?
2 Patient B has had a chest drain inserted for a pneumothorax. Bubbling has been observed in the chest drain bottle since it was inserted, but has now stopped. What could cause this?
3 What advice should you give to a patient who has a chest drain and is mobilizing?

Website

 http://www.oxfordtextbooks.co.uk/orc/ endacott

You may find it helpful to work through our short online quiz and additional scenarios intended to help you to develop and apply the skills in this chapter.

References

Allibone L (2003). Nursing management of chest drains. *Nursing Standard*, **17**(22), 45–54.

Avery S (2000). Insertion and management of chest drains. *Nursing Times Plus*, **96**(37), 3–6.

Bourke S and Brewis R (1998). *Lecture notes on respiratory medicine*, 5th edition. Blackwell, Oxford.

Clarke GM (2003). Chest injuries. In AD Bersten, N Soni, and TE Oh, eds. *Oh's intensive care manual*, 5th edition, pp. 719–29. Butterworth Heinemann, London.

Compeau C and Johnston M (1999). Chest tubes. In A Casson and M Johnston, eds. *Key topics in thoracic surgery*, pp. 42–5. Bios Scientific Publishers, Oxford.

Godden J and Hiley C (1998). Managing the patient with a chest drain: a review. *Nursing Standard*, **12**(32), 35–9.

Gomersall CD (2003). Lung infections. In AD Bersten, N Soni, and TE Oh, eds. *Oh's intensive care manual*, 5th edition, pp. 373–86. Butterworth Heinemann, London.

Laws D, Neville E, and Duffy J (2003). BTS guidelines for the insertion of a chest drain. *Thorax*, **58**(Suppl 2), 53–71.

Mallett J and Dougherty L (2000). *Royal Marsden manual of clinical nursing procedures*, 5th edition. Blackwell, Oxford.

McMahon-Parkes K (1997). Management of pleural drains. *Nursing Times*, **93**(52), 48–52.

Nelson S and Tully C (1998). Thoracic drainage. In C Shuldham, ed. *Cardiorespiratory nursing*, pp. 230–54. Cheltenham, Stanley Thornes.

Tortora GJ and Anagnostakos NP (1990). *Principles of anatomy and physiology*, 6th edition. Harper and Row, New York.

Useful further reading and websites

Griggs A (1998). Tracheostomy: suctioning and humidification. *Nursing Standard*, 13(2), 49–56 [online] **http://www.nursing-standard.co.uk/ archives/ns/vol13-02/v13w02p4953.pdf** accessed 25/10/07.

The *New England Journal of Medicine* has a video of chest drain insertion online at **http://content.nejm.org/ cgi/video/357/15/e15/**

 Answers to patient scenarios

1 Fluid in the pleural space – due to pleural effusion, haemothorax, or chylothorax.
2 The drain tubing may have become kinked or disconnected, or the pneumothorax may have resolved.
3 Make sure they keep the drain upright and below the level of their chest.

7.9 Endotracheal intubation

This is an advanced skill. You *must* check whether you can assist with or undertake this skill, in line with local policy.

Definition

Endotracheal intubation is the passing of a tube, via the mouth or nose, into the trachea. A patient with an endotracheal tube may breathe spontaneously or with support from a mechanical ventilator.

Unless you have a placement in intensive care, the emergency department, or an operating theatre, you are most likely to be involved in endotracheal intubation if your patient has suffered a cardiopulmonary arrest.

It is important to remember that:

- A patient who requires endotracheal intubation in a ward setting will be critically ill – their friends and family will need support.
- In most cases, there are warning signs that a patient is deteriorating for some hours before they become ill enough to require intubation (Department of Health 2000). Thorough assessment of the patient's vital signs, particularly respiratory rate, heart rate, blood pressure, and oxygen requirements, can alert you to this. Medical staff must be informed of signs of patient deterioration promptly.
- The ward emergency trolley should have equipment and a drugs box to use during a cardiorespiratory arrest. Emergency equipment must be available and work correctly – it should be checked daily.
- Drugs for planned intubation are usually stored separately from emergency drugs.
- The connector in the end of the endotracheal tube needs to be secure, particularly if the tube has been cut to size. If the connector is not secure it may fall out, leaving the patient disconnected from any ventilator equipment and therefore at risk of death if they are unable to breathe spontaneously.
- Sedation is almost always needed for the patient to be able to tolerate an endotracheal tube.
- A patient with an endotracheal tube will probably be moved to an intensive care unit for ongoing management.

Prior knowledge

Before becoming involved in caring for a patient requiring endotracheal intubation, make sure that you are familiar with:

- Airway anatomy and physiology.
- Signs of respiratory distress, respiratory failure, and circulatory failure.
- The local procedure to summon help in the event of a cardiopulmonary arrest or other emergency.
- The location of emergency equipment and how it works.
- The location of emergency drugs.
- The location of drugs for emergency intubation.

Background

Endotracheal intubation is undertaken to provide the patient with a secure airway, facilitate artificial ventilation, enable secretions to be cleared from their chest, and provide a degree of protection from aspiration of gastric contents or saliva (Joynt 2003). As mentioned earlier, there are several situations in which a patient may require the insertion of an endotracheal tube.

This may be an acute situation, such as:

- Respiratory failure – this could be due to either acute respiratory failure, e.g. caused by a severe pneumonia, or chronic respiratory failure, e.g. COPD. Indications for intubation would include a low arterial oxygen concentration, a high arterial carbon dioxide concentration, or both.
- Severe illness of any cause, sufficient to compromise the patient's ability to maintain spontaneous respiration.
- Airway obstruction or significant risk of inability to maintain the airway.
- Cardiorespiratory arrest.

Alternatively it may be a planned situation, such as:

- An operation or a procedure such as cardioversion that requires anaesthesia.
- A procedure such as a computed tomography (CT) scan for a patient with a significantly impaired conscious level, as they may not be able to maintain their airway.

Types of endotracheal tube

Endotracheal tubes are made from PVC and are disposable. They come in a range of sizes, from those small

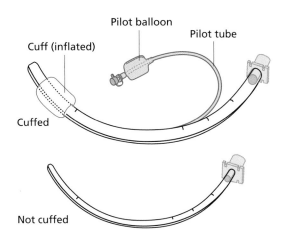

Figure 7.17 A cuffed and uncuffed endotracheal tube.

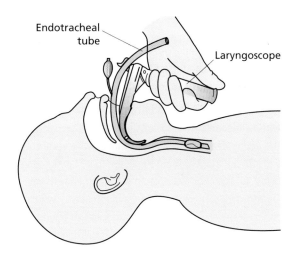

Figure 7.18 Endotracheal intubation via the oral route.

enough for neonates to those large enough for adult males. They are available in 0.5 mm increments. The size of an endotracheal tube relates to the internal diameter of the tube in mm – a size 9.0 tube has a 9 mm internal diameter. Generally, a size 7.0–8.0 tube is used for adult females and 8.0–9.0 for adult males (Joynt 2003).

Endotracheal tubes may or may not have a cuff, depending on whether the patient is a child or an adult (see **Figure 7.17**). Generally speaking, endotracheal tubes for children do not have cuffs whereas those for adults do. Pressure or damage to the mucosa of a child's trachea by the cuff of an endotracheal tube could cause swelling after the tube is taken out (Advanced Life Support Group 2005). This could lead to airway obstruction.

If the endotracheal tube is cuffed, it will have a pilot balloon and tube, as illustrated in Figure 7.17. Air is instilled through a one-way valve on the pilot balloon using an air-filled 10 ml syringe until an air-seal is achieved (approximately 5–10 ml). This means that air/gases can inflate the patient's lungs during inspiration without escaping. The pressure in the cuff should be checked using a pressure gauge and should be between 20 mmHg (Pritchard 1994) and 25 mmHg (Guyton *et al*. 1991). There may also be an indication on the tube of how much air is required.

Endotracheal tubes come with a connector attached (Figure 7.17). Sometimes the person intubating the patient will ask for the tube to be cut to size. There are markings on the tube in centimetres and also black indicators marking the length for nasal or oral intubation.

If the tube is cut, the blue connector will have to be removed from the cut piece of the tube and securely fitted to the (cut) end of the tube.

Routes for intubation

Patients may be intubated by the oral (orotracheal) or nasal (nasotracheal) route. Oral intubation is the most common route (see **Figure 7.18**). Nasotracheal intubation may be more comfortable for patients in the longer term, but is contraindicated in patients with a fractured base of skull (Joynt 2003) and those with clotting abnormalities. It is also associated with an increased incidence of sinusitis. Complications of this route include epistaxis and damage to the nasal septum (Joynt 2003).

Equipment for intubation

Equipment for emergency intubation should be kept on the ward. This should include:

- A selection of sizes of endotracheal tubes
- A laryngoscope with spare bulbs and batteries
- A self-inflating resuscitation bag plus reservoir
- An introducer
- Magill's forceps
- Catheter mount
- Lubricating jelly
- A 10 ml syringe
- Linen tape

Laryngoscope

A laryngoscope is made up of two parts – the handle and a curved blade (although straight blades may be used for infants and young children), which houses the bulb. A laryngoscope is used to move the patient's tongue to one side and pull the epiglottis forward to enable the person who is intubating to visualize the patient's vocal cords. The endotracheal tube is passed through the vocal cords and into the trachea. There should be spare laryngoscope bulbs and batteries available on the emergency trolley.

In order to check that the laryngoscope is working, either lift the blade until it clicks into place, or tighten the base of the handle until the light comes on, depending on the type of laryngoscope available. It is a good idea to familiarize yourself with whichever type of laryngoscope is available on your ward.

Resuscitation bag

A resuscitation bag is self-inflating and is used to provide artificial ventilation in a patient who has had a cardiorespiratory arrest, initially in conjunction with a mask. After the patient has been intubated, the bag is connected to the endotracheal tube using a catheter mount. It may also be used to pre-oxygenate the patient before they are intubated. Pre-oxygenation delivers a high concentration of oxygen to the patient – 98% oxygen if a reservoir bag is fitted (Advanced Life Support Group 2005). The resuscitation bag comes with an attachment for oxygen tubing. The flow of oxygen should be turned up to 15 litres/minute on the wall flow meter. A reservoir bag should be attached at the base of the resuscitation bag (most come supplied with these already attached), which fills with oxygen and, in conjunction with oxygen in the resuscitation bag, provides the patient with a high concentration of inspired oxygen.

Introducer or bougee

This is a soft, thin, flexible rod that may be used by the person intubating the patient if there is difficulty visualizing the vocal cords. It is sited first using the laryngoscope, and then the endotracheal tube is advanced over it and the introducer is removed (Joynt 2003).

Magill's forceps

These are angled forceps that may be used to remove foreign objects from the patient's pharynx (Advanced Life Support Group 2005) or to help pass a nasogastric tube once the patient has been intubated.

Catheter mount

This connects the endotracheal tube to the resuscitation bag or to ventilator tubing.

Drugs for intubation

If a patient has had a cardiorespiratory arrest, they will not require drugs for intubation, as cough and gag reflexes will be absent. In most other planned situations a selection of drugs will be required. It is important to remember that if intubation fails, the patient will need artificial ventilation using the resuscitation bag and mask.

Sedative/anaesthetic drugs

These drugs include propofol, etomidate, fentanyl, and midazolam. All drugs used for sedation or anaesthesia have the potential to cause the patient's blood pressure to fall (hypotension), particularly if the patient is hypovolaemic or has heart failure (Zimmerman 2001, Advanced Life Support Group 2005). Once the patient has been intubated, in order to tolerate an endotracheal tube, they will need a continuous infusion of a sedative and/or anaesthetic drug for a period of time to suppress cough and gag reflexes.

Neuromuscular blockers/muscle relaxants

These drugs are used to induce a temporary paralysis, which will stop the patient breathing spontaneously and eliminate a cough or gag reflex. Drugs that are commonly used include suxamethonium (succinylcholine) and vecuronium.

Suxamethonium has a very rapid onset and short duration, causes momentary muscle twitching or fasciculation (this can cause release of potassium from cells, so is contraindicated in patients with hyperkalaemia), and is a depolarizing muscle relaxant – its actions cannot be reversed. Suxamethonium must be stored in a refrigerator.

Vecuronium has a slower onset but a longer effect than suxamethonium and does not cause fasciculation. Its actions can be reversed.

Cricoid pressure

During a planned intubation, pressure is applied manually to the patient's cricoid ring (the one complete cartilaginous ring in the trachea) in order to compress the oesophagus and prevent aspiration of gastric contents. This should only be undertaken by experienced staff.

Position of the endotracheal tube

The tip of the endotracheal tube should sit approximately 1 cm above the carina, which is the point where the trachea branches into the left and right main bronchi. It is possible for the endotracheal tube to be advanced too far, so that the tip of the tube sits in the right main bronchus. This is because the right main bronchus branches off from the trachea at a less acute angle compared to the left main bronchus. If this happens, only the right lung will be ventilated. It is also possible to intubate the oesophagus rather than the trachea. It is therefore vital that the position of the endotracheal tube is checked promptly after it has been inserted. This can be done by auscultation to check that air is entering both lungs. A chest X-ray will also be required at the earliest convenient time.

Securing the endotracheal tube

It is vital that the endotracheal tube is securely tied in place to prevent it slipping further down the trachea or out through the vocal cords. Linen tape is commonly used and should be tied securely enough around the tube and the patient's neck to prevent the tube moving, but not so tightly that the patient's skin becomes damaged or venous return from the patient's head is obstructed. You should be able to insert a finger between the tape and the patient's neck (Scase 2004).

Context

 ### When to use intubation

A patient may require an endotracheal tube:

- During an operation.
- If they need ventilatory support due to severe illness.

- If they have a significantly impaired level of consciousness (a Glasgow Coma Score of 8 or less).
- Following a cardiopulmonary arrest.

Potential problems

- Hypotension
- Intubation of the oesophagus or right main bronchus
- Aspiration
- Raised intracranial pressure
- Hypoxia

Reflection and evaluation

When you have been involved with a patient who needed intubating, think about the following questions:

1 Why did the patient need intubating?
2 Were there any warning signs that alerted you to the fact that the patient might need intubating?
3 Did you know what equipment would be needed and what it would be used for?

Further learning opportunities

As this is not a skill a student nurse would perform, it is not recommended that you try to practise it. Instead, familiarize yourself with the equipment described earlier. You should be able to check that it works correctly under supervision, identify the various pieces of equipment, and locate the equipment and relevant drugs in an emergency situation.

Reminders

Don't forget to:

- Familiarize yourself with the location of the emergency trolley and how the equipment works.
- Support the patient's family.
- Alert senior colleagues/medical staff about any deterioration in a patient's condition.

 ### Patient scenarios

Consider what you should do in the following situations, then turn to the end of this skill to check your answers.

1 An adult male patient you are looking after suffers a cardiopulmonary arrest. What size endotracheal tube should be used by the arrest team to intubate him?

2 After intubation, how would you secure the tube to stop it from moving around and to ensure the patient's safety and comfort?

3 Once the patient was safe and comfortable, what would your priority be towards the man's family?

Website

 http://www.oxfordtextbooks.co.uk/orc/ endacott

You may find it helpful to work through our short online quiz and additional scenarios intended to help you to develop and apply the skills in this chapter.

References

Advanced Life Support Group (2005). *Advanced paediatric life support: the practical approach*, 4th edition. BMJ Books, Blackwell Publishing, London.

Department of Health (2000). *Comprehensive critical care*. DH, London.

Guyton D, Banner MJ, and Kirby RR (1991). High-volume, low pressure cuffs: are they always low pressure? *Chest*, **100**, 1076–81.

Joynt GM (2003). Airway management and acute upper airway obstruction. In AD Bersten, N Soni, and TE Oh, eds. *Oh's intensive care manual*, 5th edition, pp. 283–96. Butterworth Heinemann, London.

Pritchard A (1994). Tracheostomy. *Care of the Critically Ill*, **10**(2), 66–8.

Scase C (2004). Wound care. In C Russell and B Matta, eds. *Tracheostomy: a multi-professional handbook*, pp. 173–86. Cambridge University Press, Cambridge.

Zimmerman JL, ed (2001). *Fundamental critical care support, 3rd edition: a standardized curriculum of the principles of critical care*. Society of Critical Care Medicine, Des Plaines, IL.

 Answers to patient scenarios

1 An adult male patient would usually need a size 8.0–9.0 endotracheal tube.

2 After intubation, the tube would be secured with tape tied around his neck, making sure that a finger could be inserted between tape and neck to ensure comfort and safety.

3 When the patient was safe and comfortable, your priority towards the man's family would be to make sure that they were fully informed about events surrounding the resuscitation and emergency intubation, and prepared to see him unconscious and intubated. This will be a traumatic and stressful time for the family and it is part of the nurse's role to support them through it.

8 Neurological system

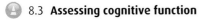
8.1 Assessing conscious level

Definition

Assessing conscious level involves examining simple but key components of a patient's neurological function, such as verbal or motor response to voice and pain. This enables an estimation of level of wakefulness and awareness at a particular time. The most commonly used tool is the Glasgow Coma Scale (GCS), which attributes a number or category to the conscious level.

It is important to remember that:

- Assessment of the patient should follow the ABCDE rule. Remember that the airway is at risk in patients with low conscious level.
- The most widely used method for assessing conscious level is the GCS because it is reproducible – scores can be compared over a period of time to gauge improvement or deterioration. It is quick and straightforward to perform and is used in a number of countries.
- The GCS was not developed to be used in isolation and should always be used in conjunction with other aspects of neurological assessment. Breathing pattern, pupils, and vital signs are often abnormal and can give a clue to where the problem lies.
- Terms such as semi-conscious and semi-coma, previously used to describe altered states of consciousness, were vague and meant different things to different people. The use of these terms should be avoided.

Prior knowledge

Before attempting to assess conscious level, make sure you are familiar with:

1 Basic neuroanatomy of structures of the brain.
2 Common causes of altered conscious level.
3 Tools in common use for assessing conscious level.
4 Breathing patterns and important pupil abnormalities.
5 ABCDE approach to assessing the critically ill patient.

Background

Being able to assess conscious level is a key skill in the initial assessment of a critically ill patient and also in determining neurological deterioration. Patients with altered conscious level are at risk of airway obstruction and respiratory and cardiovascular complications, so identifying early change is important to preserve life. You will assess patients with head injury and neurological disease on neurosurgical units who have altered conscious level. However, you will also see patients with a variety of metabolic and toxic diseases that cause altered consciousness on medical and surgical wards.

When assessing a patient who is critically ill, your assessment should follow the ABCDE rule seen in the Resuscitation Council's life support guidelines (2006). After you are sure that airway, breathing, and circulation have been assessed adequately, move on to 'D', which represents neurological assessment.

Consciousness

Consciousness is a state of wakefulness, with awareness of one's surroundings. Therefore, a conscious patient is not just awake (*normal conscious level*), but also aware and responsive to sensory stimulation such as sound and touch (*normal conscious state*).

The area of the brain that is responsible for coordinating conscious level is the brainstem reticular formation (see **Figure 8.1**). Diffuse fibres known collectively as the ascending reticular activating system (ARAS) receive and process nerve impulses from a large number of sensory sources. Visual and auditory stimuli such as a doorbell or flashing lights can influence wakefulness in this way. ARAS sends a continuous stream of impulses to the cerebral cortex, maintaining it in an awake state. ARAS can be suppressed by drugs such as inhaled general anaesthetics, sedatives, and alcohol.

Awareness

Awareness is a measure of the ability of the cerebral cortex to filter the sensory information arriving and respond accordingly. For example, a patient under partial sedation

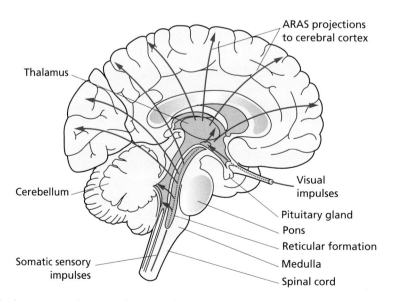

Figure 8.1 Reticular formation in relation to other parts of the brainstem and cerebral cortex.

Table 8.1 Common causes of altered levels of consciousness

Brainstem disease	Brainstem stroke (haemorrhage or infarction)
	Chronic alcoholism (Wernicke–Korsakoff syndrome)
	Trauma to brainstem
	Multiple sclerosis
Pressure effect on the brainstem	Space-occupying lesions (tumour, abscess)
	Cerebral stroke (usually haemorrhage)
Diffuse brain dysfunction (toxic and metabolic)	Drugs (e.g. general anaesthetics, sedatives, opiates, alcohol)
	Epilepsy following a seizure (post-ictal)
	Sepsis
	Hyponatraemia, hypercalcaemia
	Hypoglycaemia or diabetic Ketoacidosis
	Hypothermia
	Diffuse brain injury from head injury
	Respiratory failure (hypoxia and hypercapnia)
	Hypothyroidism
	Uraemia, dehydration
	Liver failure (lung, adrenal, pituitary, heart)
	Carbon monoxide poisoning
	Change of environment particularly in the elderly, e.g. moving the patient to another ward
	Depression and acute psychosis
	Eclampsia in pregnant women

for a procedure who responds in a confused and inappropriate way to your questions is said to be in an altered state of consciousness. Our overall consciousness is determined by complex interaction between the reticular formation, the cerebral cortex, and sensory inputs. Therefore it is important to recognize that a spectrum of altered consciousness exists that can be observed in different patterns. Patients with head injuries usually deteriorate rapidly towards low conscious level (coma), whereas patients with metabolic causes such as sepsis have a fluctuating consciousness, with episodes of low conscious level, confusion, and altered visual sensation.

Altered states of consciousness

Altered states of consciousness are produced by compression or damage to the brainstem and reticular formation. Three mechanisms of damage are seen:

1 A direct result of brainstem disease, for example a stroke affecting the brainstem itself damages the ARAS.

2 Pressure effect of a mass lesion within the cerebellum or cerebral hemisphere pressing on the reticular formation.

3 Diffuse brain failure from severe metabolic or toxic disease inhibits overall brain function, for example sepsis or hypoglycaemia.

Common causes of altered consciousness are shown in Table 8.1.

Effects on breathing

Knowledge and assessment of breathing pattern is important and can help assess the severity and the site of the underlying problem. Motor nerve fibres continuing through the reticular formation are responsible for coordinating respiratory and cardiac rhythms, so damage to this area is often associated with effects on breathing.

There are a number of abnormal breathing patterns in the unconscious patient that can be recognized from observing the patient's breathing. These can help localize the problem responsible for the coma to a particular place in the brain:

- In **Cheyne–Stokes respiration** the respiratory rate speeds up for periods of up to a minute, with intervening periods of no breathing (apnoea). This is usually seen in metabolic coma or deep cerebral lesions.
- **Central neurogenic hyperventilation** is a persistently increased rate of deep breathing and is seen in midbrain lesions.
- **Apneustic breathing** is prolonged inspiration followed by a short pause before expiration, caused usually by pontine stroke.
- **Ataxic breathing** is erratic in rate and depth and is a result of respiratory centre disease in the medulla.

Effects on pupil reaction

Pupil reaction represents activity of the IIIrd cranial nerve. This nerve supplies the small muscles that produce pupil constriction. There is one nerve for each eye. If the IIIrd nerve is dysfunctional, the pupil remains dilated and is slow to constrict when a light is shone into the eye. A pupil slow to constrict can be described as 'sluggish'. Pupil reaction should normally be 'brisk'.

The IIIrd nerve has a long course within the skull from the brain to the back of the eye. Any brain swelling or mass lesion within the skull or brain can cause dysfunction due to pressure on the nerve. Any abnormal pupil reactions should be taken in context with other parts of the neurological assessment, as abnormal pupils are usually late signs of neurological deterioration.

The Glasgow Coma Scale

The GCS is a 15-point scale originally described in 1974 by Jennet and Teasdale at the University of Glasgow. The GCS evaluates conscious level by scoring a response in three areas: eye opening, motor response, and verbal performance (see **Table 8.2**). It provides a validated global assessment and is accurate in charting change in a patient's condition. It was intended for monitoring deterioration in patients with head injuries, to try and reduce the impact of complications such as brain swelling and haemorrhage.

Table 8.2 Glasgow Coma Scale (GCS)

Response	Score (total out of 15)
Eye opening (E)	
Spontaneous	4
To speech	3
To pain	2
None	1
Verbal response (V)	
Orientated	5
Confused conversation	4
Inappropriate words	3
Incomprehensible words	2
None	1
Best motor response (M)	
Obeys commands	6
Localizes pain	5
Normal flexion (withdrawal)	4
Abnormal flexion (decorticate)	3
Extension (decerebrate)	2
None	1

Adapted from Jennet and Teasdale (1974)

Context

 When to assess conscious level

Patients can be classified according to conscious level. This skill is useful in a variety of situations:

- When briefly assessing an acutely ill patient, e.g. a patient alerted to A&E, as part of a general assessment.
- To assess whether airway may be at risk of obstruction. Altered conscious level causes unawareness of airway compromise.
- In monitoring a general medical patient who may have fallen and sustained a head injury.
- To gauge improvement in condition or response to treatment.
- To gauge prognosis in patients who are critically unwell.
- Documentation of conscious level in neurological or neurosurgical patients with chronic brain injuries.

- Regular assessment of improvement or deterioration of conscious level in intensive care patients with various metabolic diseases.
- Following general anaesthesia or sedation of patients.

Alternative interventions

AVPU

The AVPU assessment (Alert, Voice, Pain, Unresponsive) was originally taught in the American College of Surgeons Advanced Trauma Life Support (ATLS) course (American College of Surgeons 1997) as part of an assessment of trauma patients. It has now been incorporated into many Early Warning Scores for critically ill patients as a simpler tool to use than the GCS (see **Table 8.3** and **Figure 8.2**).

Deterioration of a patient's condition in hospital is frequently preceded by documented deterioration of physiological parameters. The Early Warning Score (EWS) (Morgan *et al.* 1997) is a tool for bedside evaluation based on five physiological parameters: systolic blood pressure, pulse rate, respiratory rate, temperature, and AVPU score. Many hospitals use modified Early Warning Scores that include a neurological parameter, including an AVPU score or GCS range. This can alert staff to acute deterioration so that early review by the critical care team is possible.

However, it is thought that sometimes AVPU may not identify the subtle changes in ward patients where con-sciousness may be altered by metabolic derangements rather than by a direct traumatic insult. It is also not suitable for long-term neurological observation. Mackay *et al.* (2000) compared use of AVPU to GCS and found that Voice corresponds to a GCS of 13, while a GCS of 9 was the division between Voice and Pain.

Potential problems

- Proehl (1992) stressed the need for nurses to base their GCS score on the patient's *best responses* in each category. This is to try and ensure that there is a level of standardization between different nurses undertaking the assessment.
- Students' typical mistakes are to describe people by their overall GCS score rather than the underlying components. A nearly normal score can hide a marked deficit in one category.
- Always write down the score you get, even if it is markedly different from the previous one. The change could be a sign of neurological deterioration. Ask a colleague to check your score if you think you've made a mistake.
- Patients may have other medical problems that need to be overcome such as deafness, comprehension problems, or learning disabilities. You must try to overcome these as far as possible. Strategies include ensuring the patient has their hearing aid in, and

Table 8.3 The AVPU scoring system

Score	Interpretation/meaning
Alert	Fully awake though not necessarily orientated. This patient will have spontaneously open eyes, will respond to voice (although may be confused), and will have spontaneous motor function.
Responds to voice (Voice)	The patient makes some kind of response when you talk to them, which could be in any of the three component measures of Eyes, Voice, or Motor – e.g. patient's eyes open on being asked 'Are you okay?'. The response could be as little as a grunt, moan, or slight move of a limb when prompted by the voice.
Responds to pain (Pain)	The patient makes a response on any of the three component measures when pain stimulus is used on them (see GCS procedure).
Unresponsive	Sometimes seen noted as 'Unconscious', this outcome is recorded if the patient does not give any Eye, Voice, or Motor response to voice or pain.

Early Warning Observation Chart Level 0

WARD

Name	Hospital **NHS**
	NHS Trust
	Date of Admission
Unit No.	
Attach Patient Label	OUTREACH BLEEP 5021 / 4039

Consultant

....

....

Date

| Time | | | | | | | | | | | | | | | | | | | | | |

Please enter early warning scores below

Conscious level																		Conscious level
Resps																		Resps
Pulse																		Pulse
Systolic BP																		Systolic BP
Temp																		Temp
O₂ Sats																		O₂ Sats
Urine																		Urine
EWS																		EWS

Early Warning Score

Score	0	1	2	3
Conscious level	A – Alert	V – Responds to Voice	P – Responds to Pain	U – unresponsive
Resps	8–20/min	21–24/min	25–29/min	≤8/min or ≥30/min
Pulse	61–100/min	101–110/min	41–60/min or 111–119/min	≤40/min or ≥120/min
Sys. BP	101–199 mmHg		91–100 mmHg	≤90 mmHg or ≥200 mmHg
Temp	36.0–37.9°C	35.1°C–35.9°C	38.0–39.9°C	≤35°C or ≥40°C
O₂ sats	≥85%		91–94%	≤90°C
Urine	≥30 ml/hr or ≥200 ml/6 hrs	125–199 ml/6 hours	60–124 ml/6 hours	≤30 ml/hr or ≤60 ml/6 hrs

WOE032

Figure 8.2 Typical Early Warning observation chart. Note the inclusion of AVPU alongside other vital signs. Courtesy of Walsall Hospitals NHS Trust.

standing directly in their field of vision. Language barriers cause difficulties, so any questions or phrases must be kept simple.

- Central painful stimulus by sternal rub should not be used as it causes prolonged discomfort to the patient.

Interpreting readings

Patients with head injuries or those who have suffered intracranial haemorrhage are at risk of complications that cause further deterioration in conscious level. Injury to the brain causes diffuse swelling that increases the pressure within the skull (raised intracranial pressure or ICP). This raised pressure causes a further drop in consciousness and can often only be relieved by emergency surgery. There is also a risk that the blood supply to the brain tissue will be compromised and cause an ischaemic stroke, and there is a risk of further haemorrhage within the brain tissue.

These complications are marked by a further rapid drop in conscious level usually 24 to 48 hours after the initial insult. Recognition of this should prompt a medical review of the patient. Often further brain imaging at this stage will point to the cause of the deterioration.

Pupil reaction

- A dilated and fixed pupil is a very late sign of rising intracranial pressure. One side of the brain is at risk of herniation through the skull, with death quickly ensuing.

This is an emergency, and senior help and neurosurgical opinion must be sought urgently. The GCS is always very low at this time.

■ In metabolic coma the pupils usually remain normal and reactive to light.

■ In sedated or anaesthetized patients, pupil reaction is the only sign of brain activity that can be reliably measured clinically (see **Figure 8.3**).

Motor responses

As consciousness deteriorates, responses to pain become less purposeful and the patient may not be able to localize a painful stimulus. A flexor response (also called decorticate posture) indicates damage to the corticospinal tract, the pathway between the brain and spinal cord. It is indicated by rigidity, flexion of the arms, clenched fists, and extended legs. The arms are bent inward toward the body with the wrists and fingers bent and held on the chest. It is usually more favourable than an extensor response (decerebrate posture), which is indicated by rigid extension of the arms and legs, downward pointing of the toes, and backward arching of the head. A severe injury to the brain at the level of the brainstem is a common cause. The flexor response and extensor response are illustrated in **Figure 8.4**.

Each Trust will have its own neurological observation chart for use in A&E, intensive care, and neuroscience units. Therefore, the layout will be slightly different depending on where you work. An example is seen in **Figure 8.5**. It is important to document the best response for each category on the chart, making sure you fill in all of the parts you have assessed.

Special considerations

■ Note that the GCS does not assess the patient's pupil reaction.

■ Paralysis, intubation, or anaesthetic drugs can all invalidate parts of the GCS.

■ A GCS score of less than 9 is compatible with a coma and the airway needs definitive protection by endotracheal intubation.

Patients with head injuries

■ The National Institute for Health and Clinical Excellence (NICE) has published guidelines for the management of adults and children with head injuries (NICE 2007). On arrival in the Emergency Department (ED), patients with head injuries should have a GCS score recorded. Patients presenting to the ED with a GCS score of less than 15 should be assessed immediately by a trained member of staff.

■ For head-injured patients, observations should be performed and recorded on a half-hourly basis until a GCS equal to 15 has been achieved. The minimum frequency of observations for patients with GCS equal to 15 should be as follows, starting after the initial assessment:
  – half-hourly for 2 hours
  – then once-hourly for 4 hours
  – then twice-hourly thereafter.

■ Should a head-injured patient with GCS equal to 15 deteriorate at any time after the initial 2-hour period, observations should revert to half-hourly and follow the original frequency schedule (NICE 2007).

■ A GCS of 14 or 15 signifies a mild head injury, 9 to 13 a moderate head injury, and 8 or less a severe head injury (NICE 2007).

		Description	Causes
		Normal pupils, reactive	Normal patient Metabolic coma
		Unilateral dilated pupil, fixed	IIIrd nerve palsy Uncal herniation (Neurosurgical emergency)
		Bilateral dilated pupils, fixed	Central brain herniation (Pre-terminal event)
		Unilateral constricted pupil (Horner's syndrome) Difficult to see any reaction	Sympathetic nervous system damage in the neck (neck injury)
		Bilateral constricted pupils	Opiate overdose Pontine stroke

Figure 8.3 Abnormal pupil responses seen in altered consciousness.

(a) Extensor response

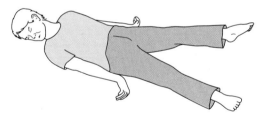

(b) Flexor response

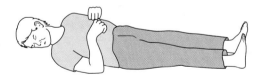

Figure 8.4 Abnormal motor responses.

Procedure

Preparation

Prepare the equipment
Make sure you have the following equipment to hand:

- A pen torch
- A neurological observation chart to record your findings (see Figure 8.5)
- Airway adjuncts
- Sphygmomanometer
- Thermometer

Discussing the procedure with the patient and family

Introduce yourself and inform the patient that you are going to assess them, whether they appear conscious or not. If the patient is conscious they must give informed consent before you assess them. This is also a good screen for whether they respond to your voice.

The procedure can be distressing for any family who might be watching. Explain to them what you are doing and the importance of recording their relative's response to a short painful stimulus.

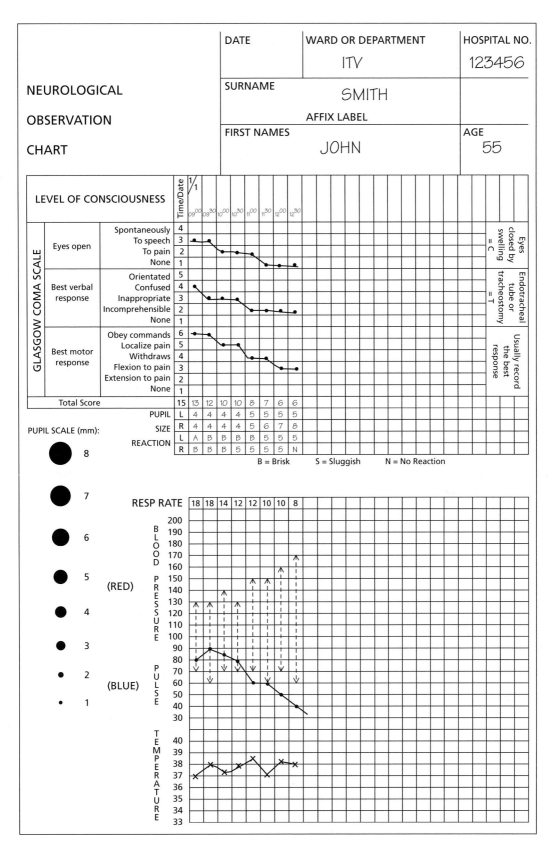

Figure 8.5 A typical neurological observation chart. Note the deterioration in GCS on the chart accompanied by an increase in blood pressure and change in pupil reaction. This is typical of the pattern of deterioration in a head injury patient.

Step-by-step guide to assessing conscious level

Step		Rationale
1	Introduce yourself, confirm the patient's identity, explain the procedure, and obtain consent.	To identify the patient correctly and gain informed consent.
2	A – Assess airway. Airway adjuncts will help protect an airway, but if the patient is likely to be unconscious for a long time, intubation by a skilled professional is needed for a definitive airway.	To ensure airway is protected.
3	B – Assess breathing patterns and respiratory rate. Count the respiratory rate and note any abnormal breathing pattern.	To assist in identifying site of injury and/or severity of the lesion.
4	C – Check pulse and capillary refill.	To identify tachycardia and bradycardia, which may complicate altered consciousness.
5	Inspect the patient: do they have a medic alert bracelet or any sign of external injury? Pay careful attention to the head and look for scalp lacerations.	To identify any known medical issues or signs of external injury.
6	Talk to the patient and say 'Can you hear me?' and 'Open your eyes'. Note whether the patient has their eyes open when you approach them and before speaking to them. If the patient opens their eyes only when you ask them to, this is 'responds to speech'. If there is no response, assess the patient's response to pain.	To assess response to verbal stimuli.
7	Assess response to pain by applying incremental pressure to the side of the patient's little finger (supraorbital ridge pressure here can cause the patient to screw up and close their eyes). Don't press the nail bed as it can cause bruising. You can press the finger between your own finger and a pencil or pen. If the patient opens their eyes, this means that the brainstem eye opening mechanism is active. It doesn't necessarily mean that the patient is aware. Note down the 'eye opening' GCS score.	To assess response to pain.
8	You will have some idea already whether there is any verbal response. Talk to the patient again: 'Can you hear me?' Spontaneous verbal response is obvious before directly questioning the patient. If there is a reduced verbal response, you need to go on and determine whether the patient is confused or not and assess the verbal response score.	Verbal response looks at comprehension of a verbal stimulus and expression and articulation of a reply. An appropriate response shows a high level of communication within the brain.

9	If the patient is conversational, ask them 'What is your name? Where are you? What day is it today?' Note occasional inappropriate words, incomprehensible responses such as grunts and groans, or no response at all. You can now note the verbal response GCS score.	To check for confusion. If the patient is confused they will respond to the questions but be disorientated in one or more of time, place, and person.
10	Observe the patient for purposeful spontaneous movement. Upper limb responses are used normally since lower limb movements are less reliable. Spinal reflexes can cause sudden movement in the lower limbs that may be mistaken for a purposeful response.	To assess motor response.
11	If there is no spontaneous movement, tell the patient 'Squeeze my fingers hard'. If there is a discrepancy on one side or other, note the response on the better side.	To help you localize the problem to one side of the brain.
12	If there is no response to voice, apply a painful stimulus to the supraorbital ridge and observe any response. There are alternative sites. Maintain this until the response is maximal. If there is no response to a central stimulus you can try a peripheral site such as squeezing the little finger.	If you try this on yourself you will find it to be more painful than pressing elsewhere on your forehead. This is because you are pressing on the supraorbital nerve, which makes it a suitable painful stimulus for this assessment.
13	Note whether there is any motor response to pain or if the patient makes an attempt to localize towards the area where you are applying the painful stimulus.	As consciousness deteriorates, the ability to do this decreases and the patient has abnormal flexion or extension responses.
14	Now make a total score for the GCS (e.g. E2, V3, M3 = GCS 8) – the range will be 3 to 15. Document this on the chart.	To provide a record of your assessment.
15	Look at the pupils. Assess size and equality. The size of the pupil will depend on the amount of light in the room; there is a guide on most neurological observation charts to help you gauge size.	Both pupils should be equal in size, but may be abnormal and unequal in altered conscious states.
16	Assess pupil constriction (response to light) by shining torchlight into each eye in turn. Bring the light in from the side directly into the eye. Normal pupils should both constrict on shining the light into one eye. If a pupil doesn't constrict it is 'fixed'.	Different patterns of abnormal pupils represent different underlying brain problems (see Figure 8.3).

Following the procedure

- Measure and record the patient's blood pressure and heart rate. It is important to record vital signs because abnormalities can indicate deterioration in the patient's condition. It will usually come after deterioration in GCS. Increasing hypertension with a wide pulse pressure (increasing systolic but low diastolic measurement) and bradycardia indicates **Cushing's response**. This is a physiological response to brain swelling and raised intracranial pressure. It predicts impending brain herniation. You can also see a tachycardia in the late stages of brain swelling.

- Take and record the patient's temperature. Hyperpyrexia (high temperature) usually means damage to the **hypothalamus**. In patients with head injury this should be treated, as it adversely affects the patient's outcome.

- Measure fingertip blood glucose. Hypoglycaemia in a diabetic initially causes arousal but as the blood glucose falls further (below 3.0 mmol/litre) it causes a lowering of conscious level leading rapidly to hypoglycaemic coma. This is a mandatory test in all unconscious patients.

- Check medications chart or patient's prescription chart for drugs that can cause drowsiness and coma. Check mainly for opiates (morphine, diamorphine, codeine, or fentanyl), benzodiazepines (midazolam, diazepam, temazepam, or lorazepam), and tricyclic anti-depressants (amitriptyline).

- If you are concerned that the patient has a deteriorating conscious level, an airway that is at risk, or medication causing decreased conscious level – call for help! You can explain to the senior nurse or doctor that you have a patient with a low GCS score. They may ask you to break the score down into its components. Also mention what is worrying you most about the patient – airway at risk, very low GCS score, pupil abnormalities.

Reflection and evaluation

When you have made an assessment of a patient's conscious level, think about the following:

1 Do the conscious level, pupil response, and breathing pattern point towards an underlying neurological diagnosis such as an intracranial haemorrhage?

2 How does the conscious level compare with previous assessments done either by you or by another nurse?

3 How will you explain to the patient's family what the problem is with their relative and why you are doing these tests on them?

Reminders

- When assessing the patient with altered conscious level, your approach should follow the ABCDE rule as with any critically ill patient.

- The GCS score should not be used in isolation, and abnormal pupil reactions, abnormal breathing patterns, and vital signs can help localize a neurological problem.

- Documenting the neurological observations accurately is important in recognizing neurological deterioration and for nursing handover.

- Always record the best possible score and follow the procedure at all times to ensure standardization between nurses' assessments.

Ⓠ Patient scenarios

Consider what you should do in the following situations, then turn to the end of this skill to check your answers.

1 You assess a 54-year-old man with a head injury in A&E. He opens his eyes when you squeeze his finger, but not when you tell him to. He does mumble a few sounds when you ask him his name. When you squeeze his little finger he moves his other arm across to try and move your hand away. What is his GCS score?

2 A 38-year-old lady was admitted to the local neurosurgical unit with a subarachnoid haemorrhage affecting her conscious level. On arrival she had a GCS score of 12 (E3, V4, M5). Twenty-four hours later her GCS drops suddenly to 7. What might have caused this deterioration?

3 It is the end of your shift in a neurosurgical unit and you need to hand over the care of a patient with a

head injury, a GCS score of 10, and a dilated and poorly responsive left pupil. Think about the information that your successor will need to be able to put their own observations in context and how you would describe the patient's current status to your colleague.

Website

 http://www.oxfordtextbooks.co.uk/orc/ endacott

You may find it helpful to work through our short online quiz and additional scenarios intended to help you to develop and apply the skills in this chapter.

References

American College of Surgeons (1997). *Advanced trauma life support course manual*, 6th edition. American College of Surgeons, Chicago.

Jennet B and Teasdale G (1974). Assessment of coma and impaired consciousness. A practical scale. *Lancet*, **2**, 81–3.

Mackay CA, Burke DP, Burke JA *et al.* (2000). Association between the assessment of conscious level using the AVPU system and the Glasgow coma scale. *Pre-hospital Immediate Care*, **4**, 17–19.

Morgan RJM, Williams F, and Wright MM (1997). An Early Warning Scoring System for detecting developing critical illness. *Clinical Intensive Care*, **8**, 100.

National Institute for Health and Clinical Excellence (2007). *Head injury: triage, assessment, investigation and early management of head injuries in infants, children and adults. Clinical Guideline No. 56*. NICE, London.

Proehl JA (1992). The Glasgow Coma Scale: do it and do it right. *Journal of Emergency Nursing*, **18**(5), 421–3.

Resuscitation Council UK (2006). *Advanced Life Support (ALS)*, 5th edition. Resuscitation Council (UK), London.

Useful further reading and websites

Adams SK and Osborne S (2005). Neurological problems. In SK Adams and S Osborne. *Critical care nursing: science and practice*, 2nd edition, pp. 290–4. Oxford University Press, Oxford.

Palmer R and Knight J (2006). Assessment of altered conscious level in clinical practice. *British Journal of Nursing*, **15**(22), 1255–9.

Waterhouse C (2005). The Glasgow Coma Scale and other neurological observations. *Nursing Standard* **19**(33), 56–64 [online] **http://www.nursing-standard.co.uk/archives/ns/vol19-33/pdfs/v19n33p5664.pdf**

The British Association of Neuroscience Nurses (BANN) provides a national benchmark for undertaking neurological observations at: **http://www.bann.org.uk/downloads/ NEURO%20OBS%20B.M.05.pdf**

 Answers to patient scenarios

1 E2, V2, M5. GCS score 9/15.
2 Commonly ischaemic stroke, hydrocephalus, or re-bleed can have this effect. The patient needs another CT scan to determine the problem.
3 You need to ensure you explain how the GCS score of 10 was reached, emphasizing the areas where the patient falls short. Don't forget to mention pupil abnormalities.

8.2 Care of the unconscious patient

Definition

Unconsciousness can be defined as a physiological state where the patient is unaware of themselves or their surroundings. Although care of the unconscious patient will depend on whether it is acute or chronic, the key priority will always be to maintain the patient's safety. In the emergency situation, care of the unconscious patient should follow the standard approach to assessing and treating the acutely ill patient, i.e. airway, breathing, circulation, disability, and exposure (ABCDE) (Smith 2000). Ongoing care involves continuing to maintain the patient's safety while attending to their daily basic needs, e.g. hygiene, elimination, nutrition, etc.

This chapter provides an overview of the care of the unconscious patient. The reader will be directed to other parts of the book for more detailed care information, e.g. nutrition (Chapter 10).

It is important to remember that:

- Unconsciousness is potentially life-threatening; such patients have reduced airway reflexes and are considered unable to protect their own airway from aspiration or obstruction. If this occurs, urgent intervention is required.
- Hearing is the last sense to fail – so it is important to communicate and speak with the patient even when there is no response.
- The Glasgow Coma Scale (GCS) is a useful tool to assess the level of unconsciousness (see Section 8.1). The GCS directly assesses the functioning of the brainstem and demonstrates to the assessor whether the reticular activating system (RAS) has or has not been stimulated, and whether the patient is aware or unaware of their environment.
- The patient's dignity and privacy should be maintained at all times.

Prior knowledge

Before attempting care of an unconscious patient, make sure you are familiar with:

1 The physiology of the neurological system, paying particular attention to the function of the reticular formation (RF), especially the RAS and its influence on levels of consciousness and arousal.
2 The common causes of unconsciousness, such as head injury, stroke, and poisons.
3 Assessment of conscious level (Section 8.1). The unconscious patient will require regular monitoring, the frequency of which will be determined by the severity of their illness.
4 Basic nursing care, e.g. hygiene requirements of a patient who is unable to wash themselves.

There may be situations in which you will find caring for an unconscious patient testing all areas of competent practice (knowledge, skill, and attitude). Review of the areas above will help you appreciate the complexities of caring for someone who is unconscious. You should also be able to prioritize your assessment and intervention in order to maintain safety and comfort.

Background

Physiological regulation of consciousness

The RF located in the brainstem controls consciousness. All sensory pathways link into the RF. The RAS is a primitive network of interconnecting nerve cells and fibres that receives input from multiple sensory pathways. It extends from the spinal cord to the lower brainstem, upward through the mese cephalon and thalamus, and is then distributed throughout the cerebral cortex (Waugh and Grant 2006). The RAS is a feature of the RF and controls our ability to be awake, to sleep, and to maintain consciousness. The level of arousal is dependent on the amount and quality of stimuli to the RAS (Pemberton 2000). The RAS receives input signals from a wide range of sources, including the five senses (visual, auditory, touch, smell, taste). Processes that disturb its function, for example reduced stimulation (sensory deprivation) or overstimulation, will lead to altered levels of consciousness.

In addition, the brain auto-regulates its own blood flows so that there is a constant flow between a mean arterial pressure of 60 and 150 (mean arterial pressure, or MAP, is the average blood pressure throughout the cardiac cycle). At higher MAP there is increased blood flow and at lower MAP there is reduced blood flow. Injured brains (e.g. head injury) are not as good at auto-regulation as healthy brains. An increased cerebral blood flow might lead to oedema; a reduced cerebral flow may lead to ischaemia (Cooper 2004). Thus it is imperative that the patient's blood pressure is maintained within normal parameters.

The unconscious patient lacks many vital and protective reflexes and depends on others for protection and maintenance of vital functions. It is the legal and professional duty of the nurse to ensure that the patient's safety is maintained during this critical period.

Levels of consciousness

There are different levels of consciousness, from being fully conscious to a state of coma. Terms used to describe the different levels include drowsiness, confusion, and comatose. An attempt has been made to categorize levels of consciousness using the Glasgow Coma Scale (see Section 8.1).

There are various insults that can alter the patient's level of consciousness. The most common reason for a reduced conscious level is critical illness (Cooper 2004). This includes hypoglycaemia, hyperglycaemia, hypoxia, hypercapnia (increased blood carbon dioxide), renal failure, and hepatic failure. Alterations can also be caused by trauma or infection, or be induced through the use of general anaesthetic. Pharmacological influences include benzodiazepines (lorazepam, midazolam, diazepam).

ABCDE

The priorities of the care of the unconscious patient should follow the systematic ABCDE approach (Airway, Breathing, Circulation, Disability, Exposure) (Smith 2000). Each stage represents a physical hierarchy. If any problems arise within a particular stage, this has to be corrected before moving to the next stage. For example, airway obstruction has to be corrected before administration of oxygen. Follow the standard 'look, listen, feel' approach to assessment (Smith 2000).

Ongoing nursing care of the unconscious patient

Ongoing nursing care of the unconscious patient, which will be determined by the situation and the length of time they have been unconscious, should include:

- Maintaining a safe environment.
- Preventing cross-infection.
- Assisting respiratory function.
- Assisting cardiovascular function.
- Maintaining nutrition and hydration.
- Maintaining gastrointestinal function.
- Maintaining genitourinary function.
- Preventing complications of immobility.
- Providing effective communication to the patient and relatives.

Communication with the unconscious patient

Effective communication is a fundamental element of nursing care (see Chapter 2). Studies suggest that skilled communication and interaction significantly influence patient satisfaction and hence quality of care (Goode 2004, Park and Song 2005).

Although verbal communication is mostly viewed as an interactive process, its importance to the unconscious patient is unquestionable. Patients have a considerable need for information and support even if they are unable to respond.

Communication typically includes verbal and non-verbal dialogue, active listening, empathy, and interviewing skills. While unconscious patients appear to be unresponsive, many are still able to receive and understand verbal communication (remember, hearing is the last sense to go). Verbal communication is a way of orientating and providing meaningful sensory input for an unconscious patient. Familiar voices, or simply using the patient's name and individualizing care, may provide better sensory input (Ashworth 1980).

Individual accounts and qualitative studies have demonstrated that verbal communication is useful, comforting, and indeed essential in unconscious patients (Elliot and Wright 1999). In one report, 100 ex-patients described how they heard, understood, and responded emotionally to what was being said even when health carers assumed they were not conscious; the patients drew strength from warm, caring verbal exchanges that were obviously directed at them as individuals (Lawrence 1995).

Information received by the unconscious patient may assist in reducing stress. They may not understand what is happening, and so verbal communication can reduce stress by facilitating the patient's use of adaptive coping mechanisms (Elliott and Wright 1999).

Communicating, particularly with the unconscious patient, has been described as a difficult and potentially stressful experience for nurses, leaving many to question their standard of communication skills. While it is initially daunting and somewhat intimidating to talk to patients who are not responsive, nurses have to overcome this barrier and talk to the unconscious patient as they would someone who is conscious.

In addition, features of the environment in health care settings can also affect the application of communication skills and the ability to communicate effectively. Environmental constraints may include other people, distracting noise, tense environments, alien environments, and interruptions (Chant *et al*. 2002).

Respecting the unconscious patient

Caring for unconscious patients requires attitudes and actions that demonstrate interest in and respect for the patient. These attitudes and actions should address the patient's concerns and values. They are generally related to patients' psychological, social, and spiritual domains (Branch *et al.* 2001). This is very difficult to achieve if the nurse does not have adequate knowledge of the patient. It is imperative that the nurse is self-aware about their own beliefs and values and views the patient as an individual.

Family involvement

The health care environment can create a barrier to human interactions, inducing dehumanization. Families may be reluctant to touch loved ones, particularly if they are connected to machines. This often results from fear of causing equipment to malfunction. Patients who are confined, restricted by, or dependent on equipment may remind family members of the loss of control that they have, not only over their loved ones but also over their own destiny. This can lead to feelings of vulnerability and helplessness. Owing to the demands of technology, nurses may become distracted from being involved in the personal emotional care of the patient, and forget that amongst the machinery there is a person who is a precious and significant part of family life (Moore 2004).

Within the care environment nurses should design and implement (where appropriate) strategies to meet the needs of the family, but only after they have accurately assessed these needs and their relative importance for family members. If nurses are to promote holistic care they must provide family-sensitive care, where nurses and relatives develop a rapport and respect for each other. This can be achieved through effective communication channels, giving new information and reinforcing information already given. Family members should not be bombarded with unnecessary jargonistic information. Content should be adequate to enable them to understand what is happening and put them in a position to be able to ask questions.

Where appropriate, family members could also be encouraged to get involved in actual care delivery at a very basic level, for example assisting with basic hygiene needs, emptying urine bags, nail care, gentle massaging, etc. They should also be encouraged to touch and talk to the patient.

The nurse as an advocate

The nurse should be the patient's advocate and should always act in the best interests of the patient (Nursing and Midwifery Council (NMC) 2008). The unconscious patient is totally dependent on the nurse to attend to all their needs, including safety. Nurses have a moral duty to protect the patient's rights and it may be difficult for the nurse to advocate for a patient they don't know (Moore 2004).

Context

 When to perform ABCDE and care for the unconscious patient

When unconsciousness is an acute problem, perform ABCDE as a priority initially; regular reassessment will then be required.

Ongoing care of the unconscious patient will be needed; airways should be checked every time the nurse attends to the patient. Other aspects of the ABCDE should be checked every 30 minutes to 4 hours depending on the severity of the patient's problems.

Vigilance is crucial to recognize changes in the patient's condition, particularly in the acute situation. The patient's airway, together with the respiratory, cardiovascular, and neurological functions, requires close observation and monitoring.

Potential problems

Potential problems when caring for an unconscious patient are numerous. Important problems to look out for include:

- Compromised airway.
- Compromised breathing.
- Deterioration in conscious level/neurological function (GCS may indicate this).
- Skin breakdown, muscle wasting, joint stiffness, and limb deformities.
- Malnutrition.
- Constipation.

Indications for assistance

- Problems identified when undertaking the ABCDE assessment.
- When changing the patient's position.

Procedure: ABCDE assessment of the acute unconscious patient

Preparation

Prepare the patient

Even though the patient may seem unresponsive, each nursing intervention should be fully explained (hearing is the last sense to deteriorate). Discuss the procedure with the patient's family, reassuring them that the patient is not being harmed.

Prepare the equipment

Ensure the necessary equipment is available when undertaking an ABCDE assessment, e.g. suction, oxygen, sphygmomanometer, temperature recording device, pulse oximeter, ECG monitor, pen torch, GCS chart.

Step-by-step guide to maintaining the patient's airway

Step	Rationale
Look	
1 Look for any signs of obvious airway obstruction.	A compromised airway can lead to asphyxia and death.
2 Look for paradoxical (seesaw) chest movement. This is caused by the patient attempting to breathe in, so that the chest wall moves out and the abdomen moves in. During expiration the chest wall moves in and the abdominal wall moves out in an attempt to remove the obstruction.	Paradoxical chest movement could indicate complete blockage.
Listen	
3 Listen for abnormal sounds during breathing: **Gurgling** – caused by vomit or excessive sputum. **Snoring** – caused by the tongue obstructing the back of the pharynx due to loss of tone in the submandibular muscles. This is more common in the unconscious patient. **Crowing** – caused by laryngeal spasm. **Inspiratory stridor** – caused by blockage above or at level of the larynx. **Expiratory stridor** – caused by bronchospasm.	To detect a compromised airway.
Feel	
4 Put your hand just below the patient's nostrils and feel for air movement.	Warm air felt during expiration shows the patient is breathing.

continued overleaf

5	If an obstruction is visible, remove it if possible, e.g. use Magill's forceps to remove a foreign body, apply suction to remove fluid in the airway (Section 7.6).	An obstructed airway can lead to asphyxia.
6	If the airway is blocked by the tongue, perform 'head tilt–chin lift' (Resuscitation Council UK 2005).	To relieve the obstruction.
7	Once an open airway has been established, consider inserting an artificial airway, e.g. oropharyngeal or nasopharyngeal airway adjunct (see Section 7.4).	To prevent occlusion of the airway by the tongue falling back against the pharyngeal wall. To help ensure an open airway and adequate ventilation and oxygenation. To promote the drainage of respiratory secretions, preventing pooling in the back of the throat.
8	Place the patient in the lateral position.	To help maintain a patent airway.
9	Administer oxygen as prescribed.	To help prevent hypoxia/hypoxaemia.

Step-by-step guide to checking the patient's breathing

Step	Rationale
Look	
1 Observe the respiratory rate and rhythm. Check for: Cheyne–Stokes breathing – rhythmic increase and decrease in depth plus periods of apnoea. Biots respirations – quick, shallow breaths followed by periods of apnoea (about 4–5 cycles). Kussmaul's respiration – rapid, deep, laboured breathing. Hypopnoea (abnormal decrease in depth of respirations).	To determine whether the patient is breathing normally.
2 Assess nasal flaring and the use of accessory muscles: sternocleidomastoid (passes obliquely across the side of the neck); scalenus (a group of three muscles in the side of the neck); trapezius (a large muscle spanning the neck, shoulders, and vertebrae).	To determine the degree of effort. More effort suggests that the patient has difficulty in breathing.
Listen	
3 Listen to breathing. Assessment of breath sounds (with and without a stethoscope) should form part of the nursing assessment (Moore 2007). Nurses listening to the patient's breath sounds through	Knowledge of the different types of breath sounds is important to aid description and diagnosis (Moore 2007). If a patient is heard to be breathing noisily this should be investigated immediately as it could indicate partial blockage.

a stethoscope should have undergone appropriate training and education. Without a stethoscope, normal breathing should be quiet.

4	Listen for wheezing – a high or low-pitched musical sound produced by restricted airflow.	May indicate patient requires bronchodilators.
5	Listen for crackles and bubbling sounds, usually indicating fluid.	Patient requires suctioning.
6	Suction when indicated, i.e. tachypnoea, decreased oxygen saturation levels, audible sounds, etc. (see Section 7.6).	To clear airways and help breathing.
7	Humidified oxygen may be indicated.	Warms and moistens lung secretions.
8	Physiotherapy as indicated.	Helps loosen secretions and facilitates lung expansion, preventing atelectasis and hypostatic pneumonia.

Measure

| 9 | Measure respiratory rate. | Widely accepted as being the most sensitive basic observation for detecting patient deterioration (Goldhill *et al.* 1999). Patient's respiratory rate/rhythm can be affected by changes in metabolic, neurological, and cardiac status. |

Step-by-step guide to assessing circulation

Step	Rationale

Look

1	Assess skin colour for signs of reduced peripheral perfusion (sweaty pallor, cool limbs).	Could indicate shock.
2	Measure capillary refill time (CRT): press on the sternum for 5 seconds and release; normal CRT is <2 seconds. If CRT >2 seconds this may indicate reduced perfusion.	To help determine whether the patient has reduced perfusion.
3	Observe for signs of haemorrhage or fluid loss both internally and externally.	To determine whether the patient has a haemorrhage.

Listen

| 4 | Record the patient's blood pressure. | To detect hypotension/hypertension. |

Feel

| 5 | Palpate the radial pulse: assess rate, rhythm, and volume. If pulse is weak and thready, consider assessing a central pulse, e.g. carotid/femoral. | To help assess the adequacy of circulation. |

Step-by-step guide to assessing disability and exposure

Step		Rationale
1	Perform bedside blood glucose measurement (see Section 10.2).	To detect hypoglycaemia/hyperglycaemia.
2	Record AVPU and GCS (see Section 8.1).	To objectively assess the level of consciousness.
3	Assess the pupils: size, shape, and reaction to light. Compare both sides (see Section 8.1).	To detect any abnormality that may indicate the cause of the unconsciousness.
4	Exposure – perform head to toe survey, maintaining the patient's dignity and temperature.	To detect any abnormalities.

Step-by-step guide to ongoing care of the unconscious patient

Step		Rationale
1	Maintain a safe environment. Ensure the patient is safe and will not fall out of bed, e.g. apply cot sides.	To maintain patient safety.
2	Take measures to prevent cross-infection, e.g. always wash and dry hands before and after caring for the patient.	To minimize the risk of cross-infection.
3	Assist and monitor respiratory function, e.g. ensure a patent airway, administer prescribed oxygen, ensure patient position does not compromise chest movement, suction as necessary.	To ensure normal respiratory function.
4	Monitor cardiovascular function, e.g. undertake routine observation, administer IV fluids as prescribed.	To ensure normal cardiovascular function.
5	Monitor nutrition and hydration, e.g. ensure IV fluids are administered as prescribed, maintain a fluid balance chart, ensure a nutritional assessment is undertaken.	To ensure normal nutrition and hydration.
6	Monitor gastrointestinal function, e.g. monitor bowel function and perform bowel care as required (see Section 10.5).	To ensure normal gastrointestinal function and prevent constipation.

7	Monitor genitourinary function, e.g. monitor urine output, insert a urinary catheter (see Section 9.1).	To ensure normal genitourinary function.
8	Attend to the patient's hygiene requirements, e.g. washing, mouth care, eye care.	To maintain patient comfort.
9	Assess the patient's skin integrity using a recognized assessment tool, e.g. Waterlow scale.	To determine the patient's risk of developing pressure sores.
10	Regularly change the patient's position.	To help prevent pressure sores.
11	Perform passive exercises (see Section 11.2).	To help prevent muscle wasting and promote muscle/joint function.
12	Monitor the patient's temperature and ensure steps are taken to avoid hyperthermia and hypothermia.	To help maintain normal body temperature.
13	Communicate with the patient.	May help reduce patient's anxiety.

Recognizing patient deterioration

A person's level of consciousness is the most sensitive indicator of brain function (Geraghty 2005). Any change in level of consciousness is often the first clue to a deteriorating condition (Morton *et al*. 2005). Sudden unconsciousness is a medical emergency (Beattie 2007). This can be a very frightening and daunting experience. As with any emergency, it is important to keep calm and not panic. You will probably feel that you are unable to deal with the situation, so it is vital that you get help immediately.

It is important to note that the unconscious patient will not be able to communicate any problems that they have. Hence it is essential that the patient is closely monitored for signs of deterioration/improvement. The nurse is in a unique position to interpret the patient's non-verbal body language and make the decision to call for additional assistance.

Wherever possible, a detailed history regarding the patient's normal pattern of behaviour should be obtained (in the first instance through family, hospital records, etc.) to act as a baseline for clinical decision-making.

Reflection and evaluation

When you have been involved in caring for a patient who is unconscious, think about the following questions:

1. Did you find performing total care for a patient difficult or straightforward? Make a list of your reasons.
2. Has this experience changed your views in any way regarding patients who are unconscious?
3. Were you able to predict potential problems for the patient? If so what were they?
4. Based on your knowledge and observations of the patient, were you able to anticipate their needs as accurately as possible? Discuss this with your mentor.

Further learning opportunities

Find a noisy, crowded place (e.g. train station, shopping centre) and close your eyes for approximately 5 minutes. Write down your experiences. Issues to think about:

- Were there any unfamiliar noises?
- Did anyone come and sit next to you? Talk to you?
- How did you feel? Did you feel exposed/ vulnerable?
- What did you want to happen to make you feel safe and secure?

Discuss your feelings with a friend or colleagues.

Reminders

Don't forget:

- Talk to the patient – hearing is the last sense to go. There are also psychological benefits for the patient, nurse, and family.
- Be careful of your own communication around the patient.
- Try to distinguish between induced unconsciousness and unconsciousness caused by the disease process.
- Caring for the unconscious patient can be a very daunting and challenging experience. It can be difficult to provide care that is individualized. Examine your own beliefs and attitudes towards patient care, particularly that of an unconscious patient.

 Patient scenarios

Consider what you should do in the following situations, then turn to the end of this skill to check your answers.

1   Samuel King is a 45-year-old gentleman who has been admitted with hyperglycaemic coma. He has been unconscious for 6 hours. You have not been involved in his care. You walk past his bed and notice that there is a noise coming from him, which sounds as though he is 'snoring'. You observe that he is lying on his back. What do you think might be the problem? What should you do?

2   Carmella Palanca is 73 years old and has recently been transferred from the high dependency unit to your ward. She has been unconscious for a total of 2 weeks following a cardiac arrest. She is self-ventilating and has a Guedel airway in place. She remains unresponsive to painful stimuli. How would you ensure her needs are met?

Website

 http://www.oxfordtextbooks.co.uk/orc/ endacott

You may find it helpful to work through our short online quiz and additional scenarios intended to help you to develop and apply the skills in this chapter.

References

Ashworth P (1980). *Care to communicate*. Royal College of Nursing, London.

Beattie S (2007). Bedside emergency: respiratory distress. *RN*, **70**(7), 34–8.

Branch WT, Kern D, Haidef P *et al.* (2001). Teaching the human dimension of care in clinical settings. *JAMA*, **286**(9), 1067–74.

Chant S, Jenkinson T, Randle J, Russell G, and Webb C (2002). Communication skills training in healthcare: a review of the literature. *Nurse Education Today*, **22**, 189–202.

Cooper N (2004). Acute care: brain failure. *Student BMJ*, **12**, 221–64.

Elliot R and Wright L (1999). Verbal communication: what do critical care nurses say to their unconscious or sedated patients? *Journal of Advanced Nursing*, **29**(6), 1412–20.

Geraghty M (2005). Nursing the unconscious patient. *Nursing Standard*, **20**(1), 54–64.

Goldhill DR, White SA, and Sumner A (1999). Physiological values and procedures in the 24 hours before ICU admission from the ward. *Anaesthesia* **54**(9), 529–34.

Goode M (2004). Communication barriers when managing a patient with a wound. *British Journal of Nursing*, **13**(1), 49–52.

Lawrence M (1995). The unconscious experience. *American Journal of Critical Care*, **4**(3), 227–32.

Moore T (2004). Suctioning. In T Moore and P Woodrow. *High dependency nursing care: observation, intervention and Support*, pp. 290–300. Routledge, London.

Moore T (2007). Respiratory assessment in adults. *Nursing Standard*, **21**(49), 48–56.

Morton G, Fontaine D, Hudak C, and Gallo B (2005). *Critical care nursing: a holistic approach*, 8th edition. Lippincott Williams and Wilkins, Philadelphia.

Nursing and Midwifery Council (2008). *The Code: standards of conduct, performance and ethics for nurses and midwives*. NMC, London.

Park E and Song M (2005). Communication barriers perceived by older patients and nurses. *International Journal of Nursing Studies*, **42**(2), 159–66.

Pemberton L (2000). The unconscious patient. In M Alexander, J Fawcett, and P Runchman, eds. *Nursing practice, hospital and home. The adult*, 2nd edition, pp. 851–71. Churchill Livingstone, London.

Resuscitation Council (UK) (2005). *Adult basic life support.* RCUK, London.

Smith G (2000). *ALERT: acute life-threatening events recognition and treatment.* University of Portsmouth, Portsmouth.

Waugh A and Grant A (2006). *Ross and Wilson anatomy and physiology in health and illness.* Elsevier, Oxford.

Useful further reading and websites

DaiWai M and Graffagnino C (2005). Consciousness, coma, and caring for the brain-injured patient. *Neurological Nursing,* **16**(4), 441–55.

Heppleston B (2008). Starting out: student experiences in the real world of nursing. Looking after an unconscious patient felt like a privilege. *Nursing Standard,* **22**(21): 27.

Sheehan M (2008). Artificial nutrition and hydration and the permanently unconscious patient. *JAMA,* **299**, 1610–11.

http://www.allnurses.com/forums/f300/ caring-unconscious-patient-299558

http://www.emory.edu/whscl/grady/inetgrp/ hplung.html (for lung sounds)

Ⓐ Answers to patient scenarios

1 Samuel has an airway obstruction caused by the tongue occluding the oropharynx. You need to open his mouth and observe quickly for any signs of obvious obstruction (vomit, etc.), then do a 'head tilt–chin lift' manoeuvre. Call for help. Assess the need for a Guedel airway. Place patient on his side. Document the event.

2

- Ensure patency of airway – position, suctioning.
- All basic care – e.g. mouth care, eye care, hygiene needs, catheter care.
- Communication needs – talk to her.
- Nutrition via enteral feed.
- Regular turning on side (to maintain airway, prevent pressure ulcers, help facilitate lung expansion).
- Continue observations, noting any improvement or deterioration in condition.

8.3 **Assessing cognitive function** Ⓐ

This is an advanced skill. You *must* check whether you can assist with or undertake this skill, in line with local policy.

Definition

Being able to assess cognitive function is an important skill both in the recognition of acute confusion (delirium) in an acutely ill patient and in determining when a patient is showing cognitive decline in dementia. This section describes the use of the Mini Mental State Examination (MMSE) and Abbreviated Mental Test (AMT) to assess cognitive function.

It is important to remember that:

- As clinical instruments, the AMT and MMSE are used to detect impairment, follow the course of an illness, and monitor response to treatment.
- While the MMSE does not give specific diagnostic answers in individual clinical syndromes, it represents a brief, standardized method by which to grade cognitive mental status.
- The AMT and MMSE assess orientation, attention, immediate and short-term recall, language, and the ability to follow simple verbal and written commands.

Prior knowledge

Before attempting an assessment of cognitive function, make sure you are familiar with:

1 The frontal, parietal, and temporal lobes of the cerebral cortex and their functions.
2 The anatomy and function of the Broca's and Wernicke's areas, concerned with speech.
3 Common causes of altered cognitive function (see Table 8.4).
4 Tools in common use for assessing cognitive function.
5 The clinical presentation of dementia.

Table 8.4 Common causes of altered cognition

Delirium (acute confusion)	Sepsis: any infection with high fever, e.g. pneumonia, UTI Metabolic disturbance, e.g. renal failure, electrolyte disturbance Hypoxia in respiratory failure Drugs: antiepileptics, sedatives Space-occupying lesions (tumour, abscess) and stroke Relocation No cause found (5–20%)
Dementia	Alzheimer's disease Lewy body dementia Multi-infarct (vascular) dementia Parkinson's disease Normal pressure hydrocephalus Genetic disease: Huntington's disease Traumatic: post-head injury Infections: Creutzfeldt–Jakob disease, HIV, syphilis Pseudodementia of depression Metabolic: vitamin B deficiency, hypothyroidism, liver disease, hyper/hypoparathyroidism, Addison's, Cushing's Cerebral lesions, e.g. subdural haematoma (especially in elderly)
Drug misuse (intoxication and withdrawal)	Alcohol Drugs of abuse (ecstasy, cannabis, opiates)

Background

Cognitive function (or cognition) is defined as the intellectual process by which one becomes aware of and comprehends ideas and situations. It includes all aspects of perception: attention, recognition, thinking, reasoning, use of memory, and imagination.

Processing sensory information is a complex task involving different areas of the brain. However, it is known that distinct areas of the brain's **cortex** are responsible for individual cognitive tasks (see **Figure 8.6**). The grooves in the brain's surface (**sulci**) divide the brain into discrete zones (**gyri**), each with a different role. It also increases the surface area of the brain and therefore the capacity for information processing; this is why humans have a greater ability for cognition than other species.

The frontal lobe is responsible for specific cognitive processes such as reasoning, judgement, insight, memory, and ability to draw shapes. It also interacts with other areas of the brain involved in sensory perception, memory, and emotion.

Cognitive impairment

Cognitive impairment is therefore a difficulty in reacting intellectually to new information or situations. For example, a patient with dementia may have a slow decline and initially be confused only in new environments. However, they may deteriorate so that they have difficulty recognizing familiar surroundings. Symptoms vary depending on the severity of the problem. In severe loss of cognitive function, symptoms may include difficulty thinking or concentrating, a drop in IQ, episodic memory loss, and episodic problems with confusion. This can interfere with activities of daily living such as shopping, working, and operating motor vehicles.

Cognitive decline is not a normal part of ageing for most people, but with age comes the increasing likelihood of developing memory loss. The mildest form, age-related memory loss, is characterized by self-perception of memory loss and a standardized memory test score showing a decline in performance compared with younger adults. About 40% of people aged 65 or older have age-related memory loss, and are able to function

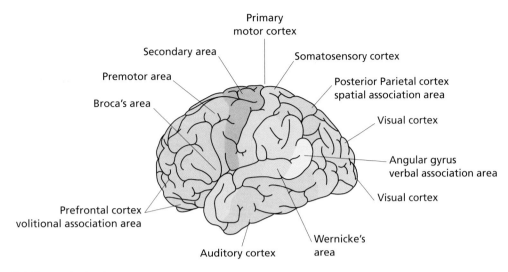

Figure 8.6 The cerebral cortex.

normally in day-to-day life. Only about 1% of them will progress to dementia each year.

Dementia can be described as the global impairment of cognition and personality but with no impairment of consciousness. There is slow deterioration in cognitive function to the extent that dementia interferes with daily life, and eventually the patient cannot live independently. There is often associated low mood, poor emotional control, and inappropriate social behaviour. Alzheimer's disease is the commonest cause of dementia in the UK, and those with the abnormal apolipoprotein E gene are more at risk. However, it is important to recognize that there are other causes of dementia, some of which are reversible. Multi-infarct dementia, resulting from multiple very small strokes in patients with cerebrovascular disease, is also common. Treatment of this disease may result in slowing of the progression of the dementia.

Acute confusional state or delirium is an acute failure of cognitive function seen in up to 20% of acutely ill hospital inpatients. Therefore, it is a presentation that you will come across virtually every day on a medical or elderly care ward. Impairment of attention and memory, and abnormal perception such as visual hallucinations are seen, and the condition classically fluctuates over time. Investigation and treatment of the underlying cause will usually help. A large number of diseases cause confusion; some of the more common ones are shown in Table 8.4.

A brain already in decline predisposes you to delirium and so the presentation commonly overlaps with dementia. As the population ages, a higher proportion of acute emergency medical admissions are elderly patients with multiple medical problems, including longstanding cognitive impairment. In some elderly care patients who are depressed, this can present as confusion, poor memory, and poor attention, without the classic symptoms of depression.

Assessing cognitive impairment

The Mini Mental State Examination (MMSE) is used to screen for the presence of cognitive impairment over a number of areas such as memory, attention, reasoning, and decision-making. It is based on a series of questions and practical tests.

The MMSE was developed by Folstein in the 1970s (Folstein *et al.* 1975) and is widely used by elderly care physicians and other health professionals worldwide. It takes 15 minutes to carry out and is based on a series of questions and tasks. Points are accrued when questions or tasks are answered or undertaken correctly. A maximum of 30 points is possible, with scores of 26 or less generally being reported by people with cognitive impairment. The

Table 8.5 The abbreviated mental test (AMT) summarized

Question	Score
What is your age?	0 or 1
What is the time (to the nearest hour)?	0 or 1
Give the patient an address ('42 West Street'), and ask them to repeat it at the end of the test. Ask the patient to repeat it to ensure they have heard it.	
What is the year?	0 or 1
What is the name of the hospital or number of the residence where the patient is situated?	0 or 1
Can the patient recognize two persons (doctor, nurse, home help, etc.)?	0 or 1
What is your date of birth?	0 or 1
In which year did the First World War begin (adjust this for a world event the patient would have known during childhood)?	0 or 1
What is the name of the present monarch (head of state, etc.)?	0 or 1
Count backwards from 20 to 1	0 or 1
Repeat address	0 or 1
	Score/10

Hodkinson (1972)

MMSE has also been used as a research tool to screen for cognitive disorders in population studies and follow cognitive changes in clinical trials.

As time is often at a premium and other clinical tasks may take priority, the Abbreviated Mental Test (AMT) is often used as a simpler alternative to the MMSE. It can be done from memory and without the need for pen and paper. The AMT was introduced by Hodkinson in 1972 to assess elderly patients rapidly for the possibility of dementia. It takes less than 5 minutes to carry out. Its uses in medicine have again become somewhat wider to include assessing for confusion, although it has mainly been validated in the elderly with dementia. Each question correctly answered scores one point (see **Table 8.5**). A score of less than seven suggests abnormal cognitive function (Jitapunkul *et al.* 1991) in delirium or dementia. In the case of dementia, further and more formal tests are necessary to confirm the diagnosis.

Full evaluation of altered cognition should include review of the onset and course of symptoms, a physical examination, and laboratory investigations to rule out treatable medical conditions. A drug history will help sort out possible drug toxicity as a cause of memory loss. Screening for low mood can often be done through a standardized anxiety and depression questionnaire. Laboratory assessments should at least include some blood tests to screen out thyroid disease, vitamin B12 deficiency, anaemia, and liver disease.

Context

 When to undertake assessment of cognitive function

Because altered cognition may signal a treatable medical condition, it is important to take any complaint seriously.

Risk factors that should trigger an assessment of cognitive function include age older than 65 years, illnesses that increase the possibility of a diagnosis of dementia (diabetes, Parkinson's disease, stroke disease, etc.), or a family history of dementia. A simple question about the patient's memory ability is often a good screen for problems, and any problems should prompt an AMT or MMSE.

An estimate of the level of a patient's cognitive function is useful in the following situations:

- When briefly assessing an acutely ill patient, e.g. a patient alerted to A&E, as part of a general assessment.
- To assess whether a patient is confused where there is some doubt over the diagnosis.
- To gauge improvement in confusion or response to treatment.
- To gauge severity of acute illness, e.g. if confusion complicates acute infection, this indicates a more severe form of sepsis.
- To contribute towards a diagnosis of dementia.
- The MMSE score can predict how well a patient will cope alone at home and may indicate social support is needed.
- To document deteriorating cognitive function over a period of time in dementia (this is done formally using a MMSE).
- To document responses to treatment in dementia (MMSE).

 When not to undertake assessment of cognitive function

A full cognitive assessment may not always be appropriate. If a patient is drowsy or unresponsive they will not be able to answer any questions, and the clinical priority should be assessment of airway, breathing, and circulation. Management of acutely unwell patients should always follow the ABCDE rule!

Potential problems

- These cognitive assessments cannot take into account very well educated people who have mild dementia. They may well score within normal range because they find the questions easy. Equally, poorly educated people may score badly simply because they find the questions difficult. Their scoring on the MMSE may indicate a diagnosis of dementia when none is present. These difficulties indicate the need for a number of different tests when diagnosing diseases such as Alzheimer's.
- The normal value for MMSE score is also corrected for degree of schooling and age. Crum *et al.* (1993) have produced tables of normal values for MMSE score depending on education and age.
- Poor attention and memory loss due to other mental disorders such as depression can also lead to abnormal findings on cognitive testing.
- The presence of purely physical problems can also interfere with interpretation if not properly noted. For example, a patient may be physically unable to hear or read instructions properly, or may have had a stroke deficit that affects writing and drawing skills.

Interpreting readings

- An AMT score of less than seven suggests abnormal cognitive function (Jitapunkul *et al.* 1991) in delirium or dementia.

- In the MMSE, scores of 27 and above are considered normal, scores of 25–27 indicate a borderline condition needing further investigation, and scores of 24 and below are abnormal and suggest cognitive impairment may be present, which may impact on day-to-day life. This loss of function will need further assessment by occupational therapists, social workers, and physiotherapists.

- Low to very low AMT and MMSE scores correlate closely with the presence of established dementia.

Special considerations

- Cognitive ability, as measured by the MMSE, varies within the population by age and educational level. There is an inverse relationship between MMSE scores and age. The average score at age 18–24 is 29; it is 25 for those older than 80 (Crum *et al.* 1993).

- The median MMSE score is 29 for individuals with at least 9 years of schooling, but 22 for those with fewer than 5 years of schooling.

Procedure

Preparation

Prepare yourself
Check the patient's notes.

Prepare the patient
Assessing cognitive function can be a sensitive subject for patients and their families, who may be fearful of the outcome of wrong answers and poor performance.

Prepare the environment
Find a quiet area away from the distractions of a busy ward – ideally a side room or quiet office. You need a pen and a piece of paper, and make sure there is a firm surface to lean on so that you can write down the responses. If your department has copies of the MMSE for use with patients you can use the back for AMT or drawing on, and this also provides evidence when filed in the medical notes.

> **Discussing the procedure with the patient and family**
>
> Anxiety and depression can produce poor outcomes on cognitive assessments, so explain to the patient and family what you are doing – that you are just going to test their memory with a few simple questions.

A guide to using AMT to assess cognitive function is presented in the following step-by-step guide.

Step-by-step guide to assessing cognitive function

Step	Rationale
1 Introduce yourself, confirm the patient's identity, explain the procedure, and obtain consent.	To identify the patient correctly and gain informed consent. It is also a good screen for whether they recognize your role or appear to be very confused.
Orientation	
2 'What is the time?' to the nearest hour. 'What day is it today?' 'What is the date today?' Ask the patient *two* questions about time, date, or location. There is one mark for each correct answer, and no marks for incorrect answers.	To test orientation in time.
3 Ask the patient the name of the hospital or number of the residence where they are currently situated. Score one point for a correct answer.	To test orientation in place.
4 Can the patient recognize two persons nearby (doctor, nurse, home help, etc.)? Score one point for a correct answer.	To test orientation in person.
Memory – short term	
5 Give the patient an address ('42 West Street'). Ask them to repeat it to ensure they have heard it. There are no points scored here. If the patient fails, repeat the address until it has been remembered.	To test immediate recall.

6 Ask 'What is the name of the present monarch?' You could also ask about the Prime Minister. Score one point for a correct answer.

To test short-term memory.

Memory – long term

7 Ask 'How old are you?' or 'What is your age?' Score a point for the correct answer.

To test memory.

8 Ask 'What is your date of birth?' Score a point for the correct answer.

To test memory.

9 Ask 'In which year did the First World War begin?' You can adjust this for a world event the patient would have known during childhood, for example the Second World War instead. Score one point for a correct answer.

To test memory.

Attention and calculation

10 Ask 'Can you count backwards from 20 to 1?' Alternatively: 'Spell W-O-R-L-D backwards'. To score a single point, the person must count backwards from 20 correctly, i.e. 19, 18, 17, 16, 15, etc. (or spell word backwards correctly).

To test the ability to concentrate.

Memory – recall

11 Ask 'Can you repeat to me the address I asked you to remember earlier?' Give one point if the patient can remember the correct address.

To test recall.

Following the procedure

Record the patient's AMT score in their current medical notes. This will then be available for all health care professionals to see on a day-to-day basis. If taking a more formal MMSE, file the completed MMSE score sheet in the medical notes in the results section. Write down any factors that you think may compound the results – such as 'patient became drowsy', 'patient seemed disinterested' or 'low in mood'.

Reflection and evaluation

When you have undertaken a cognitive assessment with a patient, think about the following questions:

1 Was the score consistent with your expectations for that particular patient? If not, why not?

2 Were you able to answer any questions that the patient asked you?

3 Were you able to interpret the score in light of the patient's medical conditions?

Further learning opportunities

- Discuss the results or any difficulties with the test with more senior nursing staff.
- You will need to practise asking the questions in order to remember them. It will probably be necessary to carry a small reminder card to prompt you.
- The score you get may be different to a previously documented score. This may be because the patient's condition has changed. However, if you think you have made a mistake, ask a senior colleague to check for you.

Reminders

Don't forget to:

- Give the patient the correct number of points for each task.
- Record the AMT or MMSE score in the patient's notes.
- Consider other causes of cognitive impairment before assuming a patient has dementia.

Patient scenarios

Consider what you should do in the following situations, then turn to the end of this skill to check your answers.

1 You meet a 76-year-old lady who has had a steady decline in her short-term memory over the preceding 2 years. Her family are concerned that she is too forgetful to live on her own any more, particularly as she was found wandering round the local village late at night. Lately she becomes tearful about the death of her husband, an event that happened over 20 years ago. What do you think is happening? What would her AMT or MMSE show?

2 You meet a 60-year-old man on a medical ward whose wife tells you he was completely normal prior to admission with confusion. His MMSE score is 12/30. What conditions may be causing his low MMSE score?

Website

 http://www.oxfordtextbooks.co.uk/orc/ endacott

You may find it helpful to work through our short online quiz and additional scenarios intended to help you to develop and apply the skills in this chapter.

References

Crum RM, Anthony JC, Bassett SS, and Folstein MF (1993). Population-based norms for the mini-mental state examination by age and educational level. *Journal of the American Medical Association*, **18**, 2386–91.

Folstein MF, Folstein SE and McHugh PR (1975). Mini-Mental State: a practical method for grading the state of patients for the clinician. *Journal of Psychiatric Research*, **12**, 189–98.

Hodkinson HM (1972). Evaluation of a mental test score for assessment of mental impairment in the elderly. *Age and Ageing* **1**, 233–8.

Jitapunkul S, Pillay I, and Ebrahim S (1991). The abbreviated mental test: its use and validity. *Age and Ageing*, **20**, 332–6.

Useful further reading and websites

Cockrell JR and Folstein MF (1988). Mini Mental State Examination (MMSE). *Psychopharmacology*, **24**, 689–92.

Small GW (2002). What we need to know about age related memory loss. *British Medical Journal*, **324**, 1502–5.

Tombaugh TN and McIntyre NJ (1993). The mini-mental state examination: a comprehensive review. *Journal of the American Geriatric Society*, **41**(3), 346.

Home of the Folstein Mini Mental State Examination (Psychological Assessment Resources Inc. hold the copyright): **http://www.minimental.com/**

Resource for carers and patients including explanation of the MMSE: **http://www.alzheimers.org.uk/**

Answers to patient scenarios

1 This lady has a slow cognitive decline typical of Alzheimer's disease (also consider depression). Her MMSE score would be less than 25 and possibly very low at this stage.

2 Sepsis, renal failure, electrolyte disturbance, respiratory failure, stroke, and drugs would be the common ones.

8.4 Pain assessment and management

Definition

Pain is described by the International Association for the Study of Pain as 'an unpleasant sensory and emotional experience associated with actual or potential tissue damage or described in terms of such damage' (Merskey 1979). Its subjective nature and lack of objective methods of measurement mean that there is a heavy reliance upon 'whatever the experiencing person says it is, existing wherever they say it does' (McCaffery 1979).

It is important to remember that:

- Pain can mean different things to different people at different times in their lives.
- Individual patient requirements for pain relief can vary. This necessitates the need for a thorough initial pain assessment as part of the overall assessment of the patient's general condition.
- As the patient's medical condition changes, so can their pain experience. A dynamic individualized approach to pain assessment and management is therefore needed, which includes regular review of the patient's condition and treatment.
- Not all patients will need or benefit from the use of analgesic drugs. Other non-pharmacological means of providing pain relief may therefore be useful and as effective as pain-relieving drugs.
- Nurses have a key role to play in the assessment of pain, education of patients with pain, and administration of pain relief.
- The successful management of pain is frequently an amalgam of skills, which when combined result in the provision of individualized patient care.

Prior knowledge

Before undertaking assessment and management of pain, make sure you are familiar with:

1   The physiology of the nervous system. In particular, look at the normal functioning of the nervous system and how information is transmitted along nerves to the brain.
2   The pharmacology of drugs. This is a large subject so try and limit your focus to the different methods of administration, how drugs are absorbed by the body, their actions within the body (including both desired and unwanted effects), and how they are metabolized and excreted from the body. You can then apply this to the commonly used analgesic drugs such as opiates, paracetamol, non-steroidal anti-inflammatory drugs, and local anaesthetics.
3   Policies and procedures (including legal restrictions) governing the use of drugs for the management of pain. Of particular importance are the storage, prescription, and administration of controlled drugs.

Background

At its simplest level, pain may be thought of as a process whereby sensory nerve endings detect a noxious event such as excessive pressure, heat, cold, or chemical irritation. Information is then passed via peripheral nerves to the spinal cord and the brain. Various centres within the brain are then activated that in turn provoke a physical and emotional response. This pain pathway can be influenced by the use of a variety of therapeutic interventions, such as the use of analgesic drugs to limit the amount of information passing to the brain or to alter the perception of pain within the brain. In reality pain is much more than the detection of a noxious event; it is a complex interplay of physiological and psychological processes that modulate the perception of and reaction to pain. The pain experience can therefore differ considerably between individuals with seemingly similar causes of pain, for example following a surgical procedure.

The importance of the psychological component of pain is underlined when factors such as anxiety, previous pain experiences, and cultural factors that enhance the perception of pain are considered. Likewise relief of anxiety and use of cognitive techniques such as relaxation therapy and distraction can reduce the feeling of pain. Such factors can be influenced by the therapeutic relationship between the patient and the nurse, as well as the patient's wider social context. In short, pain is a bio-psycho-social phenomenon.

Pain is a common feature of many medical conditions. Hence, the nurse will encounter patients who require pain assessment and management on an almost daily basis. It is therefore important that nurses appreciate its effects upon their patients and the different ways in which pain can be:

- **Assessed** by the use of observation, questioning, and assessment tools.
- **Managed** using a variety of physical, pharmacological, and psychological strategies in order to improve patient comfort and optimize clinical outcome.

Pain is such an important aspect of clinical practice that it has been termed the 'fifth vital sign' (Joint Commission on Accreditation of Healthcare Organisations 2001). It is an important symptom of many medical conditions, informing both the sufferer and the health care provider that something is wrong. In this respect pain is beneficial to our health, forming part of the body's natural defence system.

Pain can, however, be counterproductive with regard to the restrictions it places upon normal activity. For example, sleep can be disturbed, preventing adequate rest. In hospital there are also important clinical considerations, particularly following surgery, as severe pain can impair mobility and contribute to the development of complications such as chest infections and deep vein thrombosis. The stresses it places upon the body can also increase the risk of a myocardial infarction and delay wound healing. Such problems have a human and financial cost as they impact upon the patient's recovery and increase length of stay in hospital.

Long-term pain is a frequent cause of disability with significant psychological, social, and economic effects on the sufferer (Pain Coalition 2007). In Europe it is estimated that one in seven adults experience some form of chronic pain (see **http://www.painineurope.com**). This has an impact on society as a whole due to problems such as loss of employment and claims for incapacity benefits (Pain Coalition 2007).

Evidence shows that pain is often poorly addressed, despite being a particular concern for patients (Health Care Commission 2006). Studies have also found that nurses significantly underestimate the intensity of pain in patients (Sloman *et al.* 2005).

Specialist pain management services are available to deal with different forms of pain (Royal College of Anaesthetists and The Pain Society 2003). However, the management of pain needs to be viewed as a fundamental component of normal nursing practice and not left solely to the specialists. It is therefore an issue for nurses in both primary and secondary care.

Knowledge of the need for and difficulties involved in pain assessment and the bio-psycho-social influences that can affect it has assisted in the development of various physical, psychological, and pharmacological treatments. These can be termed 'the **four Ps** of pain', which the nurse can apply during day-to-day clinical practice.

Causes and classification of pain

Pain has many causes and treatments and is usually classified in two ways: acute or chronic, and nociceptive or neuropathic.

- **Acute pain** is typically of sudden onset, occurring as a result of tissue injury or disease. It usually resolves over time as tissue healing occurs.
- **Chronic pain** often begins with an episode of acute pain, but does not resolve over time. The most common causes of chronic pain are degenerative conditions such as diabetes or osteoarthritis. A small number of patients experience chronic pain without a clearly defined medical cause.

Patients can experience acute and chronic pain at the same time. An example of this is an older person with arthritic pain who sustains an acute injury. They experience acute pain from their injury as well as their chronic arthritic pain.

- **Nociceptive pain** is caused by the activation of nerve receptors by a noxious stimulus. This may be caused by excessive heat, cold, stretching, or chemical irritation. It is commonly seen in clinical practice as a result of tissue damage following injury, surgery, or disease. It typically resolves following tissue healing, but, if caused by a chronic condition such as arthritis, it can be continuous. This form of pain is sometimes termed inflammatory pain. Patients may describe this form of pain as *sharp, aching, crushing*, or *throbbing* in its nature.
- **Neuropathic pain** results from a malfunction of the peripheral or central nervous system. It is therefore often called nerve pain. Shingles (*Herpes zoster* infection) is a condition that can produce severe *peripheral* neuropathic pain. *Central* neuropathic pain arises from a condition of the brain and most commonly results following a stroke (cerebrovascular accident). Patients may describe this form of pain as *hot, burning, stabbing, jumping, shooting* (like an electric shock), and *tingling* (pins and needles). It can be accompanied by changes in sensation and colour of the skin in the affected area.

It is important to be aware of these different forms of pain, as they often require different treatment strategies. Some patients can have both forms of pain. For example, a person with diabetes can have peripheral neuropathic pain caused by degeneration of peripheral nerves, and nociceptive (inflammatory) pain caused by an infected venous leg ulcer. As a consequence they may require a combination of drugs to treat both forms of pain.

Pain commonly results from injury or disease. However, pain also often occurs as a result of medical and nursing procedures. The undertaking of dressings, insertion and removal of drains, and manipulation of a fracture site are some examples of **procedural** pain. Although generally short lived, procedural pain can pose a significant problem for patients and their carers. For example, severe pain associated with the changing of a leg ulcer dressing can limit the choice and effectiveness of the dressing used (Hollinworth 1997). The need to control procedural pain, for example post-operative pain, has led to the development of various pain management techniques and creation of acute pain services.

Cancer pain

Pain is often associated with cancer and can manifest as either an acute or chronic problem that may be nociceptive, neuropathic, or a combination of both in its nature. Cancer pain should therefore not be viewed as a distinct form of pain in its own right but as a cause of the previously mentioned forms of pain.

Assessing pain

The way the patient describes their pain can vary. Therefore, always allow time for the patient to describe the way their pain feels, as this can be particularly important in helping to determine the nature of the pain. Special arrangements such as the provision of an interpreter may also have to be made if there are language difficulties.

Your interview skills and the quality of information obtained will be enhanced if you keep in mind the following:

- Seek to establish a relationship with the patient.
- Encourage the patient to do most of the talking.
- Begin with a wide-angle, open question before clarifying and focusing with more specific ones (see below).
- Watch the patient for clues regarding pain.
- Avoid jumping to conclusions.

When interviewing the patient, try to obtain the following information:

- **The time of the onset of pain** – Did the pain follow a particular event such as an injury or infection, or did it develop over time?
- **The site or sites of the pain** – Some patients may have pain in more than one area.
- **Frequency of pain** – Does the pain come and go or is it constant?
- **Description of the pain** – This is important in determining the type of pain experienced. Also note if there are any accompanying symptoms, such as altered sensation, numbness, or increased sensitivity in a particular area.
- **Intensity of the pain** – How bad the pain feels. This can be quantified using a simple pain scale (see Box 8.1).
- **Factors that aggravate the pain** – E.g. is it worse after standing, walking, or eating certain foods?
- **Factors that make the pain appear better** – E.g. changing position, taking rest, use of drugs or complementary therapies. If taking drugs, note the dose and frequency.
- **Success or failure of previous treatment** – Has the patient used any drugs, etc. before? If so, did they have any effect? In particular, make a note of any drug-related side effects that may have occurred, such as stomach upset, nausea, vomiting, constipation, or sedation.
- **Effects on day-to-day physical activity, sleep, and emotional state** – Is the patient having enough sleep? Are there any problems with friends and family as a result of their condition?
- **Use of other medications** – The use of other drugs should be noted as some may have implications for the use of certain analgesics. E.g. non-steroidal anti-inflammatory drugs have a risk of causing gastric irritation and bleeding, which can be dangerous for patients taking anticoagulant drugs such as warfarin.

Documentation

Initial information should be recorded in the patient's assessment documentation. A repeat assessment may be needed if the nature or site of the pain changes. Subsequent assessments of pain intensity and other symptoms may be recorded on an assessment chart that makes use of an assessment tool.

Pain assessment tools

Box 8.1 Examples of simple assessment tools used to describe pain intensity and other symptoms at ward level

Numerical scales

Pain assessment scale
0 = No pain
1 = Mild pain
2 = Pain
3 = Severe pain

Sedation scale
0 = None
1 = Mild (occasionally drowsy, easy to rouse)
2 = Moderate (frequently drowsy, easy to rouse)
3 = Severe (difficult to rouse)
S = Sleep (normal sleep, easy to rouse)

Visual analogue pain scale

No pain _____ Unbearable pain
Patients mark a point along a 10 cm line that best equates to their pain. This can then be measured to derive a numerical record. Small differences in pain intensity can then be identified.

Faces scale

| No pain | Mild discomfort | Pain | Severe pain | Unbearable pain |

Primarily used to assess children's pain but can also be useful for adults with learning difficulties or those whose first language is not English; it has also been successfully used to assess pain in adult intensive care units.

Assessment charts have an important role in providing:

- A measure of the patient's clinical condition and pain intensity.
- A measure of the effectiveness of treatment being given to the patient.
- A measure of the quality of care for the purposes of a nursing or medical audit.
- A record of the assessment and outcome of treatment should a patient or family member raise concerns regarding standards of care at a later date.

Key points to remember when using assessment charts and tools are:

- It is the assessment process, not the tool being used, that is important.
- To be effective, patients need to receive education on their use and the reasons behind it.
- The tool needs to be simple to use and meaningful to both patient and assessor.
- Assessment, particularly after surgery, needs to be done regularly.
- The measurement of pain should be a record of what the patient says their pain is, and not a subjective assessment by the nurse or doctor, as health care professionals tend to underestimate the intensity of patients' pain (Klopfenstein *et al.* 2000). However, some tools particularly designed for use in assessing patients unable to communicate their feelings (such as the very young or cognitively impaired) rely on observation and subjective judgements by the assessor.
- A key goal of pain management is to enable the patient to undertake activities that would otherwise be limited by their pain. Therefore, it is useful to measure pain both at rest and during activities (Hobbs and Hodgkinson 2003).
- It may also be difficult for patients whose first language is not English to find a suitable word or phrase to describe their pain. For example, words such as *minimal*, *moderate*, or *intense* may be used rarely by patients in daily life, and as such do not have as much meaning for them as for health care professionals (Thomas 1998). Cultural influences can also affect the perception of and reaction to pain and so need to be taken into account when making initial and subsequent assessments (Horn and Munafo 1998).

Management of pain

The care setting can have a significant influence upon the patient's perception of pain and the way in which pain is managed. For example, a patient's pain management needs can differ considerably between an intensive care unit and a nursing home. This should therefore be taken into consideration when devising a plan of care to address the patient's nursing needs with regard to the management of their pain. We can, however, adopt a common approach to all situations by addressing the remaining three **Ps** of pain (physical care, psychological care, and pharmacology).

Physical care

The normal physical and emotional response to the presence of pain is to take measures to avoid its causes and prevent or limit tissue damage. This in turn can cause restrictions in normal activity. For example, we avoid further pain and injury by resting a sprained ankle and allowing healing to occur. Nurses can assist this normal response by allowing patients to rest and by providing aids such as cushions or splints to help support or immobilize an affected area, or a rolled-up towel or pillow held against the abdomen to assist respiratory exercises following abdominal surgery.

A variety of physical therapies can also be used to help reduce pain. The application of heat or cold, hydrotherapy, or massage can be useful, according to the individual patient's circumstances and needs. Physiotherapists and other physical therapists often make use of these techniques in order to maximize physical activity.

Transcutaneous electrical nerve stimulation (TENS) is a self-contained portable system that involves the passage of an electrical current between two self-adhesive electrodes, which are placed on the skin either side of a painful area or close to a sensory nerve supplying the area of pain. The resulting stimulation of subcutaneous nerves has a blocking effect upon pain sensations. The more sophisticated TENS units have variable modes of stimulation that can alter the frequency and strength of the current. This can be controlled by the patient.

TENS units are now freely available for sale to the public. Some degree of education and support from someone familiar with the use of TENS, i.e. a pain nurse specialist or physiotherapist, may be required in order to maximize the chances of success. Because the system is battery powered, it is portable and allows the user to carry on day-to-day activities. Ease of use and lack of side effects (some mild skin burning is possible at the electrode sites) makes TENS potentially useful for a variety of pain conditions. It is also popular for the management of pain during childbirth.

Psychological care

A patient's personal attitude towards pain is of great importance, affecting both their perception and subsequent reaction to pain. This is illustrated by studies that have demonstrated the negative effects of anxiety, neuroticism, and depression on the perception of pain (Caumo et al. 2002, Kalkman et al. 2003).

For some patients, the hospital environment is an alien and threatening place. This, combined with concerns over their diagnosis, its treatment, and potential outcome, can increase levels of patient anxiety. This is perhaps the most commonplace emotion associated with pain, raising awareness of the patient's environment and their perception of pain. This can lead to a fear of pain and the development of avoidance behaviours, such as refusing to mobilize after surgery or the development of long-term disability (Viaeyen and Linton 2000). Anxiety can be induced by the pain itself (pain meaning something is wrong), or other concerns relating to the patient's treatment, family, or social circumstances. Taking one's mind off things with distractions such as reading, watching television, or other activities that occupy the mind can therefore be useful (Heafield 1999).

Anxiety can increase with the anticipation of a painful event such as a dressing change. Techniques that help to distract and calm the patient can be useful in such circumstances. Relaxation training has been shown to be of benefit to patients undergoing medical treatment (Luebbert et al. 2001). However, patients need training and support if this is to be effective.

Studies have shown that simple measures, such as the provision of information, can help reduce anxiety, level of pain, and need for analgesia (Haywood 1975, Suls and Wan 1989). However, patient information may not be welcomed by all, as the provision of too much information and the need to make too many decisions can themselves be a source of increased anxiety and pain (Miro and Raich 1999).

An additional fear among some patients and health care staff is the risk of drug addiction when using drugs such as Morphine. In reality, the likelihood of addiction occurring in patients with genuine pain is extremely low (World Health Organization 1986).

Pharmacology of pain relief

Analgesic drugs are our most important tools for the management of pain. The following drugs are commonly used to treat the two forms of pain.

Drugs used to treat nociceptive pain

- **Paracetamol** may be used singularly, in combination with other drugs such as codeine, or in over-the-counter cold and flu remedies.
- **Non-steroidal anti-inflammatory drugs** (NSAIDs), e.g. Ibuprofen, diclofenac, require caution due to their potential gastrointestinal, renal, and respiratory side effects.
- **Weak opiates** (e.g. codeine phosphate) are not considered controlled drugs when taken orally. However, when given intravenously they have a much more powerful effect and are therefore considered to be controlled drugs.
- **Strong opioids**, e.g. morphine sulphate and fentanyl, are considered controlled drugs. However, morphine sulphate in a solution of less than 13 mg in 5 ml is not a controlled drug when taken orally. Controlled drugs require two Registered Nurses to check and administer them to a patient, regardless of the route used. Patient-controlled analgesia is a commonly used method of providing pain-relieving intravenous opiates under the control of the patient. Hospitals should have specific protocols regarding the care of patients receiving this form of pain relief.
- **Local anaesthetics** are commonly used to provide pain relief via an epidural infusion by blocking sensory information along nerves. Hospitals should have specific protocols regarding the care of patients receiving these forms of pain relief.
- **Nitrous oxide/oxygen mixture** (Entonox®) is a mixture of 50% oxygen and 50% nitrous oxide gas. When inhaled, it produces a powerful analgesic effect. It is commonly used for the control of pain during childbirth, its great advantage being the speed with which it takes effect. Its effects also wear off quickly should any side effects occur. Delivery of the gas mixture is via a mouthpiece or mask. As the patient inhales, a valve is opened, allowing the release of gases from a gas cylinder. Entonox® is particularly suitable for the management of procedural pain, such as changing of a painful dressing or removal of a wound drain. Users of the system need to be aware of the health and safety issues of using Entonox® in a confined space and its lack of suitability for long-term use (BOC Medical 2006).

Drugs used to treat neuropathic pain

- **Anticonvulsant drugs**, e.g. gabapentin and pregabalin.
- **Antidepressants**, e.g. amitriptyline and duloxetine.

Adjuvant drugs are drugs used to treat conditions that in turn provoke pain. For example, Diazepam may be used for its muscle relaxant qualities, so easing painful muscle spasm.

It is now commonplace to see a patient receiving a variety of analgesic drugs in order to provide a multimodal approach to their pain management. This approach is based on the concept that a synergistic effect occurs between each analgesic drug, the sum of the whole being greater than the sum of the individual parts. Lower doses of a single drug can then be used, resulting in fewer drug-related side effects. This approach is often used for the management of post-operative pain. However, longer-term administration of multiple drugs (so-called polypharmacy) may prove burdensome to some patients.

The way drugs are prescribed and administered is often key to the success or failure of treatment. Nurses therefore need to develop knowledge regarding the use, actions, and side effects of analgesia drugs in order to administer them safely and address any patient concerns. This knowledge can help improve the chances of successful treatment for the patient by helping them to understand how their drugs work and addressing any concerns they may have.

Context

 When to undertake pain assessment

Pain assessment should be included in any initial nursing assessment, i.e. when the patient is admitted to hospital or seen for the first time in the community. Subsequent assessments will depend upon the nature of the patient's condition and anticipated treatment.

Any complaint of pain by the patient should be assessed and documented. In particular, the nurse should always inform medical staff of the presence of unexpected or increasing pain, as this can signify a deterioration in the patient's condition.

Regular assessment of pain is important because it leads to improved pain management (ANZCA and FPM

2005). However, assessment is very much dependent upon what the patient is capable of communicating to the assessor. Assessment of the very young, the cognitively impaired (such as the unconscious or heavily sedated patient in an intensive care unit), and those with a communication problem such as lack of speech (aphasia) following a stroke can pose particular problems. A variety of assessment tools have been developed in order to overcome the problems associated with communication difficulties in these groups of patients. For the majority, self-reporting of pain by the patient remains the most important factor in assessing pain.

Initial assessment of a patient's pain is important, as it helps to establish a medical diagnosis and guides subsequent treatment. For example, pain in the lower right side of the abdomen may indicate the presence of appendicitis and a need for urgent medical attention. Less urgent is the presence of constant hip pain, which may indicate the need for a hip replacement.

Step-by-step guide to managing pain

Step	Rationale
1 Introduce yourself, confirm the patient's identity, explain the procedure and obtain consent.	To identify the patient correctly and gain informed consent.
2 Undertake patient assessment, taking into account factors mentioned previously.	To assess the level and nature of the patient's pain.
3 Formulate a plan of care based on the patient's physical, psychological, and pharmacological needs. This can vary according to the care environment and the patient's overall clinical condition. For example, a patient with an epidural infusion following major surgery will have different needs from those of a patient with chronic pain in the home environment. If appropriate, plan the administration of pain relief before the undertaking of painful procedures such as dressing changes, ensuring enough time is allowed for the drug to take effect.	So that an adequate level of pain relief can be provided, tailored to the individual patient's needs.
4 Implement the planned care, including the use of prescribed medication. Some forms of pain relief will require specific monitoring, involving the use of dedicated assessment charts.	To provide the patient with pain relief. To ensure safe and effective care and correct use of controlled substances.
5 Evaluate care and treatment given. Important measures of care outcome should include the level of pain intensity, ability to carry out activities of daily living, and incidence of adverse effects caused by treatment.	So that care can be adjusted as necessary.

Following the procedure

Recognizing patient deterioration

Any unexpected change in the severity or nature of a patient's pain or their overall condition must be reported. Frequent assessment of the patient's condition will ensure early detection of a change in their medical condition or development of adverse effects caused by treatment. For example, patients receiving strong opiates for the relief of post-operative pain should be frequently monitored for the presence of sedation and respiratory depression alongside observations of pain. Another example is advising patients of the risks and symptoms associated with taking NSAIDs, i.e. risk of developing gastric irritation potentially leading to the formation of a gastric ulcer. This highlights the importance of informing patients about potential concerns in order that they may be addressed at an early stage.

Patients with chronic pain often have a degree of day-to-day variability in the intensity of their pain. Patient education in how best to manage their pain themselves can help reduce this variability and prevent acute exacerbations in their pain intensity, which may necessitate hospital admission. The patient may then become an '**expert patient**', capable of managing their condition themselves without the need to resort to medical help frequently.

Reflection and evaluation

When you have undertaken pain assessment and management, think about the following:

Pain is a feature of many medical conditions and as such plays an integral part in many patients' day-to-day care. The use and application of nursing care plans and clinical pathways therefore need to reflect any actual or potential pain issues that may arise. With this in mind, do you feel pain management is given sufficient priority in patients' care? For example, consider how often patients have their pain assessed and recorded.

Many hospitals now have specialist pain services, which can help with understanding and appreciating the importance of good pain control. They can also provide help and support in developing a range of clinical skills related to the management of pain that can be applied to daily practice. Should pain management therefore be the responsibility of pain specialists only, or do all members of the multidisciplinary team have a role to play?

Finally, try to remember that good pain management is a key feature in achieving a favourable outcome for the patient, resulting in fewer physiological and psychological adverse effects. It is also rewarding for staff to be able to manage a patient's discomfort, enhancing their recovery period (Simmonds 2007).

Reminders

When caring for a patient with pain, remember the following:

- Think of pain as being the fifth vital sign. An unexpected increase in pain intensity may mean deterioration in the patient's condition.
- Always report to medical staff any unexpected new source of pain, as this might be a sign of the development of a new medical problem.
- Analgesic drugs can have side effects that may require the patient to undergo specific monitoring. For example, the use of epidural pain relief will require the undertaking of specific observations, according to a hospital's policies and procedures.
- The use of analgesic drugs may require the use of other drugs to overcome side effects. For example, the use of morphine may require the use of antiemetics to counteract nausea and a laxative to prevent constipation.
- Never focus solely on one aspect of a patient's care. Take into account all possible factors that may be affecting the patient's pain management.

Ⓠ Patient scenarios

Consider what you should do in the following situations, then turn to the end of this skill to check your answers.

1 John is a 68-year-old who is to undergo elective surgery for cancer of the large bowel. He is normally in good health. However, he is a little anxious about some aspects of his treatment.
   a) How can John's anxiety about his condition and surgery be reduced?
   b) What options might be offered to John to control his pain during the first 3 days of the initial post-operative period?

c) How should John's pain be assessed following surgery?

2 Joan is 56 years old and has breast cancer. This has spread to her spine, lungs, and liver. She is admitted to a hospice for nursing care and symptom control. She is assessed as having two main sources of pain. The first is severe back pain that radiates into her legs, is often shooting in nature, and worsens upon standing. It is felt to be neuropathic and caused by a tumour compressing the spinal nerves supplying her legs. The second is a constant, right-sided abdominal pain. It is felt to be related to her liver tumour causing pressure on the liver capsule and is a nociceptive pain. She has been told that no further active treatment of her condition is possible.

a) How should Joan's pain be assessed?

b) What is the aim of pain management in Joan's case?

3 John is a 25-year-old student, admitted to hospital with excruciating 'gnawing' pain in his hips and back. His chest is also painful and feels 'tight'. He is very anxious as he has had frequent admissions to hospital with sickle cell crisis. He is quite knowledgeable about his condition and knows that his pain is caused by occlusion of small blood vessels due to clumping together of abnormal red blood cells.

a) How should John's pain be assessed?

b) How should John's pain be treated?

4 Sally has severe rheumatoid arthritis and is under the care of a rheumatologist. Her condition and treatment needs are assessed regularly by a rheumatology nurse specialist. Sally prefers not to use analgesic drugs due to their side effects. In particular she becomes easily constipated. She is admitted to a nursing home for respite care.

a) How should Sally's pain be assessed?

b) How can Sally be helped to manage her pain without the use of analgesic drugs?

Website

 http://www.oxfordtextbooks.co.uk/orc/ endacott

You may find it helpful to work through our short online quiz and additional scenarios intended to help you to develop and apply the skills in this chapter.

References

Australian and New Zealand College of Anaesthetists and Faculty of Pain Medicine (2005). *Acute pain management: scientific evidence*, 2nd edition. ANZCA and FPM, Melbourne.

BOC Medical (2006). *Entonox: controlled pain relief. A reference guide*. BOC, London.

Caumo W, Scmidt AP, Schnieder CN *et al.* (2002). Preoperative predictors of moderate to intense acute pain in patients undergoing abdominal surgery. *Acta Anaesthesiologica Scandinavica*, **46**, 1265–71.

Haywood J (1975). *Information: a prescription against pain*. Royal College of Nursing, London.

Heafield R (1999). The management of procedural pain. *Professional Nurse*, **15**(2), 127–9.

Health Care Commission (2006). *National survey of adult inpatients 2006* [online] **http://www. healthcarecommission.org.uk/nationalfindings/ surveys/healthcareprofessionals/ surveysofnhspatients/acutecare/ surveyofadultinpatients2006.cfm** accessed 02/09/08.

Hobbs GJ and Hodgkinson V (2003). Assessment, measurement, history and examination. In DJ Rowbotham and PE Macintyre, eds. *Clinical pain management – acute pain*, p. 103. Arnold, London.

Hollinworth J (1997). Wound care – less pain more gain. *Nursing Times*, **93**, 89–91.

Horn S and Munafo M (1998). *Pain: theory, research and intervention*. Open University Press, Buckingham: 8.

Joint Commission on Accreditation of Healthcare Organisations (2001). *Pain: current understanding of assessment, management and treatments.* JCAHO and the National Pharmaceutical Council, Inc. [online] **http://www.jcho.org** accessed 01/07/07.

Kalkman CJ, Visser K, Moen J et al. (2003). Preoperative prediction of severe postoperative pain. *Pain*, **105**, 415–23.

Klopfenstein CE, Herrman FR, Mamie C, van Gessel E, and Forster A (2000). Pain intensity and pain relief after surgery. A comparison between patients' reported assessments and nurses' and physicians observations. *Acta Anaesthesiologica Scandinavica*, **44**, 58–62.

Leubbert K, Dahme B, and Hasenbring M (2001). The effectiveness of relaxation training in reducing treatment related symptoms and improving emotional adjustment in acute non surgical cancer treatment: a meta analytical review. *Psychooncology*, **10**, 490–502.

McCaffery M (1979). *Nursing management of the patient with pain*. Lippincott, Philadelphia.

Miro J and Raich RM (1999). Preoperative preparation for surgery: an analysis of the effects of relaxation and information provision. *Clinical Psychology and Psychotherapy*, **6**: 202–9.

Pain Coalition: **http://www. paincoalition.org.uk/challenge.html**

Royal College of Anaesthetists and The Pain Society (2003). *Pain management services good practice* [online] **http://www.britishpainsociety.org/** accessed 01/07/07.

Simmonds T (2007). Pain management in the critically ill patient. In P Jevon, ed. *Treating the critically ill patient*, pp. 147–67. Blackwell Publishing, Oxford.

Sloman RG, Rosen M, and Rom Y Shir (2005). Nurses' assessment of pain in surgical patients. *Journal of Advanced Nursing*, **52**(2), 125–32.

Suls J and Wan CK (1989). Effects of sensory and procedural information on coping with stressful medical procedures and pain. A meta analysis. *Journal of Clinical Psychology*, **57**, 372–9.

Thomas VN (1998). *Pain. Its nature and management*. Bailliere Tindall, London: 86.

Viaeyen JWS and Linton SJ (2000). Fear avoidance and its consequences in chronic musculoskeletal pain: a state of the art. *Pain*, **85**, 317–32.

World Health Organization (1986). *Cancer pain relief*. WHO, Geneva.

Useful further reading and websites

Cancer Backup: **http://www.cancerbackup.org.uk/ Resourcessupport/Symptomssideeffects/Pain**

The Oxford Pain Internet site: **http://www. jr2.ox.ac.uk/bandolier/booth/painpag/**

Pain Concern: **http://www.painconcern.org.uk/**

The British Pain Society: **http://www. britishpainsociety.org/**

Paineurope.com: **http://www.paineurope.com/ index.php?q=en/book_page/ the_pain_in_europe_report**

 Answers to patient scenarios

1

a) John should be offered an opportunity to discuss his care with his surgeon and/or a colorectal nurse specialist. This may help relieve some of his fears concerning his treatment, which can have a positive effect upon his post-operative pain.

b) John should be assessed by an anaesthetist before his operation who will discuss the different options available, e.g. epidural or patient-controlled analgesia. Note that these options should only be offered if nursing staff caring for John after surgery are known to be competent in management of the different techniques.

c) John will require frequent monitoring of vital signs during the post-operative period. His pain score at rest and during movement should be assessed. This will ensure the provision of continuous pain relief, which in turn can assist in early mobilization and prevention of post-operative complications.

2

a) Joan has two main sources of pain that require different forms of treatment, so each should be assessed separately. She should have her pain assessed frequently in order to maximize her pain relief and to detect any side effects of the drugs being used.

b) The primary aim of Joan's care is quality rather than quantity of life. It is therefore important to explore Joan's wishes and concerns, and develop a plan of care that meets her needs and desires. This may mean an acceptance of a certain degree of pain in order to avoid some of the side effects of analgesics, e.g. nausea and vomiting or excessive drowsiness. It may be necessary to explore a variety of therapeutic options before settling on a treatment regime acceptable to Joan. The nurse should provide regular feedback to the palliative care specialists.

3

a) John is experiencing a severe sickle cell disease crisis. It is also a serious medical condition characterized by excruciating pain. He will therefore require frequent monitoring of his vital signs and pain severity using a pain assessment tool.

b) Initially an intravenous bolus dose of opiate will be required until John's pain is controlled. Patient-controlled analgesia using a strong opiate drug such as morphine can then be used, allowing

John to self-administer as much or as little pain relief as he needs. This also relieves nursing staff of the need to check and administer controlled drugs frequently. It will help John maintain a degree of control over his pain without the need to rely on others who may have conflicting assumptions about the nature and treatment of his pain.

Sickle cell pain is so severe that John may require large amounts of pain relief. This should *not* be affected by fears about developing addiction, although tolerance to opiates can develop over time. Any patient receiving strong opiates should be closely monitored for opiate-related side effects, e.g. nausea and vomiting, sedation, respiratory depression. As John's pain eases he will be able to manage his pain with oral analgesia.

4

a) Sally's rheumatology nurse specialist should assess her level of pain at each review. The character of her pain should be noted as well as its severity in order to help identify any changes in her disease progression. This may also help identify any new pathology that may be developing. It is important that she undergoes a comprehensive assessment of her pain upon admission to the nursing home. This should include documentation of any specific care needs associated with the management of her pain, e.g. does she need limb splints or supportive cushions when sitting or asleep in bed?

b) Disease modification drugs used to treat rheumatoid arthritis (i.e. steroids) can help relieve pain by treating the cause. Attention to physical and psychological issues is very important in this case. The help of an occupational therapist may be useful. Additional therapy could be used to counteract side effects of analgesia, e.g. regular use of a laxative to prevent constipation. Advice on this and other ways of avoiding constipation should be offered.

Could there be some other reason behind Sally's reluctance to take analgesic drugs? Take time to explore this issue but always respect the patient's wishes.

8.5 **Lumbar puncture**

This is an advanced skill. You *must* check whether you can assist with or undertake this skill, in line with local policy.

Definition

Lumbar puncture is a specialist skill that involves withdrawing cerebrospinal fluid (CSF) by the insertion of a hollow needle with a stylet into the lumbar subarachnoid space (Hickey 1997). It is carried out when certain types of infection are suspected such as bacterial meningitis, subachrioid haemorrhage (SAH), or Guillain–Barré syndrome. Lumbar puncture may also be used as a route to deliver drugs and medication such as chemotherapy or local anaesthetic (often used for Caesarean section).

Lumbar puncture is usually performed by a registered doctor or other competent health care professionals who have developed this as an extended role (Waterhouse 2003). Nursing students will only ever assist in this procedure. Performance of a lumbar puncture is most likely to occur in neurological areas, A&E, ITU, HDU, or acute medical and paediatric wards.

It is important to remember that:

- Lumbar puncture can be a painful and difficult procedure to perform. Some patients may require light sedation with an intravenous benzodiazepine, e.g. midazolam.
- This is a specialist skill that requires strict aseptic (sterile) techniques.
- Lumbar puncture is usually performed to confirm or refute a diagnosis such as meningitis, so thorough explanations to the patient and family before and after the procedure are essential.

Prior knowledge

Before attempting to assist with lumbar puncture, make sure you are familiar with:

1 Musculoskeletal and central nervous system anatomy.
2 The principles and measurement of the Glasgow Coma Score/Scale.

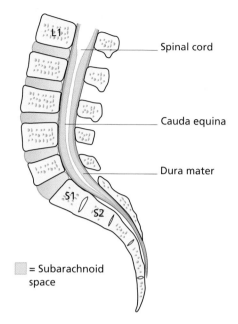

Spinal cord

Cauda equina

Dura mater

= Subarachnoid space

Figure 8.7 Saggital section through lumbosacral spine.

3 The principles of aseptic technique.
4 The principles of infection control and safe disposal of sharps.

Background

The spinal cord lies within the spinal column, beginning at the foramen magnum and terminating about the level of the first lumbar vertebra as conus medullaris (**Figure 8.7**). Like the brain, the spinal cord is enclosed and protected by the meninges, i.e. the dura mater, arachnoid mater, and pia mater. The dura and arachnoid mater are separated by the subdural space; the arachnoid and pia mater are separated by a potential space known as the subarachnoid space, which contains the CSF. Below the first lumbar vertebra, the subarachnoid space contains the CSF, the filum terminale, and the cauda equina. To avoid any damage to the spinal cord, it is imperative that the lumbar puncture is performed below the first lumbar vertebra where the cord terminates (Figure 8.7).

Cerebrospinal fluid (CSF)

CSF is a clear, straw-coloured fluid that surrounds the brain and spinal cord, and offers support and protection to these delicate structures in the manner of a shock absorber. It is composed of water, mineral salts such as sodium, potassium, calcium, and magnesium, and small amounts of protein. CSF is secreted by specialist cells located in the choroid plexuses within the brain, and approximately 0.5 ml is secreted every hour. Abnormalities in the CSF may include presence of infection, blood, raised glucose levels, increased levels of protein, or increased intracranial pressure.

Investigations of CSF

It may be possible to see some abnormalities in the CSF with the naked eye, for example it may be bloodstained, xanthochromic (yellow), or cloudy due to increased white blood cells. Laboratory investigations may include Gram staining, Ziehl–Nielsen stain, and cultures (placing the sample in a warm environment and then examining any bacterial growth under a microscope).

Context

When to perform a lumbar puncture

● As a diagnostic aid to confirm the presence of infectious disease such as meningitis.
● To measure CSF.
● As a delivery route for certain medications such as antibiotics or chemotherapy.
● To administer regional or spinal anaesthesia.
● To administer X-ray contrast media in order to perform a myelogram, i.e. an X-ray exam of the spinal cord and nerves using a special dye to highlight problem areas.

When not to perform a lumbar puncture

● If there is raised intracranial pressure (Harrison and Daly 2001) or presence of tumours or masses (in these circumstances the patient should be referred for radiological opinion and assessment following MRI or CT scan prior to a lumbar puncture being performed).
● When there is evidence of local infection around the potential puncture site, as this may introduce infection into the spinal canal.

- If there are spinal joint problems, e.g. previous spinal surgery or previous problems with attempted lumbar puncture, as there may be a greater risk of nerve damage.
- In patients on anticoagulation therapy or with thrombocytopenia, as these may cause excessive bleeding and further problems such as headache.

Indications for assistance

Lumbar puncture is usually performed by a doctor. Any member of staff undertaking lumbar puncture must be familiar with the technique, and it is recommended that they should undertake a period of supervised practice before performing the procedure.

Lumbar puncture ideally requires three people:

- One performing the lumbar puncture.
- Second person assisting the operator by assembling and opening the equipment required, as the operator will be wearing sterile gloves.
- Third person to support the patient, both in the correct position and emotionally. As lumbar puncture is often performed as an emergency investigation, this role is often overlooked or delegated to students or very junior members of staff.

Potential problems

There are four main adverse reactions to observe for during or following lumbar puncture:

1. Nerve stimulation during the procedure

As lumbar puncture is usually a 'blind' technique (i.e. the needle is being advanced without any direct confirmation of its location), it is sometimes possible to place the needle very close to or into a nerve, which may cause pain or a jolt to the patient. In the event of a nerve being touched, the operator must stop advancing the needle and withdraw, then either try a different angle of approach or abandon the procedure. The use of ultrasound to assist with the placement of needles and catheters for nerve blocks and intravascular access is increasing and this technique has also been described as being of benefit when performing lumbar puncture (Cummings and Jones 2007, Stiffler *et al.* 2007).

2. Reduction in CSF surrounding the brain

Performing lumbar puncture in the presence of raised intracranial pressure (ICP) may cause CSF to be forced out. This sudden reduction of pressure in the CSF may cause the brain to be 'sucked' downwards and forced through the foramen magnum (the hole at the base of the skull where the brainstem and spinal cord come through), and may lead the patient to suffer rapid neurological compromise and injury (Harrison and Daly 2001).

3. Cushing's triad

This consists of hypertension, bradycardia, and respiratory depression (slowing of respiratory rate and/or shallow breathing). It is a sign of increased intracranial pressure and possible imminent herniation of the brain.

4. Anaphylaxis

May occur as a reaction to skin cleaning solutions, local anaesthetics, or any medications being given via this route. Signs and symptoms include:

- Breathing difficulties including shortness of breath.
- Swelling around the lips, tongue, and eyes.
- Rash (urticaria and/or erythema).
- Tachycardia.
- Hypotension.
- Nausea and vomiting.
- Collapse and cardiorespiratory arrest.

Special considerations

- A clean, well-lit environment is required, e.g. side room, operating theatre, or anaesthetic room.

- A comfortable trolley or surface for patient to be positioned on is needed. Ideally it should be a tilting trolley with height adjustment.

- Family or carers may be present to offer support to the patient but must not be allowed to interfere with the conduct of the procedure, especially interference with the sterile field.

- All the required equipment, including spares, should be assembled prior to starting the lumbar puncture.

- An established method of labelling the samples and transporting them safely to the lab is needed, e.g. porter or air tube.

The procedure

Preparation

Prepare yourself (as second assistant)

Ensure that you are familiar with the procedure and the equipment required, including how to open items using an aseptic technique. It is prudent to have additional items to hand in case of equipment failure or items being dropped or desterilized.

The second assistant should be fully briefed on their role – this includes helping the patient get into the correct position and helping them maintain this position. The second assistant may also be responsible for monitoring the patient's vital signs by visually inspecting their skin, observing any monitors that may be attached to them (e.g. pulse oximeter), and observing any oxygen being delivered to them.

Ensure there is close access to a sink to wash your hands.

Prepare the patient

Both physical and emotional preparation are crucial to the success of lumbar puncture. Lumbar puncture is usually performed under local anaesthesia with the patient awake or mildly sedated. While lumbar puncture may be uncomfortable, it should not be excessively painful. Positioning of the patient is also very important in ensuring successful placement of the needle, and you must ask the patient to try and stay as still as possible during the procedure.

The doctor will obtain consent from the patient, explaining the benefits and risks associated with lumbar puncture before obtaining consent. It is helpful if the patient is given the opportunity to use the toilet before the procedure, if practical.

The doctor will also secure intravenous access and administer sedation or analgesia as required prior to the procedure.

Prepare the equipment

Ensure that all the equipment required by the doctor is available, including spare items in case of equipment failure or if they become desterilized. The choice of needle used will be made by the doctor and a selection should be available. Often a size 22g or smaller needle is used. A specific needle such as a Sprotte™ or Whitacre type has the advantage of parting rather than cutting through tissue and therefore may reduce the risk of post-dural puncture headache (Turnbull and Shepherd 2003).

Equipment required:

- Personal protective equipment for the operator, including hat, face mask, sterile handtowels, gloves, and gown.
- A trolley to lay the sterile equipment on.
- Sterile drapes including a fenestrated (with a hole) drape to cover the patient and the trolley.
- Selection of sterile needles, e.g. 25g, 21g, 18g, a blunt filter needle, and a filling quill.
- Spinal or lumbar puncture needle with or without an introducer needle. A larger bore spinal needle may allow faster flow of CSF. Usual sizes include 27g, 26g, 25g, 24g, and 22g (the smaller the 'g' number, the wider the diameter of the needle).
- 1% or 2% Lidocaine as local anaesthetic.
- 2 ml and 5 ml syringes. Larger or specialist syringes may be required to inject medications into the spinal space.
- Small gallipot for a suitable antiseptic solution, e.g. chlorhexidine.
- Swabs or sponges to apply the antiseptic to the patient's skin. Forceps or sponge holders may also be required.
- Three small, sterile specimen bottles to collect the CSF.
- Adhesive dressing with or without dressing spray for the puncture wound.
- Clinical waste bag and sharps container.
- An oxygen wall pipeline point or cylinder.
- Appropriate resuscitation equipment.

(A special spinal pack may be available that will contain many or all of the items required.)

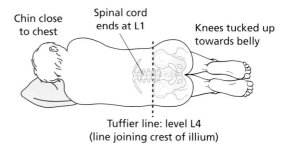

Chin close to chest

Spinal cord ends at L1

Knees tucked up towards belly

Tuffier line: level L4 (line joining crest of illium)

Figure 8.8 Patient lying on their side curled up into the 'foetal position'.

Step-by-step guide to assisting with lumbar puncture

Step	Rationale
1 Introduce yourself, confirm the patient's identity, explain the procedure and obtain consent (some of this may be done be the doctor).	To identify the patient correctly and gain informed consent.
2 Secure intravenous access.	To allow rapid administration of emergency drugs or fluids, if required.
3 Attach monitoring equipment to the patient. A pulse oximeter and automatic non-invasive blood pressure cuff should be sufficient for most patients; 3-lead ECG may also be useful if indicated.	Patient monitoring with alarms may alert the staff to subtle changes in the patient's condition and may allow swift action to prevent critical incidents.
4 Position the patient. There are two commonly used positions: patient lying on their side curled up into the 'foetal position' (**Figure 8.8**) or sitting up with chin drawn down onto chest. It may also be useful to ask the patient to arch their back out towards the operator, 'like an angry cat'.	To help spread or 'open up' the spinal spaces to make needle placement easier.
5 Take baseline readings of blood pressure and pulse rate and give oxygen if indicated.	To establish the physiological readings that are 'normal' for that patient. Supplemental oxygen may be useful to raise the patient's oxygen saturation levels.
6 Assist the doctor to feel the patient's back in the area of needle insertion and to mark the relevant landmarks on the skin before scrubbing up. The most common approach is spaces in between either L3–4 or L4–5 (see Figure 8.7).	To identify the appropriate landmarks to aid correct placement of the needle. To avoid damage to spinal cord with needle as cord ends at L1–2 level and only meninges filled with CSF and nerve endings (cauda equina) extend below to S1–2 level.
7 Assist the doctor to don sterile gown, mask, and gloves using a strict aseptic technique.	To reduce the risk of introducing infection into the wound.
8 Assist the doctor to lay out the required equipment.	To minimize the time the patient has to spend in a position that may be uncomfortable and to reduce the possibility of errors.
9 With the patient in the appropriate position, the skin should be cleaned with an antiseptic solution. Application of the antiseptic solution is often very cold and may make the patient jump, so it is important to warn the patient	To reduce the risk of introducing infection into the wound. To minimize discomfort to the patient during application.

continued overleaf

before prepping the skin. Placing the bottle or sachet of solution in warm water beforehand may reduce this shock.

10	Expose the adhesive section on the fenestrated drape and apply to the cleaned area on the patient's back.	To provide a sterile area around the wound and to reduce the risk of introducing infection into the wound.
11	Inject the local anaesthetic into the skin using a fine gauge needle and into the deeper tissues.	To provide local anaesthesia and reduce the discomfort experienced by the patient.
12	Insert an introducer needle (if used) through the skin and towards the spinal space.	An introducer needle may reduce damage and buckling of the spinal needle and prevent its contact with skin bacteria.
13	The spinal needle is advanced, with reliance on interpretation of the pressure felt to indicate when dura is reached and punctured. Stylet withdrawal shows CSF flashback.	This provides an indication that the needle is following the correct path.
14	If there is no CSF, reposition slightly and advance once again until the 'pop' is felt when the dura is punctured.	To reduce the discomfort experienced by the patient. The 'pop' indicates the needle is now in the correct place.
15	Withdraw the stylet and wait as the CSF should start to flow from the needle. The wider the needle used, the faster the CSF will flow.	This will confirm if the needle is in the correct place.
16	Attach a manometer and measure the CSF pressure (recorded in cmH_2O, normal is 6–15 cm).	Diagnose increased pressure conditions, e.g. hydrocephalus.
17	Collect the CSF in the sterile specimen bottles as it flows. Be prepared to hand the bottles quickly in succession to the doctor. It is useful to label the bottles 1, 2, 3, as the first sample may be bloodstained due to needle trauma and it is useful to distinguish this from blood that may appear in the CSF from subarachnoid haemorrhage.	To aid diagnosis of the patient's condition and support appropriate treatment.
18	Remove needle, clean skin, and apply appropriate dressings to the puncture wound.	To reduce the risk of introducing infection into the wound.
19	Remove any drapes from the patient and dispose of sharps in an appropriate container. All other non-sharp items should be disposed of in a clinical waste bag as per local policy.	To reduce the risk of injury or infection to the patient and members of the care team.
20	Take the patient's blood pressure and pulse rate to monitor for hypotension, and take venous blood to measure glucose level.	To ensure the patient's parameters are within the expected limits.

21	Document the procedure: Complexity of procedure. Amount of local anaesthetic used. Opening pressure. Closing pressure. Colour of CSF.	To provide accurate record of procedure.
22	Label the specimen bottles, complete the appropriate laboratory forms, and send the samples complete with form to the appropriate laboratory.	To allow correct identification in the laboratory and correct results to be sent to the relevant ward/department.
23	If performing spinal anaesthesia or administering other medications such as antibiotics, inject the medication.	Administration of the medication to aid the patient's treatment.

Following the procedure

Observation of vital signs should be carried out following lumbar puncture. These will include: heart rate, blood pressure, respiratory rate, temperature, sedation, and pain scores, as well as wound observation and care. Neurological observations may also be recorded. This could include the use of the Glasgow Coma Scale and observation of pupil size and reactivity to light.

Advise patient to mobilize gradually. Suggest that they lie down flat for at least half an hour, possibly longer, until they feel able to stand. Ensure that the patient is able to get up and walk around before they leave. Remind them that they should not drive for the next 24 hours and recommend that they drink 3 litres of fluid a day for the next 48 hours. The patient should remove the plaster on their back after 24 hours. Some patients experience a headache after a lumbar puncture. Very occasionally the headache can last for up to 5 days, and even more rarely for 10 days, following the procedure. Recommend that the patient contact their local GP or the hospital for further advice if necessary. Ask them to report if they feel any pain in their legs during or after the procedure, headache, backache, or neurological deterioration.

Reflection and evaluation

When you have assisted with or observed a lumbar puncture, think about the following questions:

1 Did the laboratory results of the CSF reflect the results you were expecting given the patient's condition?
2 Were you able to answer the patient's questions?
3 Did your visual assessment of the patient's condition alert you to any changes in their condition before the monitors did?
4 Were you able to interpret the laboratory results in light of the patient's medical condition?

Further learning opportunities

At the next available opportunity, try to put yourself in the patient's position for lumbar puncture.

- How comfortable or uncomfortable is it to be in that position?
- What effects did being in that position have on your breathing?
- How long could you comfortably stay in that position?

Reminders

- Reassure the patient during all stages of the procedure.
- Make sure any specimen bottles are labelled correctly, accompanied by the appropriate request forms, and sent to the correct department.

Patient scenarios

Consider what you should do in the following situations, then turn to the end of this skill to check your answers.

1 Patient A is having a lumbar puncture performed but is becoming restless. What should you do?
2 Patient B underwent a lumbar puncture 20 minutes ago and has noticed some blood seeping from the dressing over the puncture site. What action should you take?
3 Patient C had a lumbar puncture performed 1 hour ago and now complains of a very bad headache. What action should you take?

Website

 http://www.oxfordtextbooks.co.uk/orc/endacott

You may find it helpful to work through our short online quiz and additional scenarios intended to help you to develop and apply the skills in this chapter.

References

Cummings T and Jones JS (2007). Use of ultrasonography for lumbar puncture. *Emergency Medicine Journal*, **24**, 492–3.

Harrison and Daly (2001). *Acute medical emergencies – a nursing guide*. Churchill Livingstone, Edinburgh.

Hickey J (1997). *The clinical practice of neurology and neurosurgical nursing*, 4th edition. JB Lippincott, Philadelphia.

Stiffler KA, Jwayyed S, Wilber ST, and Robinson A (2007). The use of ultrasound to identify pertinent landmarks for lumbar puncture. *American Journal of Emergency Medicine*, **25**(3), 331–4.

Turnbull DK and Shepherd DB (2003). Post-dural puncture headache: pathogenesis, prevention and treatment. *British Journal of Anaesthesia*, **91**(5), 718–29.

Waterhouse C (2003). *Lumbar puncture procedure policy*, Sheffield Teaching Hospitals NHS Trust [online] **http://www.bann.org.uk/downloads/Lumbar%20Puncture.pdf** accessed 03/09/08.

Useful further reading and websites

Ferre RM and Sweeney TW (2007). Emergency physicians can easily obtain ultrasound images of anatomical landmarks relevant to lumbar puncture. *American Journal of Emergency Medicine*, **25**(3), 291–6.

Toft B (2001). *External Inquiry into the adverse incident that occurred at Queen's Medical Centre, Nottingham, 4th January 2001*. Department of Health [online] **http://www.dh.gov.uk/en/Publicationsandstatistics/Publications/PublicationsPolicyAndGuidance/DH_4010064**

Department of Health (2008). *Intrathecal chemotherapy: keeping up the pressure for safe administration* [online] **http://www.dh.gov.uk/en/Publicationsandstatistics/Publications/AnnualReports/Browsable/DH_4875362**

Woods K (2001). *The prevention of intrathecal medication errors: a report to the Chief Medical Officer*. Department of Health [online] **http://www.dh.gov.uk/prod_consum_dh/idcplg?IdcService=GET_FILE&dID=27988&Rendition=Web**

Royal Free lumbar puncture patient information leaflet 2007: **http://www.royalfree.org.uk/pip_admin/Docs/lumbar_puncture_938.pdf**

Website with information for health care professionals and students: **http://www.inmed.co.uk**

 Answers to patient scenarios

1 You need to monitor the patient closely: check level of consciousness by AVPU response, also monitor BP and pulse rate. Early signs of increased intracranial pressure (ICP) are reduced GCS score, and Cushing's response. Inform the operator as the lumbar puncture may have to be postponed until patient has urgent CT scan to rule out increased ICP.
2 Apply sterile dressing with pressure and advise bed rest. There could be some blood or CSF leakage which should stop after some time. Check all vital signs and note any signs of infection such as raised temperature. If leakage persists, prophylactic antibiotics may be needed.
3 Check for signs of postural dural puncture headache, which is worsened by sitting up. Advise bed rest and plenty of oral fluids: 2 to 3 litres over the next day. Drinks such as coffee and Coca-Cola are helpful because of their caffeine content. Reassure the patient and give them an explanation of the cause. Oral analgesics such as paracetamol and NSAIDs (e.g. diclofenac) with caffeine tablets could be prescribed.

   Continue regular observations; if headache does not improve in 24 hours, autologous epidural blood patch (EBP) might be needed to seal dural leak of CSF.

Renal system

9

Skills

9.1 Insertion of a urinary catheter

Definition

Insertion of a urinary catheter is an invasive procedure involving the placement of a Foley catheter (flexible self-retaining hollow tube) via the urethra, resulting in the immediate drainage of urine from the bladder for short- or long-term use. The procedures for urinary catheterization in male and female patients are very similar; however, there are a few small differences to accommodate the anatomical differences (see **Figure 9.1**). A urinary catheter can also be placed suprapubically, but this can only be done in a secondary care facility by a clinician. Non-self-retaining catheters may also be placed, but these are for patients to empty the bladder themselves (this should only be taught by a qualified nurse).

It is important to remember that:

- An appropriate reason for catheterization should be determined by the doctor responsible for the patient's care as a result of clinical need according to local catheterization protocol. Patient consent should be obtained.
- This procedure should only be carried out by a trained health care professional proficient in catheterization.
- At no point in the procedure should force be used.
- A pre-catheterization assessment must be carried out as per local protocol to determine if it is appropriate and safe to catheterize (Addison and Mould 2000).

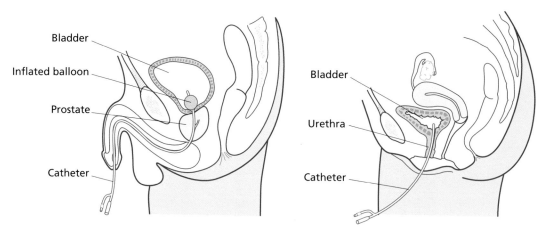

Figure 9.1 Side view of catheter insertion (male and female).

- Students should only catheterize under the direct supervision of a qualified member of staff.

Prior knowledge

Before undertaking catheter insertion, make sure you are familiar with:

1 Male and female urological anatomy and physiology, including mechanism of urine transport.
2 Factors influencing normal and abnormal urine transport.
3 Pathophysiology of urinary retention and intractable incontinence.
4 The principles of aseptic technique.

Background

Urine transport

To understand why catheterization may be necessary, it is useful to understand the mechanism of urine transport. There are four main areas in this pathway:

1 Kidneys.
2 Ureters.
3 Bladder.
4 Urethra.

Waste products and excess water are filtered from the blood by the kidneys. The urine produced passes from the kidneys down through the ureters via peristalsis (wave-like movements that push urine down the ureters) to the bladder. Urine accumulates in the bladder until the volume of urine it contains causes the bladder wall to stretch. Stretch receptors in the wall trigger relaxation of the internal sphincter – the first of the two sphincters that are normally contracted to prevent urine from leaving the bladder. The stretch receptor also sends a signal to the brain causing the conscious awareness of a need to urinate. While the internal sphincter relaxes involuntarily, relaxation of the external sphincter can be inhibited by healthy adults so that micturition (passing urine) is delayed until a suitable opportunity (e.g. in a toilet), when urine passes down the urethra and out of the body.

Disorders that may lead to catheterization

It is important to have an understanding of the disorders that may result in catheterization (see **Table 9.1**).

Choice of catheter

The choice of catheter is important, because using an inappropriate catheter could reduce the patient's mobility and comfort and increase the risk of infection, trauma and encrustation, or allergy. The choices of catheter are as follows:

- Short term – these catheters can only be left in for up to 7 days. They are usually made of PVC (plastic) and can be used for bladder drainage or irrigation.

Table 9.1 Reasons/disorders that may lead to catheterization

Disorder/problem	Probable cause/reason	Side effects/complications
Acute urinary retention (sudden onset of bladder's inability to pass urine, painful)	Bladder outflow obstruction (physical obstruction to bladder flow) due to: benign prostatic hyperplasia in men; bladder neck stenosis (build up of scar tissue at bladder neck); or urethral stricture (narrowing of urethra) Women in labour (during labour the urethra can be squeezed closed)	Abdominal pain Palpable bladder (swelling of abdomen due to retention of urine) Anuria (kidneys stop producing urine)
Chronic urinary retention (slow onset of bladder's inability to empty completely, painless) with renal impairment	Bladder outflow obstruction (see above) Neuropathic bladder (bladder does not empty properly due to diseased nerve supply caused by diabetes, multiple sclerosis, spinal injury, spina bifida, or other neurological condition)	Inability of bladder to empty itself, increasing amounts of urine unable to pass whatever is causing the obstruction (e.g. enlarged prostate, tight bladder neck, urethral stricture, bladder stone) Possible overflow incontinence (leaking of urine without intent) Possible recurrent urinary tract infections Possible stone formation Hydronephrosis (swelling of kidneys due to inability to drain urine)
Intravesical drug administration (placing of drugs into the bladder via a urethral catheter)	For treatment of superficial bladder cancer (insertion of chemo- or immunotherapeutic drugs) For treatment of interstitial cystitis (non-bacterial cystitis causing bladder inflammation)	Frequency and urgency when passing urine, with or without pain
Intractable incontinence (constant uncontrolled loss of urine, resistant to cure, relief, or control)	Terminal disease (cancer causing death or cancer causing comobidities that lead to death) Physical impairment that may make the patient unsuitable for surgery or intervention	Excoriation (deterioration of skin integrity causing ulceration) Dribbling incontinence (constant dribbling of urine) Inability to store urine
Post-surgical urinary drainage	Urological surgery: Irrigating bladder to wash out blood Acting as drain To rest bladder and promote healing of an anastomosis (join) in urethra, ureter, or bladder Accurate measurement of fluid output or to diagnose anuria	
Terminal disease (any abdominally placed cancer leading to death)	Cancer	Physical inability to mobilize to pass urine Obstructive mass (mass that obstructs passage of urine)
For investigation (urodynamics – test to check function of bladder by filling and then measuring activity – or to obtain sterile urine specimen)	Bladder dysfunction disorders (such as overactive bladder): For the diagnosis of bladder dysfunctions and bladder outflow obstruction For the diagnosis of urinary infection	

- Medium term – these can be left in for up to 28 days. They are usually made of PTFE (polytetrafluoroethylene) or Teflon-coated or uncoated latex.
- Long term – these can be left in for up to 12 weeks. They are usually made of hydrogel-coated latex, 100% silicone, silicone-coated latex, hydrogel-coated silicone, or silicone elastomer-coated latex. Silicone-only catheters should be used for patients with a latex allergy.

Usually, short-term and medium-term catheters are used for patients after surgery or procedures, while long-term catheters are usually used if the patient is going to go home with the catheter.

Catheter size

The decision about catheter size should be made by the medical team or to suit the purpose of catheterization and allow adequate drainage and maximum comfort. It is commonplace to suggest using size 14–16 Ch for permanent indwelling catheters as they provide better drainage long term and are less prone to blockage.

Catheter length

Catheters for men are typically 40–45 cm in length. Catheters for women are typically 20–26 cm in length. However, male-length catheters may be used for obese or wheelchair-bound women.

Selection of drainage system

The drainage system should be chosen to encourage patient independence. It is important to assess the patient's manual dexterity and mobility, and there are also different taps to aid this decision. The choices are as follows:

1. Two litre drainage bag with stand

This allows observation of the urine's colour, consistency, and volume for post-operative observation. It can be attached to the leg bag for drainage at night, and can also be used if the patient is unable to use a leg bag. It must be changed every 5–6 days as specified by the manufacturer's guidelines (Department of Health (DH) 2001). Bags are available with or without a drainage tap, but only those without a drainage tap should be used in hospitals and the bag should be discarded when detached. Patients may use this type of bag at home for up to 7 days, providing they wash it out with soapy water on a daily basis.

2. Leg bag

Leg bags are available in the following sizes: 350 ml, 500 ml, 750 ml. They ensure dignity and mobility. They also come in different tube lengths (long, attaching to shin, or short, attaching to thigh), according to the patient's needs. Leg bags must not be used if diuresis (passage of large amounts of urine) is expected. The bags must be placed below the level of the bladder to encourage urine flow (Dieckhaus and Garibaldi 1998) and must be changed every 5–7 days (DH 2001).

3. Urometer

This is used for the accurate measurement of urine (usually hourly) after major surgery, trauma, or if medically indicated.

4. Catheter valve

A catheter valve may be used instead of a drainage bag as they maintain bladder capacity and reduce erosion. This choice must be made by the medical team or after an appropriately trained health care professional makes a complete pre-catheterization assessment. They should be changed every 5–7 days (DH 2001). The choice of valve should depend on the patient's dexterity. Valves should not be used in the following circumstances: reduced bladder capacity, cognitive impairment, during diuresis, no bladder sensation, poor manual dexterity, nocturnal polyuria (passing large amounts of urine at night), if patient chooses not to, and if attempting to relieve a hydronephrosis (swelling of renal pelvis and calyces).

Use of antibiotics

In some cases, prophylactic antibiotics will be administered before the procedure to prevent infection. This must be checked against local urological and cardiac protocol/guidance and agreed by the clinician ordering the catheterization. The most common reasons for using antibiotics are if the patient:

- Has had rheumatic fever (used as prophylaxis to prevent infection).
- Has an artificial or other heart valve, septal defect, patent ductus, or heart valve lesion (National Institute for Health and Clinical Excellence (NICE) 2003).
- Has had an abdominal aortic aneurysm (check local cardiac policy).
- Has had a long-term catheter.
- Has a urine infection or history of infection after change – this must be discussed with medical team prior to catheterization or use local protocol (NICE 2003).

If the patient is found to have an infection after catheterization has been carried out, medical staff must be consulted to consider commencing antibiotic treatment.

Context

 ## When to catheterize

This procedure is carried out for many reasons (see also Table 9.1), including:

- Acute retention.
- Chronic urinary retention.
- Drug administration into the bladder.
- Intractable incontinence, allowing excoriated skin to heal (where other interventions have failed).
- Post-urological surgery.
- Drainage of hypotonic bladder.
- Accurate measurement of urine output in critical illness.
- Bladder irrigation.
- Urodynamic investigations.
- Terminal illness.

 ## When not to catheterize

This procedure should not be carried out unless considered carefully and, within the hospital setting, requires the input of the medical team looking after the patient. Catheterization should not be considered the first choice for patients who are incontinent or for patients who have a urinary tract infection (UTI). It should not be done if a patient refuses to give consent.

There are situations that may make catheterization difficult, such as previous urological, orthopaedic, or gynaecological surgery, congenital defects, or traumatic urological injury (as these may alter patient anatomy, meaning the urethral opening may not be in the correct anatomical position). An attempt at catheterization in these patients could cause a fistula (abnormal passage created between areas not normally joined). These situations may not prevent catheterization, but mean the position of the urethral opening must be ascertained before the attempt. Patients with neutropenia should not be catheterized unless specifically requested by the consultant (to avoid bacteraemia).

Alternative interventions

Alternative interventions to catheterization are limited to clean intermittent self-catheterization (CISC), insertion of a suprapubic catheter, medication, or surgery.

Insertion of a suprapubic catheter may be necessary if urethral catheterization is not possible; however, students may only assist with this procedure. Only a clinician is permitted to place a suprapubic catheter and this is only done in a secondary care facility. Changing of suprapubic catheters does, however, go on in the community, and the procedure is the same for males and females.

CISC can be an alternative for patients with bladders that do not empty completely. The factors limiting this choice are the patient's manual dexterity and body size (it may be difficult for obese patients, particularly women, to self-catheterize). Only qualified nurses with training in teaching CISC may teach a patient how to carry out intermittent self-catheterization.

For acute urinary retention in men, surgery may be the best option if the patient has had symptoms prior to the episode of retention and is fit for an anaesthetic. However, a trial of alpha blockers may be carried out (once the patient is catheterized to enable trial of voiding) prior to making the decision for surgery in men who have not had symptoms prior to the episode. For men who are unfit for surgery, single or combination medical therapy (alpha blocker and 5-alpha reductase) may be sufficient to prevent catheterization or re-catheterization. A plan of care for these patients once catheterized is important to avoid unnecessary catheterized periods.

Surgery can also be employed for men with bladders that do not empty completely due to benign prostate hyperplasia (BPH), if their bladders are otherwise functioning and if medical therapy fails.

Potential problems

Resistance is a common potential problem in male catheterization (this occurs as there is a natural bend in the male urethra and an enlarged prostate or bladder neck can cause obstruction). This is recognized by the inability to advance the catheter any further; it can also feel like there is an obstruction in the way. Should this occur, ask the patient to try to relax (deep breathing helps). If resistance continues despite this, ask him to try to initiate micturition (passing urine). Also, a very gentle twist of the catheter can allow it to become disentangled from mucosal folds.

Lidocaine (a local anaesthetic gel) must be used when catheterizing (Bardsley 2005). Catheterizing without it may cause trauma to the urethra. It may sometimes be difficult to locate a woman's urethra. This may be due to unusual anatomy (due to genetic reasons or surgery) or to prolapse of the bladder or vagina (where the bladder or vagina drops lower than usual). Use of lidocaine may help to identify the urethra, as it slightly opens when gel is poured over the area, before trying to place the catheter. KY jelly must not be used for lubrication in catheterization because it is not sterile. Packs of sterile KY jelly have been developed; however, it would be difficult to place this gel into a sterile syringe for instillation. If a woman is being catheterized when in labour and has had an epidural, assistance must be sought from two others to support her legs in the lithotomy position (patient flat on back with legs held in the air with knees bent) to prevent back injury. This approach should also be used for patients with paraplegia or who are confused (such as in dementia or Alzheimer's disease). Special care and supervision should be sought for spinal-injured patients.

Indications for assistance

You may need assistance when trying to catheterize a patient; never be afraid to ask for help. If you still find catheterization difficult after a reasonable attempt, call a senior urologist (registrar or above), nurse specialist (if available), or senior colleague rather than risking further trauma to the patient's urethra.

Observations and monitoring

The patient should be observed while inserting the catheter for unreasonable pain or deterioration in condition such as fainting or onset of chest pain. In the event a patient experiences a bladder spasm while catheterizing, one should stop the procedure and wait until it abates before proceeding. Helping the patient to relax will help the spasm to pass. If an inpatient, the patient's urine output should be monitored and the patient observed for signs of infection or sepsis. If an outpatient, the patient should be advised what action to take if they become unwell or feel they have an infection after going home. They should be advised an infection may present with bloody and/or cloudy or smelly urine, possibly accompanied by a temperature. They would contact their district nurse or GP to obtain antibiotics if deemed necessary after providing a urine specimen. A district nurse should be arranged to see the patient at home and provide follow-up care, supplies, support, and assistance.

Special considerations

In the community it is rare to have access to a trolley, therefore extra care must be taken to provide the cleanest space possible to lay out your equipment, choosing an enclosed private place. Catheterizations in the community mean less immediate access to aid, so it is good practice to contact the nearest urology facility for advice and to arrange a visit if necessary.

Procedure

Preparation

Prepare yourself

Ensure you understand the procedure for catheterization and are familiar with the manufacturer's instructions concerning use of the catheter. A pre-catheterization assessment must be carried out. This is to ensure catheterization is safe to carry out and to help anticipate any problems that may impede the procedure or occur after it. The assessment should include checking:

- Medical history.
- Normal fluid intake.
- Bowel habits (constipation/diarrhoea).
- Patient dexterity and ability to self-care (or ability of carers).
- Psychological acceptance and understanding of outcome of catheterization.
- Allergies (latex/rubber/lidocaine).
- Patient support.
- Sexual function and activity.
- Patient preferences.

Prepare the patient

The procedure should be fully explained to the patient (Lloyd and Bor 2004) and carer if present (see Discussing the procedure box).

Prepare the equipment

Equipment needed includes:

- Yellow clinical waste bag.
- Disposable apron.
- Catheter (male or female, of appropriate size).
- Lidocaine gel (Bardsley 2005).
- Syringe and 10 ml of sterile water for injection (unless catheter contains water for balloon within pack).

- Two pairs sterile gloves.
- Drainage bag or catheter valve (depending on indication for catheterization).
- Catheter stand (as necessary).
- Catheterization pack.
- Cleansing solution (e.g. normal saline).

Including extra sterile equipment such as another catheter, gloves, and catheterization pack is good practice to ensure the patient is not abandoned during the procedure.

> **Discussing the procedure with the patient and family**
>
> - Explain why the catheter is necessary.
> - Assure the patient that they may feel some discomfort but not undue pain.
> - Advise the patient on how they can assist with the procedure.
> - Explain the consequences of having a catheter *in situ* and the importance of caring for it.
> - Answer any questions they may have.

Step-by-step guide to female catheterization

Procedure	Rationale
1 Introduce yourself, confirm the patient's identity, explain the procedure, and obtain consent.	To identify the patient correctly and gain informed consent.
2 Wash and dry hands.	To minimize the risk of cross-infection.
3 Prepare the trolley, placing all equipment on the bottom shelf.	To avoid leaving the patient mid-procedure.
4 Screen the bed.	To ensure patient privacy.

continued overleaf

5	Assist the patient into the supine position, ensure that the bed is at a comfortable height, and ensure adequate light. If in the community, use most appropriate available furniture to ensure safety for you and the patient.	To facilitate the procedure. For health and safety.
6	Put on plastic apron and take trolley to patient. In primary care use most appropriate table.	To minimize the risk of cross-infection and contamination.
7	Expose patient's pelvis and place incontinence pad under patient. Cover patient while preparing trolley. Position patient with legs abducted and knees flexed.	Maintain patient dignity at all times and allow ease of access.
8	Wash and dry hands again.	To minimize skin flora.
9	Open catheterization/dressing packs and arrange sterile field. Open the supplementary packs and cleansing solution.	To ensure an aseptic procedure.
10	Check all expiry dates.	To ensure safe use of equipment (Medical Devices Agency (MDA) 2000).
11	Wash hands, put on sterile gloves (either one or two pairs). Draw up appropriate amount of water to instil in the balloon if not already included (some catheters may have syringe with water already included).	Hands may have become contaminated by handling the outer packaging.
12	Place sterile drape over the pubic area.	To minimize contamination of catheter on insertion.
13	Clean the vulval area with gauze and saline, using single strokes and wiping from front to back.	To provide clean area for catheterization and prevent bacteria being transferred to the urethral meatus. Inadequate cleansing of the urethral orifice is a major cause of UTI.
14	Isolate the urethral opening and insert the instillagel or lidocaine gel; leave for 3–5 minutes (as per manufacturer's instructions).	Ensures least amount of trauma to the urethra, easing catheter passage along it. Allows lidocaine time to take effect, minimizing discomfort to the patient (Bardsley 2005, Woodward 2005).
15	Remove first pair of gloves and put on second pair (if not double-gloved) after using alcohol gel or washing hands between.	To prevent contamination of the catheter.
16	Place sterile receiver between the patient's legs.	For urine to drain into.
17	Separate the vulva, indentify the urethral opening, and insert the catheter gently	To avoid trauma to the vulva and allow easy access.

18	Once urine has begun to flow, advance catheter up to the level of the bifurcation.	This ensures balloon is not inflated in the urethra.
19	Inflate the balloon with sterile water as per the manufacturer's instructions.	Ensures adequate inflation of the balloon.
20	Once balloon is inflated, withdraw the catheter until resistance is felt.	This ensures draining all of the bladder.
21	Collect a urine specimen if indicated.	For microscopy, culture and sensitivity.
22	Connect the catheter to an appropriate drainage bag or catheter valve.	To allow free drainage of urine and to maintain a closed system to avoid infection.
23	Help the patient get clean and comfortable. Explain how to care for catheter. Instruct her in catheter hygiene.	To reduce anxiety over catheterization and reduce risk of infection.
24	Complete relevant records: reason for catheterization, residual volume, date, time of catheterization, make and size of catheter, volume of water in balloon, material and batch number, amount and type of gel used, cleansing agent used, any problems encountered.	To be accountable and maintain patient safety (Nursing and Midwifery Council (NMC) 2008).

Step-by-step guide to male catheterization

Procedure   Rationale

1	Introduce yourself, confirm the patient's identity, explain the procedure, and obtain consent.	To identify the patient correctly and gain informed consent.
2	Wash hands.	To minimize the risk of cross-infection.
3	Prepare trolley, placing all equipment on the bottom shelf. Check all equipment expiry dates.	To avoid leaving the patient once prepared. To ensure safe use of equipment.
4	Screen the bed.	To ensure patient privacy and dignity.
5	Assist the patient into the supine position, ensure that a good light source is available, and make sure the bed is at a comfortable working height.	Correct positioning and use of light ensures optimum vision and adheres to health and safety rules.
6	Put on apron. Take trolley to patient or prepare useable surface.	To minimize contamination.

continued overleaf

7	Expose the patient's pelvis and place incontinence pad under them. Cover patient while preparing trolley or work surface.	To maintain patient dignity.
8	Wash and dry hands.	To minimize skin flora and prevent cross-infection.
9	Open catheterization/dressing packs and arrange sterile field. Open supplementary packs and cleansing solution.	Procedure is aseptic.
10	Draw up amount of water for balloon as per manufacturer's instructions before touching patient, and place cleansing solution into gallipot.	For safe balloon inflation and to maintain sterility.
11	Again wash hands and put sterile gloves on (one or two pairs).	Hands may have become contaminated by handling the outer packs.
12	Place sterile drape over pubic area.	To minimize contamination of catheter on insertion.
13	Wrap a piece of sterile gauze around shaft of penis and hold with non-dominant hand.	To avoid contamination with skin flora and cross-infection.
14	Retract foreskin if uncircumcised and clean glans penis and meatus using cleansing solution.	Provides clear access to the urethral orifice and prevents contamination of catheter. Inadequate cleansing of the urethral orifice is a major cause of UTI (Gray 1992).
15	Insert the nozzle of the lidocaine gel into the urethra and gently squeeze in the gel. There must be at least 11 ml of 2% anaesthetic gel inserted (Clinimed 2004). The gel may need to be massaged down the urethra to ensure that it travels beyond the bulb of the penis. Hold the shaft of the penis firmly for 3–5 minutes.	Adequate lubrication helps to prevent urethral trauma and eases catheter passage along the urethra. The use of local anaesthetic minimizes patient discomfort (Bardsley 2005).
16	Remove gloves and gel or wash hands before putting on second pair of sterile gloves (if not double-gloved).	To prevent contamination of the catheter.
17	Place sterile receiver on or between the patient's legs.	For collection of urine.
18	Place a fresh piece of gauze around the shaft of the penis.	To maintain clean hold of the penis.
19	Hold penis in an upright position with non-dominant hand, and gently insert the catheter down the urethra.	Enables more control of the catheter.

20	Once the catheter has travelled approximately 8–12 cm, stretch and move the penis downwards while continuing to insert the catheter gently.	This helps to negotiate the anterior curve of the urethra, leaving only the posterior curve to be negotiated (Sokeland 1989).
21	If resistance is felt at the bladder neck, instruct the patient to breathe deeply and relax. Continue to pass the catheter until urine begins to flow.	Deep breathing will help the sphincter relax.
22	Once urine has begun to flow, advance catheter up to the level of bifurcation of catheter. Inflate the balloon as per specification, using sterile water not normal saline or another solution. Once inflated, withdraw the catheter until resistance is felt.	This prevents the inflation of the balloon inside the urethra. Stop inflation if pain or discomfort felt. Inflating to the manufacturer's specifications ensures the balloon is adequately filled. Saline solutions can rot and seep out of the catheter balloon.
23	Collect urine specimen if indicated. Connect to sterile catheter drainage bag.	If urine looks infected, to identify microbe sensitivity. To ensure clear urine drainage.
24	Ensure that the glans is clean and then reposition the foreskin.	Prevents paraphimosis (swelling of foreskin) (Laker 1994).
25	Help the client get comfortable and instruct them in catheter hygiene.	To reduce anxiety over catheterization. To reduce risk of infection and ensure patient able to look after catheter safely at home.
26	Complete relevant records: reason for catheterization, residual volume, date, time of catheterization, make and size of catheter, volume of water in balloon, material and batch number, amount and type of gel used, cleansing agent used, any problems encountered.	Accountability, and to be able to trace catheter in the event of failure (NMC 2008).

Following the procedure

- Patients should be taught how to look after their catheter and given a leaflet with written instructions (Getliffe 1995).
- They should also be given guidance on suitable drinking habits to try to avoid infection.
- Patients should be advised of the possibility of bladder spasms – this is irritation caused by the physical presence of the catheter inside the bladder. It can result in feeling the urge to pass urine, bypassing (passage of urine around the sides of the catheter), and discomfort.
- They should also be given advice about what action to take should they get an infection or haematuria (blood in the urine).

Reflection and evaluation

When you have undertaken catheter insertion, think about the following:

1 Did the patient experience any pain on insertion?

2 Was the pain avoidable?

3 Did you cause any bleeding?

4 If there was bleeding what was the cause?

5 Was the patient relaxed and cooperative?

6 If the patient was not cooperative, what could you have done to improve the situation?

7 Did you have to leave the patient once the procedure started?

8 If you had to leave the patient, could this have been avoided?

9 Did you have any problems with the actual procedure?

10 If you did have problems, what were they and could they have been avoided through better preparation?

Further learning opportunities

Practise regularly on patient dummies to improve catheterization skills.

Reminders

Don't forget to:

- Replace a man's foreskin.
- Monitor the patient's urine output.
- Record the catheterization procedure in the patient's notes, including the amount of water in the balloon and any difficulties experienced.

Patient scenarios

Consider what you should do in the following situations, then turn to the end of this skill to check your answers.

1 Your patient is a 66-year-old woman receiving intra-vesical therapy. She has come to her appointment to have her third treatment and says she has had no symptoms over the last week. Her urine looks cloudy. What should you do and why?

2 Your patient is 80 years old and has been admitted because his district nurse was unable to remove his urethral catheter to change it. What should you do and what should you consider?

3 A patient has been admitted with haematuria and complains of discomfort and difficulty in passing urine. What should you consider and why?

Website

 http://www.oxfordtextbooks.co.uk/orc/ endacott

You may find it helpful to work through our short online quiz and additional scenarios intended to help you to develop and apply the skills in this chapter.

References

Addison R and Mould C (2000). Risk assessment in suprapubic catheterisation. *Nursing Standard*, **14**(36), 43–6.

Bardsley A (2005). Use of lubricant gels in urinary catheterization. *Nursing Standard*, **20**(8), 41–6.

British Association of Urological Nurses (2001). *Guidelines for female catheterisation*. BAUN, London.

British Association of Urological Nurses (2001). *Guidelines for male catheterisation*. BAUN, London.

Clinimed (2004). *Instillagel, anaesthetic, antiseptic, lubricant* [online] **http://www.clinimed.co.uk/ cl/products/uk** accessed 04/09/08.

Department of Health (2001). Guidelines for preventing infections associated with the insertion and maintenance of short term indwelling urethral catheters in acute care. *Journal of Hospital Infection*, **47**(Suppl), S39–S46.

Dieckhaus KD and Garibaldi RA (1998). Prevention of catheter associated urinary tract infections. In E Abrutytn, DA Goldmann, and WE Scheckler, eds. *Saunders infection control reference service* pp. 169–73. WB Saunders, Philadelphia.

Getliffe K (1995). Care of urinary catheters. *Nursing Standard*, **10**(1), 25–9.

Lloyd M and Bor R (2004). *Communication skills for medicine*, 2nd edition. Harcourt, London.

Medical Devices Agency (2000). *Equipped to care. The safe use of medical devices in the twenty-first century*. DH, London.

National Institute for Health and Clinical Excellence (2003). *Infection control – prevention of healthcare-associated infection in primary and community care*. NICE, London.

Nursing and Midwifery Council (2008). *The Code: standards of conduct, performance and ethics for nurses and midwives*. NMC, London.

Woodward S (2005). Use of lubricant in female urethral catheterisation. *British Journal of Nursing*, **14**(19), 1022–3.

Useful further reading and websites

Gupta S and Shergill I (2004). Managing the non-deflating Foley catheter balloon: deflating the undeflatable! *Urology News*, **8**(2), 12–15.

Simpson L (2001). Indwelling urethral catheters: reducing the risk of potential complications through proactive management. *Primary Health Care*, **11**(2), 57–64.

Tew L, Pomfret I, and King D (2005). Infection risks associated with urinary catheters. *Nursing Standard*, **20**(7), 55–61.

Ⓐ Answers to patient scenarios

1 The patient may have a UTI. Do not catheterize: obtain urine, dipstick specimen, then send for culture and sensitivity. Provide patient with antibiotics if dipstick positive for nitrites. You should never catheterize a person suspected of having a UTI as it may lead to septicaemia. Also the solution being given could be systemically absorbed and cause the patient harm. The fact that the patient is asymptomatic does not make any difference; catheterization should still not take place. Consider giving preventative advice.

2 Determine why the catheter could not be changed. Has the patient had a history of frequent infections or blockages, has he been bleeding, what efforts have been made to remove catheter, and what was experienced during this? Is catheter blocked or does patient have infection? Then assess patient catheter status, state of urine (bloody, cloudy, presence of debris), balloon inflated or not. If blocked, attempt to unblock using usual methods as described in Section 9.3. If this fails, call for medical assistance. If catheter not blocked but still unable to remove, call for medical assistance. Once cause known, consider giving advice for future prevention (hygiene, drinking).

3 Obtain history of haematuria. How long has patient been bleeding, has anything precipitated it (such as trauma), are there any other relevant symptoms (pyrexia, frequency, urgency), has patient had any urological surgery recently? Consider if patient is going into retention due to infection, post-operative complication, constipation, or clots. Once cause determined or considered, catheterize and treat as per medical advice. Take urine specimen to send for culture.

9.2 **Removal of a catheter**

Definition

The removal of a urinary catheter (urethral or suprapubic) from a patient's bladder.

It is important to remember that:

- You should only perform this procedure if competent to do so.
- Catheter removal can be painful; great care should be taken to reduce discomfort and physical trauma to the urinary tract.
- Patients must receive instructions about what to expect once the catheter has been removed, and advice on how to manage any problems (e.g. keep containers close by to pass urine into after prostate surgery, as the need to pass urine may become frequent and urgent). If it was a suprapubic catheter, explain when to change dressings and how to arrange them.
- Although removal of a catheter is a fairly simple procedure, the aftercare varies depending on the site of the catheter (urethral or suprapubic). Urethral removal leaves the body in its original state. Removing a suprapubic catheter leaves an open wound that will need a wound dressing to help it heal properly.
- Urine should be measured to ensure that the amount of urine being passed is adequate.
- If you are unsure why the catheter is to be removed or of post-removal plans, it is best to find out before starting to remove it.
- The patient must not be constipated as this can cause obstructive pressure on the urethra leading to urinary retention.

Prior knowledge

Before attempting removal of a catheter, make sure you are familiar with:

1 Bladder and urethral anatomy.
2 Aseptic wound dressing (for suprapubic catheters).
3 The manufacturer's guidelines on the use of its catheters.

You should have had appropriate training in urethral and suprapubic catheter removal.

Background

Prior to removing a catheter, it is important to know when and why the catheter was placed as this will dictate the post-removal instructions for the patient. It is also relevant to know if the patient is constipated as this can lead to urinary retention and the need to replace the catheter. See Section 9.1 for more information on catheters – Table 9.1 shows some common reasons for catheterization.

Context

 ## When to remove a catheter

A catheter must only be removed:

- If the catheter is not draining urine.
- When instructed to do so by the medical team responsible for the patient.
- With full knowledge of why the catheter was placed and the plans post-removal.

The medical team may instruct catheter removal:

- For permanent removal after surgical treatment if the patient is already able to pass urine naturally.
- For a trial period after surgical treatment.
- In order to replace the catheter if it is blocked and cannot be unblocked.
- To allow the patient to be taught selfcatheterization.

 ## When not to remove the catheter

A catheter must not be removed under the following circumstances:

- If there is not a clinical reason for catheter removal.
- If the patient has a symptomatic UTI, because this could lead to sepsis. To confirm whether this is the case, take a sterile urine specimen to send for microscopy, culture and sensitivity tests.
- If the patient is constipated, as they may find it difficult to pass urine (Getliffe and Dolman 2003).
- If the patient is male and taking anticholinergic medication, check with the team looking after them

before removing, as this may lead to worsening of prostatic hyperplasia and precipitate difficulty micturating (Joint Formulary Committee 2008).

Alternative interventions

There are no alternative interventions. If the catheter cannot be removed (in primary care), medical assistance must be sought as the patient will need to be seen in a secondary care facility. Further attempts to remove the catheter once the procedure has failed must not be carried out in primary care. The procedure can only be deferred to a later date if the catheter is draining and must be arranged in a secondary care facility as soon as possible. In a secondary care facility, if you are unable to remove a catheter you must call for medical assistance as more drastic measures (such as removal in theatre under anaesthetic) may be needed.

Potential problems

Potential problems include:

- Trauma to the urethra or suprapubic channel on removal (can be caused by an encrusted catheter tip); this can lead to infection or bleeding.
- Urethral bleeding post-removal; patient must be observed until bleeding stops.
- Haematuria post-removal; patient must be observed until bleeding stops.
- If the patient does not pass urine after catheter removal it is reasonable to give them water to drink to encourage this; if this does not work medical assistance must be sought.

There may be several reasons why a catheter is difficult to remove; encrustation of the catheter tip or intussusception of the balloon (deflated the balloon does not go back to original size and excess balloon forms a folded rim) are the most common. The catheter may still be removable with gentle twisting, or after leaving for 5 minutes until balloon settles (as recommended by the manufacturer). If this does not work it is best to call for assistance from a more experienced practitioner. If the catheter cannot be removed without causing physical trauma to the patient, medical assistance will be needed to employ more drastic measures such as removal under general anaesthetic or with the aid of a flexible cystoscope (flexible telescope designed to enter the bladder via the urethra while patient is awake) in a secondary care facility.

Indications for assistance

Indications for assistance include:

- If you have difficulty removing the catheter and are causing undue discomfort to the patient (experience in catheter removal will improve awareness of this).
- If the balloon cannot be deflated.
- If bleeding caused does not resolve.

Special considerations

Anticholinergic medication can cause urine retention (Joint Formulary Committee 2008). This could lead to inability to pass urine, so this information should be obtained before removing the catheter and used to determine if it should be removed. Although constipation does not necessarily stop micturition, it can impair ability to pass urine and therefore should be resolved before removing the catheter. It is important to be aware that some natural seepage occurs from the balloon and the amount of water withdrawn may not be the amount of water used to inflate it; it is therefore only relevant to ensure that the balloon is empty. Resistance to removal indicates that the balloon may not be properly deflated – reinflate it and deflate again; if resistance persists seek assistance.

Procedure

Preparation

Prepare yourself

Ensure you understand the procedure for catheter removal, are familiar with the manufacturer's instructions concerning use of the catheter, and know how much water was instilled into the balloon.

Prepare the patient

Explain the procedure fully to the patient (see Discussing the procedure box).

Prepare the equipment

Equipment needed includes:

- Disposable gloves and apron.
- Clinical waste disposal bag.
- Appropriate size syringe (10 ml, or 20 ml and 10 ml) for size of balloon.
- Incontinence pad.
- Urine jug.
- If catheter is being replaced, ensure equipment is gathered for catheterization process.
- Extra equipment to ensure patient is not abandoned during the procedure should equipment become contaminated.

When removing a suprapubic catheter, also prepare:

- Sterile gloves (plus extra pair should contamination occur).
- Dressing pack.
- Cleansing solution (e.g. normal saline or Hibisept solution).
- Gauze and tape for dressing.

Discussing the procedure with the patient and the family

- Explain why removal of the catheter is necessary.
- Assure the patient that they may feel some discomfort but not undue pain.
- Advise the patient on how they can assist with the procedure.
- Explain the consequences of catheter removal and what is expected of them.
- Explain that it may be necessary to re-catheterize if they are unable to pass urine.
- Answer any questions they may have.

Step-by-step guide to removing a urethral catheter

Procedure	Rationale
1 Introduce yourself, confirm the patient's identity, explain the procedure, and obtain consent.	To identify the patient correctly and gain informed consent.
2 Screen the bed.	To ensure patient privacy and dignity.
3 Ask patient to remove garments below waist completely, or at least down to below the knees.	To allow ease of access and keep clothes dry and unsoiled.
4 Cover the patient while preparing equipment.	To ensure patient dignity.
5 Observe the urine in the catheter bag.	To detect UTI and decide if catheter specimen of urine (CSU) is required, and whether the catheter can still be removed.
6 Remove leg straps.	To ease removal of catheter.
7 Place incontinence pad under catheter exit site.	To protect patient and keep area clean.
8 Don non-sterile gloves and apron.	To avoid cross-infection.
9 Insert appropriately sized syringe into the balloon channel and remove water from balloon (most catheters have 10 ml of water; irrigation catheters have 30 ml). The amount of water listed on balloon cuff may not equal the amount removed (see Special considerations box). Water should empty automatically, but a gentle pull may be needed to ensure complete drainage.	To deflate the balloon.
10 Remove syringe from balloon channel.	To prevent water being pulled back into balloon.
11 Inform patient and then remove catheter by pulling gently, slowly, and steadily until it is removed.	To prepare patient and prevent trauma to catheter tract.
12 If catheter is being changed, follow the instructions in Section 9.1.	To insert a new catheter correctly.
13 Dry vulval or meatal (urethral) opening.	For patient comfort.
14 Assist patient in redressing as necessary.	To maintain patient dignity and safety.
15 Dispose of equipment and catheter into clinical waste bag.	For health and safety, and infection control.

16	Remove gloves and apron, disposing of them in clinical waste bag.	For infection control.
17	Wash and dry hands.	For infection control.
18	Give patient post-removal advice; this will depend on reason catheter was placed.	To ensure patient knows what to expect and is prepared.
19	Advise patient to drink 2 litres of fluid over the next 24 hours.	To reduce possibility of infection post-removal.
20	Ensure district nursing services in place or book these.	To ensure patient has appropriate support, supplies, and advice.

Following removal of a urethral catheter

Observe for bleeding and haematuria; if these occur, monitor until they resolve.

It is important to monitor the patient's urine output:

- The patient should be instructed to drink an amount of fluid sufficient to fill their bladder (this amount is usually dictated by a local protocol or guidelines, and is dependent on the patient's other medical conditions, which may limit the amount of fluid they can drink).
- The patient should pass their urine into a jug for measuring at each micturition. They should pass approximately 150–200 ml or more (depending on bladder capacity) on three occasions for removal to be considered successful.
- If the procedure is carried out in hospital, the bladder must be scanned to ensure that the amount of residual urine (urine left in bladder) is also reasonable. This acceptable residual volume is usually indicated by the clinician.

If removal is successful, the patient must be given information about what to expect, such as frequency, urgency, and dysuria after removal, and what they may do to ease these symptoms. Advice for helping to resolve these issues may include:

- Pelvic floor exercises.
- Bladder retraining.
- Cutting out caffeinated or fizzy drinks.
- Drinking at least 1.5 litres of fluid.

If the catheter has been removed following radical retropubic prostatectomy (an operation to remove the prostate in men with prostate cancer), the patient must be advised that incontinence is possible. They should be advised (both verbally and with supporting written leaflets) to commence pelvic floor exercises and be given fluid intake advice, as these measures will aid a return to continence. The patient must then be given sufficient pads to take home and referred to a district nursing service to support him and provide appropriate further supplies and advice.

Step-by-step guide to removing a suprapubic catheter

	Procedure	Rationale
1	Introduce yourself, confirm the patient's identity, explain the procedure, and obtain consent.	To identify the patient correctly and gain informed consent.
2	Screen the bed.	To ensure patient privacy and dignity.
3	Ask patient to remove garments below waist completely, or at least down to below the knees.	To allow ease of access and keep clothes dry and unsoiled.
4	Cover patient while preparing equipment.	To ensure patient dignity.
5	Observe urine in catheter bag.	To detect UTI and decide if CSU required and if catheter can still be removed.
6	Remove leg straps.	To ease removal of catheter.
7	Place incontinence pad under catheter exit site.	To protect patient and keep area clean.
8	Put on apron.	To protect self and prevent contamination.
9	Wash and dry hands.	Hands may have become contaminated by outer packaging.
10	Put on one or two pairs of sterile gloves.	This is an aseptic procedure.
11	Clean insertion site with normal saline.	To clean any debris that may make it difficult to remove catheter and reduce possibility of infection.
12	If replacing catheter, remove catheter bag and replace with a spigot or a Flip-Flo valve to stop flow of urine. Place 50 ml of sterile water into empty bladder.	To ensure fluid present in bladder to drain through new catheter, ensuring proper placement.
13	Insert syringe into balloon channel and allow water to empty into appropriately sized syringe. Most catheters have 10 ml of water; irrigation catheters have 30 ml. The amount of water is listed on balloon cuff but may not be equal to water removed (see Special considerations box). Water should empty automatically, but a gentle pull may be needed to ensure complete drainage.	To allow safe removal of catheter as per manufacturer's instructions.
14	Remove syringe from balloon channel when deflated.	To prevent water being pulled back into balloon.

15	Inform patient and then gently twist catheter and pull gently, slowly, and steadily until all of catheter is out.	To prepare patient and prevent trauma to catheter tract.
16	Clean suprapubic wound site.	To maintain asepsis and remove debris.
17	If catheter is being replaced, remove dirty gloves and replace with fresh sterile gloves from opened catheterization pack. Apply only a small amount of lidocaine gel to site and gently insert catheter into the same track until urine starts to flow. Push catheter into bladder up to bifurcation and inflate balloon, gently pull catheter out until resistance felt, then attach appropriate drainage bag or valve and secure. Place a plain gauze dressing on site. There should be a delay of no more than 10–20 minutes between removal and replacement. *This procedure should only be carried out by a health care professional trained and competent to do so.*	After 10–20 minutes the risk for suprapubic site closure is high.
18	Place and firmly secure gauze dressing (a pressure dressing is recommended).	To protect wound site and prevent urine leakage from suprapubic site.
19	Dispose of all equipment and catheter into clinical waste bag.	For health and safety, and infection control.
20	Remove gloves and wash hands.	To preserve infection control.
21	Advise patient to drink 2 litres of fluid over the next 24 hours.	To reduce possibility of infection.
22	Ensure district nursing services in place or book these.	To ensure arrangements made for dressing change and observation of wound healing.

Following removal of a suprapubic catheter

The patient needs to be supplied with an appropriate number of replacement dressings at home. They need to be referred to the district nursing service, which will apply further dressings as necessary until the site has healed, support the patient, and provide supplies for catheter care. If the catheter removal is successful, the patient must be given information about what to expect after removal: dressing to be left in place for 48 hours before being changed by district nurses, then further dressings to be applied at the discretion of the district nurse depending on healing of the wound. If the catheter is replaced, the dressing may be removed at home once the site has healed sufficiently – district nurses may advise on this. The patient should be advised to drink at least 1.5 litres of fluid (NICE 2005). Ensure that the patient is given a leaflet regarding care of catheter, fluid intake, and bowel advice.

Recognizing patient deterioration

Identifying deterioration is important as it may lead to re-catheterization:

- Is the amount of urine passed increasingly less?

- Is the patient able to pass urine at all?

Reflection and evaluation

When you have undertaken removal of a catheter, think about the following questions:

1 Did the removal cause pain?
2 If pain was caused on removal, what could you have done to prevent it?
3 Was it necessary to remove the catheter?
4 Was any bleeding caused?
5 If bleeding was caused, what did you do about it?
6 If bleeding was caused, was it preventable?
7 Was the removal difficult?
8 If the removal was difficult, why was it and could it have been made easier?

Further learning opportunities

Every attempt must be made to observe this skill. It should only be done autonomously if you are signed off to do so.

Reminders

Don't forget to:

- Ensure the patient has a district nurse or refer them for this service (give the patient a referral form to take with them).
- Discuss good drinking habits and ways to avoid constipation.
- Ensure the patient goes home with adequate supplies to last them until the district nurse visits.
- Ensure the patient understands exactly what to do when they get home.

 Patient scenarios

Consider what you should do in the following situations, then turn to the end of this skill to check your answers.

1 You are trying to remove a urethral catheter when it gets stuck. What should you do?
2 If a patient starts to bleed when their catheter is removed or replaced, what should you do?
3 If a patient has gross haematuria after their catheter is removed or replaced, what should you do?
4 You are replacing a suprapubic catheter and are unable to insert the new one. What should you do?
5 You have replaced a catheter and no urine comes out on insertion. What should you do?

Website

   http://www.oxfordtextbooks.co.uk/orc/ endacott

You may find it helpful to work through our short online quiz and additional scenarios intended to help you to develop and apply the skills in this chapter.

References

Joint Formulary Committee (2008). *British national formulary*, 55th edition. British Medical Association and Royal Pharmaceutical Society of Great Britain, London.

Getliffe K and Dolman M (2003). *Promoting continence: a clinical and research resource*, 2nd edition. Bailliere Tindall, London.

Useful further reading and websites

Evans A, Painter D, and Feneley R (2001). Blocked urinary catheters: nurses' preventive role. *Nursing Times*, **97**(1), 37–8.

Evans A and Feneley R (2000). A study of current nursing management of long-term catheters. *British Journal of Community Nursing*, **5**(5), 240–5.

Winn C (1996). Basing catheter care on research principles. *Nursing Standard*, **10**(8), 38–46.

A **Answers to patient scenarios**

1 Ensure balloon is properly deflated. Gently twist the catheter while pulling. If it becomes impossible to remove, call for medical assistance.
2 Keep patient in the department until bleeding stops. If bleeding continues unabated, call for medical assistance.

3 Provide patient with fluid to flush bladder until it resolves. If haematuria continues unabated, call for medical assistance.

4 Call for specialist or senior nurse or medical assistance within 20 minutes.

5 If you are certain catheter is in right position, give patient fluid to drink and within half an hour urine should flow. If it is not flowing after this time, call for medical assistance or senior or specialist nursing advice (they may suggest you try inserting catheter again).

9.3 Bladder lavage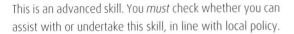

This is an advanced skill. You *must* check whether you can assist with or undertake this skill, in line with local policy.

Definition

The terms bladder lavage and bladder washout seem to be interchangeable in the literature but this skill also includes the use of catheter maintenance solutions. Bladder lavage is the insertion of a solution into the bladder that is then immediately drained (Robinson 2004). The term bladder washout is also used to describe the washing out of a catheter in hospital patients using a different method for different reasons (Castledine 2006). Bladder lavage is a skill for which there are no clear protocols for how to do it, how often to do it, and what to use. The clearest evidence that exists relates to the use of catheter maintenance solutions to prevent and treat catheter blockage in patients with long-term indwelling catheters (Gray 2001, Getliffe 2003). This section therefore concentrates on this use of the term in this context.

It is important to remember that:

- There is no evidence to support the use of water for this purpose.
- It is an aseptic procedure.
- Drainage in the catheter bag should mirror the amount of fluid instilled.
- This procedure should only be undertaken by a qualified nurse with the appropriate experience.

- It is important for student nurses to understand the procedure itself, why it is done, how your institution undertakes it, and how to support a nurse and patient adequately during the procedure. Students may only undertake this skill under direct supervision of an experienced, qualified member of staff.
- Preparing extra sterile equipment before the procedure is good practice, to ensure the patient is not abandoned during the procedure should any equipment become contaminated.

Prior knowledge

Before undertaking bladder lavage, ensure that you are familiar with:

1 Universal infection control practice.
2 Anatomy of the urinary system.
3 The patient's urinary catheter and catheter drainage system.

Background

Please refer to Section 9.1 for more information on catheterization. A urinary catheter may be inserted into the bladder to facilitate drainage of urine or instillation of medicine for a number of reasons. If the catheter becomes fully or partially blocked, urine may be prevented from draining out of the bladder or may bypass around the catheter. This can be painful and/or distressing for the patient (Pomfret 2000), and even though the bladder can stretch somewhat (this differs from patient to patient) to accommodate more urine than it is used to, it will eventually rupture if the blockage is not relieved. The normal bladder can accommodate around 500–600 ml. The causes of a blocked catheter are varied, and it is important to identify the cause correctly. Examples include:

- Drainage bag above the level of the bladder.
- Drainage bag more than two-thirds full.
- Twisted drainage tubing.
- Constipation causing pressure on the urethra from a full bowel.
- Bladder spasm.
- Bladder calculi.
- Catheter encrustation by mineral deposits.

It is important to identify the cause in order to manage the patient appropriately and hopefully prevent the problem from recurring (Getliffe 2003).

The most common cause of a blocked catheter is encrustation (particularly in the community setting), with an incidence of 40–50% of affected patients (Getliffe 2003). This occurs when bacteria (such as *Proteus mirabilis*, *Pseudomonas aeruginosa*, and *Klebsiella*) enter the bladder and release urease, an enzyme that causes the urine to become alkaline and form calcium phosphate and magnesium ammonium phosphate salts (Getliffe 2003, Pomfret *et al.* 2004, The Cochrane Collaboration 2008).

Traditionally, nurses have advised patients with indwelling catheters to maintain a high fluid intake to promote the flow of urine through the catheter. Although this will not prevent or reduce UTI or encrustation (Getliffe 1993), it does result in diluted urine output, reducing the risk of urethritis, constipation, and stagnant urine. These are all possible contributory factors in causing leakage and bypass of urine (Rees-Williams *et al.* 1988) and blockage of the catheter (The Cochrane Collaboration 2008).

Sodium chloride 0.9% solution is usually used for bladder washouts in inpatients (McCarthy and Hunter 2001). Being an isotonic solution, it does not alter the body's fluid and electrolyte levels, and large volumes can be used. Water should not be used for bladder washout because it can be absorbed by the process of osmosis.

Context

 ### When to undertake a bladder lavage lavage

A bladder lavage should be undertaken to clear debris, clots, or encrustation from a catheter that is blocked in order to enable urine drainage (Dougherty and Lister 2005).

 ### When not to undertake a bladder lavage

A bladder lavage is not undertaken if the catheter is not blocked and is draining urine. It is also important to remember that bladder washout in patients who have had major urinary surgery must be done carefully and under supervision to avoid rupturing of stitches or anastomoses.

Alternative interventions

The only other intervention possible would be to replace the catheter with a new one; however, this should only be done if instructed by the doctor and is not a common occurrence.

Potential problems

If the catheter has been in place for more than 3 months or the patient's urine is full of debris, there is a possibility of encrustation. It may then be difficult to perform the procedure and urine may not drain freely out of the bladder, meaning it is necessary to change the catheter (if removal of the catheter is difficult, this may indicate that significant encrustation has developed, in which case medical assistance should be sought). It has been suggested that one or two instillations of a recommended catheter maintenance solution (40 ml) may be used first to dispel the encrustation, reducing trauma caused on removal of the catheter or avoiding the need to change the catheter too soon (Gray 2001, Getliffe 2003).

Other potential complications include:

- Urinary infection – ensure an aseptic technique in order to prevent this.
- Retention of injected solution – monitor the input and output out of the catheter as this can cause inflammation of the bladder mucosa.
- Insertion of air into the catheter, which would cause discomfort and pain for the patient.

Indications for assistance

If the bladder washout fails to unblock the catheter, seek medical assistance. The patient should be observed during bladder washout for unreasonable pain or adverse effects such as abdominal or chest pain. If these occur, the procedure should be stopped and medical assistance sought.

Procedure

Preparation

Prepare the equipment

- Yellow clinical waste bag
- Disposable apron

- Bladder syringe
- One litre bottle of sterile normal saline
- Pair of sterile gloves
- Replacement drainage bag or Flip-Flo valve
- Two sterile jugs and kidney dish
- Sterile drape

Step-by-step guide to bladder lavage

Procedure	Rationale
1 Introduce yourself, confirm the patient's identity, explain the procedure, and obtain consent.	To identify the patient correctly and gain informed consent.
2 Wash and dry hands.	To minimize the risk of cross-infection.
3 Prepare the trolley, placing all equipment on the bottom shelf.	To avoid leaving the patient during the procedure.
4 Screen the bed. Assist the patient into the supine position and ensure that a good light source is available and the bed is at a comfortable working height.	To ensure privacy. Correct positioning and adequate light ensure optimum vision.
5 Put on a plastic apron. Take the trolley to patient, positioning it on the patient's right side.	To minimize contamination. To facilitate the procedure.
6 Expose the patient's pelvic region. Place an incontinence pad under them. Cover the patient while preparing equipment. Position patient with legs abducted and knees flexed.	To facilitate the procedure. To avoid the need to change the sheet post-procedure. To maintain patient dignity. To facilitate the procedure and allow ease of access.
7 Wash and dry hands again. Open sterile drape and arrange sterile field, opening the jug, syringe, and kidney dish.	To minimize skin flora (the procedure is aseptic). To prepare equipment for procedure.
8 Check the solution and expiry date. Pour sterile saline into jug.	To ensure that the solution is the correct one and is not out of date.
9 Again wash hands, put on sterile gloves.	Hands may have become contaminated by handling the outer packaging.
10 Place sterile drape under the catheter. Place the kidney dish between the patient's legs.	To minimize contamination of catheter on detaching the catheter bag for insertion of bladder syringe. To collect urine.

continued overleaf

11	Draw up 30 ml of solution into the bladder syringe and expel any air.	To prepare the solution for the procedure. Injecting large volumes of air into the bladder would cause discomfort and distension for the patient.
12	Disconnect catheter bag and place in yellow waste bag.	To minimize the risk of cross-infection.
13	Connect the bladder syringe nozzle to the catheter and insert 30 ml of solution into the bladder.	To unblock the catheter.
	Disconnect the bladder syringe and allow the bladder contents to drain into the kidney dish. Repeat the above procedure until the urine drains clear.	To allow the contents of the bladder to be drained.
14	If urine does not start draining, gentle aspiration using the bladder syringe should be applied.	To try to dislodge the blockage.
15	When urine starts to drain clear, connect a new catheter drainage bag.	To collect draining urine.
	Ensure the patient is covered up before removing the bed screen.	To maintain the patient's dignity.
16	Remove apron and gloves and dispose of all equipment as per local protocol.	To prevent cross-contamination.
17	Document the procedure and update the patient's fluid balance chart.	To maintain accurate records.

Following the procedure

The patient's urine output should be monitored for a repeat occurrence or for blood clots or debris if this were the cause of the blockage. Maintain a fluid balance and monitor for blood clots and haematuria. If necessary, remember to recommence irrigation. Thought should be given to prevention.

Reflection and evaluation

When you have undertaken bladder washout, think about the following:

1 Was the washout being carried out in primary or secondary care?
2 What did you use to carry out the washout?
3 Was the washout successful?
4 If the washout was not successful, why wasn't it?

5 Were you able to determine the reason for the blockage?
6 What steps did you take to prevent further blockages?

Reminders

Don't forget to:

- Record bladder washout in notes.
- If blood clots caused the blockage, inform medical staff if clotting continues.
- Advise patient to have a good fluid intake of at least 1.5 litres (as instructed by medical staff) to help prevent recurrence of the blockage.

Patient scenarios

1 Patient A is 57 years old and is 1 day postcystectomy (bladder removal) with bladder reconstruction. You

have observed that the patient has become hypertensive, complains of a severe headache and palpitations, and is pale and sweating profusely. What may help resolve this problem and what may be the cause?

2   Patient B is 68 years old and diabetic. He has had a transurethral resection of the prostate and is 4 hours post-operative. He has irrigation running and is complaining of abdominal pain; his urine is bright red and he is pyrexial. What do you do to resolve this problem and what do you need to take into consideration?

Website

 http://www.oxfordtextbooks.co.uk/orc/ endacott

You may find it helpful to work through our short online quiz and additional scenarios intended to help you to develop and apply the skills in this chapter.

References

Castledine G (2006). Nurse whose inexperience and negligence in bladder washout put her patient at risk. *British Journal of Nursing*, **15**(3), 141.

Getliffe K (1993). Care of urinary catheters. *Nursing Standard*, **3**(8), 16–18.

Getliffe K (2003). Managing recurrent urinary catheter blockage: problems, promises and practicalities. *The Journal of Wound, Ostomy and Continence Nursing*, **30**(3), 146–51.

Gray M (2001). Managing urinary encrustation in the indwelling catheter. *Journal of Wound, Ostomy and Continence Nursing*, **28**(5), 226–9.

McCarthy K and Hunter I (2001). Importance of pH monitoring in the care of long term catheters. *British Journal of Nursing*, **10**(19), 1240–5.

Pomfret I (2000). Catheter care in the community. *Nursing Standard*, **14**(27), 46–51.

Pomfret I, Bayait F, Mackenzie R, Wells M and Winder A (2004). Using bladder instillations to manage indwelling catheters. *British Journal of Nursing*, **13**(5), 261–7.

Rees-Williams C, Meyrick M, and Jones M (1988). Urinary catheters. *Nursing Times*, **84**(40), 46–7.

Robinson J (2004). A practical approach to catheter-associated problems. *Nursing Standard*, **18**(31), 38–42.

Useful further reading and websites

Cruikshank J and Woodward S, eds (2001). *Management of continence and urinary catheter care: evidence based practice (BJN Monograph)*. Quay Books, Pinton.

Pratt R, Pellow EC, Loveday H *et al.* (2001). The EPIC project: developing national evidence based guidelines for preventing healthcare associated infections. *Journal of Hospital Infection*, **47**(Suppl), 53–54.

Wilson J (2001). *Infection control in clinical practice*, 2nd edition. Bailliere Tindall, Edinburgh.

http://www.patient.co.uk/leaflets/urinary_ catheterization.htm

http://www.nhs.uk/conditions/ urinary-catheterization

http://www.nursing-standard.co.uk/archives/ns/ vol14-27/pdfs/p4651w27.pdf

http://www.icna.co.uk/default.asp

http://www.nhshighland.scot.nhs.uk/ Health%20Services/Pharmacy/Formulary/ Prescribing%20Guidelines/Catheter%20pat

http://www.library.nhs.uk/Theatres/ ViewResource.aspxresID=238622

http://www.touchbriefings.com/pdf/2808/ Getliffe.pdf

http://www.nursing-standard.co.uk/archives/ns/ vol17-27/pdfs/v17n27p3338.pdf

http://www.dh.gov.uk/en/Publicationsandstatistics/ Publications/PublicationsPolicyAndGuidance/ Browsable/DH_4879467

http://www.sglos-pct.ns.uk/ClinGov/Policy %20PDS%20Oversions/04.Clinical%20 Guidelines%20use%20of%20catheter%20mai

http://www.jcn.co.uk/journal.asp?MonthhNum=07 &YearNum=2006&Type=backissue&ArticleID=950

http://www.patient.co.uk/showdoc/40001972/

http://www.nhshealthquality.org/nhsqis/files/ urinary_cath_COMPLETE.pdf

 Answers to patient scenarios

1   Call for medical assistance urgently. Check if catheter is blocked as this may be causing autonomic dysreflexia. With medical help, positively identify source of problem. If catheter blocked, change catheter and treat symptoms as instructed. If patient has UTI, treat with antibiotics as advised by medical practitioner.

2 Check catheter for blockage; if blocked stop irrigation and wash out bladder. Observe urine to check for infection and take urine sample; if infection found administer antibiotics as instructed by medical staff. If clots present, recommence irrigation after washout. If washout unsuccessful, inform medical staff as patient may need catheter changed. This will need to be carried out by a doctor as the surgery may necessitate a guide wire to prevent perforation of prostate capsule. Check blood sugar as infection may derange, and take necessary action as per medical instruction.

9.4 **Monitoring renal replacement therapy** 🅐

This is an advanced skill. You *must* check whether you can assist with or undertake this skill, in line with local policy.

Definition

Renal replacement therapy (RRT) replaces some of the functions of the kidney that have been lost due to acute or end stage renal disease (Thomas 2002). When the kidneys fail to function correctly, RRT is required to remove waste products and to restore electrolytes and fluid balance. RRT is a term used to describe haemodialysis (HD) (Figure 9.2), peritoneal dialysis (PD) (Figure 9.3), and renal transplantation, as well as haemofiltration and continuous veno-venous haemofiltration (CVVH). They are all treatment options used to provide care for patients with acute and chronic kidney disease. Patients receiving RRT require close monitoring, e.g. vital signs, weight, and fluid balance.

It is important to remember that:

Not all renal units allow students to be actively involved in RRT. However, you will find it helpful to understand the principles of the skill so that when you come into contact with a patient receiving any RRT you will be able to assist in the care provided by the multiprofessional members of the renal team. Please make sure you check with your individual placements before taking part in any RRT skills.

Prior knowledge

Before attempting any RRT skill, make sure you are familiar with:

1 Renal anatomy and physiology (particularly osmosis, ultrafiltration, and convection).
2 Basic renal processes of glomerular filtration, tubular reabsorption, and secretion.
3 Conditions causing chronic kidney disease (CKD) and the classification of such diseases as stages 1–5 (depending on the presence of kidney damage and glomerular filtration rate, e.g. stage 5 describes established renal failure).

Background

In order to understand fully how RRT is carried out it will be useful for you to consider electrolyte and fluid balance, RRT access, the range of symptoms that can develop due to uraemia, and fluid and dietary allowances.

The aim of any dialysis is to replace the excretory functions of the kidney by artificial means to remove excess solutes and fluid from the blood. Haemodialysis and peritoneal dialysis utilize the basic principles of **osmosis** (movement of solutes down a concentration gradient across a semi-permeable membrane) and **ultrafiltration** (movement due to pressure changes across a semi-permeable membrane).

Solute removal uses the principle of osmosis, where solutes move (or diffuse) from an area of higher concentration to an area of lower concentration across a semi-permeable membrane until equilibrium is achieved. **Fluid removal** or ultrafiltration is achieved by transmembrane pressure, so fluid is pushed out of the blood compartment across the semi-permeable membrane into the dialysate compartment (Kendall 2005). As fluid is moved through the membrane, smaller solutes are dragged along; this solute drag is known as convection (Levy *et al.* 2001). A visit to a renal unit will help you to see how the principles are applied to the different treatment options.

Complications of dialysis include fatigue, hypotension, and bacterial infections. Particular to peritoneal dialysis are the possibility of constipation, abdominal pains, 'cloudy bags', fever, nausea, and vomiting and diarrhoea.

For patients who suffer from haemodynamic instability there are other strategies, namely continuous renal replacement therapies including CVVH, usually seen on intensive care units. Haemofiltration is where blood is filtered across a highly permeable membrane, facilitating the removal of waste products by convection. These therapies allow gentler fluid and solute removal, minimizing complications such as electrolyte disturbances and fluid shifts, as well as hypotension.

Indications for RRT in kidney disease include:

- Fluid overload (principally pulmonary oedema in acute renal failure).
- Uncontrolled hyperkalaemia (causes cardiac arrhythmias).
- Metabolic acidosis.
- Uraemia.

(Leach 2004)

It is worth remembering that RRT can only partly replace kidney function; for example, it cannot mimic the kidneys' natural endocrine functions.

Context

 ## When to monitor patients receiving RRT

All patients receiving RRT will require close monitoring, and the frequency of such monitoring will be dictated by local policy. Vital signs should be recorded at least 4-hourly, though sometimes more frequent recording will be required. Fluid balance should be continually monitored, with input and output recorded on an ongoing basis to help ensure accuracy. Weight is generally recorded on a daily basis, at the same time each day to ensure consistency.

 ## When not to monitor RRT

The only reason for not monitoring a patient receiving RRT is if this contravenes local policy. In some renal units, only the senior nurses care for these patients (check local policy). Note that where patients are performing their own exchanges on PD or APD (automated peritoneal dialysis, commonly used at night-time), monitoring is less urgent and will be carried out at regular intervals according to local policy (this may be adapted for patients who need to sleep).

Specific observations

Specific observations are documented according to individual unit policy; however, they will generally include the patient's weight, fluid balance, clinical observations, and blood chemistry. Dialysis treatments are very dependent on the correct recording of these. Please refer to your clinical area's policy for the frequency of recording and documenting of clinical observations/fluid balance.

Special considerations

Haemodialysis

- What fluid allowance has been prescribed for the patient?
- Is there any special diet allowance?
- Before carrying out any clinical observations, check where the patient's HD access is sited. You will not be able to take a blood pressure reading on the limb where the access is.
- Avoid tight, restricting clothing or wristbands on the access limb.
- Always check when the patient is due for their next dialysis session. The sessions are usually set to the same appointment times; check with the HD unit.
- On return from dialysis the patient may complain of feeling 'washed out'; this is normal.
- Always wear protective equipment and adhere to infection control polices when dealing with blood products/bodily fluids.

Special considerations

Peritoneal dialysis

- Does the patient need assistance in collecting the equipment required to carry out their PD exchanges?
- What fluid allowance has been prescribed for the patient?
- Is there any special diet allowance?
- Before carrying out any clinical observations, check to see if the patient has a HD access sited in any of their limbs. Many PD patients also have HD access, and you will not be able to take a blood pressure reading on the limb where the access is.

- Does the patient need assistance to weigh?

- If the patient complains about constipation, ensure you inform the Registered Nurse in your team. Constipation can prevent PD working efficiently.

- Does the patient need assistance to perform their PD catheter care?

- Always wear protective equipment and adhere to infection control polices when dealing with blood products/bodily fluids.

Procedure

Preparation

Prepare the patient
Even though the patient may be familiar with the monitoring procedures associated with RRT, a full explanation should still be provided. Discuss the monitoring procedure with the patient and provide reassurance as necessary.

Prepare the equipment
Ensure the necessary equipment is available, e.g. sphygmomanometer, temperature recording device, and scales.

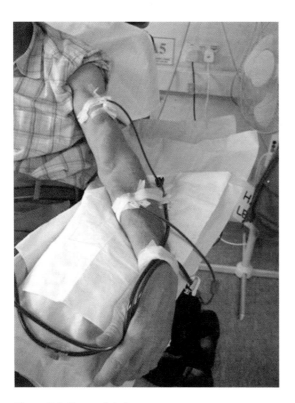

Figure 9.2 Haemodialysis.

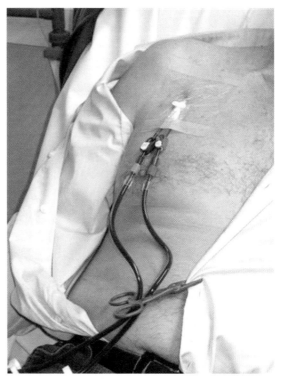

Figure 9.3 Peritoneal dialysis.

Step-by-step guide to monitoring an inpatient on dialysis

Step	Rationale
1 Introduce yourself, confirm the patient's identity, explain the procedure, and obtain consent.	To identify the patient correctly and gain informed consent.
2 Undertake regular observations as stipulated by local policy: pulse rate, blood pressure, temperature, respiratory rate, blood sugar levels if diabetic.	Clinical observations are closely linked to fluid balance and therefore provide a constant assessment of the patient before, during, and after RRT treatments. Tachypnoea, tachycardia, and hypertension suggest fluid overload; pyrexia suggests possible infection.
3 Strictly monitor fluid balance.	To minimize the risk of fluid overload and hypertension.
4 Provide fluid/dietary allowances. There should be close collaboration with other members of the multiprofessional team such as dieticians.	Many patients have different diet and fluid allowances. Non-adherence with these can cause problems such as fluid overload/dehydration, electrolyte disturbance, and poor adequacy of dialysis.
5 Record the patient's weight on a daily basis. Use the same scales and weigh the patient at the same time each day to allow a more accurate assessment of weight.	Dry weight is the patient's weight minus any fluid overload/dehydration. Patients need to reach their dry or target weight at the end of a HD session. PD patients are encouraged to try and remain on or closely around their prescribed dry weight.
6 Monitor RRT access site.	It is impossible to perform any RRT without a functioning access site. Checks are made to ensure that the access remains patent and free from infection. Patients are educated in the care of their renal access.
7 Monitor blood chemistry. Most HD units monitor the patient's bloods every month, while PD patients will have their blood tested according to their individual prescriptions. This can be carried out during an outpatient appointment or in the patient's home by the community renal team.	As the kidneys are unable to regulate electrolytes, it is vitally important that the patient's blood chemistry is checked.

Following the procedure

Following the intervention it will be necessary to document the findings accurately, e.g. on the patient's observation chart. It is important to compare the findings with previous findings, looking for signs of deterioration during RRT. For example, a rising blood pressure could indicate circulatory overload. Report any changes to the senior nurse/doctor as appropriate.

Recognizing patient deterioration

- Are the respiratory rate, blood pressure, and pulse rising?

- Has the patient developed pyrexia that could indicate infection?

- Is the access site red, inflamed, or tender? These are signs of local infection.

- Is the patient's weight increasing and the fluid balance showing a positive balance?

Reminders

Don't forget to notify the Registered Nurse about any problems regarding the patient's dialysis access.

 Patient scenarios

Consider what you should do in the following situations, then turn to the end of this skill to check your answers.

1 Patient A is undertaking their PD exchange and notifies you that they feel hot, have abdominal pain, and that the fluid they are draining out into their PD bag looks cloudy. What might the problem be and what action do you think needs to be taken?

2 Patient B has returned from their HD treatment feeling lightheaded. Handover from the HD nurse indicates that the patient's post-dialysis blood pressure is lower than normal and they are slightly under their post-dialysis dry weight. (Note that 'dry weight' is the post-dialysis weight that allows pre-dialysis blood pressure to remain normal – Turner 2006.) What do you think happened during their treatment that contributed to the patient having these problems?

3 While you are carrying out Patient C's clinical observations, they inform you that they can no longer feel the buzz in their arteriovenous fistula. What do you think could be the problem?

4 Patient D is unable to carry out their PD exit site care and asks for your assistance. What should you check before undertaking the task?

Website

 http://www.oxfordtextbooks.co.uk/orc/ endacott

You may find it helpful to work through our short online quiz and additional scenarios intended to help you to develop and apply the skills in this chapter.

References

Kendall G and Shiu KY (2005). *Medicine and surgery: a concise textbook*. Blackwell Publishing, Oxford.

Leach R (2004). *Critical care medicine at a glance*. Blackwell Publishing, Oxford.

Levy J, Morgan J, and Brown E (2001). *Oxford handbook of dialysis*. Oxford University Press, Oxford.

Thomas N (2002). *Renal nursing*, 2nd edition. Bailliere Tindall, London.

Turner N (2006). *Dry weight*. EdRen (the website for the Renal Unit at the Royal Infirmary Edinburgh) [online] **http://renux.dmed.ed.ac.uk/EdREN/ Handbookbits/HDBKdryweight.html** accessed 04/09/08.

Useful further reading and websites

Department of Health (2004). *The national services framework for renal services. Part one dialysis and transplantation*. DH, London.

Redmond A and Doherty E (2005). Peritoneal dialysis. *Nursing Standard*, **19**(40), 55–65.

Renal Association (2002). *Treatment of adults and children with renal failure, standards and audit measures*, 3rd edition. Royal College of Physicians of London and the Renal Association, London.

Springhouse (2002). *Fluids and electrolytes made incredibly easy*, 2nd edition. Springhouse, Pennsylvania.

EDTNA/ERCA: **http://www.edtna-erca.org**

National Kidney Federation: **http://www.kidney.org.uk**

Renal Association: **http://www.renal.org**

http://www.nephronline.org

http://www.renaladvances.com

http://www.renalweb.com

http://www.doh.gov.uk

Answers to patient scenarios

1 These are signs and symptoms of peritonitis; you need to notify the Registered Nurse. Action must adhere to the unit's peritonitis protocol.

2 Too much fluid has been removed during the dialysis session. Encourage the patient to limit mobilizing until they no longer feel lightheaded. Check with the nurse regarding their fluid regime and recheck the clinical observations according to local policy and patient need.

3 The bruit or buzzing indicates that there is blood flow through the arteriovenous fistula (HD access).

If you can no longer hear the bruit, the blood flow to the access may have been interrupted and the fistula is at risk of clotting. Notify the nurse, who will need to inform the renal team.

4 Most renal units will have a PD catheter care policy or protocol. The policy will inform you of the required resources, explain how to check the site for signs of infection, and give the correct way to clean and dress the site. Check with the nurse or individual clinical area regarding the local policy and whether you are allowed to carry out the skill.

10 Gastrointestinal system

Skills

10.1 **Nutritional assessment**

Definition

Nutritional assessment is an in-depth analysis of a patient's nutritional status (Dudek 2006). The term nutritional assessment is often used interchangeably with the term nutritional screening. Nutritional screening is an initial stage of a nutritional assessment and identifies patients who require, or who potentially will require, more comprehensive nutritional assessment.

It is important to remember that:

- Any chronic/acute illness will impact on a patient's nutritional status and requirements.
- Basic nutritional assessment is an essential component of initial nursing assessment.
- This assessment combined with a simple screening tool can easily identify patients who have actual or potential problems with nutrition, and this should be the first step leading to multi-disciplinary nutritional assessment and care.
- Most nurses are not nutritional specialists and must work closely with specialist practitioners in this field to ensure that patients' needs are identified and met. These practitioners will include dieticians, nutritionists, and nurse specialists in nutrition. Often speech and language therapists liaise closely with dieticians in the care of patients who have difficulty swallowing, e.g. many stroke patients.

- Any assessment over and above basic level should be undertaken by an appropriately skilled and trained practitioner such as a dietician or nutrition specialist. However, it is a fundamental and invaluable nursing role to ensure that all patients have access to good nutrition, regular meals, and accessible bedside fluids as required.

Prior knowledge

Before attempting nutritional assessment, make sure you are familiar with:

1 The relevant anatomy and physiology of the **alimentary tract** (see Figure 10.1).

2 The normal processes involved in the acquisition of nutrients.

3 The processes involved in the assimilation of nutrients.

4 Socio-economic factors that influence nutrition.

5 The effects of malnutrition.

Background

In order to understand why nutritional assessment is important, it is helpful to understand the scale of malnutrition in health care and the negative effects that this can have on patient outcome and management.

There is evidence that malnutrition occurs in different societies; there is also evidence of malnutrition occurring

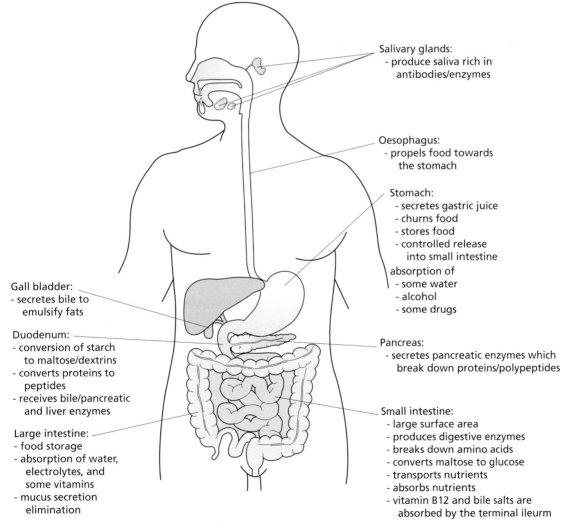

Figure 10.1 Basic anatomy and physiology of the alimentary tract.

in hospitals in the UK. It has been reported that 40% of patients admitted to hospital are undernourished and that the nutritional status in these patients often continues to deteriorate during the course of their hospital stay (McWhirter and Pennington 1994, Elia and Stratton 2000). This figure may be an underestimation as malnutrition is often unrecognized and untreated in hospitals (both inpatients and outpatients), nursing homes, and in the community (Elia 2003).

The detrimental effects of malnutrition, present at admission or developing during hospital stay, are also undeniable. Poor nutrition can have a negative impact on wound healing, immunological response, and muscle strength (Leather *et al*. 2003). Lack of optimal nutrition can also increase patients' physical and psychological stress and can affect almost every body system (Horan and Coad 2000). Malnourished patients cope poorly with modern medical and surgical interventions and, on average, stay in hospital for approximately 5 days longer than the normally nourished, incurring approximately 50% greater costs (Reilly *et al*. 1988).

There is widespread recognition of malnutrition in UK hospitals. The *Essence of Care* framework (Department of Health (DH) 2003) clearly states that nutritional screening and further assessment will help to reduce the incidence of malnutrition in hospitals. To this effect many nutritional screening tools have been devised, including the Subjective Global Assessment (Sacks *et al*. 2000) and the Short Nutritional Assessment questionnaire (Kruizenga *et al*. 2005).

Green and Watson (2005) reviewed 35 tools for nursing use, and in a separate study (Green and Watson 2006) reviewed tools specifically designed for the older population. As a result of these studies, it has been suggested that many assessment tools have not been subject to evaluation and consequently may not demonstrate sensitivity and/or specificity in clinical use.

The Malnutrition Universal Screening Tool (MUST) was developed and published in 2003 by the Malnutrition Advisory Group, part of the British Association for Parenteral and Enteral Nutrition (BAPEN). It has been designed for use in a wide variety of patients and comprises a five-step approach to nutritional screening (Elia 2003). This tool is enjoying widespread recognition as a valid tool.

Any screening tool used must make the screening process simple, acceptable to the patient, accurate, pre-cise, and sensitive to the effects of good and bad nutrition (Bond 1998).

Assessment criteria

Assessment involves communication with the patient to establish how they meet their nutrition needs normally. It should be remembered that most of the information about nutrition will be gathered through listening to the patient and analysing answers. Open and closed questions may be used, and may include:

- What is the patient's normal dietary intake?
- Have the patient's eating habits/appetite changed recently/since the onset of illness?
- Has the patient experienced any nausea or vomiting?
- Does the patient have any problems with eating, swallowing, or chewing?
- Does the patient have any food allergies or specific dietary requirements?
- Is the patient's diet influenced by cultural/ethnic/ religious factors? What does the patient prefer to eat?
- Is the patient's ability to eat and drink hindered by any physical limitation, for example arthritis of the fingers?
- How do social factors influence nutritional status (e.g. shopping habits/limitations, etc.)?
- Does the patient receive any nutritional support at present (e.g. medication such as pancreatic enzymes, or sip feeds/vitamin supplementation)?

The way in which the patient responds to these questions may provide invaluable data about nutritional status. Basic psychological assessment and observation of mental state should go hand in hand with nutritional assessment. A depressed patient may be less inclined to consider their own health/nutrition and thus neglect their needs. Likewise emotional relationships with food may be discovered, for example binge eating or eating disorders.

Visual assessment of the patient may also provide clues about nutritional status and indicate recent weight gain or loss, for example loose-fitting clothes. Arthritic fingers/reduced manual dexterity or poorly fitting dentures may indicate that a patient's ability to achieve good nutritional status is hindered. Oral hygiene may also provide an indication of the patient's nutritional status, so oral assessment should be performed in partnership with nutritional assessment.

Assessment in the community may allow the practitioner to observe eating and shopping habits (e.g. what foodstuffs are kept in the house). Consent must be obtained to explore any patient's private property (including their refrigerator).

Factors associated with the current illness or its management that will impact on nutritional needs should be identified. This can include gastrointestinal surgery, pre-operative starving, or any reduced oral intake over three or more days. Also, a patient who is bedbound and needs a bedpan or commode, rather than being able to use a toilet in the conventional way, may be reluctant to eat or drink. There are instances where they may need physical help in urinating or opening their bowels and, if this help is delayed, they become reluctant to eat or drink in case of 'accidents'. This is seen countless times on wards.

Calculation of body mass index (BMI)

Body mass index (BMI) is a measure of body fat based on height and weight that is applicable to the adult population. The calculation used to work out BMI is shown in **Box 10.1**. This measurement allows classification of patients into certain groups (see **Table 10.1**). BMI may have limitations as a diagnostic tool, and all other data and information must be considered when assessing nutritional status (Johnstone *et al.* 2006). Examples of the limitations of BMI include patients with large muscle

---

Box 10.1 Calculating BMI

- Measure patient's height in metres and multiply the figure by itself (to give height squared).
- Measure patient's weight in kilograms.
- Divide the weight by the height squared:

$$\frac{\text{weight (in kg)}}{\text{height (metres)}^2}$$

For example if a man is 1.64 m high and weighs 72 kg:

$1.64 \times 1.64 = 2.69$

$72/2.69 = 26.7$

This patient's BMI = 26.7

Box 10.2 Calculating percentage weight loss

% weight loss
$$= \frac{\text{usual weight} - \text{actual weight}}{\text{usual weight}} \times 100$$

Therefore, for a patient who was 110 kg and who now weighs 95 kg:

$$\frac{110 - 95}{110} \times 100 = 13.6\% \text{ weight loss}$$

---

mass such as weightlifters and fit athletes who have a very low body fat content, or people with missing limbs.

Estimating patients' unplanned weight loss

The estimated weight loss may be calculated and expressed as a percentage over the last 3–6 months. This calculation is demonstrated in **Box 10.2**. This figure may be scored, classified, and incorporated into nutritional screening scores. This should be complemented by visual indication of weight loss.

Anthropometric measurements

Anthropometric measurements such as hip to waist ratio, mid upper arm circumference, and skin fold thickness have been used to measure fat distribution, muscle mass, and subcutaneous fat content. These tools, while not commonly used in nursing assessments, may play a role in more complex assessment. They may also be useful in patients who are difficult to weigh. These measurements are only undertaken if the practitioner has been specifically trained to do so.

Context

 When to undertake nutritional assessment/screening

A comprehensive nursing assessment should include nutritional assessment for all patients. It will include visual assessment of the patient as well as gathering data about other factors influenced by nutritional status such as oral hygiene and ability to perform activities of daily living. The process should be performed on presentation,

Table 10.1 BMI classifications

Classification	BMI (kg/m²)	
	Principal cut-off points	Additional cut-off points
Underweight	<18.50	<18.50
Severe thinness	<16.00	<16.00
Moderate thinness	16.00–16.99	16.00–16.99
Mild thinness	17.00–18.49	17.00–18.49
Normal range	18.50–24.99	18.50–22.99
		23.00–24.99
Overweight	≥25.00	≥25.00
Pre-obese	25.00–29.99	25.00–27.49
		27.50–29.99
Obese	≥30.00	≥30.00
Obese class I	30.00–34.99	30.00–32.49
		32.50–34.99
Obese class II	35.00–39.99	35.00–37.49
		37.50–39.99
Obese class III	≥40.00	≥40.00

Reproduced with permission from WHO

to hospital or otherwise. Nutritional needs and status are dynamic, and any care plan derived from the assessment should reflect this, with regular reassessments. If a nutritional screening tool/assessment indicates that a patient is not malnourished and is at low risk of developing malnutrition, this, again, should be reviewed regularly.

 When not to undertake nutritional assessment/screening

There are no absolute contraindications to nutritional assessment. However, assessment should take into account the patient's physical, religious, cultural, and age-related needs, requirements, and requests (DH 2003). Assessment should be undertaken non-judgementally.

Alternative methods of nutritional assessment

Biometrical impedance

Biometrical impedance is an electrical measurement of total body water compared to body fat. It may be used to complement nutritional assessment, but may be unreliable as patients frequently have water retention as part of the disease process. This test is performed by specialist staff.

Biochemical investigations

Body proteins may be measured to assess nutritional status, but again this has limitations in the sick patient or those with ongoing disease processes.

If malnutrition or a risk of malnutrition is suspected, a referral to a multidisciplinary group is essential. This will include dieticians, nutritional nurse specialists, medical staff, and members of other professions allied to medicine.

Potential problems

As with all assessment, subjectivity should be avoided, e.g. a higher BMI may be the norm in some population groups and BMI may also decrease naturally with age. In addition, as with all patient assessment, singular values or scores will be of limited use; any data obtained must be analysed in conjunction with all other clinical data and history to provide accurate information.

Observations and monitoring

A patient who is deemed malnourished or at risk of malnutrition will also be at risk of other problems such as tissue viability risk and increased risk of infection. All patients at risk of malnutrition should have their vital signs monitored regularly to detect complications and should have related assessments such as oral hygiene and pressure areas assessment undertaken regularly.

Special considerations

Patient's age

The elderly are a high risk category for malnutrition; 20–65% of older hospitalized patients may be malnourished (Hajjar *et al.* 2004).

Pregnancy

During pregnancy a weight gain of approximately 12.5 kg is expected. If a pregnant woman's diet is varied and provides adequate energy for sufficient weight gain, the increased requirements for most nutrients will be met (Barker 2002).

Pregnancy may also cause nausea and vomiting and in severe cases hyperemesis.

Chronic illness

Patients with chronic body system failure/disease will require dietary modification, for example low potassium diets in patients with established/end stage renal disease.

Patients with liver disease may also become malnourished because of abnormalities in protein and energy metabolism (Wicks 2001).

Patients with chronic respiratory disease may have increased nutritional requirement because of an increased energy expenditure related to an increased work of breathing (Felbinger *et al.* 2001).

The critically ill patient

The acutely ill or critically ill patient often experiences ongoing continued physiological stress related to injury and/or body system(s) failure. They may also be in a hypercatabolic state. This will significantly increase nutritional requirements.

Procedure

Preparation

Prepare yourself

Ensure that you have any assessment criteria either written down as an *aide memoir* or clear in your mind. Ensure you have the correct documentation to record your findings. Ensure that you are familiar with any mathematical calculations you may have to make.

Prepare the patient

Explain to the patient the reasons for undertaking a nutritional assessment and reassure them that all data will be kept confidential as appropriate. Explain the rationale and the technique of any physical measurements. Obtain informed consent for undertaking the assessment.

Prepare the equipment

Make sure that weighing scales are clean and have been calibrated to zero. If a BMI calculator is to be used, ensure that the tool has been agreed for use by the Trust/organization.

Step-by-step guide to nutritional assessment

Step	Rationale
1 Introduce yourself, confirm the patient's identity, explain the procedure and obtain consent.	To identify the patient correctly and gain informed consent.
2 Communicate with the patient to establish normal nutritional status/needs.	To assess for factors that may indicate good or bad nutrition. To identify risk factors for potential malnutrition. To identify indicators for further, more advanced nutritional assessment. To assess impact any illness and planned treatment will have on nutritional needs.
3 Weigh the patient and if necessary convert weight unit to kg (see Box 10.3).	To provide a baseline weight for further assessment/trend analysis. To allow calculation of BMI.
4 Measure the patient and if necessary convert the height unit to metres (see Box 10.4).	To allow calculation of BMI.
5 Using the calculation in Box 10.1, calculate BMI.	To provide a baseline BMI for further assessment/trend analysis.
6 Communicate with the patient to establish any unplanned weight loss within the last 3–6 months; if necessary calculate percentage weight loss (see Box 10.2).	To identify indicators for more advanced nutritional assessment.
7 Identify any high risk factors for increasing nutritional needs.	To allow specialist referral/care planning that will assist patient in meeting nutritional needs.
8 Observe for factors that may suggest poor nutrition: Clinical impression – underweight/overweight, muscle wasting, loose jewellery/clothes.	To support other clinical data.
9 Document findings. If a scoring tool is used, calculate score according to specific criteria and document this.	To provide a baseline and provide written communication for further referral as necessary.
10 Based on findings, develop care plan to meet patient's needs.	To ensure that ongoing care meets patient's requirements.
11 Referral to multidisciplinary team as required.	To access more advanced nutritional assessment and multidisciplinary care planning.
12 If no referral is required, plan reassessment at appropriate intervals for ongoing assessment. Document this plan.	To highlight and act upon changes in patient's nutritional status/needs.

Box 10.3 Conversion formula: stones – kilograms

First convert stones to pounds: stones × 14 plus
remaining pounds.
To convert pounds to kilograms: total pounds × 0.4536
For example, a patient weighs 12 stone 3 pounds:

$$(12 \times 14) + 3 = 171 \text{ pounds}$$

$$171 \times 0.4536 = 77.5 \text{ kg}$$

Box 10.4 Conversion formula: feet – metres

First convert feet to inches: feet × 12 plus remaining inches.
To convert inches to centimetres: total inches × 2.54
Divide by 100 to give height in metres.
For example, if a patient is 5 feet 8 inches:

$$(5 \times 12) + 8 = 68 \text{ inches}$$

$$68 \times 2.54 = 172 \text{ cm}$$

$$172/100 = 1.72 \text{ m}$$

Following the procedure

- All findings of the nutritional assessment should be
  discussed with the patient. The limitations of some of
  the tools used (such as BMI) should be discussed and
  patients should be provided with the opportunity to
  ask questions and make any comments.
- Any equipment used in the assessment such as
  weighing scales should be cleaned to reduce the risk
  of infection.
- A date for reassessment should be set. Assessment
  data and any score should be documented clearly and
  concisely in accordance with organization guidelines.

Recognizing patient deterioration

If the process highlights deficits in nutritional status,
action should involve referral to appropriate specialists
who may include dieticians, occupational therapists, and
other specialist staff. However, certain actions may be
indicated and form part of that particular patient's care
plan. These actions may include responding to particular
dietary needs, initiating a food chart, providing
assistance with eating and drinking, and offering
nutritional supplementation such as high calorie drinks
or high protein diets.

Reflection and evaluation

When you have undertaken a nutritional assessment with
a patient, think about the following questions:

1 Did the assessment provide data that you expected
   for that particular patient?
2 Were you unable to answer any of the patient's
   questions?
3 Did you highlight any key risks to nutrition presented
   by any underlying medical conditions or planned
   treatment?
4 Were there any socio-economic, cultural, or religious
   factors influencing nutritional status?

Further learning opportunities

At the next available opportunity and with their consent,
undertake a nutritional assessment with a colleague and
vice versa:

- When being assessed, does the process make you
  uncomfortable?
- If assessing a colleague of different ethnic origin to
  yourself, do your findings differ?

Undertake a nutritional assessment on a patient in a
supervised capacity. Discuss your findings with your
supervisor and ask for the process to be constructively
criticized.

Reminders

Don't forget to:

- Document the findings of your assessment.
- Plan for reassessment.
- Initiate any strategies to meet nutritional needs such
  as assistance with eating and drinking, education,
  sip feeds.
- Make appropriate referrals for those patients
  identified as having problems/risks.

Ⓠ Patient scenarios

Consider what you should do in the following situations, then turn to the end of this skill to check your
answers.

1   Patient A is admitted electively for major gastrointestinal surgery for gastric/oesophageal cancer. What would you expect his nutritional status to be and how will his nutritional needs change pre- and initially post-surgery?

2   Patient B is 85 years old and on nutritional assessment. Her BMI is 16.5, despite describing an unchanged balanced diet, no weight loss, and a healthy appetite. Would you consider this patient malnourished?

3   Patient C has been newly diagnosed as having gluten intolerance/coeliac disease and has approached you to discover what foods to avoid. What is the best way to manage this situation?

Website

 http://www.oxfordtextbooks.co.uk/orc/ endacott

You may find it helpful to work through our short online quiz and additional scenarios intended to help you to develop and apply the skills in this chapter.

References

Barker HM (2002). *Nutrition and dietetics for health care*, 10th edition. Churchill Livingstone, London.

Bond S (1998). Eating matters: improving dietary care in hospitals. *Nursing Standard*, **12**(17), 41–2.

Department of Health/NHS Modernisation Agency (2003). *Essence of care: patient-focused benchmarks for clinical governance*. S.F. Taylor and Co. Ltd, Stockport.

Dudek SG (2006). *Nutrition essentials for nursing practice*, 5th edition. Lippincott Williams and Wilkins, Philadelphia.

Elia M (2003). *Screening for malnutrition: a multidisciplinary responsibility. Development and use of the Malnutrition Universal Screening Tool ('MUST') for Adults*. BAPEN, Redditch.

Elia M and Stratton R (2000). How much undernutrition is there in hospitals? *British Journal of Nutrition*, **84**, 257–9.

Felbinger TW, Suchner U, Klaus P, and Askanazi J (2001). Nutrition support in respiratory disease. In J Payne-James, G Grimble, and D Silk. *Artificial nutrition support in clinical practice*, pp. 537–52. Greenwich Medical Media Limited, London.

Green S and Watson R (2005). Nutritional screening and assessment tools for use by nurses: literature review. *Journal of Advanced Nursing*, **50**(1), 69–83.

Green S and Watson R (2006). Nutritional screening and assessment tools for older adults: a literature review. *Journal of Advanced Nursing*, **54**(4), 477–90.

Hajjar RR, Kamel HK, and Denson K (2004). Malnutrition in ageing. *Internet Journal of Geriatrics and Gerontology*, **1**(1).

Horan D and Coad J (2000). Can nurses improve patient feeding? *Nursing Times*, **96**(50), 33–4.

Johnstone C, Farley A, and Hendry C (2006). Nurses' role in nutritional assessment and screening. *Nursing Times*, **102**(49), 28–9.

Kruizenga HM, Seidell JC, de Vet HCW, Wierdsma NJ, and van Bokhorst-de van der Schueren MAE (2005). Development and validation of a hospital screening tool for malnutrition: the short nutritional assessment questionnaire. *Clinical Nutrition*, **24**, 75–82.

Leather A, Bushell L, and Gillespie L (2003). The provision of nutritional support for people with cancer. *Nursing Times*, **99**(46), 53–5.

McWhirter JP and Pennington CR (1994). Incidence and recognition of malnutrition in hospital. *British Medical Journal*, **308**, 945–8.

Reilly JJ Jr, Hull SF, Albert N, Waller A, and Bringardener S (1988). The economic impact of malnutrition: a model system for hospitalised patients. *Journal of Parenteral and Enteral Nutrition*, **12**(4), 371–6.

Sacks GS, Dearman K, Replogle WH, Cora VL, Meeks M, and Todd C (2000). Use of subjective global assessment to identify nutrition-associated complications and death in geriatric long-term care facility residents. *Journal of the American College of Nutrition*, **19**(5), 570–7.

Wicks C (2001). Nutrition and liver disease. In J Payne-James, G Grimble, and D Silk. *Artificial nutrition support in clinical practice*, pp. 499–511. Greenwich Medical Media Limited, London.

Useful further reading and websites

Age Concern (2006). *Hungry to be heard: the scandal of malnourished older people in hospital*. Age Concern, London.

Ng WQ and Neill J (2006). Evidence for early oral feeding of patients after elective open colorectal surgery: a literature review. *Journal of Clinical Nursing*, **15**(6), 696–709.

Stratton RJ, King CL, Stroud MA, Jackson AA, and Elia M (2006). 'Malnutrition Universal Screening Tool' predicts mortality and length of hospital stay in acutely ill elderly. *British Journal of Nutrition*, **95**, 325–30.

British Association for Parenteral and Enteral Nutrition website: **http://www.bapen.org.uk**

 Answers to patient scenarios

1 This patient has a disease process that may have been detrimental to his nutritional status over the last 3–6 months. His ability to consume nutrients may have been compromised. In particular he may have had problems swallowing, which would limit oral intake. Also, pre-operative therapy such as radio-therapy or chemotherapy may have induced nausea and/or vomiting.

   The malignancy may well have affected other body systems, notably the liver, which would reduce the patient's ability to metabolize nutrients, mobil-ize energy stores, and produce plasma proteins and vitamins. Thus his pre-admission nutritional status is likely to be poor.

   During the pre-operative period the patient will require starvation as a pre-requisite to general anaesthesia. This will limit nutritional intake further. Post-operatively his nutritional requirements will increase significantly, not least because of the phys-iological stress associated with major surgery and the increased requirements for tissue healing and repair. Oral intake will be avoided because of poten-tial gastric stasis/intestinal ileus and because of delicate anastomoses. This will severely reduce his ability to acquire nutrients in the initial post-operative period.

2 This patient's BMI indicates that she is undernour-ished but this may not be the case. The BMI may be low because of numerous factors including a natural decrease with age and an active lifestyle. Good communication and history taking may well indicate that the patient's nutritional intake is sufficient to meet her needs. This may be a situation where other anthropometrical measurements may have a role in assessing nutritional status.

3 Unless your clinical speciality is food allergy, it is likely that the level of information this patient

requires should be provided by referral to nutritional specialists, gastroenterologists, and specialist dieti-cians. These referrals should have already been made when the condition was diagnosed/suspected. You may consider introducing the patient to specific groups/organizations for further advice/support. The patient, if hospitalized, will also need a gluten-free diet while an inpatient.

10.2 Blood glucose measurement

Definition

Bedside blood glucose measurement is a rapid and rel-atively simple way of gaining an indication of a patient's blood glucose concentration, thereby allowing diagnosis and treatment of specific conditions. The aim of the pro-cedure is to obtain a blood glucose level, also known as a blood sugar level.

Measuring a patient's blood glucose level involves obtaining a small sample of blood, usually from the patient's fingertip, and applying it to a test strip inserted into an electronic meter commonly known as a glucome-ter. The unit of measurement for blood glucose values is millimoles per litre (mmol/litre), which is the standard international method for recording a substance's mole-cular concentration. In the case of blood glucose level, this is measuring millimoles of glucose per litre of blood.

It is important to remember that:

- Bedside blood glucose measurement is an important method of assessment with the diabetic patient, but in cases of abnormal readings further investigations may be warranted. For instance, in acutely ill patients a venous blood sample should be obtained by a registered, competent practitioner for accurate laboratory analysis.

- There are now a number of glucometers on the market manufactured by different companies, but they all work in a very similar manner. It is still vitally important that you follow the manufacturer's instructions for the blood glucose measurement device you are using in your clinical area, as there are sometimes subtle differences in how the procedure should be carried out. Always ensure that you have received the correct training and have been assessed as competent in using the device according to your organization's policy before using any blood glucose measurement device in the clinical setting.

- Always remember to use your clinical assessment skills to make an assessment of the patient's condition. If a patient is displaying clinical signs of hypoglycaemia (e.g. reduced levels of consciousness or confusion) but has a normal blood glucose reading, always act upon the clinical signs and seek assistance.

- Prior to the advent and popularity of bedside blood glucose measurement, testing a patient's urine with a reagent strip was the common way of obtaining a measurement of glucose within the body. However, urinalysis only measures glucose that has exceeded the renal threshold (ability to be absorbed by the kidneys) and has been excreted into the urine. Urinalysis will not detect low levels of glucose in the body, and has no value in determining hypoglycaemia (low blood glucose).

Prior knowledge

Before engaging in bedside blood glucose measurement you must have received the correct training in use of the equipment. Both equipment and procedures will vary with individual Trusts, and you *must* have been assessed as competent within the Trust in which you work. Students should always seek the advice of local policy before undertaking this skill, as some employers may require that students only practise this skill under the supervision of a registered practitioner.

Before attempting blood glucose measurement, make sure you are familiar with:

1 The correct operation of the model of glucometer used in your clinical area.
2 Physiology of glucose metabolism within the body.
3 Pathophysiology of common disorders affecting blood glucose metabolism, e.g. diabetes mellitus.

4 The normal range of blood glucose, which is 4–7 mmol/litre, and the significance of readings outside of this range (see the Interpreting readings box later in the section for further information).
5 The indications for blood glucose measurement (see the 'When to use blood glucose measurement' section for further information).

Background

In order to understand how blood glucose measurement works, it is helpful to consider how and why glucose is transported around the body.

Glucose is an essential form of energy used for the normal function of cells within the body (Sherwood 2005). It is derived from eating carbohydrates in our diet. The monosaccharides (known commonly as simple sugars) are transported to the liver following absorption through the intestinal wall. Excess carbohydrates not immediately used are stored in the muscles and liver as glycogen for when the body requires extra energy, such as during exercise (Montague *et al.* 2005)

The brain in particular is sensitive to levels of glucose, and, when the body's supply of glucose is reduced to about half of its normal levels or below, the brain's function becomes impaired. If this condition is not rectified, it can lead to adverse symptoms, coma, and even death.

Insulin is a hormone produced by the pancreatic beta cells. It is required in order to allow the glucose molecule to enter the cell and be effectively metabolized. It also stimulates the conversion of glucose to glycogen as mentioned above.

Diabetes mellitus is the most common condition that impairs glucose metabolism and has a prevalence in the general population of Europe and the USA of about 8% (British Medical Association 2004). It is generally classified as type 1 and type 2. Type 1 is where the pancreas has lost its ability to regulate glucose efficiently due to autoimmune destruction of the pancreatic cells that produce insulin. It is more common in the under forties, often appearing in childhood. Type 2 diabetes is related to a resistance to insulin at a cellular level, or a secretory deficit by the pancreas failing to release sufficient insulin. It is more common in the over forties age group, with a link to obesity (National Institute for Health and Clinical Excellence (NICE) 2002).

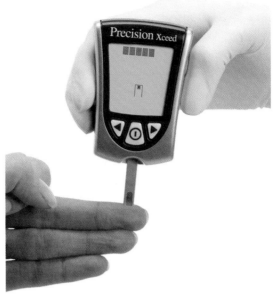

Figure 10.3 Applying the blood sample to a glucose test strip.

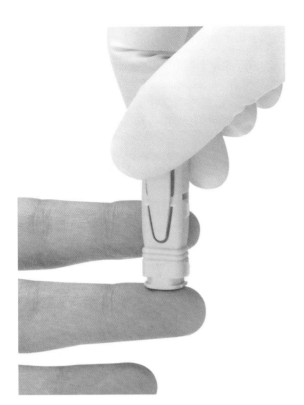

Figure 10.2 Obtaining a drop of blood from the fingertip with a single-use sampling device.

Bedside blood glucose measurement involves pricking the skin of the patient with a small needle or lancet to draw blood. It is important to differentiate between a single-use lancing device and a multiuse lancing device. Multiuse devices are more commonly used by patients carrying out self-sampling, as they are easier to carry around and can be more cost-effective than single-use devices. If a multiuse device is to be used on multiple patients, then this *must* be one that is intended for that purpose, used only with disposable single-use lancets (Medicines Healthcare Regulatory Agency (MHRA) 2006).

Single-use devices are more commonly used when health care professionals are carrying out the sampling, as single-use devices generally minimize the risk of cross-infection (see **Figure 10.2**). In this case the blood that appears at the surface is drawn from the capillaries and is whole blood. This is in comparison to laboratory measurement of glucose, where blood is drawn from a vein, and the process is known as plasma glucose measurement. Some studies have shown that there can be a difference of up to 10–15% in the values measured by

capillary (whole) and venous (plasma) glucose (Schrot *et al.* 2007), hence the need to obtain a venous sample in the acutely ill patient.

Once a drop of blood is obtained, it is placed on the sample strip of the glucometer for analysis (**Figure 10.3**). Blood glucose measurement is particularly important in the management of the diabetic patient as it gives an indication of **glycaemic** (glucose in the blood) control, and can allow health care staff or the patient themselves to alter their medication or diet accordingly to achieve optimal blood glucose levels.

It is important to be aware that a medical condition called **diabetic ketoacidosis** (DKA) can occur within diabetics. When the body is unable to utilize glucose effectively due to a lack of insulin, other forms of energy are sought and fats are broken down to provide this. This fat metabolism produces ketones, which can quickly make the **pH** of the blood become acidic, hence the term 'acidosis' (Montague *et al.* 2005).

In turn the high level of glucose in the blood, which is unable to enter the cells due to a lack of insulin, is retaining water osmotically. The diuresis of this excessive water and electrolyte load by the kidneys can lead to **dehydration**, electrolyte depletion (particularly potassium), and loss of circulating volume, resulting in circulatory collapse, shock, and death if left untreated. DKA is a medical emergency requiring intravenous fluid to replace the lost fluid volume and insulin therapy to reduce blood glucose.

Another diabetic emergency called hyperosmolar non-ketotic (HONK) coma exists. This is a rarer complication of type 2 diabetes, and is caused by massive fluid and electrolyte loss resulting in dehydration, confusion, and possibly coma. This is due to the high levels of glucose causing a shift of water out of the cells into the bloodstream and then into the urine. In HONK, insulin is still produced, so severe ketosis as seen in DKA is avoided. HONK can be characterized by hyperglycaemia, signs of dehydration, generalized weakness, altered conscious levels, and nausea and vomiting. Any patient suspected to be suffering from HONK should be immediately referred to medical staff.

Context

 When to use bedside blood glucose measurement

Bedside blood glucose measurement is indicated in a range of patient conditions, which can all affect blood glucose concentrations (Ferguson 2005), including:

- Diabetes (diagnosis and ongoing monitoring).
- Seizures.
- Liver disease or pancreatitis.
- Suspected head injury or any patient with an altered level of consciousness.
- Alcohol or drug intoxication.
- Infection.

 When not to use bedside blood glucose measurement

It is important to remember that there are certain conditions that may affect the accuracy of bedside capillary blood glucose testing (see **Table 10.2**). In these conditions, bedside testing is contraindicated and a venous blood sample must be obtained by a competent person to send for laboratory measurement (MHRA 2005). In these conditions there can be a significant discrepancy between capillary (finger-prick) and venous (blood drawn from a vein) measurements.

Potential problems

It is extremely unusual for patients to experience an adverse reaction while undergoing capillary blood glucose measurement, but staff should be particularly cautious with patients who have coagulation disorders or who are taking anticoagulant medication, in order to ensure that bleeding has fully ceased after the procedure has been carried out.

Indications for assistance

If a patient fails to respond to initial oral treatment for hypoglycaemia then it is important to seek urgent medical review, as prolonged hypoglycaemia can result in seizures, coma, and long-term brain damage. Hyperglycaemia should always be reported to an appropriate member of staff to enable patient review and to establish the cause as a high priority. If you suspect a glucometer may be malfunctioning or is displaying incorrect readings, then you should inform a member of staff with responsibility for arranging servicing of medical equipment.

Interpreting readings

The normal fasting (between meals) blood sugar level for adults is generally accepted to be 4–7 mmol/litre. However, this reading can rise to 8 or 9 mmol/litre for up to 90 minutes after a meal. The current recommendation detailed by the Joint British Societies' (comprising British Cardiac Society, British Hypertension Society, Diabetes UK, HEART UK, Primary Care Cardiovascular Society, and The Stroke Association) *Guidelines for prevention of cardiovascular disease* (2005) is that people with diabetes should aim to keep their blood glucose between 4–6 mmol/litre (follow local guidelines) before eating (preprandial).

Ensure that your meter is displaying readings in mmol/litre, which is the measurement system used for blood glucose monitoring in the UK. In other countries the units of milligrams per decilitre (mg/dl) are used. However, mg/dl gives a reading *18 times higher* than mmol/litre, and could lead to confusion over diagnosis and treatment (MHRA 2005).

If a patient's blood glucose is below 4 mmol/litre, then this is referred to as hypoglycaemia.

Table 10.2 Conditions affecting the accuracy of blood glucose measurement

Condition	Rationale	Example
Dialysis treatments	Some CAPD (continuous ambulatory peritoneal dialysis) fluids contain maltose, which may give elevated readings.	Patients undergoing CAPD.
Peripheral circulatory failure	The result obtained from finger-prick testing may be much lower than actual value.	Patients suffering hypovolaemic shock.
Severe dehydration	Falsely low results can be obtained from finger-prick testing.	Prolonged diarrhoea and vomiting.
Variations in blood oxygen tensions	This can affect capillary blood glucose levels and give an inaccurate reading.	Patients receiving intensive oxygen therapy.
High concentrations of non-glucose reducing substances in the blood	Ascorbic acid may depress blood glucose readings.	Patients receiving ascorbic acid therapy for acute vitamin C deficiency.
High bilirubin values	Can give falsely elevated readings.	Jaundiced patients/liver failure.
Extremes of haematocrit	Can give falsely low readings if levels elevated, or falsely high readings if haematocrit levels low.	Chronic obstructive pulmonary disease (COPD) can cause high haematocrit levels. A severe haemorrhage could cause a low haematocrit.
Hyperlipidaemia (abnormal fat concentrations in the blood)	Can give falsely elevated readings.	Patients with hyperlipidaemia.

Adapted from MHRA (2005)

Signs of hypoglycaemia

- Confusion or altered conscious level.
- Pallor.
- Clammy skin.
- Tachycardia.
- Headache.

If a patient's blood glucose is over 7 mmol/litre, then this is referred to as hyperglycaemia.

Signs of hyperglycaemia

- Polydipsia (increased thirst).
- Polyuria (increased urine output).
- Confusion or altered levels of consciousness.

Special considerations

- Always follow your local infection control policy when carrying out procedures that carry a risk of contact with bodily fluids.
- Be aware that some glucometers now offer 'alternative site testing' where the patient can use areas other than the finger for pricking, e.g. the forearm. Note that while this may be useful for diabetics monitoring their glucose regularly at home, it is not recommended for patients in the acute setting as there can be discrepancies between blood taken from the forearm and finger (Ellison *et al.* 2002). In the hospital setting and in the ill patient, *always* use the fingertip for bedside blood glucose measurement.
- Remember that certain conditions can affect the accuracy of bedside blood glucose measurement (see Table 10.2).

Procedure

Note: blood glucose meters vary between clinical areas and you must have had training and been assessed as competent in the use of the specific meter in your clinical area before proceeding with this skill.

Preparation

Prepare yourself

- Wash and dry your hands in accordance with clinical hand washing guidelines, then don appropriate personal protective equipment (gloves and apron) in order to minimize risks of cross-contamination and protect you, your patient, and your uniform from contamination.
- Ensure you are familiar with the operating instructions for the glucometer.

Prepare the patient

- Explain the procedure to your patient in order to minimize patient anxiety and allow the patient to cooperate with the procedure.

- Ensure that consent is gained from the patient before you commence the procedure.
- Discuss with the patient their normal blood glucose measurement regime where possible, as they may be able to inform you of the best location for obtaining a blood sample.
- Ask the patient where the blood sample was taken from last time their blood glucose was measured (if appropriate) in order to avoid repeated testing at the same site, which can cause discomfort.

Prepare the equipment

- Blood glucose testing meter (check that a current high/low quality test has been carried out in accordance with the manufacturer's instructions and local policy).
- Finger-pricking device (e.g. lancet).
- Sharps bin.
- Container of test strips that are in date and match the calibration code for the meter.
- Gauze swab/cotton wool ball to stop bleeding (depending upon local policy).

Step-by-step guide to measuring blood glucose

Step	Rationale
1 Introduce yourself, confirm the patient's identity, explain the procedure, and obtain consent.	To identify the patient correctly and gain informed consent.
2 Select an area for testing, preferably on the patient's fingertip (the side of the fingertip, not the centre).	The most accurate readings will be obtained from blood drawn from the patient's fingertips, as this will be the freshest supply and give a true indication of blood glucose. Taking the sample from the side of the fingertip will ensure minimal discomfort after the procedure.
3 Ensure that the hand to be tested is clean and dry. If necessary, assist patient to clean and dry their hand.	Substances such as food matter, fruit juice, or soft drinks may contribute to a false reading because of their sugar content. Washing the hands with warm water will encourage vasodilatation of blood vessels in the hand and improve the blood flow on testing.

4	Using an appropriate disposable device, prick side of patient's fingertip and allow blood to form into a droplet. Gentle squeezing of the finger above the puncture site may be necessary if blood is not immediately forthcoming. Note: it is important to rotate the testing site if blood glucose monitoring is to be repeated frequently.	It is necessary that pricking devices are single-use to minimize risks of cross-infection. The side of the finger is used as it is less painful than the centre. It is important that a sufficient amount of blood is obtained to ensure the accuracy of the result. Repeated pricking of the same site will become painful, and may affect testing and patient compliance with the procedure.
5	Apply the drop of blood to the test strip, following the manufacturer's instructions and local guidelines.	Some test strips require the blood to be applied to the side; others require it to be dropped onto the centre of the strip.
6	Immediately and safely dispose of the sharp used in the finger-pricking device. *Do not* put used pricking devices back into the meter's carrying/storage case.	To minimize risk of needlestick injury. This poses a risk of sharps injury to the next person to use the meter.
7	Ensure that the patient is comfortable and bleeding has stopped (apply pressure with cotton wool or gauze, or encourage patient to do so themselves if able).	To prevent unnecessary blood loss and promote patient comfort.
8	Wait for the meter to provide digital readout of the result, then record on an appropriate chart.	Recording the result as soon as it appears will ensure that this step is not forgotten, or the result mislaid.
9	Dispose of waste appropriately, remove gloves and apron, and wash your hands.	To avoid risk of cross-infection.
10	Report any abnormalities to appropriate staff and take necessary action (e.g. treating hypoglycaemia).	So appropriate action can be taken if readings are out of normal range.

Step-by-step guide to measuring blood glucose

Recognizing patient deterioration

Hypoglycaemia (low blood sugar level) needs to be treated rapidly to prevent further deterioration. The *British national formulary* (Joint Formulary Committee 2008) suggests the following actions for the treatment of the hypoglycaemic patient:

■ Ensure patient and scene safety, as the patient may be confused, aggressive, or in a collapsed state.

■ If the patient is conscious and able to swallow safely then 10–20 g of glucose ('simple' sugar) can be administered orally. Examples of this include: two teaspoons of sugar, three sugar lumps, Coca-Cola® 90 ml, Ribena original®

15 ml, or Lucozade® 50 ml. Note that diet versions of these drinks should not be used as they contain little or no simple sugars and will not deliver the recommended 10–20 g of glucose. Wait 10–15 minutes and repeat the blood glucose measurement. If the measurement is over 4 mmol/litre and the patient's symptoms have subsided then a 'complex' carbohydrate should be offered, e.g. a sandwich, fruit, milk, or biscuits. This ensures a more sustained release of glucose to prevent reoccurrence of hypoglycaemia.

■ If the patient is unconscious or unable to tolerate liquids safely then this should be considered a medical emergency. Glucagon (a polypeptide hormone that increases blood glucose by mobilizing glucose stores from the liver, converting glycogen back to glucose) should be administered intramuscularly or intravenously by a competent registered practitioner.

- If there is no response to glucagon within 10 minutes, 50 ml of 20% dextrose solution should be administered intravenously (Joint Formulary Committee 2008), again by a competent practitioner.

If you detect hyperglycaemia when undertaking blood glucose measurement, consider urinalysis to check for the presence of ketones, which could indicate DKA. You should always report and discuss an episode of hyperglycaemia

with senior staff to determine its cause and any further action to be taken. *Note:* DKA is an acute medical emergency, and, if suspected, medical staff should be informed immediately.

The cause of the episode of hypo/hyperglycaemia should be explored once treatment has been administered. For instance, has the patient recently had a change to their medication, or missed a dose or a regular meal? Note that patients whose hypoglycaemia was suspected or known to have been caused by an oral antidiabetic agent should be transferred to hospital even if their symptoms have resolved, as the action of this type of medication can often last for many hours.

Reflection and evaluation

When you have undertaken blood glucose measurement with a patient, think about the following questions:

- Have you recorded the result and taken appropriate action if necessary?
- Did you notice any unusual signs or symptoms in the patient that might reflect the result you obtained (e.g. hypo/hyperglycaemia) and take appropriate action?
- Have you prepared the meter for its next use (i.e. left it clean and replaced test strips if necessary)?
- Were you able to answer any questions from your patient or mentor?
- If the patient is to undertake blood glucose measurements on themselves in the future, consider the need to deliver any advice or education on correct technique and interpretation of results.

Further learning opportunities

When you have undergone appropriate training and assessment in using the blood glucose meter in your clinical area, carry out the procedure as per your local guidelines. Remember that if you move to another clinical area where a different blood glucose measurement device is used, you should receive training and assessment on that device before attempting to use it.

Reminders

- Remember to verify that the meter has had a recent quality control check. Ensure that the test strips are in date and the code on the strips matches the code on the meter before use.
- Remember to collect all of the equipment you require in a clean tray before you attempt the procedure, in order to minimize disruption to the patient and ensure that the procedure goes smoothly.
- Ensure that you fully explain the procedure to the patient and gain consent where necessary, also allowing the opportunity for the patient to ask any questions.
- Ensure that all sharps and clinical waste are disposed of safely after the procedure and that you record the result appropriately and act upon any abnormalities found.

Patient scenarios

Consider what you should do in the following situations, then turn to the end of this skill to check your answers.

1 You have carried out bedside blood glucose measurement on Patient A, and the reading is 19 mmol/litre. Patient A is not exhibiting any clinical signs of hyperglycaemia. What would your course of action be?

2 You receive an abnormally high capillary blood glucose reading from Patient B, who has been receiving 60% oxygen for the past 3 hours. What should you do?

3 Patient C is known to be a type 1 diabetic, has a blood glucose level of 2.3 mmol/litre, and is complaining of a headache. What would your course of action be?

Website

 http://www.oxfordtextbooks.co.uk/orc/ endacott

You may find it helpful to work through our short online quiz and additional scenarios intended to help you to develop and apply the skills in this chapter.

References

British Medical Association (2004). *Diabetes mellitus: an update for healthcare professionals*. BMA, London.

Ellison J, Stegmann J, Colner S *et al.* (2002). Rapid changes in post prandial blood glucose produces concentration differences at finger, forearm and thigh sampling sites. *Diabetes Care*, **25**(6), 961–4.

Ferguson A (2005). Blood glucose monitoring. *Nursing Times*, **101**(28), 28–9.

Joint British Societies (2005). Joint British Societies' guidelines on prevention of cardiovascular disease in clinical practice. *Heart*, **91**(Suppl 5), 1–52.

Joint Formulary Committee (2008). *British national formulary*, 55th edition. British Medical Association and Royal Pharmaceutical Society of Great Britain, London.

Medicines Healthcare Regulatory Agency (2005). *Point of care testing, blood glucose meters. Advice for healthcare professionals*. DH, London.

Medicines Healthcare Regulatory Agency (2006). *Medical device alert: lancing devices used in nursing homes and care homes*. DH, London.

Montague S, Watson R, and Herbert R (2005). *Physiology for nursing practice*, 3rd edition. Elsevier, London.

National Institute for Health and Clinical Excellence (2002). *Managing blood glucose: a guide for adults with type 2 diabetes*. HMSO, London.

Schrot R, Patel K, and Foulis OP (2007). Evaluation of inaccuracies in the measurement of glycaemia in the laboratory, by glucose meters, and through measurement in haemoglobin. *Clinical Diabetes*, **25**(2), 43–9.

Sherwood L (2005). *Human physiology: From cells to systems*. Brooks/Cole, California.

Useful further reading and websites

British Diabetic Association:
   http://www.diabetes.org.uk

Answers to patient scenarios

1 Clean the patient's fingers with warm water, dry, and try a different digit. If the reading is still high, seek appropriate help.

2 A venous sample of blood should be obtained for laboratory plasma glucose measurement, as high concentration of oxygen can affect capillary blood glucose levels.

3 This patient is hypoglycaemic and requires simple sugar (glucose) to raise the blood glucose level. Document the hypo and the timing carefully; if a trend becomes apparent, the information is very useful to the diabetes team.

10.3 Nasogastric tube insertion

Definition

A nasogastric tube is a tube inserted through the nose into the stomach, via the oesophagus, for the purpose of administering fluids, feed, or drugs for absorption by the gastrointestinal tract (see Figure 10.4). It may also be inserted to facilitate the drainage of gastric contents as a part of surgical or medical management.

Accessing the gastrointestinal tract via a nasogastric tube may provide a relatively inexpensive and uncomplicated method of providing nutritional support. It is particularly useful in those patients with compromised swallowing mechanisms and those with altering levels of consciousness.

It is important to remember that:

● The incorrect placement of a nasogastric tube with subsequent administration of fluids/feed may lead to

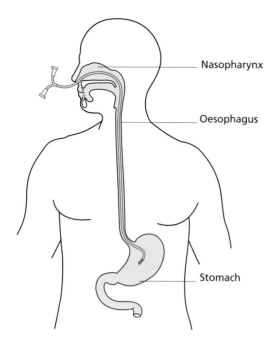

Figure 10.4 Nasogastric tube *in situ*.

serious patient harm, even death (National Patient Safety Agency (NPSA) 2005).

- A nasogastric tube may move out of the stomach at a later stage following insertion (NPSA 2005).
- The insertion of a nasogastric tube may be contraindicated in certain patients.
- Insertion may be complicated in the unconscious patient and particular caution will be required.

- The procedure can cause considerable distress to patients.

Prior knowledge

Before attempting nasogastric tube insertion, make sure you are familiar with:

- The relevant upper gastrointestinal and upper airway anatomy and physiology.
- Pathophysiology of the upper airway and upper gastrointestinal tract.
- The physiology associated with swallowing.
- The differences in sizes/types of nasogastric tubes and their appropriateness for the intended therapy (Table 10.3).

Background

On insertion, the nasogastric tube follows the passage from the nostril of the nose, through the nasopharynx, oropharynx, and laryngopharynx, to enter the oesophagus, and then moves down past the gastro-oesophageal junction to sit in the stomach.

Passing the tube requires a certain amount of skill and experience. It is important to emphasize that the procedure causes some distress and discomfort to patients, particularly as the tube tip comes into contact with the delicate structures around the nasopharynx. Verbal,

Table 10.3 Choosing the right nasogastric tube

Tube type	Uses	Duration of therapy	Disadvantages/comments
Fine bore tube (polyurethane or silicone elastomer) Size 6–8 (Ch)	Administration of feed/ water/liquid-based drugs	Less than 4 weeks	Materials not affected by gastric acid. May be difficult to aspirate due to small internal diameter. Limited use in gastric decompression. Better tolerated by patients. Metal stylet tubes may increase risk of pneumothorax (Olbrantz *et al.* 1985).
Large bore tube (Ryles tube) PVC Size 10–16 (Ch)	Gastric decompression May be used for short-term feeding (10–12 days)	10–12 days	Increased risk of tube cracking (Payne-James 2001). Increased risk of rhinitis/oesophagitis and erosion-related gastric haemorrhage (Payne-James 2001).

Image labels: Nasopharynx, Oesophagus, Stomach

Table 10.4 Procedures for confirming correct nasogastric tube placement

Recommended tests	Comments
Testing pH of aspirate with pH indicator strips	The pH of any aspirate must be 5.5 or lower. This must be easy to distinguish from the strips. Consideration must be given to any gastric pH-lowering drugs that the patient may have taken. This may be difficult to ascertain, particularly with fine bore tubes where it may be difficult to aspirate.
Chest/upper abdominal X-ray	Provides radiological confirmation of tube position. This must be documented in multidisciplinary notes. Recommended in certain patient groups such as critical care patients. The individual confirming position on X-ray must be qualified in radiological interpretation. Concerns regarding radiological exposure promote the use of pH indicator strips as an initial test.

informed consent should always be obtained in the conscious patient and all attempts should be made to allay anxiety and reduce any distress. Where verbal consent is not possible, a multidisciplinary discussion should occur to ensure that the therapy is in the best interests of the patient.

Incorrect tube placement, notably into the pulmonary tree, occurs in a proportion of patients (NPSA 2005). There is also reported evidence of inadvertent intracranial (into the cranial space) placement (Metheny 2002). The nasogastric tube, once inserted, must have its position confirmed as correct prior to the administration of any solutions via the tube. The procedures for determining correct tube placement are outlined in **Table 10.4**.

Previous traditional methods of confirming tube position are no longer recommended. These include:

- Auscultation of air insufflated through the feeding tube (the 'whoosh' test).
- Testing acidity/alkalinity of aspirate using blue litmus paper (Medicines and Healthcare Products Regulatory Agency 2004).
- Interpreting absence of respiratory distress as an indicator of correct positioning.
- Monitoring bubbling at the external end of the tube when immersed in water.
- Observing the appearance of feeding tube aspirate.

These tests should *not* be used to confirm nasogastric tube position.

Nasogastric tube position should be confirmed:

- Prior to the commencement of each feed/medication dose.
- Following any evidence suggestive of tube displacement, i.e. loose dressings, obvious tube movement (as noted by measurements on the tube), respiratory distress.
- In the event of excessive gagging/vomiting.

Obtaining aspirate for testing, particularly from fine bore tubes, may be difficult. A large volume syringe may assist in obtaining aspirates, as may positioning the patient on their side. It may also be useful to inject 10 ml of air into the tube as its tip may be resting against the gastric mucosa (NPSA 2005). Likewise, advancing the tube forward by a few centimetres may have the same effect.

If difficulty obtaining the correct aspirate pH is experienced in a recently fed patient, a time lapse of 1 hour should allow the gastric contents to empty and pH to return to normal (NPSA 2005). The pH of the gastric contents may be altered by certain drugs such as antacids or histamine H2 receptor agonists. If a pH of less than 5.5 cannot be achieved, a chest X-ray must be performed.

The procedure is routinely performed as a clean procedure. This requires universal infection control precautions as well as precautions to protect against inoculation injury.

How does a nasogastric tube work?

A nasogastric tube is a hollow catheter approximately 100 cm in length. The external diameter of the tube can vary in size and may be measured in 'French' Charriere units or the British Gauge system. Selection of an appropriate gauge is largely dependent on the intended use for the tube and the anticipated duration of therapy (see Figures 10.5 and 10.6). Feed or liquids are administered via the tube using a peristaltic pump, gravity, or pushing via a syringe (Figure 10.7).

Gastric fluid and gas may also drain passively into a collecting bag attached to the external end of the tube, or be actively aspirated out of the stomach via the tube using a syringe. Aspirating the tube may also be performed in the nasogastric-fed patient to assess feed absorption.

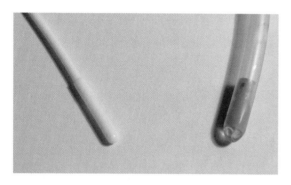

Figure 10.5 Fine bore and 'Ryles' type tubes allowing size comparison.

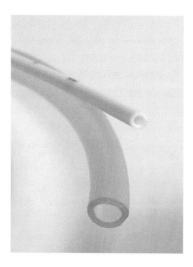

Figure 10.6 Fine bore and 'Ryles' type tubes allowing size comparison.

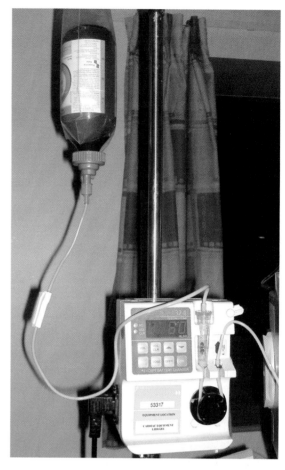

Figure 10.7 A peristaltic feeding pump.

Context

When to insert a nasogastric tube

- Following nutritional assessment, to support nutrition partially or totally where a patient's ability to meet their own requirements using the oral route is compromised and the gastrointestinal tract is functional.
- To facilitate the drainage of gastric fluid or gas.

A nasogastric tube can be used for the administration of drugs if the oral route is compromised and the gastrointestinal tract is functional. However, most medication is not licensed for nasogastric use (Smith 1997) and advice from a pharmacist should be sought. There are occasions where drugs that are not licensed for nasogastric administration are prescribed, and this may be covered by local agreement; however, practitioners are recommended to review the advice regarding unlicensed administration in the Nursing and Midwifery Council (NMC) publication *Guidelines for the administration of medicines* (NMC 2004a).

⊗ When not to insert a nasogastric tube

- If a patient does not consent. For many patients the concept of having a nasogastric tube passed will cause some anxiety, possibly related to previous insertions. Nurses should be aware that exploring any anxieties and discussing previous experiences should be a central component in psychological support for these patients. Explaining the rationale, any potential alternatives, and the 'pros and cons' of having the tube inserted will allow them to make an informed decision on whether or not to accept the procedure.
- If the patient has a known allergy to any material used in the manufacture of the tube.
- If nutritional assessment deems that a patient's nutritional needs can be adequately met using the oral route (including the use of sip feeds).
- If any contraindication exists, such as basal skull fracture, maxillo-facial surgery, or upper gastrointestinal surgery/disease. In these situations expert advice should be sought.
- To support nutrition in patients with a dysfunctional gastrointestinal tract such as patients with pancreatitis or short bowel syndromes.
- Where longer-term nutritional support is indicated and another route may be appropriate (such as endoscopic tube placement). However, short-term nasogastric nutritional support may be required while awaiting these procedures.

Alternative interventions

While nasogastric tubes are invaluable in allowing drainage of gastric contents, the underlying cause for any gastric stasis must be explored, and any treatment directed at this cause. This may include dietary modification, the optimization of mobility, and pharmacological treatment. With delayed gastric emptying the risk of pulmonary aspiration is high; correct patient positioning, e.g. a semi-recumbent position in an immobile patient, may facilitate gastric emptying and reduce this risk.

If a nasogastric tube is being inserted to support nutrition, full consideration must be given to ascertain that the nasogastric route of enteral feeding is the optimal approach to nutritional support for the particular patient. A patient may be at risk of suboptimal nutrition simply because the appropriate foods are not available, for example vegetarian options not being provided on hospital menus or a patient newly diagnosed with a food allergy not being provided with the necessary information regarding foods to be avoided.

Potential problems

- The nasogastric tube is a potential route for transmission of bacteria (Padula *et al*. 2004). All interventions involving the tube, such as the changing of feed bottles, should be done as a clean procedure with strict adherence to hand washing.
- There is a risk of tissue damage from securing nasogastric tubes. The dressings also become dirty frequently. Dressings should be changed regularly and the area inspected for tissue damage/soreness.
- The position of a nasogastric tube may alter once *in situ*, particularly following vomiting or violent coughing. If tube displacement is suspected, the feed must be stopped and not recommenced until the position of the tube is confirmed. This can only be achieved by chest X-ray or aspirate less than pH 5.5 (see Background section).
- If aspirate cannot be obtained: most tubes have distance markers, and the length of the tube at the fixation point must be noted and clearly documented as a reference point should tube misplacement be suspected. However, a tube being at the same fixation point cannot rule out misplacement.
- Trauma bleeding to the nostrils may occur during insertion, and erosion of delicate mucosa may occur as a result of the tube being *in situ*. These should be observed for, and appropriate fixing of the tube should reduce the risks.
- A common problem where nasogastric tubes are used for enteral feeding or drug administration is tube blockage/occlusion. This is discussed in detail in Section 10.4, *Administering enteral nutrition*.

Indications for assistance

Expert assistance in passing a nasogastric tube may be sought from a nutritional nurse specialist or senior medical/nursing staff. It is advisable that if two insertions are attempted without success, a referral to a more experienced practitioner is made.

Passing a tube in an unconscious patient is particularly complicated because the patient cannot swallow on command. Expert advice should always be sought in these cases.

Observations and monitoring

- The date of insertion, type of tube, and length of tube at the fixation point must be clearly documented in patient notes/care plans.
- All patients with nasogastric tubes should have their vital signs monitored regularly (particularly respiratory observations) as an indicator of pulmonary aspiration/tube misplacement.
- The amount of fluid/gas aspirated or drained from the tube must be clearly recorded and incorporated into the patient's fluid balance calculations for that 24 hour period. The characteristics of the fluid drained must also be noted, for example bile-stained fluid, faecal fluid, etc.

Special considerations

- If inserting a nasogastric tube in a patient's home environment, access to radiology is not realistic. If all techniques to confirm a pH of less than 5.5 fail, expert advice should be sought.

- Patients with altered mental state and possibly confusion are likely to remove nasogastric tubes; fixing the tube so that it is 'out of the line of sight' may help. Remember that the replacement of any removed tube should not be undertaken against the patient's wishes.

- In patients who are independent in the use of their nasogastric tube, education should reinforce good infection control practice.

- Passing a tube in an unconscious patient is particularly complicated because the patient

---

cannot swallow on command. Tubes can be correctly positioned in these patients using a blind insertion technique. However, expert advice should always be sought in these cases. Some organizations recommend radiological confirmation of tube position in all tube insertions in unconscious patients.

Procedure

Preparation

Prepare yourself
Ensure you have washed your hands and put on a plastic apron.

Prepare the patient
Explain the procedure to the patient (see Discussing the procedure box). Position the patient so they are semi-recumbent/sitting up. The head should be in a midline position. The head being flexed slightly forward may facilitate the swallow mechanism and ease passage. The head flexed back should be avoided as swallowing is difficult in this position.

Prepare the equipment
Select the appropriate tube for the patient. Collect lubrication, patient drink if required, syringes, and pH indicator strips. Check all equipment is within expiry and that packaging is intact. Ascertain the tube's radio-opacity as this may influence the timing of guide wire removal if radiological confirmation is required.

Discussing the procedure with the patient and family

- Explain the need for the tube to be inserted.

- Explain how the tube will be inserted.

- Explain that while the procedure is not pleasant, with good communication the unpleasantness will be short-lived.

- Agree a signal that the patient can use if the procedure becomes unpleasant and they wish it to stop. This may reduce anxiety.

- Obtain verbal consent.

Step-by-step guide to nasogastric tube insertion

▶ **Step**   **Rationale**

	Step	Rationale
1	Introduce yourself, confirm the patient's identity, explain the procedure, and obtain consent.	To identify the patient correctly and gain informed consent.
2	Assess the patency of the patient's nostrils; clean if necessary.	To identify the most suitable nostril through which to pass the tube.
3	Using either a tape measure or the measurements on the nasogastric tube, measure the distance from the patient's nostril to the earlobe and then to the xiphoid process.	To provide an indication of the distance to insert the tube.
4	If local aerosol anaesthesia is indicated and prescribed, administer according to local guidelines. Allow sufficient time for this to work.	To reduce sensitivity in the nasal cavity.
5	Ensure that any guide wire/stylet (if being used) is seated correctly.	To ensure correct guide wire position.
6	Lubricate the distal 20 cm of the tube with water or a lubricating jelly as indicated.	To aid insertion.
7	Insert the tube into the patent nostril, easing it along the floor of the nasal passage in a horizontal plane. If resistance is felt, adjust the direction slightly and attempt gentle reinsertion. Using the natural curve of the tube to mirror the natural curve of the anatomical pathway may assist in successful placement.	To allow the tube to follow the normal anatomical passage.
8	At 12–20 cm insertion depth, a small amount of resistance may be felt. Ask the patient to swallow while gently advancing the tube to the predetermined measure. Allowing the patient a drink of water (if their swallowing mechanism is competent) may facilitate the tube's passage.	To allow the passage of the tube into the oesophagus.
9	If signs of respiratory distress are noted, remove the tube to the nasopharynx.	To remove the tube from potential bronchial placement. Removing the tube to the nasopharynx may make a further attempt more acceptable to the patient (Higgins 2005).
10	If insertion is successful, secure the tube according to the organization's policy.	To ensure tube is not removed.

continued overleaf

11	Confirm the tube position, aspirating from the tube with a large volume syringe and testing with pH sticks.	To confirm tube position.
12	If an aspirate cannot be obtained, consider the following: Advancing the tube 5–10 cm. Injecting a small amount of air. Altering patient position. Asking the patient to drink a small amount of coloured water (squash, etc.). Only do this in the presence of competent swallowing. Wait 1 hour and reattempt aspiration. Consider X-ray.	To move the tube tip into any gastric fluid. To move the tip away from the mucosa. To provide easily identifiable gastric contents. To allow gastric contents to accumulate.
13	Remove guide wire if used (if radiological confirmation is not required).	To facilitate feeding.
14	Connect tube to drainage bag as required.	To allow drainage of gastric contents.
15	Document the procedure.	To comply with NMC (2004b) requirements.

Following the procedure

- If used for gastric drainage, observe any gas or fluid drained and document on the patient's fluid balance chart, reporting as necessary.
- If used for feeding, commence feeding as indicated by nutrition team and in line with organizational policy.

Reflection and evaluation

When you have inserted a nasogastric tube, think about the following questions:

1 Was the patient anxious about the procedure and how did you allay any anxieties?
2 Did the patient find the procedure distressing?
3 If the tube was inserted for gastric drainage, what were the characteristics of this drainage? What would be considered normal?
4 If you were unsuccessful at passing the tube on the second attempt, what would your course of action be?
5 How would the procedure differ in the unconscious patient?

Further learning opportunities

Anatomical models are available to help you practise this skill.

Reminders

- Always communicate fully with the patient and allow them the option to stop the procedure if they become too distressed.
- For nutritionally supported patients, the 'normal' oral route of nutrition is the optimal route and care should be directed towards this goal.

ⓠ Patient scenarios

Consider what you should do in the following situations, then turn to the end of this skill to check your answers.

1 A patient refuses to have a nasogastric tube passed for the purposes of gastric drainage because he has a painful abdomen. What might be the problem?

2 You are asked to pass a nasogastric tube in a patient suffering from a cerebrovascular accident (stroke) whose swallowing mechanism is questionable. How might you manage this situation?

3 You attempt to pass a nasogastric tube and are unable to enter the nasal passage on one side. What would your course of action be?

Website

 http://www.oxfordtextbooks.co.uk/orc/ endacott

You may find it helpful to work through our short online quiz and additional scenarios intended to help you to develop and apply the skills in this chapter.

References

Higgins D (2005). Practical procedures: inserting nasogastric tubes. *Nursing Times*, **101**(37), 28–9.

Medicines and Healthcare Products Regulatory Agency (2004). *Enteral feeding tubes (nasogastric)*, Medical Device Alert Ref. MDA/2004/026. MHRA, London.

Metheny NA (2002). Inadvertent intracranial nasogastric tube placement. *American Journal of Nursing*, **102**(8), 25–7.

National Patient Safety Agency (2005). *Reducing the harm caused by misplaced nasogastric feeding tubes*, Patient Safety Alert. NPSA, London.

Nursing and Midwifery Council (2004a). *Guidelines for the administration of medicines*. NMC, London.

Nursing and Midwifery Council (2004b). *The NMC code of professional conduct: standards for conduct, performance and ethics*. NMC, London.

Olbrantz KR, Gelfand D, Choplin R, and Wu WC (1985). Pneumothorax complicating enteral feeding tube placement. *Journal of Parenteral and Enteral Nutrition*, **92**(2), 210–11.

Padula CA, Kenny A, Planchon C, and Lamoureux C (2004). Enteral feeding: what the evidence says. *American Journal of Nursing*, **104**(7), 62–9.

Payne-James J (2001). Enteral nutrition: tubes and techniques of delivery. In J Payne-James, G Grimble, and D Silk. *Artificial nutrition support in clinical practice*, pp. 281–303. Greenwich Medical Media Limited, London.

Smith A (1997). Inside story. *Nursing Times,* **93**(8), 68–70.

Useful further reading and websites

Payne-James J, Grimble G, and Silk (2001). *Artificial nutrition support in clinical practice*. Greenwich Medical Media Limited, London.

Rolandelli R (2005). *Clinical nutrition: enteral and tube feeding*, 4th edition. Elsevier Saunders, Pennsylvania.

British Association for Parenteral and Enteral Nutrition website: **http://www.bapen.org.uk**

National Patient Safety Agency website: **http://www.npsa.nhs.uk**

 Answers to patient scenarios

1 The patient is obviously apprehensive about the tube insertion, and particularly the fact that it may cause him more pain. Achieving the best outcome for him is reliant on excellent communication. Allowing the patient to express his fears and anxieties may aid in allaying them. The patient may be experiencing pain because of abdominal distension/gastric stasis. While the procedure may be unpleasant initially, the decompression of the stomach may contribute to alleviating the pain. Effective pain control is of paramount importance, and this will incorporate the administration of analgesia as well as utilizing other possible therapies. Remember that informed consent should be obtained prior to any procedure.

2 The ideal approach to managing this situation would be to facilitate a formal swallowing assessment; this may be via referral to speech and language therapists or practitioners with specific swallowing assessment training. This will not only be of benefit in tube insertion, but if swallowing is deemed competent, may actually negate the need for insertion as the patient's nutritional needs may be met more appropriately. Ultimately, however, access to swallowing assessment is not realistic in a 24 hour period. If a nasogastric tube is deemed appropriate, the tube should be passed without using the sips of water technique. The risk of insertion into the pulmonary tree may be higher and this should be observed for rigorously using all the checking procedures as outlined previously. The threshold for radiological confirmation may be lower.

3 The nostril may be blocked with nasal debris and secretions. Inserting the tube into the other nostril may be appropriate; however, respiration may then be compromised in the patient who breathes 'nasally'. All attempts should be made to clear the nostril prior to attempting either side.

10.4 **Administering enteral nutrition**

Definition

Enteral nutrition is the delivery of nutrients into the gastrointestinal tract. While the term refers to normal oral nutrition, and can incorporate eating normally, it refers specifically to the administration of nutrient solutions (feeds) into the upper gastrointestinal tract via a tube for the purposes of nutritional support. A nasogastric tube is the most common device for the administration of enteral nutrition (Best 2005).

It is important to remember that:

- The initiation of enteral feeding should only occur as a result of a comprehensive nutritional assessment and multidisciplinary discussion.
- Care and therapy should be directed towards meeting patients' nutritional needs via normal mechanisms, which can have significant advantages over artificial support.
- The risk of pulmonary aspiration in patients receiving enteral nutrition is high, particularly in the unconscious patient, and patients should be monitored accordingly.
- Administering enteral nutrition may impact on other health care needs, for example oral hygiene and elimination. These needs will require assessment, and care to be planned and evaluated based on the findings.

Prior knowledge

Before administering enteral nutrition, make sure you are familiar with:

1 The relevant anatomy of the gastrointestinal tract.
2 The normal processes involved in the acquisition of nutrients.
3 Normal nutritional requirements.
4 Pathophysiology of common gastrointestinal diseases.
5 Factors influencing nutrition in health care.

Background

McWhirter and Pennington (1994) suggest that 40% of patients admitted to hospital are undernourished and that nutritional status in these patients often continues to deteriorate during the course of the hospital stay. The detrimental effects of malnutrition are well documented (Leather *et al.* 2003). Nutritional assessment and the institution of support where necessary can improve patient outcome (NICE 2006).

Nutritional support may take the form of dietary advice or oral supplementation, such as the provision of nutritionally fortified fluids/foods; it may also take the form of a liquid-based feed delivered into the gastrointestinal tract. Alternatively, in certain circumstances feeds can be prepared and delivered intravenously (parenteral nutrition). Decisions on route, content, and management of nutritional support are best made by multidisciplinary nutrition teams (Stroud *et al.* 2003).

When the gastrointestinal tract is functional and accessible, the enteral route of support is the preferred choice (Clinical Resource Efficiency Support Team (CREST) 2004).

Routes of enteral feeding

Enteral feeding may be administered in different ways.

The nasogastric route

The administration of a liquid-based feed via a nasogastric tube – a tube inserted through the nose into the stomach via the oesophagus. This route is appropriate for total or supplemental support in the short term (4 weeks). Fine bore tubes should be used unless there is a need for repeated gastric aspiration (Stroud *et al.* 2003). The presence of a nasogastric tube may interfere with the function of the lower oesophageal sphincter (Holmes 2004), which may lead to oesophageal reflux.

Occasionally orogastric tubes are inserted in ventilated patients, particularly those with actual/potential basal skull fracture. These may be used for enteral feeding in the short term only.

The nasojejunal/nasoduodenal route

The administration of a liquid-based feed via a nasojejunal tube, inserted through the nose into the jejunum or duodenum via the oesophagus, stomach, and the pyloric sphincter. This route is appropriate for total or supplemental support in the short term (4 weeks). It may be useful for patients with gastric stasis or gastric reflux. It may also have a role in patients with specific conditions such as pancreatitis.

Nasojejunal tubes are inserted either with endoscopic/radiological guidance or with direct vision during surgery. Tubes are available that are inserted using patient position, natural or promoted gastric motility, and tube design to induce tube migration from the stomach into the jejunum; research to support their use is in its infancy. Nasojejunal tubes may also be of dual lumen design with a shorter gastric aspiration port.

The gastrostomy route

The administration of a liquid-based feed through a tube that is inserted via the skin and the stomach wall to sit in the stomach. This route is appropriate where nasogastric feeding is not possible, or when nutritional support is likely to be long term (more than 4 weeks) or permanent. The procedure is undertaken with radiological/endoscopic guidance or with direct vision during surgery.

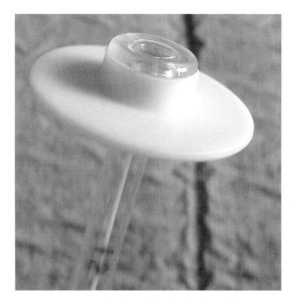

Figure 10.8 A PEG feeding tube, distal end with flange.

Although percutaneous gastrostomy tube placement has a low immediate morbidity, the overall mortality within a few weeks of the procedure is very high (Stroud *et al.* 2003); this may be related to the underlying medical condition. In some cases the tube is held in place with a small balloon or flange situated in the stomach (**Figure 10.8**). There is also a fixation device attached to the skin to prevent tube movement (**Figure 10.9**). Gastrostomy tubes are collectively called PEG tubes (percutaneous endoscopic gastrostomy tubes).

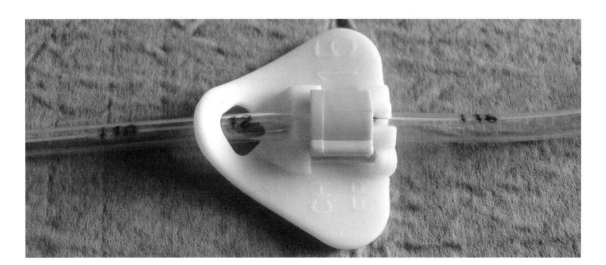

Figure 10.9 A PEG feeding tube, skin fixation device.

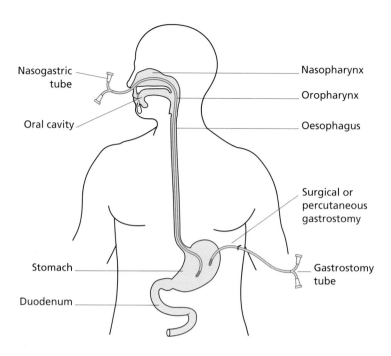

Nasogastric tube

Oral cavity

Nasopharynx

Oropharynx

Oesophagus

Surgical or percutaneous gastrostomy

Gastrostomy tube

Stomach

Duodenum

Figure 10.10 Nasogastric and gastrostomy feeding tube positions.

The jejunostomy or duodenostomy route

The administration of a liquid-based feed through a tube that is inserted via the skin to sit in the jejunum or duodenum (jejunostomy/duodenostomy). This route is appropriate where nasogastric feeding is not possible, or where nutritional support is likely to be permanent/long term (more than 4 weeks). It is used in the management of long-term gastric stasis/paresis. Jejunostomy tubes may also have a role in providing support for patients with gastric reflux and specific conditions such as pancreatitis.

Insertion is undertaken with radiological/endoscopic guidance or with direct vision during surgery. Anatomical tube positions are shown in **Figures 10.10** and **10.11**.

Types of enteral feed

There are many different types of feed available to meet differing needs. These are outlined in **Table 10.5**. This list is not exhaustive, and feeds are in use that have a variety of properties.

The decision on what feed is suitable for each patient should be made by a health care professional skilled and trained in nutritional requirements and methods of nutritional support (NICE 2006). The prescribed feed should

take into account nutritional requirements, activity levels, medical condition, potential metabolic instability, and the likely duration of nutritional support (NICE 2006).

Most enteral feeds are listed under the borderline substances section of the *British national formulary* (Joint Formulary Committee 2008). A full medical or dietetic prescription will be required for a feed to be administered.

Feeding techniques

Enteral feeds can be administered via bolus, intermittent, or continuous infusion methods. There does appear to be controversy over the best method.

Bolus feeds

Bolus feeds delivered drip fed by gravity may have a role in delivering small feed volumes (200–300 ml) over 20–40 minutes on a regular basis. This is a relatively cheap method of administering feed but may cause bloating and diarrhoea (Stroud *et al*. 2003). The 'open' syringe system (**Figure 10.12**) may carry an increased risk, as frequent manipulations and decanting will increase the risk of contamination/infection (Payne-James *et al*. 2001, Padula *et al*. 2004).

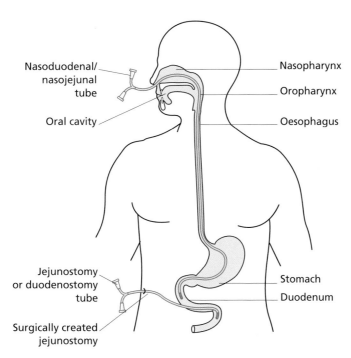

Figure 10.11 Positions of nasojejunal/nasoduodenal and jejunal/duodenal feeding tubes.

Table 10.5 Different types of nasogastric feeds

Feed type	Comments
Standard feed	Usually 1 Kcal/ml solution suitable for supplemental or total nutrition.
Standard feed with extra fibre	Usually 1 Kcal/ml solution suitable for supplemental or total nutrition. Extra fibre is added – fibre may be beneficial for maintaining gut ecology and function (Dougherty and Lister 2008).
High energy feed	Usually 1.5 Kcal/ml – allows equivalent calorific intake in a smaller volume. May have a use in fluid-restricted patients or those with increased energy requirements. The feed is hypertonic and may draw water into the gut lumen.
Medium chain triglyceride (MCT) feed	Medium chain triglycerides are more readily metabolized by the liver than long chain triglycerides (St-Onge and Jones 2002). MCT feeds may be more suitable for patients with fat malabsorption/gastrointestinal dysfunction. MCT feeds also have a reduced osmolality.
Peptide-based feed	The amino acid content in the feed is available as short chain peptides, which may be easier to absorb. These feeds may be useful in patients with gastrointestinal disease.
Low sodium feed	Standard feed with reduced sodium. May be useful in reducing sodium load.
High fat, low carbohydrate feed	May be of use in patients with chronic lung disease as carbon dioxide production is reduced.
Low electrolyte, moderate protein, low volume feed	May have a role in supporting nutrition in patients with renal disease.
Soya-based feed	For patients with lactose intolerance.

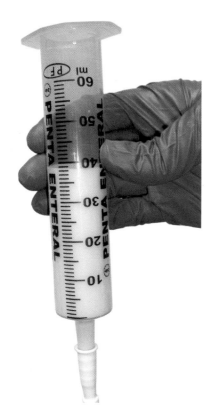

Figure 10.12 Open gravity method of feeding.

Administering feed via bolus injection is generally not undertaken as the risk of bloating is again high. This technique is reserved for administration of drugs via enteral tubes, although this practice should be avoided if at all possible and governed by best practice/policy if not. Administration of bolus feeds may also cause dumping syndrome (Stroud *et al.* 2003). This is a situation where gastric contents are rapidly moved into the duodenum, causing unpleasant gastrointestinal effects such as abdominal cramps and nausea. The bolus method may also cause spikes in blood glucose, which may be poorly tolerated in the diabetic or sick patient.

If the bolus feeding method is to be used, an electronic, volumetric pump may be indicated. This allows the administration of bolus feeds from a closed system and may be time and cost-effective. Practitioners should ensure that they are competent in using the particular pump, as operator error could have clinical consequences. The feeding tube should also be flushed as indicated. Bolus feeding is not appropriate for post-pyloric (nasojejunal or jejunal) feeding as the stomach reservoir is not utilized.

Intermittent feeding

Intermittent feeding may be useful as it allows periods of time when feeding is not occurring. The obvious example of this is overnight feeding, although this should be avoided in patients with high aspiration risk. The method may improve body image issues and allow the independent patient to work during the day. In hospitalized patients it may allow for enhanced mobility and rehabilitation plans. As with bolus feeding it may cause problems with blood sugar control, particularly in the diabetic or sick patient.

Continual feeding

Continual feeding allows a constant flow and delivery of nutrients into the route; peak and trough levels of blood glucose are avoided. This method may reduce the incidence of 'dumping' effect and diarrhoea (Stroud *et al.* 2003). However, the natural bacteriostatic properties of the stomach are reduced as the gastric acid is decreased by the continual delivery of feed. Many organizations recommend a continual infusion with a 6–8 hour overnight rest period to allow natural acidity to return to normal, particularly for critically ill patients.

Thirty per cent of feeds are contaminated with a variety of microorganisms, largely due to poor preparation or poor administration of feeds (NICE 2003). Regardless of feeding method, minimal handling and an aseptic non-touch technique should be used to connect the feed container administration system and enteral feeding tube (DH 2006).

Context

 When to use enteral feeding

- Enteral feeding should be instituted following comprehensive nutritional assessment when a patient's nutritional needs cannot be met via the normal oral route and they have a functioning gastrointestinal tract.
- Enteral feeding should also be considered when a patient is likely to be at risk of malnutrition as a result of treatment/disease process.

While ethical and legal positions with regard to enteral nutrition vary slightly from country to country (Korner *et al.* 2006), the provision of enteral nutrition via a tube is considered a medical treatment. The commencement, discontinuation, and withholding of this support are medical decisions.

The commencement of enteral nutrition as a therapy should be made in the patient's best interests and should involve multidisciplinary discussion.

When not to use enteral nutrition

- When the patient does not consent.
- Where the gastrointestinal tract is severely compromised or dysfunctional. In these cases other forms of nutritional support, such as parenteral nutrition, should be considered.
- An enteral feed should not be administered unless the feeding tube has been confirmed as being in the correct position. Please see notes below:

The confirmation of the position of nasojejunal and jejunostomy tubes is achievable through radiological means. This, however, would be unrealistic prior to the commencement of each feed. The practitioner should therefore ensure that the tube has not moved in any way. This can be ascertained by observing distance markers on the tube at the point of fixation. Any concerns about tube position should be directed to medical staff/nutritional specialists.

The position of nasogastric and gastrostomy tubes can be confirmed by testing the pH of the gastric aspirate using pH indicator sticks. Aspirate pH of 5.5 or less will indicate gastric placement (NPSA 2005). Obtaining aspirate for testing, particularly from fine bore tubes, may be difficult. A large volume syringe may assist in obtaining aspirates, as may positioning the patient on their side. It may also be useful to inject 10 ml of air into the tube, as its tip may be resting against the gastric mucosa (NPSA 2005). Advancing the tube forward by a few centimetres may have the same effect. If difficulty in obtaining the correct aspirate pH is experienced in a recently fed patient, a time lapse of 1 hour should allow the gastric contents to empty and pH to return to normal (NPSA 2005).

Alternative interventions

- Remember that the optimal way of providing nutrition is through the oral route. Can the patient's nutritional needs be met by supplementing their oral

intake? For example, encouraging dietary intake or providing fortified drinks and sip feeds?
- If the enteral route of providing nutritional support is not appropriate, the parenteral route should be considered.
- There are certain situations, particularly near the end of life, where the commencement (or withdrawal) of enteral feeding may be appropriate. These decisions should be made by senior, experienced, multidisciplinary teams.

Potential problems

Blocked tubes

Enteral feed tubes often become blocked with feed. Feeding tubes must be flushed with water before and after feeding and before and after administration of any medication in order to prevent tube blockage. The volume, frequency of flushing, and type of flush solution should be specified in the patient's individual feeding regimen/prescription (CREST 2004).

Reising and Scott Neal (2005) recommend flushing with 30–50 ml of sterile water using a large volume (50 ml) syringe. Tap water may be used but sterile water should always be used in the immunosuppressed patient (DH 2006) and those considered at risk. It has been suggested that using warm water may be beneficial (Reising and Scott Neal 2005); however, this may not be practical. If this technique is used the temperature of the water should not be greater than body temperature.

The criteria for tube flushing are shown in **Box 10.5**.

Unblocking enteral feeding tubes A blocked enteral feeding tube may be the result of failure to flush the tube at regular intervals (Marcuard *et al.* 1989). Many approaches to unblocking tubes have been described (Reising and Scott Neal 2005); these include carbonated drinks and sodium bicarbonate solutions. Water should be

Box 10.5 When to flush enteral feeding tubes

- Every 4 hours.
- Before, between, and after medication administration.
- Before and after bolus feedings.
- Before and after checking for gastric residuals.

used in the first instance. The use of carbonated drinks and bicarbonate solutions is controversial; practitioners should refer to local policies or seek specialist advice. However, if either of these approaches are used and are successful, they should be followed by a water flush.

Certain pancreatic enzymes may be administered into the tube to break down blockages, but again this should only be done according to prescription and organizational policy. Specialist nutrition nurses and/or dietetic staff should be consulted. Under no circumstances should an intubating stylet (guide wire) be inserted back into the tube and into the patient, as this may cause tube/anatomical perforation.

A blocked feeding tube refractory to all these interventions should be removed and a new tube inserted as necessary. Any resistance noted on attempting to remove the tube may indicate knotting; the procedure should then be abandoned and expert opinion should be sought.

Tube movement

Tube movement/migration may occur, particularly with nasogastric tubes, with resultant administration of feed into the incorrect place. Nasogastric/gastrostomy tube position must be confirmed prior to commencing a feed; however, migration may occur while the feed is in progress.

Episodes of vomiting or regurgitation may indicate tube movement into the oesophagus; in this situation the feed should be stopped and tube position checked. Any sudden respiratory distress may alert the practitioner to potential tube movement into the pulmonary tree. Should this occur, the feed should be stopped immediately, a respiratory assessment undertaken, and a position check performed; senior assistance may be required.

Abdominal X-ray is the only confirmatory mechanism to establish post-pyloric tube position. Administration of feed into the abdominal cavity could occur if a gastrostomy/post-pyloric tube is dislodged. Observations should be made for signs of any inflammatory response. Distance markers on the tube should be documented and the tube length checked against this documentation.

Gastrointestinal problems

Diarrhoea, constipation, and nausea and vomiting can be caused by enteral feeding (Pancorbo-Hidalgo *et al.* 2001). The incidence may be as high as 95%, although differ-

ences in classifying and reporting diarrhoea and identifying the cause make accurate assessment of incidence difficult (Whelan *et al.* 2004). Enteral feeding-related diarrhoea may be related to the type of feed and/or its method of delivery. Hyperosmolar feeds may increase the amount of water drawn into the gut; bolus feeding may cause intermittent movement of large volumes of water.

Advice from a nutritional specialist/dietician can lead to the alteration of feeding regime to attempt to reduce diarrhoea. The administration of fibre-enhanced feeds may play a role (Stroud *et al.* 2003). An infective cause of diarrhoea should always be considered and microbiological sampling should be initiated at the earliest opportunity.

Nausea and vomiting may be caused by gastric stasis, and bloating may also be experienced as a result of feed delivery; this will again be influenced by underlying disease. Feed delivery should be reviewed to select the most appropriate method. Pharmacological enhancement of gastric motility may play a role in reducing nausea and vomiting. Simple measures such as positioning the patient in a semi-recumbent/sitting position can aid gastric drainage. Specific drugs should be administered to treat nausea. Again, advice should be sought from the nutrition team/specialist.

Refeeding syndrome

This is a syndrome where providing nutritional support to previously malnourished patients precipitates hypophosphataemia with resultant cardiac failure (Hearing 2004). Fat and protein metabolism (part of the starvation process) results in a loss of intracellular electrolytes, in particular phosphate. Renewed carbohydrate metabolism as a result of nutritional support causes electrolyte movement, particularly the movement of phosphate into the intracellular compartment, causing hypophosphataemia. This can have detrimental effects on cardiac function. Understanding of refeeding syndrome and its treatment is limited (Hearing 2004); however, management of fluid and electrolyte balance is of paramount importance.

Infection risks

The tube entrance site should be inspected regularly for signs of localized infection and tissue damage. Any dressings should be performed with strict asepsis.

Drug errors related to enteral feeding

There are reported cases of drug errors and clinical incidents causing severe harm and death as a result of confusion between enteral and intravenous (IV) fluid/feed/drug administration (NPSA 2007). This is most probably as a result of similar equipment (such as syringes and three-way taps) being used for both enteral and IV devices. The NPSA (2007) suggest that the following practice should be in place to reduce these errors:

- Using only labelled oral/enteral syringes that cannot be connected to IV catheters or ports to measure and administer oral liquid medicines.
- Using only IV syringes to administer parenteral drugs/fluids.
- Enteral feeding systems should not contain ports or proximal connections that can be connected to IV syringes.
- Enteral feeding systems should be labelled to indicate the route of administration.

Indications for assistance

Any concerns about administering an enteral feed should be addressed initially to a senior nurse. Nutritional specialist nurses and dietetic staff should be available to provide specialist advice/opinion.

Observations and monitoring

Fluid balance monitoring and vital signs monitoring should be instituted for all hospitalized, enterally fed patients. Observations of bowel movements should also occur. For the patient in the community on an established feeding programme, the frequency of these observations may be reduced; observations for symptoms of infection and tube migration should occur and the patient should be educated to undertake this if appropriate. Blood glucose monitoring will be required in the diabetic/sick patient (see Section 10.2).

Special considerations

- If administering feed using a post-pyloric tube in the patient's home, tube confirmation will be difficult. The tube should be inspected for migration and the patient/carers educated to detect signs of tube movement.
- Patients with specific disease processes may have individualized feeds that require reconstitution. This procedure should be performed using a non-touch technique to reduce infection risk.
- Independence in managing enteral feeding is desirable for the patient, particularly in the community setting. This goal will only be achieved through good patient education and support. Particular areas of education will include infection control and management of feeding tubes.

Procedure

Preparation

Prepare yourself
Ensure you know how any equipment works. Ensure you are competent to confirm tube position. Wash your hands, don a plastic apron.

Prepare the patient
See Discussing the procedure box.

Prepare the equipment
Ensure any disposable equipment is in intact packaging and within expiry date. Ensure that electrical equipment is clean, plugged in, and working.

Discussing the procedure with the patient and carers

- Explain why enteral feeding is necessary.
- Discuss the advantages of the selected feeding method.
- Discuss potential complications and ask the patient to report if any are experienced.
- Encourage any questions.

Step-by-step guide to administering enteral nutrition

Step	Rationale
1 Introduce yourself, confirm the patient's identity, explain the procedure, and obtain consent.	To identify the patient correctly and gain informed consent.
2 Confirm tube position.	To ensure delivery of feed into correct place.
3 Note the distance of the tube at fixation point.	As a reference to detect future tube movement.
4 Check feed type/delivery method against medical prescription/dietetic regime.	To ensure the correct feed is administered to the correct patient using the correct method.
5 Reconstitute feed if required using manufacturer's recommended guidelines and a sterile/non-touch technique.	To ensure feed is made to correct concentration. To reduce the risks of bacterial contamination.
6 Assess tube access site; clean and dress as necessary.	To observe for signs of localized inflammation and prevent bacterial contamination.
7 Flush the tube with 30–50 ml of sterile water.	To prevent tube blockage.
For bolus administration using gravity/syringe method:	
8 Using non-toothed clamp or integral tube device, close off the tube at the proximal end. Remove the tube closure device.	To prevent air or feed entering the patient.
9 Remove plunger from catheter-tipped/specific syringe and attach to tube.	To provide a feed reservoir.
10 Decant desired amount of feed into syringe and, holding the device above the level of the patient, open the tap.	To allow gravitational flow of feed into patient.
11 Turn the tap off to the patient and refill syringe as necessary. Open tap to deliver feed.	To allow prescribed amount of feed to be delivered.
12 Flush the tube with 30–50 ml of sterile water.	To prevent tube blockage.
For bolus administration using a volumetric pump:	
8 Prime the administration set using gravity or a priming facility on the pump.	To purge any air from the administration set.
9 Using non-toothed clamp or integral tube device, close off the tube at the proximal end. Remove the tube closure device.	To prevent air entering the patient.

10	Using a non-touch technique, attach the distal end of the administration set to the proximal end of the feeding tube.	To reduce the risk of bacterial contamination.
11	Programme the pump to bolus mode.	To administer the correct bolus volume over an appropriate time period.
12	Set the prescribed bolus volume.	To administer the correct bolus volume over an appropriate time period.
13	Set the prescribed bolus rate in ml/hour and press run.	To administer the correct bolus volume over an appropriate time period.
14	Flush the tube with 30–50 ml of sterile water.	To prevent tube blockage.

For continuous or intermittent administration:

8	Prime the administration set using gravity or a priming facility on the pump.	To purge any air from the administration set.
9	Using non-toothed clamps, tap, or integral tube device, close off the tube at the proximal end. Remove the tube closure device.	To prevent air entering the patient.
10	Using a non-touch technique, attach the distal end of the administration set to the proximal end of the feeding tube.	To reduce the risk of bacterial contamination.
11	Programme the pump to continuous mode. Set the prescribed volume to be infused and the prescribed rate in ml/hour. Press run.	To administer the correct bolus volume over an appropriate time period.

Following the procedure

- Observe the patient for any detrimental effects such as nausea/vomiting.
- Document feed delivery.

Reflection and evaluation

When you have administered an enteral feed, think about the following questions:

1 Was the feeding method the most appropriate one for that particular patient?
2 Did the patient experience any physical effects of feed delivery?
3 Did the patient experience any ongoing effects?

4 Is enteral feeding the optimal form of nutrition for this patient? What are the barriers to normal oral feeding?

Further learning opportunities

At the next available opportunity, discuss with dietetic and specialist nutrition staff why certain feeds and feeding methods are chosen for particular patients.

Reminders

Don't forget to:

- Sign for feed administration in the appropriate documentation.

- Document tube position.
- Note and record the tube distance marker at fixation point.

 Patient scenarios

Consider what you should do in the following situations, then turn to the end of this skill to check your answers.

1 Patient A is receiving bolus feeds into a gastrostomy tube via a volumetric pump. The tube flushed easily prior to administration but the pump is alarming 'occlusion'. What do you suspect has happened and how would you remedy this?

2 Patient B is being fed continually via a nasogastric tube following discharge from critical care. His swallowing has been assessed as competent and he may now eat and drink. He is taking small amounts of fluid but complains of lack of appetite and bloating. How might you manage this situation?

3 A junior colleague reports that patient C, who has recently suffered a stroke and is fed via a nasogastric tube, has a large volume of feed in his mouth. What would your course of action be?

Website

 http://www.oxfordtextbooks.co.uk/orc/ endacott

You may find it helpful to work through our short online quiz and additional scenarios intended to help you to develop and apply the skills in this chapter.

References

Best C (2005). Caring for the patient with a nasogastric tube. *Nursing Standard*, **20**(3), 59–65.

Clinical Resource Efficiency Support Team (2004). *Guidelines for the management of enteral tube feeding in adults*. CREST, Belfast [online] **http://www.crestni.org.uk/tube-feeding-guidelines.pdf** accessed 08/09/08.

Department of Health (2006). *Essential steps to safe, clean care. Enteral feeding: reducing healthcare-associated infections in Primary care trusts; Mental health trusts; Learning disability organisations; Independent healthcare; Care homes; Hospices; GP practices and Ambulance services*. DH, London.

Dougherty L and Lister S (2008). *The Royal Marsden Hospital manual of clinical nursing procedures*, 7th edition. Blackwell Publishing, Oxford.

Hearing SD (2004). Refeeding syndrome is underdiagnosed and undertreated, but treatable. *British Medical Journal*, **328**(7445), 908–9.

Holmes S (2004). Enteral feeding and percutaneous endoscopic gastrostomy. *Nursing Standard*, **18**(20), 41–3.

Joint Formulary Committee (2008). *British national formulary*, 55th edition. British Medical Association and Royal Pharmaceutical Society of Great Britain, London.

Korner U, Bondolfi A, Buhler E *et al.* (2006). Ethical and legal aspects of enteral nutrition. *Clinical Nutrition*, **25**, 196–202.

Leather A, Bushell L and Gillespie L (2003). The provision of nutritional support for people with cancer. *Nursing Times*, **99**(46), 53–5.

Marcuard SP, Stegall KL, and Trogdon S (1989). Clearing obstructed feeding tubes. *Journal of Parenteral and Enteral Nutrition*, **13**(1), 81–3.

McWhirter JP and Pennington CR (1994). Incidence and recognition of malnutrition in hospital. *British Medical Journal*, **308**, 945–8.

National Institute for Health and Clinical Excellence (2003). *Infection control. Prevention of healthcare associated infection in primary and community care*. DH, London.

National Institute for Health and Clinical Excellence (2006). *Nutrition support in adults: oral nutrition support, enteral tube feeding and parenteral nutrition, National Institute for Health and Clinical Excellence Clinical Guideline 32*. DH, London.

National Patient Safety Agency (2005). *Reducing the harm caused by misplaced nasogastric feeding tubes, Patient Safety alert*. NPSA, London.

National Patient Safety Agency (2007). *Promoting safer measurement and administration of liquid medicines via oral and other enteral routes*. NPSA, London.

Padula CA, Kenny A, Planchon C, and Lamoureux C (2004). Enteral feeding: what the evidence says. *American Journal of Nursing*, **104**(7), 62–9.

Pancorbo-Hidalgo PL, Garcia-Fernandez FP, and Ramirez-Pérez C (2001). Complications associated with enteral nutrition by nasogastric tube in an internal medicine unit. *Journal of Clinical Nursing*, **10**(4), 482–90.

Payne-James J, Grimble G, and Silk D (2001). *Artificial nutrition support in clinical practice*. Greenwich Medical Media Limited, London.

Reising DL and Scott Neal R (2005). Enteral tube flushing: what you think are the best practices may not be. *American Journal of Nursing*, **105**, 358–63.

St-Onge MP and Jones PJH (2002). Physiological effects of medium-chain triglycerides: potential agents in the prevention of obesity. *Journal of Nutrition*, **132**, 329–332.

Stroud M, Duncan H, and Nightingale J (2003). Guidelines for enteral feeding in adult hospital patients. *Gut*, 52(Suppl 7), 1–12.

Whelan K, Judd PA, and Taylor MA (2004). Assessment of faecal output in patients receiving enteral tube feeding: validation of a novel chart. *European Journal of Clinical Nutrition*, 58, 1030–7.

Useful further reading and websites

Lee JSW and Auyeung WT (2003). A comparison of two feeding methods in the alleviation of diarrhoea in older tube-fed patients: a randomised controlled trial. *Age and Ageing*, **32**, 388–93.

Answers to patient scenarios

1   The tube has possibly become blocked. Firstly the feed set should be checked to ensure it is loaded into the pump correctly. The tube should be flushed; if patent the feed should be recommenced. If the pump still alarms, the troubleshooting guide for the particular pump should be consulted. If pump malfunction is suspected, another pump should be used. If the feeding tube is blocked, attempts should be made to unblock it according to organization policy. If all of the above fails, senior/nutritional staff should be consulted.

2   A continual feeding regime in this patient may no longer be appropriate. His lack of appetite and bloating are possibly related to the volume of feed in his stomach, and attempted oral nutrition. However, he is still in a recovery stage of acute illness, and good nutrition must be ensured. After consultation with a dietician, a low volume feed may be administered with the same calorific value. Or it may be more appropriate to change the feeding regime to inter-

mittent feeding, overnight if not contraindicated. This will allow time for gastric emptying and stimulation of appetite during the day. As the patient's oral intake increases, supplemental nutrition can decrease. The patient's oral intake should be encouraged with small meals that he likes, and supplemental sip feeds should be encouraged to increase calorie intake.

3   First the feed should be stopped and a baseline assessment of vital signs undertaken. The patient should also be assessed for signs of pulmonary aspiration. If any signs of compromise are noted, medical staff should be consulted immediately. Nasogastric tube position should be checked. If the tube is not in the correct position a new tube should be passed, checked, and therapy recommenced. If the tube is in the correct position, factors such as feeding method/volume of feed and patient position should be considered. A smaller volume feed may be required and a continuous delivery method may be more appropriate. The patient may also be experiencing some reflux. Feeding in the semi-recumbent position may aid gastric emptying, as might the administration of gastro-kinetic drugs. Feed should only be restarted after discussion with medical staff/ nutritional specialists.

10.5 Administration of suppositories and enemas

Definition

A suppository is a solid or semi-solid pellet that is inserted into the bowel. Suppositories are usually torpedo-shaped (see Figure 10.13). An enema is the introduction of a solution into the rectum and/or colon. Enemas and suppositories can be administered for local or systemic action.

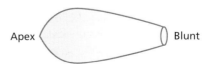

Figure 10.13 Torpedo-shaped suppository.

It is important to remember that:

- Administration of rectal medication is invasive and embarrassing for the patient and may involve some discomfort. Consideration should be given to providing a supportive and conducive environment (Price 2001).
- Patients should have cognitive function in order to understand the procedure and offer consent.
- Rectal medication can be administered for local or systemic action. Prior to administering a treatment for evacuant action, the nurse should undertake a full assessment that considers the patient's medical history, surgical history, and lifestyle factors.

Prior knowledge

Before undertaking administration of suppositories and enemas, make sure you are familiar with:

1 The principles of informed consent.
2 Gastrointestinal anatomy and physiology.
3 Mechanisms of defecation.
4 Common bowel illnesses.
5 Factors influencing bowel function (**Box 10.6**).
6 Symptoms of constipation (**Box 10.7**).
7 The use, action, dose, contraindications, and side effects of the medication.
8 Correct drug administration procedure.
9 Safe manual handling principles.
10 Infection prevention and control policy and procedure.

Box 10.6 Factors influencing bowel function

- Change in diet, e.g. reduced fibre intake.
- Change in fluid intake.
- Reduced mobility.
- Underlying pathology.
- Medication.
- Anorectal pain, e.g. anal fissure.
- Reduced abdominal pressure.
- Oral health.
- Social status, e.g. poor financial state.
- Lack of privacy.
- Over-riding the urge to defecate.

Box 10.7 Symptoms of constipation

- Altered frequency of bowel movement.
- Altered consistency of bowel movement.
- Altered quantity of bowel movement.
- Incomplete evacuation.
- Faecal impaction.
- Overflow diarrhoea.
- Coated tongue.
- Halitosis.
- Headache.
- Nausea.
- Malaise.
- Abdominal bloating.
- Abdominal distension.
- Abdominal pain.

Background

Normal bowel function is influenced by factors that include physical, psychosocial, and environmental elements (see Box 10.6). Constipation can be defined as the passage of hard stools, less frequent than the individual's normal bowel pattern. Constipation can be grouped into three classifications:

- Primary constipation can be attributed to lifestyle changes with no underlying pathophysiology.
- Secondary constipation can occur as a result of diseases or conditions affecting bowel function.
- Iatrogenic constipation can occur as a result of taking medication.

Individuals suffering from constipation can present with a variety of symptoms (see Box 10.7).

Individualized assessment is required to determine the patient's normal bowel function in order to achieve successful management (DH 2003). The nurse should utilize an assessment tool to assist in identifying patients at risk of developing constipation (Richmond and Wright 2005 (**Figure 10.14**), Kyle 2007). Patient assessment should also consider the use of tools that determine the extent of constipation (Heaton *et al.* 1992, Downing *et al.* 2007) – see **Figure 10.15**.

The nurse's role in managing constipation should focus on health education and preventative measures. Treatment of constipation should incorporate a range of approaches and address lifestyle factors (Denby 2006),

<u>Circle risk factors in table and total</u>

GENDER:

Male	1
Female	2

MOBILITY:

Independently mobile	0
Dependent on walking aids/assistance from others	1
Restricted to bed/chair	2
Spinal cord injury/spinal cord compression	3

FIBRE INTAKE:

5 pieces fruit/veg or more consumed daily	0
3 or 4 pieces fruit/veg consumed daily	1
2 pieces fruit/veg or less consumed daily	2
Bran products consumed daily Yes	0
No	2

FLUID INTAKE:

10 cups/glasses or more consumed daily	0
6 to 9 cups/glasses consumed daily	1
5 cups/glasses or less consumed daily	2

PERSONAL BELIEFS:

Does patient believe they are prone to constipation?   Yes/No

Have laxatives ever been used for constipation?   Yes/No _____

Current bowel habit: _____

SECTION SUB TOTAL ☐

WARD PATIENTS ONLY:

Does patient have difficulty evacuating bowels in hospital toilets?

No	0
Yes	2

PATIENTS REQUIRING COMMODE/BEDPAN:

Does patient anticipate problems using a commode or bedpan?

No/Not applicable	0
Yes	2

SECTION SUB TOTAL ☐

Conditions which increase risk of constipation.

From medical notes, patient history and blood results, assess presence of the following:

PHYSIOLOGICAL CONDITIONS

Metabolic disorders:	
Hypokalaemia/uraemia/hypothyroidism poisoning	2
Pelvic conditions:	
Hysterectomy/ovarian tumour/uterine prolapse/pregnancy	3
Neuromuscular disorders:	
Parkinson's disease/Multiple sclerosis/Systemic sclerosis/Hirschsprung's disease/ Cerebrovascular accident/Spina bifida/Rheumatoid arthritis/Cerebral tumour	3
Endocrine disorders:	
Diabetes Mellitus/hypothyroidism/hypopituitarism/hypercalcaemia	3
Colorectal/abdominal disorders:	
Irritable Bowel Syndrome/Crohn's disease/Diverticulitis/Ulcerative Colitis/colorectal tumour/anorectal stricture/anorectal fissure/anorectal prolapse/haemorrhoids/hernias	3

PSYCHOLOGICAL CONDITIONS

Psychiatric illness:	
Depression/Anorexia Nervosa/Bulimia Nervosa	2
Learning disabilities or dementia (as evidenced by lack of understanding of speech or situations)	2

SECTION SUB TOTAL ☐

Medications which increase risk of constipation.

Is patient presently taking any of the following medications on a regualr basis?

Antiemetics	2	**Analgesia:**	
Calcium channel blockers	2	Non-opioid analgesia	3
Iron supplements	2	OR continuous opioid therapy	5

Anticholinergic containing medication:		**Cytotoxic chemotherapy:**	
Anticonvulsants	2	Cytotoxic chemotherapy	3
Antidepressants	2	OR Vinca alkaloid agents	5
Antiparkinson drugs	2		
Antispasmodics	2		

SECTION SUB TOTAL ☐

TOTAL SCORE ☐

Figure 10.14 Constipation risk assessment scale. Richmon and Wright (2005)

before pharmacological interventions. Rectal medication is indicated for acute, short-term treatment of constipation.

How do suppositories and enemas work?

Depending on the medication prescribed, suppositories and enemas work either by absorption or by stimulating peristalsis. Suppositories achieve this effect by dissolving in the rectum.

Rectal medications work in a variety of ways:

- Delivering medication directly onto the rectal mucosa for absorption into the bloodstream (systemic action).
- Stimulating the lower colon resulting in the expulsion of faeces (evacuant action).
- Remaining in the bowel for specific action (retention action).

Context

 ### When to use suppositories and enemas

Suppositories and enemas may be prescribed for the following reasons:

- To empty the bowel before certain types of surgery and investigation. Abdominal surgery requires a clear bowel in order to reduce the risk of post-operative peritonitis.
- For the treatment of short-term constipation. They can relieve constipation by lubricant or stimulant action.
- To introduce medication for systemic action, as the rectum is highly vascular and drugs are absorbed quickly (Addison *et al.* 2000). Examples include: analgesics, sedatives, and anti-inflammatory drugs. The rectum is an alternative route for the

	−4	−3	−2	−1	0	+1	+2	+3	+4
		Constipation ⟵					Diarrhoea ⟶		
Characteristic	Impacted or obstructed (−/+small leakage)	Formed Hard with pellets	Formed Solid Hard	Formed Solid	Formed Semi-solid	Formed Soft	Unformed Loose or paste-like	Unformed Liquid +/−mucus	Unformed Liquid +/−mucus
Pattern	No stool produced	Delayed ≥ 3 days	Delayed ≥ 3 days	Pt's usual		Pt's usual	Usual or frequent	Frequent	Frequent
Control	Unable to defecate despite maximal effort or straining	Major effort or straining required to defecate	Moderate effort or straining required to defecate	Minimal or no effort required to defecate	Minimal or no effort to defecate	Minimal or no effort required to control urgency	Moderate effort required to control urgency	Very difficult to control urgency and may be explosive	Incontinent or explosive – unable to control or unaware

1. BPS is a 9-point numerical scale. It is a **single score**, based on the overall '**best vertical fit**' among the above three parameters [characteristics, pattern, control] and is recorded for example as: BPS +1, BPS −3 or BPS +2

2. Look vertically down each BPS level to become familiar with how the three parameters of **characteristics, pattern & control** change in gradation from constipation to diarrhoea

3. The 'usual' bowel pattern for a patient may be in the 0, −1 or +1 columns. For any of these, the actual frequency of bowel movements may vary among patients from one or more times daily to once every 1–2 days but the patient states as being their usual pattern

4. Patients with a surgical intervention (colostomy, ileostomy, short loop bowel) may have a more frequent 'usual' bowel pattern than above. BPS is still overall graded by combining all three parameters (eg. BPS +2 or BPS +3 with ileostomy) to ascertain a 'best fit'

5. Patients may use different words than above to describe their bowel activity. One must use clinical judgment in deciding which boxes are most appropriate

6. In potential confounding cases, determination of the most appropriate BPS score is made using the following methods:
   • Two vertically similar parameters generally outweigh the third;
   • Single priority weighting among parameters is Characteristics > Pattern > Control

Figure 10.15 Victoria Bowel Performance Scale (BPS). Bowel performance scale, copyright Victoria Hospice Society, BC, Canada. www.victoriahospice.org or *Medical care of the dying* (2006) p. 345.

administration of drugs when a person is unable to take the drug orally because of nausea or vomiting, unconsciousness, nil by mouth, or being unable to swallow for other reasons. If the medication is being administered for systemic action, it is important to reassure the patient that they will not experience the need to evacuate the bowel.

- Suppositories can be used to soothe and treat haemorrhoids or anal pruritus. These preparations act locally and contain anaesthetics and/or corticosteroids.
- To soothe or lubricate the rectal mucosa in cases of inflammatory bowel disease.
- To soften, lubricate, and increase the volume of impacted faeces for treatment of constipation.

When not to use suppositories and enemas

Suppositories and enemas are contraindicated in the following situations:

- **Chronic constipation:** suppositories and enemas are indicated for short-term use only. Chronic constipation should not be treated with repeated rectal preparations as this can, over time, lead to an atonic bowel.

- Paralytic ileus: the action of suppositories and enemas is dependent on the peristaltic action of the bowel. Handling the bowel during surgery can cause relaxation of the smooth muscle leading to the absence of peristalsis.
- **Gastrointestinal obstruction:** gastrointestinal obstruction inhibits natural bowel motility and can cause spasm.
- **Gastrointestinal, colorectal, or gynaecological surgery:** post-operatively, there is a risk of ruptured suture lines (Dougherty and Lister 2008).
- **Malignancy or other pathology of the perineal and perianal areas:** if malignancy is present, administering a suppository or enema could cause damage to the bowel and increase the risk of bleeding.
- **Low platelet count:** a low platelet count could predispose patient to bleeding.
- **Anal fissure:** administering a suppository or enema when an anal fissure is present is extremely painful.
- **Rectal prolapse:** a prolapse can alter sphincter muscle control, which may affect the ability to retain medication.
- **Sexual, emotional, and other types of abuse:** patients who have experienced abuse may not consent to treatment. A sensitive approach is necessary.

Alternative interventions

Comprehensive assessment will enable the nurse to establish lifestyle and dietary factors that may influence bowel function. It is preferable to address these concerns prior to or alongside treatment. There are various treatment options for acute and chronic constipation; these include both oral and rectal intervention.

Potential problems

- There are a number of circumstances that may lead to potential problems (see 'When not to use suppositories and enemas').
- Not all patients have the ability to retain rectal medication.

Indications for assistance

It is important to be aware of the reasons for treatment. If the patient experiences any pain or discomfort during the procedure, stop immediately and seek help from your supervisor, the Registered Nurse, or a member of the medical staff.

Observations and monitoring

- Prior to administration, it is necessary to make a visual assessment of the patient's perianal area to identify abnormalities.
- During and after insertion, it is necessary to observe the patient for signs of discomfort or distress (see Box 10.8)

Special considerations

- Before administration, the nurse should be aware that in the case of unresolved constipation, a digital rectal examination (DRE) must be performed by a competent Registered Nurse. A DRE will determine the presence of faeces in the rectum (Royal College of Nursing (RCN) 2008). The patient's personal, religious, and cultural sensitivities should be considered prior to performing the DRE. There may be situations when the procedure is inappropriate or dangerous.

- Microenemas contain smaller volumes of concentrated solution, resulting in less discomfort and distress on administration.

- If undertaking these skills in the patient's home, remember to ensure that the patient has clear access to their toilet and is capable of a safe transfer.

- The nurse should be aware that there is conflict within the literature regarding whether a suppository should be inserted apex or blunt end first (Bradshaw and Price 2006). Trust policies should take into account this dilemma and advise staff accordingly. The Registered Nurse and the student nurse should act in accordance with Trust policy.

- There is also conflicting information within the literature regarding where the suppository should rest within the rectum after insertion. There is evidence to suggest that a suppository can be inserted either alongside the rectal wall (Campbell 1993, Kyle 2006) or directly into the faeces (Dougherty and Lister 2004). The Registered Nurse and the student nurse should act in accordance with Trust policy.

Box 10.8 Signs and symptoms of discomfort/distress

- Pale, cold, clammy.
- Confusion.
- Dizziness.
- Nausea.
- Impatience.
- Rapid speech.
- Dry mouth.
- Sweating.
- Panic attacks.
- Palpitations.
- Shaking/trembling.
- Irritability.
- Flushed face.
- Lack of concentration.

Procedure

Preparation

Prepare yourself

- Undertake a manual handling risk assessment (performed by a suitably qualified person) (Health and Safety Executive 1992a).
- Wash hands.
- Don protective clothing. Non-sterile single gloves and single-use disposable aprons should be worn to minimize the risk of cross-infection/ contamination during the procedure (Health and Safety Executive 1992b).
- Assess the patient for allergies, e.g. to medication and equipment.
- Allow the patient to empty the bladder as a full bladder may cause discomfort during the procedure.

Prepare the equipment

- Clean trolley/tray.
- Prescribed medication and prescription chart.
- Protective waterproof bed covering.
- Water-soluble lubricant.
- Disposable gloves and apron.
- Wipes or tissue paper.
- Bedpan/commode/access to toilet facilities.
- Bag to dispose of used equipment.

Discussing the procedure with the patient

- Explain the procedure to the patient. The patient may wish to see the suppository or enema. An explanation will ensure that the patient understands the procedure and provides informed consent. It can also provide the patient with a sense of control and encourage cooperation.

- Revise information regarding last bowel movement: the date; time; amount; the character of the stool; and the patient's ability to mobilize and retain the medication. Check the patient's history for any previous rectal problems that may help to identify risk.

- Remind the patient that if the medication is being used for systemic action, they will not experience the urge to defecate.

- Remind the patient to let a nurse know if they become uncomfortable at any time during or after the procedure.

- Explain what toilet facilities are available and remind the patient that the nurse is available.

Step-by-step guide to administration of a suppository

Step	Rationale
1 Introduce yourself, confirm the patient's identity, explain the procedure, and obtain consent.	To identify the patient correctly and gain informed consent.
2 Safeguard the patient's privacy and dignity throughout the procedure.	To avoid unnecessary embarrassment. Privacy and dignity are important to every individual (Amnesty International 1999, Matiti *et al.* 2007, NMC 2008).

3	Check the prescription and the identity of the patient in accordance with drug administration procedure.	To minimize the risk of error and comply with legal requirements (NMC 2007).
4	Wash and dry hands. Put on disposable apron.	To reduce the risk of cross-infection.
5	Prepare the medication and equipment.	To ensure there is no need to leave the patient during the procedure.
6	Provide access to toilet facilities.	To reassure the patient that toilet facilities are readily available.
7	Reiterate the procedure to the patient and confirm consent.	To ensure the patient understands the procedure and to comply with professional/legal requirements (NMC 2008).
8	Ask the patient to lie in the left lateral position with knees flexed (see **Figure 10.16**).	This position follows the natural anatomy of the colon, allowing gravity to aid the insertion. Keeping the knees flexed ensures more comfortable passage of the medication (Campbell 1993).
9	Place the protective sheet under the patient's buttocks.	To avoid cross-contamination by unnecessary soiling of linen and to reduce embarrassment.
10	Wash and dry hands or use bactericidal hand rub. Put on disposable gloves.	To reduce the risk of contamination and cross-infection.
11	Open the suppositories onto clean tissue and lubricate the ends of the suppositories with gel.	To maintain a clean procedure. Lubrication eases entry into the rectum and prevents trauma by reducing friction.
12	Gently part the patient's buttocks and insert the suppositories using the index or middle finger. Advance them approximately 2–4 cm along the anal canal (see **Figure 10.17**).	Parting the buttocks eases insertion. Advancing the suppositories 2–4 cm ensures that they are resting in the rectum.
13	Dry the patient's perianal area. Change any soiled linen/clothing. Remove gloves.	To promote patient comfort and avoid excoriation and perianal infection.
14	Ask the patient to retain the suppositories for approximately 10–15 minutes or in accordance with the manufacturer's instructions. Ensure the patient has the means to summon assistance.	To enable the suppositories to dissolve and be effective. Ensuring the patient can summon assistance will reduce the patient's anxiety.
15	Ensure the patient is as comfortable as possible.	To reduce stress and anxiety.
16	The protective bed covering should be left in place.	To prevent accidental soiling of bedding.
17	Discard equipment according to clinical waste procedure. Wash and dry hands.	To reduce the risk of cross-infection.
18	Record the procedure, documenting any effects of the administration.	To conform with professional and legal requirements (NMC 2005) and to monitor the patient's bowel function.

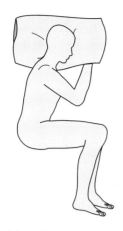

Figure 10.16 Left lateral position.

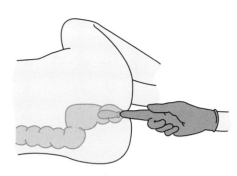

Figure 10.17 Insertion of a suppository.

Step-by-step guide to administration of an enema

Step		Rationale
1	Introduce yourself, confirm the patient's identity, explain the procedure, and obtain consent.	To identify the patient correctly and gain informed consent.
2	Safeguard the patient's privacy and dignity.	To avoid unnecessary embarrassment. Privacy and dignity are important to every individual (Amnesty International 1999, Matiti *et al.* 2007, NMC 2008).
3	Check the prescription and the identity of the patient in accordance with drug administration procedure.	To minimize the risk of error and comply with legal requirements (NMC 2007).
4	Wash and dry hands. Put on disposable apron.	To reduce the risk of cross-infection.
5	Prepare the medication and equipment.	To ensure there is no need to leave the patient during the procedure.
6	Provide access to toilet facilities.	To reassure the patient that toilet facilities are readily available.
7	Reiterate the procedure to the patient and confirm consent.	To ensure the patient understands the procedure and to comply with professional/legal requirements (NMC 2008).
8	Ask the patient to lie in the left lateral position with knees flexed (see Figure 10.16).	This position follows the natural anatomy of the colon, allowing gravity to aid the insertion. Keeping the knees flexed ensures more comfortable passage of the medication (Campbell 1993).
9	Place the protective sheet under the patient's buttocks.	To avoid cross-contamination by unnecessary soiling of linen and reduce embarrassment.

10	Wash and dry hands or use bactericidal hand rub. Put on disposable gloves.	To reduce the risk of contamination and cross-infection.
11	Enemas must be at room temperature or should be warmed.	To minimize shock and prevent bowel spasms.
12	Lubricate the nozzle of the enema.	To reduce friction, thereby easing entry into the rectum and preventing trauma.
13	Expel excessive air by squeezing a small amount of fluid down the nozzle.	The introduction of air into the colon can cause distension resulting in unnecessary discomfort and increased peristalsis.
14	Gently part the patient's buttocks and slowly insert the nozzle into the rectum in an upward and slightly backward direction to a depth in accordance with the manufacturer's instructions (see **Figure 10.18**). Instruct the patient to take deep breaths and exhale slowly during insertion.	Follows the natural anatomy of the colon and minimizes discomfort. Helps to facilitate the relaxation of the external anal sphincter and reduces discomfort on insertion of the enema.
15	If administering an evacuant enema, introduce the fluid slowly by rolling the container from the bottom to the top until empty.	Ensures that all contents are delivered and prevents backflow and premature ejection of solution. Rapid administration should be avoided as this stimulates immediate peristalsis by increasing the pressure on the rectal walls.
16	Retention enemas should be administered slowly. The foot of the bed may be elevated to an angle of 45°.	Slower administration produces less pressure on the intestinal wall. Elevating the foot of the bed can facilitate retention of the solution by force of gravity.
17	Withdraw the nozzle slowly.	To avoid reflex emptying of the rectum.
18	Dry the patient's perianal area. Change any soiled linen/clothing. Remove gloves.	To promote patient comfort and avoid excoriation and perianal infection.
19	Ask the patient to retain the enema for approximately 10–15 minutes or in accordance with the manufacturer's instructions. Ensure the patient has the means to summon assistance.	To enable the enema to be effective. Ensuring the patient can summon assistance will reduce the patient's anxiety.
20	Ensure the patient is as comfortable as possible.	To reduce stress and anxiety.
21	The protective bed covering should be left in place.	To prevent accidental soiling of bedding.
22	Discard equipment according to clinical waste procedure. Wash and dry hands.	To reduce the risk of cross-infection.
23	Record the procedure, documenting any effects of the administration.	To conform with professional and legal requirements (NMC 2005) and to monitor the patient's bowel function.

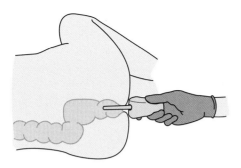

Figure 10.18 Insertion of an enema.

Recognizing patient deterioration

■ If the patient becomes unwell or experiences discomfort during the procedure, stop immediately and inform the Registered Nurse or medical staff.

■ The patient may experience abdominal discomfort as a result of the treatment.

■ Inform the Registered Nurse or medical staff if the patient does not experience a successful bowel movement following the procedure.

Reflection and evaluation

When you have administered a suppository/enema, think about the following questions:

1 Were you able to prepare the patient for this procedure by providing relevant information?
2 Were you able to answer the patient's questions?
3 How did you feel about the intimate nature of this skill?
4 How did you think the patient felt about having the treatment?
5 Where and why did you document this episode of care and what information did you record?

Further learning opportunities

At the next available opportunity:

● Examine the literature in relation to:
  – inserting a suppository apex or blunt end first
  – where a suppository should rest when inserted into the rectum
  – the introduction of air when administering an evacuant enema

  – the optimum temperature of an enema prior to administration.
● There are anatomical models designed to assist in the acquisition of these skills. Make arrangements to practise these skills in a simulated environment.
● Observe the Registered Nurse performing these skills in order to gain a deeper understanding of the procedures.
● After observing the Registered Nurse performing the skills, elicit the patient's perspective through sensitive communication.
● Carry out the procedure under supervision.
● Consider how you would adapt your practice to accommodate the biopsychosocial and cultural needs of different patients.
● Identify different types of enemas and suppositories.

Reminders

Don't forget to:

● Ensure that an individualized, holistic assessment has been performed prior to the procedure.
● Document the episode of care (NMC 2008).

Patient scenarios

Consider what you should do in the following situations, then turn to the end of this skill to check your answers.

1 Aito has expelled the suppositories before the recommended time period. There has been no bowel movement. What action should you take?
2 Gloria has received suppositories and would like to mobilize. What would you advise?
3 Donald has been prescribed a phosphate enema for acute constipation. He is unable to lie in the left lateral position due to pain in his hip. What action should you take?

Website

 http://www.oxfordtextbooks.co.uk/orc/ endacott

You may find it helpful to work through our short online quiz and additional scenarios intended to help you to develop and apply the skills in this chapter.

References

Addison R, Ness W, Abulafi M *et al.* (2000). How to administer enemas and suppositories. *Nursing Times NT Plus: Continence*, **96**(6), 3–4.

Amnesty International (1999). *Universal Declaration of Human Rights*. Amnesty International UK, London.

Bradshaw A and Price L (2006). Rectal suppository insertion: the reliability of the evidence as a basis for nursing practice. *Journal of Clinical Nursing*, **16**, 98–103.

Campbell J (1993). Skills update: suppositories. *Community Outlook*, **3**(7), 22–3.

Denby N (2006). The role of diet and lifestyle changes in the management of constipation. *Journal of Community Nursing*, **20**(9), 20–4.

Department of Health (2003). *Essence of care. Patient-focused benchmarks for clinical governance. Benchmarks for continence and bladder and bowel care*. DH, London.

Dougherty L and Lister S (2008). *The Royal Marsden Hospital manual of clinical nursing procedures*, 7th edition. Wiley-Blackwell Publishing, Oxford.

Downing GM, Kuziemsky G, Lesperance M, Lau F, and Syme A (2007). Development and reliability testing of the Victoria Bowel Performance Scale (BPS). *Journal of Pain and Symptom Management*, **34**(5), 513–21.

Health and Safety Executive (1992a). *Manual handling operations regulations*. The Stationery Office, London.

Health and Safety Executive (1992b). *The personal protective equipment at work regulations*. The Stationery Office, London.

Heaton KW, Radvan J, Cripps H, Braddon FE, and Hughes AO (1992). Defaecation frequency and timing, and stool form in the general population: a prospective study. *Gut*, **33**(6), 818–24.

Kyle G (2006). Assessment and treatment of older patients with constipation. *Nursing Standard*, **21**(8), 41–6.

Kyle G (2007). Norgine risk assessment tool for constipation. *Nursing Times*, **103**(47), 48–9.

Matiti M, Cotrel-Gibbons E, and Teasdale K (2007). Promoting patient dignity in healthcare settings. *Nursing Standard*, **21**(45), 46–52.

Nursing and Midwifery Council (2005). *Guidelines for records and record keeping*. NMC, London.

Nursing and Midwifery Council (2007). *Standards for medicines management*. NMC, London.

Nursing and Midwifery Council (2008). *The Code: standards of conduct, performance and ethics for nurses and midwives*. NMC, London.

Price B (2001). Tackling embarrassment. *Nursing Standard*, **16**(13), 47–53.

Richmond JP and Wright ME (2005). Development of a constipation risk assessment scale. *Clinical Effectiveness in Nursing*, **9**, 37–48.

Royal College of Nursing (2008). *Bowel care including digital rectal examination and manual removal of faeces*. RCN, London.

Useful further reading and websites

Kyle G (2007). Developing a risk assessment tool for constipation. *Continence UK*, **1**(1), 38–43.

Richmond J (2003). Prevention of constipation through risk management. *Nursing Standard*, **17**(16), 9–46.

Royal College of Nursing (2005). *Good practice in infection prevention and control*. RCN, London.

http://victoriahospice.org/ed_tools.html

http://www.nmc-uk.org/

http://www.romecriteria.org

http://www.ibsgroup.org/main/bristolstool.shtml

 Answers to patient scenarios

1 An inability to retain rectal medication implies that the patient may have poor muscle tone. The medical staff should be informed and an alternative treatment should be considered.

2 There are no contraindications to mobilizing following the administration of rectal medication. Assuming that Gloria is safe to mobilize (a manual handling risk assessment should be performed), you should offer reassurance and reiterate that she may suddenly experience an urge to defecate.

3 It is possible to administer an enema safely with the patient adopting an alternative position. However, care must be taken to prevent injury or trauma to the bowel. A referral regarding Donald's hip pain should be considered.

10.6 **Stoma care**

Definition

The three main types of stoma are colostomy, ileostomy, and urostomy. 'Stoma' is a Greek word for mouth or opening. The term in this context refers to an artificial opening on the abdominal surface created surgically to divert the passage of urine and faeces. Colostomy is an opening from the colon or large bowel, ileostomy is an opening from the ileum or small bowel, and urostomy is an opening from the urinary tract.

Stoma care is the term used to describe the nursing care that the patient will need because they have (or will have) a stoma to enable them to resume the kind of lifestyle that they define as normal and acceptable.

It is important to remember that:

- Patients with a stoma may feel ashamed and have low self-esteem that is probably due to the resulting uncontrollable diversion of the body waste. This change in body image requires sensitive and empathetic support from the nurse.
- A well-informed nurse can advise and educate the patient to enable them to come to terms with this change and adapt their lifestyle accordingly. Every patient is an individual and will react differently to their situation.
- A flexible approach to care planning is necessary to meet these individual concerns and anxieties and ensure a successful outcome. This can be very challenging but also very rewarding for the nurse.
- It is essential that there is a clinical nurse specialist in stoma care to provide a focus of expertise in the care of these patients, as most nurses do not possess the necessary specific skills.

Prior knowledge

Before attempting stoma care, make sure you are familiar with:

1 Anatomy of the small and large bowel and urinary tract.
2 Physiology of the digestive system and urinary system.
3 Pathophysiology of common colorectal and urology disorders.

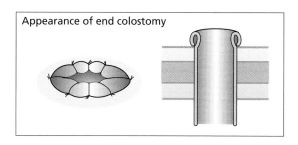

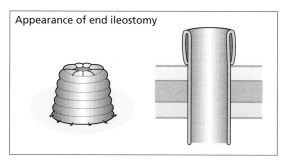

Figure 10.19 A terminal colostomy and a terminal ileostomy. Reproduced with permission of Coloplast Ltd from An Introduction to Stoma Care (2000).

Background

To form a stoma, the bowel (ileum or colon) is surgically divided and the ends brought to the surface of the abdomen as a loop or end stoma (**Figure 10.19**).

A loop stoma is formed when a loop of bowel is brought to the surface of the abdomen and opened. It can be supported by a rod (**Figure 10.20**). The loop has two ends, the non-functional or distal end and the functional or proximal end. Stomas may be temporary or permanent. A temporary stoma is formed to divert faeces from the anastomosis to allow it to heal or to bypass an obstruction in the distal bowel. The stoma can be reversed when the anastomosis has healed or after further surgery to remove the obstruction.

A permanent stoma cannot be reversed when there has been loss of normal function, most commonly with cancer of the rectum and inflammatory bowel disease, or when the rectum and anus have been removed.

Psychosocial aspects

Patients undergoing surgery involving a stoma may face various problems and uncertainties. The stoma surgery may be required for many reasons and this will have

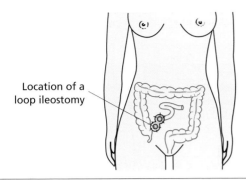

Location of a
loop ileostomy

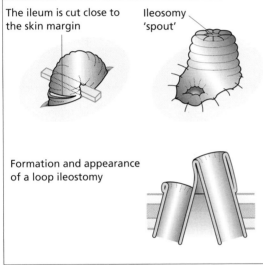

The ileum is cut close to
the skin margin

Ileosomy
'spout'

Formation and appearance
of a loop ileostomy

Figure 10.20 Loop ileostomy. Reproduced with permission of Coloplast Ltd from An Introduction to Stoma Care (2000).

implications on psychological recovery. The stoma may be temporary or permanent, the underlying condition curative or palliative, and it may even have been an emergency procedure with minimal pre-operative preparation.

The patient is in a position where they have to cope with a complex 'rollercoaster' of emotional, social, and physical problems associated with the newly formed stoma (Williams 2005). Psychological adaptation and successful rehabilitation are potentially achievable through careful and comprehensive assessment, facilitating further understanding of individual patient, family, and community needs (Borwell 2006).

Bowel function in many cultures is considered to be private and the patient may learn self-care very quickly, finding it unbearable for the nurse to deal with such a personal function. Conversely, some patients may be reluctant to learn, viewing bag changing as a medical matter. In Western society, children are often taught

Box 10.9 Main psychological concerns of stoma patients

- Not being complete as a person.
- General impact of stoma on life (e.g. 'rules my life').
- Feeling in control of body.
- Whether other people will hear or smell stoma.
- Effect on personal relationships and sexual function.
- Being able to deal with stoma care.

Adapted from White (1999). Courtesy of *Nursing Times*.

that body waste is 'dirty'. In later life when the patient is faced with the situation of having an artificial anus on the abdomen and having to deal actively with body waste, this is contrary to previous learning and requires a vast alteration in body image (Virgin-Elliston and Williams 2005).

White (1999) emphasizes that nurses should routinely screen for the most commonly occurring psychological concerns (**Box 10.9**), and should not assume that a patient will mention concerns as this is not always the case. Patients may actively avoid discussing them for fear that it is not appropriate or that this will result in a waste of a busy member of staff's time.

Radical pelvic surgery can create difficulties with sexual function in both men and women (Philips 1998). Physical problems are often compounded by the psychological impact of stoma formation (Fillingham 2006). Surgery can result in damage to the nerves that control ejaculation and erection, and cause sexual dysfunction in men. In women undergoing this type of surgery, dyspareunia or painful intercourse can be a problem. Human beings have the need for sexual expression throughout life, despite disabilities and major illness. What appears to concern many stoma patients is the issue of when and how to disclose that they have a stoma to others without the fear of rejection by individuals who are close to them (Williams 2005).

A patient who has experienced a change in body image will need much support and encouragement from the nurse. They may need to discuss their thoughts and concerns continually in order to come to terms with this change. The nurse should enlist the help of the patient's family to encourage acceptance (Virgin-Elliston and Williams 2005). Developing strategies to enhance personal appearance and achievement will help to improve self-confidence, self-esteem, and body presentation, and is a positive helping technique (Borwell 2006).

Types of stoma

There are three main types of stoma:

1 Colostomy.
2 Ileostomy.
3 Urostomy.

Colostomy

This is an opening into the colon. A colostomy is usually sited in the left iliac region and usually protrudes 0.5–1 cm above the abdominal wall.

The output will depend on the portion of the colon that has been utilized; flatus will appear initially followed by faecal fluid. The output will have a typical faecal odour and must be drained frequently to prevent overfilling and leakage. It may take 5–6 days before a formed stool is passed, usually around the time the patient has resumed a full diet, and an opaque or clear closed appliance with a filter can be used at this stage.

If there is a rod *in situ*, it may be removed after 6–10 days on instruction from the surgeon. The plastic rod is positioned under the loop of bowel and prevents retraction of the bowel back into the abdomen. It is easily removed; one end of the rod swivels and can be straightened and pulled gently from beneath the stoma. This should be painless; if there is any resistance, medical advice should be sought.

Ileostomy

This is an opening into the ileum. An ileostomy is usually situated in the right iliac region and will be everted to form a spout (Brook 1952) to a length of 3–5 cm to avoid skin excoriation.

The output will be green and copious initially and will usually commence within the first 48 hours. The output will be 1000–1200 ml per day and will then reduce to 600–800 ml within 24 hours. The appliance must be drained frequently and all output must be observed, measured, and recorded to avoid dehydration. There will be little or no odour. An opaque/clear drainable appliance will be used for an ileostomy. The output will eventually have a 'porridge-like' consistency.

If there is a bridge *in situ*, ensure the appliance fits under the plastic rod and around the stoma, protecting the peristomal skin from the effluent. The effluent from an ileostomy contains enzymes that will cause skin breakdown on contact, therefore careful skin hygiene is very important.

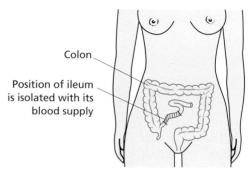

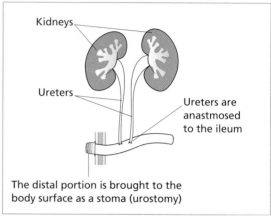

Figure 10.21 Formation of an ileal conduit. Reproduced with permission of Coloplast Ltd from An Introduction to Stoma Care (2000).

Urostomy

This is an opening into the urinary tract. There are two common types of urostomy, ileal conduit and ureterostomy. The most popular type is the ileal conduit (**Figure 10.21**). The procedure involves diverting the ureters into a segment of ileum with its blood supply, approximately 10–15 cm in length. This acts as a passageway to the abdominal surface. Urine will immediately flow and output must be observed, measured, and recorded.

Stents are often used to ensure urine drainage in case of oedema of the ureters post-operatively. The stents are normally held in place by a dissolvable suture and can be gently removed after 6–10 days on the instruction of the surgeon. The urine will contain mucus produced by the bowel and this is normal. A drainable appliance with a tap is used and another larger capacity drainage bag can be connected at night to prevent sleep disturbance. All stoma sutures that are not dissolvable are usually removed on the tenth post-operative day.

Reasons for stoma formation

- Carcinoma of the rectum or bowel.
- Diverticular disease.
- Obstruction.
- Inflammatory bowel disease.
- Radiation enteritis.
- Familial adenomatous polyposis.
- Carcinoma of the bladder.
- Traumatic injury.
- Ischaemic bowel.
- Faecal or urinary incontinence.
- Congenital conditions (e.g. necrotizing enterocolitis, Hirschsprung's disease).

Stoma siting

The choice of position for a stoma is extremely important if the patient is to live a full and active life after surgery. Pre-operative siting is essential as a badly positioned stoma can make subsequent appliance management difficult and thus have severe repercussions on patients' lifestyles (Breckman 2005). A clinical nurse specialist should site the stoma or, if unavailable, a Registered Nurse with agreed competencies (RCN 2002).

The site is located within the rectus abdominus sheath as this reduces the risk of developing a parastomal hernia (Blackley 1998). Most colostomies are sited on the left iliac fossa and ileostomies and urostomies on the right iliac fossa.

The site should be on a flat area of the abdomen, avoiding abdominal contours and previous scars, and be accessible and visible to the patient. It is important to explain the procedure to the patient and involve them in the process. Various positions should be adopted to evaluate the site: sitting, standing, bending, and lying flat.

Areas to avoid

- The waistline.
- Bony prominences.
- Previous scars, skin creases, and folds.
- Umbilicus.
- Pendulous breasts.
- Groin areas.
- Straps or belts for attachment to prosthesis.
- Incision site.

The stoma should be sited away from these areas (**Figure 10.22**), as they will impair the secure fitting of an appliance. It should be remembered that the patient may gain or lose weight following surgery, or develop further if a child. The stoma should be sited higher on a protuberant abdomen.

Other considerations include:

- Physical ability.
- Eyesight.
- Occupation.
- Hobbies.
- Position of waistband.
- Wearing of prosthesis.
- Wheelchair users.
- Skin conditions, e.g. psoriasis.
- Cultural beliefs.

Patients from certain ethnic minorities may wish to have their stoma sited above the waistline. Muslim patients

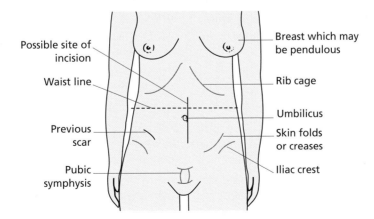

Figure 10.22 Stoma siting.

tend to be very particular about cleanliness, and faeces are considered unclean; a stoma sited above the waistline is considered food content and therefore acceptable for the patient to self-care. It is essential that full discussion (with an interpreter if necessary) is organized to assess patient wishes (Black 2000).

Selection of appliance

The aim of supportive stoma care is to maximize the individual's potential for independent living. To achieve this aim, the selection of an appropriate, safe, and secure pouch is fundamental to building confidence and re-establishing social activities (Winney 2006).

The range of appliances can be confusing for both nurse and patient when choosing a suitable appliance. Advances in technology have revolutionized the range and choice of appliances now available (Black 2000). A stoma pouch is more than a receptacle for the collection of body waste; it plays an important part in psychological adjustment to stoma surgery. Comprehensive clinical assessment is the key to success (Winney 2006). The point at which stomal diversion occurs in the bowel pathway should first be ascertained. The amount of effluent produced will largely be determined by the amount of bowel above that diversion (Breckman 2005).

Appliances are generally divided into drainable or non-drainable (closed) types. These may also be one-piece or two-piece. One-piece pouches incorporate an adhesive flange to secure to the skin. Two-piece pouches have a separate adhesive flange or base plate that is secured to the skin. The pouch is then either clipped into position on the base plate or secured with an adhesive on the pouch. The pouches are available in clear and opaque versions. A clear version is preferable in the immediate post-operative period in order to visualize the stoma.

There are three main types:

- Closed pouches are worn where the output is formed. These pouches have charcoal filters to release and deodorize flatus. Usually worn by colostomists and changed once or twice per day.
- Drainable pouches are worn in the immediate post-operative period and where the output is liquid or semi-formed. The outlet can be secured with a clip or clamp or an integral closure mechanism. These

pouches also have filters. Usually worn by ileostomists and changed every 2–3 days.
- Urostomy pouches are worn where the output is urine or fluid effluent from an enterocutaneous fistula. Most types incorporate a non-return valve to prevent back flow and a tap outlet for emptying. Frequency of change varies but is usually every 2–3 days. It is important to remember that the pouch selected should be easy to apply, safe and skin-friendly, and leak and odour proof.

Context

 When to perform stoma care

Stoma care should be used to inform and support patients with a stoma pre- and post-operatively in the hospital setting, and also afterwards in the community setting to help them achieve physical and psychological rehabilitation.

Potential problems

Potential problems with stomas post-operatively include:

Ischaemia
Ischaemia may compromise the stoma as a result of an impaired blood supply. The stoma will appear a dusky purple or black when necrotic. Necrosis is due to an inadequate blood supply to the stoma. This may have occurred during surgery, or the skin opening may be too small, resulting in the oedematous stoma being constricted or the bowel being under tension. This may be due to obesity, distension of the abdomen, or surgical technique. If the ischaemia is superficial the tissue will 'slough' off the stoma and the stoma will function normally. Deeper ischaemia will need surgical revision.

Paralytic ileus
This is the absence of bowel sounds and failure to pass flatus. It is a temporary paralysis of a portion of the bowel, typically after abdominal surgery due to bowel handling. It should resolve within 48–72 hours.

High output from the stoma
High output from the stoma may cause electrolyte imbalance and pouch leakage. Large volumes of effluent

of up to several litres may be lost over the first few days following the initial action of the stoma. The sodium concentration of an ileostomy secretion is around 100–120 mmol/litre and this must be replaced to prevent dehydration (Nicholls 1996). An overfull pouch will also pull the appliance from the skin (Myers 1996).

Mucocutaneous separation

Mucocutaneous separation is the breakdown of the suture line securing the stoma to the abdominal wall; it can be partial or total. Apply protective powder if superficial, or hydrocolloid paste and stoma seals (available on prescription) as directed by the specialist nurse if deeper separation has occurred. This will provide protection from further faecal contamination and therefore promote healing. Larger areas of deep separation may require a wound assessment by the nurse specialist and also the tissue viability nurse specialist, and surgical correction may be necessary if granulation of tissues does not occur. Oedema is common in the immediate post-operative period and this should subside over the following 7 days. Careful measurement of stoma and application of appropriately sized pouch is important.

Retraction of stoma

This is when the stoma descends back into the abdominal cavity and does not protrude above the level of the skin (McCahon 1999). This is usually due to the bowel being under tension or weight gain. Leakages can be a major problem and stomahesive paste, seals, skin protective wafers, and use of convexity should be considered as advised by the specialist nurse. Convexity produces an outward curve on the flange and when applied to the stoma has the effect of pushing the stoma out and helping the stoma to go into the pouch rather than leaking onto peristomal skin (Black 2000).

Skin excoriation

This is not an uncommon problem. The cause of the skin excoriation should be assessed by the specialist nurse and rectified. It may be due to leakage of effluent onto the peristomal skin, possible allergy, or patient technique. The patient's pouch change technique should be examined for possible causes of the problem; to correct poor technique it is imperative to listen to the patient and pick up key points in what they are saying (Myers 1996). The use of

barrier cream or protective wipes may be helpful, and the pouch should be checked to make sure it is the right size and fits correctly. The aperture of the pouch should fit snugly around the stoma, ensuring no peristomal skin is left exposed. A referral to the dermatologist may be necessary if there is no improvement.

Other complications

Other complications that may occur following discharge into the community:

Prolapse of stoma is when a length of bowel prolapses out of the abdominal wall (Taylor 1999). The patient can be taught to reduce the prolapse in order to apply a pouch; a larger aperture and pouch may be necessary. This is most commonly seen in transverse loop colostomies. Surgical intervention may be necessary.

Herniation is when the abdominal muscle is not strong enough and the bowel pushes against the abdomen causing a spherical bulge around the stoma (McCahon 1999). The size of herniation varies from patient to patient and can cause considerable distress. A surgical support can be fitted for patient comfort and the appliance needs to be flexible to mould around the hernia. Surgical intervention may be necessary.

The introduction of integrated care pathways with both professionals and voluntary support agencies working together would help to ease the new stoma patient through the transition of rehabilitation (Black 2000).

Special considerations

Choosing a pouch

When choosing a pouch, think about:

- Type of stoma.
- Nature of output and stoma function.
- Mental ability.
- Physical ability (to include visual ability).
- Peristomal skin condition.
- Personal choice/lifestyle.
- Abdominal shape.
- Stoma length, size, shape.

Post-operative care

In the immediate post-operative period the physical care of the patient is the priority and the responsibility of the

Box 10.10 Aspects of physical care

Ewing identified key aspects of physical care of the stoma, from the literature, as requirements for self-management of the stoma pouch:

- Preparation of equipment.
- Preparation of patient.
- Removal of old appliance.
- Skin care.
- Skin protection.
- Selection of the new appliance.
- Preparation of the new appliance.
- Disposal.

Adapted from Ewing (1989)

nurse until they feel well enough to participate and learn the procedure. Ewing (1989), in her study of nursing preparation of stoma patients, concluded that if ostomates are not given the opportunity to practise skills while in hospital, their competence of stoma pouch management will be compromised and so delay their return to their previous lifestyle.

The main difficulty for ostomates is adjusting to their loss of control over elimination. This may be regained in some way through proficient management of the stoma bag, which needs a coordinated approach of support and guidance from nursing staff in hospital. Information in the form of a chart may be helpful for the patient and staff to aid teaching and self-management (see **Box 10.10**) and can be used in conjunction with nursing care plans.

This framework encourages the patient to take a step-by-step approach to stoma care and takes into account the changing needs of the patient with regard to management of the pouch. It is also necessary to consider ways in which nursing care can be provided to meet these changing needs. This was accomplished using Orem's nursing model.

Orem's (1991) five helping methods can be utilized to develop a care plan:

1   *Acting for another* – nurse performs care.
2   *Teaching* – nurse performs task, explaining how it is done.
3   *Guiding* – patient takes over care with nurse supervision.

4   *Supporting* – patient performs care with nurse providing psychological support.
5   *Providing a developmental environment* – a safe, private environment to maintain patient dignity and an empathetic approach by nurse.

The helping methods increase self-care from a high level of nursing intervention to a low level prior to discharge. Patient motivation should be improved with a more coordinated approach to care by the nurse. Patients should be involved in care planning, and stoma care should be broken down into basic tasks for the patient to complete (Box 10.10), beginning with equipment preparation and moving through the tasks.

Patients should be encouraged to be involved in stoma care at their own pace and not coerced to move on before they are physically and mentally ready to do so. Consideration should also be given to patients' lack of knowledge, skills, motivation, and any behaviour limited by social and cultural norms. Anxiety can be a barrier to learning. Information retention is poor if patients are anxious about their illness and its effects. Anxious patients commonly deny receiving teaching or information although it has been provided.

Patient attitudes to post-operative care Kelly and Henry (1992) conducted a study examining stoma patients' perceptions of the help they received in preparing for surgery and coping afterwards. They concluded that patients became angry and frustrated due to lack of support post-operatively to help them cope with the many anxieties experienced both physically and psychologically. They felt, on comparison with other studies, that the negative behaviours were due to lack of knowledge and skills in coping with pouch changes, and not necessarily fear of disease or stoma.

Specific tasks in post-operative care Post-operative aims and objectives, and preparation for discharge into the community:

- It is important that the stoma is monitored in the immediate post-operative period. The condition of the stoma (it should be pink and moist) and its function should be recorded.

- Ensure a suitable, comfortable, leak-proof pouch is fitted to contain effluent.
- Supply a stock of pouches and accessories for use.
- Encourage the patient to look at the stoma and accept its existence.
- Discuss the outcome of the surgery with the patient.
- Teach the patient to care for the stoma.
- Provide opportunities for counselling and confidential discussion of problems; explore potential psychological problem areas.
- Inform the patient how to obtain future supplies of pouches and accessories.
- Explain the dietary principles to the patient, including what foods may result in alteration in stoma function.
- Discuss rehabilitation and explain any restrictions in activity.
- Explain to patient what help and support is available after discharge and how this may be obtained.
- Ensure patient is in possession of all the information required prior to discharge.
- Liaise with the colorectal/stoma care nurse specialist.

Complications of stomas

Research has demonstrated that approximately 15% of ostomists experience complications of one form or another during the first year following surgery (Wade 1988). Stomal problems not only cause management difficulties but also affect the patient's psychological well-being and create lifestyle issues (Pringle and Swan 2001).

Procedure

Preparation

Prepare yourself

Ensure you understand how the equipment works, and how to remove and position the new appliance.

Prepare the patient

The procedure should be fully explained to the patient. Psychological support and active listening are vital before, during, and after this procedure.

These procedural guidelines contain the basic information needed for changing a stoma appliance. Modifications may be made according to the following factors:

- Place of change, which may be bathroom or bedside, preferably bathroom if possible.
- Person changing the appliance, which may be nurse or patient.
- Type of appliance used, which may be one- or two-piece, closed or drainable.
- Any accessories used, such as protective wafers, powder, paste, or barrier creams/wipes, etc.

Prepare the equipment

- Container holding tissues, new appliances, disposal bags for used appliances and tissues, relevant accessories.
- Measuring guide.
- Bowl of warm water.
- Jug for contents of appliance.

Step-by-step guide to stoma care

Step	Rationale
1 Introduce yourself, confirm the patient's identity, explain the procedure, and obtain consent.	To identify the patient correctly and gain informed consent.
2 Ensure privacy. The patient should be in a suitable and comfortable position where they will be able to watch the procedure.	To respect patient dignity. To enhance patient understanding of procedure.

continued overleaf

3	Wash and dry hands or use antibacterial hand rub. Put on a disposable apron and disposable gloves.	To reduce the risk of contamination and cross-infection.
4	Place disposable absorbent towel over patient's clothing.	To protect patient's clothing and avoid unnecessary soiling.
5	If the bag is of the drainable type, empty the contents into a jug before removing the bag.	To avoid spillage of appliance contents.
6	To remove the appliance, peel the adhesive away from the skin with one hand while exerting gentle pressure on the skin with the other.	To avoid unnecessary discomfort for patient and avoid skin stripping.
7	Remove excess faeces or mucus from the skin with a dry tissue.	To facilitate cleaning of the stoma.
8	Wash the skin and stoma gently until they are clean with warm tap water and unscented soap. Dry thoroughly.	To avoid skin irritation and ensure adhesion of new appliance to skin.
9	Examine the skin and stoma for soreness, ulceration, or other unusual phenomena. If the skin is unblemished and the stoma is a healthy pink/red colour, proceed.	To identify any problems to report to the specialist nurse.
10	Apply a clean appliance, checking that it is the correct size for the stoma using the measuring guide.	To avoid skin irritation.
11	Dispose of used appliance and other equipment in a clinical waste bag and place in an appropriate plastic bin according to hospital policy. Wash and dry your hands.	To ensure safe disposal and reduce the risk of cross-infection.

Following the procedure

Ensure the procedure is recorded in the relevant patient case notes. The level of patient participation should also be noted.

Prior to discharge into the community

The transition from hospital to home can be daunting for the patient. Ensure patients are proficient in stoma care and have the information they need to feel confident.

- Self-care – patient should be competent and able to change appliance, or carer taught to manage care.
- Disposal – stoma pouches should be emptied if drainable type prior to removal, and then sealed in a plastic bag and disposed of in the household waste.
- Supplies – GP and patient are informed of details of surgery and of stoma equipment for ongoing prescription purposes. Patients with permanent stomas are exempt from prescription charges. Initial supplies are given from hospital to allow for transition to home. Further stoma equipment supplies are obtained with a prescription from the local chemist or from specialist suppliers who will deliver directly to the patient's home.
- Help available – if patient/carer unable to manage self-care of stoma, liaison with community services to arrange ongoing care of stoma.

- Written information given – regarding care of stoma and possible problems that may occur, obtaining supplies, disposal, physical activity, and diet. A well-balanced diet and fluid intake should be encouraged. The specialist nurse will have discussed specific information needs with the patient.
- Specialist nurse – details given regarding further contact for ongoing care, telephone number for advice and information, stoma clinic dates and times, and home visits as necessary.
- Voluntary organizations – for further information and support.

Reflection and evaluation

When you have undertaken stoma care with a patient, think about the following questions:

1 Did you anticipate the patient's reaction to the procedure?
2 Were you able to reassure the patient?
3 Did your assessment of the stoma alert you to any potential problems?
4 Were you able to make an evaluation of the patient's level of participation with the procedure?

Further learning opportunities

At the next opportunity, arrange to 'shadow' the clinical nurse specialist to gain a more in-depth understanding of stoma care.

Reminders

Don't forget:

- Provide the patient with a clear explanation of the procedure.
- A flexible approach to care planning is necessary to meet the individual needs of the patient.
- Select an appropriate, safe, and secure pouch to contain effluent.

Patient scenarios

Consider what you should do in the following situations, then turn to the end of this skill to check your answers.

1 Patient A has been informed that they will need to have stoma formation surgery. How would you address the patient's concerns?
2 Patient B, who has had an end colostomy formed following cancer surgery, has been fitted with a clear, drainable pouch. What is the purpose of a clear pouch and what specific observations of the stoma are necessary?
3 Patient C is recovering from stoma formation surgery. How would you prepare them for discharge home?

Website

 http://www.oxfordtextbooks.co.uk/orc/ endacott

You may find it helpful to work through our short online quiz and additional scenarios intended to help you to develop and apply the skills in this chapter.

References

Black PK (2000). *Holistic stoma care*. Bailliere Tindall, London.

Blackley P (1998). *Practical stoma wound management*. Research Publications, Victoria, Australia.

Borwell B (2006). Psychological aspects of care for the stoma patient. In CREST. *Caring for stoma patients*. Clinimed, High Wycombe.

Breckman B, ed (2005). *Stoma care and rehabilitation*. Elsevier Churchhill Livingstone, London.

Brook BN (1952). The management of an ileostomy including its complications. *Lancet*, **2**, 102–4.

Ewing G (1989). The nursing preparation of stoma patients for self care. *Journal of Advanced Nursing*, **14**, 411–20.

Fillingham S (2006). Post operative sexual function. In CREST. *Caring for stoma patients*. Clinimed, High Wycombe.

Kelly M and Henry T (1992). A thirst for practical knowledge. *Professional Nurse*, **7**(6), 350–6.

McCahon S (1999). Faecal stomas. In T Porrett and N Daniel, eds. *Essential coloproctology for nurses*, pp.165–87. Whurr Publishers Ltd, London.

Myers C, ed (1996). *Stoma care nursing*. Arnold, London.

Nicholls RJ (1996). Surgical procedures. In C Myers, ed. *Stoma care nursing*, pp. 90–122. Arnold, London.

Orem D (1991). *Nursing: concepts of practice*. McGraw Hill, New York.

Philips RKS, ed (1998). *Colorectal surgery*. WB Saunders Company Ltd, London.

Pringle W and Swan E (2001). Continuing care after discharge from hospital for stoma patients. *British Journal of Nursing*, **10**(19), 1275–88.

Royal College of Nursing (2002). *Colorectal and stoma care nursing*, 2nd edition. RCN, London.

Taylor P, ed (1999). *Stoma care in the community*. Emap Healthcare Ltd, London.

Virgin-Elliston T and Williams L (2005). Psychological considerations in stoma care. In C Elcoat, ed. *Stoma care nursing*, 2nd edition, pp. 55–63. Hollister Ltd, Reading.

Wade B (1988). *A stoma is for life.* Scutari Press, Middlesex.

White C (1999). Psychological aspects of stoma care. In P Taylor, ed. *Stoma care in the community*, pp. 89–109. Emap Healthcare Ltd, London.

Williams J (2005). Psychological issues in stoma care. In T Porrett and A McGrath, eds. *Stoma care*, pp. 157–68. Blackwell Publishing Ltd, Oxford.

Winney J (2006). Novice-Stoma Appliance Selection. In CREST. *Caring for stoma patients*. Clinimed, High Wycombe.

Useful further reading and websites

Jones DJ, ed (1999). *ABC of colorectal diseases*, 2nd edition. BMJ books, London.

Royal College of Nursing (2002). *Caring for people with colorectal problems.* RCN, London.

Salter M (1997). *Altered body image*, 2nd edition. Bailliere Tindall, London.

White CA (1997). *Living with a stoma*. Sheldon Press, London.

British Association of Cancer Unit Patients: **http://www.cancerbacup.org.uk**

Colostomy Association: **http://www.bcass.org.uk**

Core (formerly known as Digestive Disorders Foundation): **http://www.corecharity.org.uk**

Ileostomy and internal pouch support group: **http://www.the-ia.org.uk**

National Association for Colitis and Crohn's Disease (NACC): **http://www.nacc.org.uk**

Urostomy Association: **http://www.uagbi.org**

Ⓐ Answers to patient scenarios

1 Advise and educate the patient about the surgery and the implications for their lifestyle in a sensitive manner, answering their questions and concerns, and reassuring them that more help, support, and information will be given throughout their hospital stay. It is important not to overwhelm patients with too much information; it should be given in stages when the patient is able to absorb it.

2 To facilitate observation of the stoma. Colour of stoma, size, output, and condition of surrounding skin.

3 Ensure patient is able to perform stoma care independently and has had the opportunity to discuss any concerns. A nurse specialist should be involved to make discharge arrangements. Liaison and transfer of care to nursing team as necessary, and GP with ordering information details regarding stoma equipment.

10.7 **Administering parenteral nutrition** Ⓐ

This is an advanced skill. You *must* check whether you can assist with or undertake this skill, in line with local policy.

Definition

Parenteral nutrition is the delivery of a nutritionally complete solution directly into a vein.

It is important to remember that:

- The initiation of parenteral feeding should only occur as a result of comprehensive nutritional assessment and multidisciplinary discussion.
- Care and therapy should be directed towards meeting patients' nutritional needs via less invasive mechanisms, which can have significant advantages over artificial support.
- While parenteral nutrition is an effective method of meeting certain patients' nutritional needs, it carries a high complication risk and can be fatal.
- The administration of parenteral nutrition will usually involve the use of a **central venous catheter** (CVC). These devices create significant risks to the patient, both on insertion and throughout the duration of

therapy. Nurses should only care for these devices and provide therapy using them after training and demonstrated competence.

Prior knowledge

Before administering parenteral nutrition, make sure you are familiar with:

1 Universal infection control practice.
2 The normal processes involved in the acquisition of nutrients.
3 Normal nutritional requirements.
4 Factors influencing nutrition in health care.
5 The relevant vascular anatomy.
6 You also need to be competent in the administration of intravenous drugs and in the care of a patient with a centrally placed venous access device (CVC).

Background

McWhirter and Pennington (1994) suggest that 40% of patients admitted to hospital are undernourished and that nutritional status in these patients often continues to deteriorate during the course of hospital stay. The detrimental effects of malnutrition are well documented (Leather *et al.* 2003). Nutritional assessment and the institution of support where necessary can improve patient outcome (NICE 2006).

While enteral feeding is the preferred route of nutritional support in terms of cost and mechanical, septic, and metabolic complications (Mercadante 1998), parenteral nutrition should be considered if this route is unavailable or contraindicated.

Parenteral nutrition (PN) may be short term, long term, or permanent. It may be targeted to meet total nutritional requirements or be used to supplement nutritional requirements while other methods of support are being established.

Route of administration

PN is predominantly administered via a large central vein. This is because the solution is hyperosmolar and can be irritant to small peripheral veins, causing thrombophlebitis. Common veins used include the internal jugular and subclavian veins. Femoral vessels are avoided

for PN as they carry an increased risk of infection, possibly due to bacterial colonization of this area (Merrer *et al.* 2001, McGee and Gould 2003). Subclavian vein lines are favoured as the patient's head and neck movement is not restricted, although the risk of pneumothorax on insertion may be higher.

Some devices are tunnelled under the skin (tunnelled line). This means that the insertion site through the skin, the portal for bacterial contamination, is away from the point at which the catheter enters the blood vessel, reducing the risk of contamination/infection. Tunnelled subclavian lines are recommended for long-term use (more than 30 days) (NICE 2006). Certain catheters are made from special hypoallergenic materials that allow them to remain *in situ* for many months.

For short-term use a single lumen catheter may be used. The flow of infusion fluid must not be interrupted for the administration of drugs/fluid, etc., as this will lead to an increased infection risk. This has led to the use of multiple lumen access devices (see **Figure 10.23**) to allow concurrent central venous pressure monitoring or administration of drugs/fluids. When using these lines it is essential that the PN lumen is used only for PN. Many organizations label the PN lumen as 'PN feed only' to avoid access into that lumen. Access ports (three-way taps) should not be used on a PN lumen. It is also essential that access into or any handling of the line is performed with strict asepsis (EPIC 2001).

The use of peripherally inserted central catheters (PICCs) (see **Figure 10.24**) for the administration of PN is growing in popularity. Complications of central venous catheterization are many, and the use of these lines will

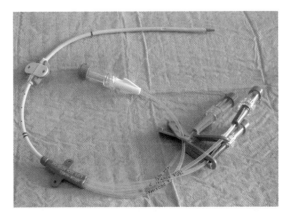

Figure 10.23 A multiple lumen central venous catheter.

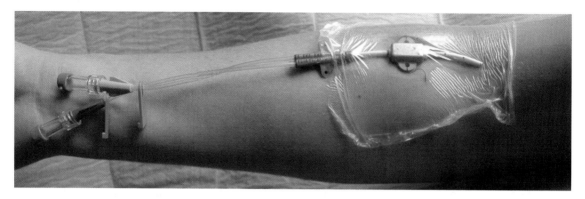

Figure 10.24 A double lumen peripherally inserted central catheter *in situ*.

Box 10.11 Potential complications with use of PICCs

- Mechanical phlebitis.
- Thrombophlebitis.
- Infection.
- Catheter blockage.
- Haemorrhage.
- Catheter malposition.

significantly reduce these risks (EPIC 2001). PICCs are inserted peripherally, usually through the basilic or cephalic veins, and threaded through the axillary vein into the lower third of the superior vena cava (Todd and Hammond 2004). The device can be inserted in the ward, outpatient clinic, or during a home visit (Brown 1989), although it should be inserted under aseptic conditions. Though PICCs are relatively easy to insert and carry significant cost advantages, they are not without complications. These are outlined in **Box 10.11**.

PN has been administered using peripheral venous access. However, this carries a large risk of phlebitis and should only be used in exceptional circumstances for short term (less than 14 days) provision of nutrition.

Storage of PN solutions

Storage of PN should be aimed at reducing bacterial contamination and maintaining solution stability. This may include refrigeration and/or protection from light. Protection from light may also be required during administration. Manufacturer's guidelines/pharmacy advice should be used.

Context

 When to administer PN

PN should be administered, following nutritional assessment, to the patient who is malnourished or at risk of becoming malnourished, where:

- The oral/enteral route is unsafe/inadequate.
- The gastrointestinal tract is dysfunctional.

This group may include:

- Patients in whom the intestine is compromised following major abdominal surgery.
- Patients with severe paralytic ileus.
- Patients with specific gastrointestinal conditions such as severe mucositis, perforation, intestinal fistulae, and severe acute pancreatitis where jejunal feeding is contraindicated.
- Patients with inflammatory bowel disorders such as Crohn's disease and ulcerative colitis refractory to treatment or during acute episodes.
- Patients with high output intestinal fistulae.
- Patients with high output stomas.

An electronic infusion device must be used during the administration of this PN.

 When not to administer PN

- When the patient does not give consent (or in the case of inability to provide consent, when it is not in the patient's best interests).

- Allergy to PN solution or any of its contents.
- There are no absolute contraindications to PN.

Alternative interventions

The enteral route of nutritional support is the preferred route. This is because of the lower complication risk, reduced complexity of management, and reduced need for highly invasive therapies. Unless contraindicated, attempts should be made to utilize the enteral route. These attempts should continue, if appropriate, following the commencement of PN, and the treatment goal should be providing all of the patient's nutritional requirements enterally.

Potential problems/complications

Infection

The incidence of catheter-related bloodstream infection as a result of central venous catheterization is difficult to quantify, as classification differs from study to study. However, it may be as high as 15%. Up to 25% of patients with catheter-related sepsis die (Pittet et al. 1994). PN fluid is an excellent environment for bacterial colonization, and is a significant risk factor in the development of catheter-related sepsis (Beghetto et al. 2005).

Many PN prescriptions are individualized, based on specific nutritional requirements, and are thus prepared in a pharmacy department. PN bags should be compounded under sterile conditions and great care must be taken to ensure that they are contamination free and that there is no risk of incompatibility problems (Colagiovanni 1997).

Pre-prepared bags may avoid contamination, but the components may not be suitable for specific patient needs. These bags will require reconstitution prior to administration; this usually requires breaking a seal within the bag and ensuring that the fluid is thoroughly mixed. Basic components of PN fluid are outlined in **Box 10.12**.

Access into the bags, for the purpose of adding supplementary additives following initial preparation, should be avoided. The administration of PN must occur under the most rigorous aseptic conditions, and once connected to the patient, no access should be made into the line or bag. Three-way taps/multiple infusion taps should

Box 10.12 Basic PN fluid composition

- Nitrogen source (amino acids).
- Carbohydrate source (glucose).
- Fats.
- Trace elements.
- Electrolytes.
- Vitamins.

not be used. Administration sets used for PN must be changed every 24 hours and immediately upon suspected contamination or when the integrity of the product or system has been compromised (RCN 2005).

Some organizations recommend the use of specifically designed inline filters to prevent particulate contamination of the infused fluid.

If catheter-related sepsis is suspected, urgent referral to senior nutritional/medical staff should be made.

Fluid overload

Most complete PN solutions will be 2–3 litre volumes, but this will differ based on nutritional requirements and fluid needs; for example, patients with end stage renal disease will require low volume solutions. Fluid overload may occur from the concurrent administration of fluids/blood products (Dougherty and Lister 2008).

Glucose imbalance (hyper/hypoglycaemia)

Hyperglycaemia may be a result of the glucose content of the infusion fluid. The administration of insulin may be required, particularly in diabetic patients, those with ongoing physiological stress, and those with pancreatic/metabolic dysfunction. Glucose control should be maintained using the intravenous route initially, although long-term established diabetic PN patients may return to subcutaneous administration.

Hypoglycaemia may occur as a result of discontinuing PN (rebound hypoglycaemia). This may be avoided by reducing the infusion rate gradually, or if not applicable the temporary administration of dextrose solutions.

Uraemia

A high blood level of urea may occur because of a high nitrogen content in the PN fluid. This may be complicated further by dehydration and renal dysfunction.

Hepatic dysfunction

Research suggests that artificial nutrition in critically ill patients can be associated with alterations in liver dysfunction biomarkers such as enzymes and serum bilirubin (Stehle 2007). This necessitates regular monitoring of liver function and enzymes for the duration of therapy.

Electrolyte imbalance

This may occur because of electrolyte concentrations in the PN fluid and any underlying disease process. Any electrolyte supplementation on top of PN administration should be discussed with the nutritional team.

Refeeding syndrome

This is a metabolic syndrome seen in the malnourished patient once feeding commences. The malnourished patient decreases insulin production in response to reduced carbohydrate load and utilizes fat and protein for energy with a resultant loss in intracellular electrolytes, particularly phosphate. The introduction of high glucose solutions stimulates the release of insulin and glucose; potassium and phosphate then move rapidly into the intracellular space with potentially disastrous effects. Gradual introduction of nutrition support in the severely malnourished patient and phosphate replacement have been discussed as ways to reduce the systemic effects of the syndrome (Hearing 2004, Dougherty and Lister 2008).

Mechanical problems

Catheter blockage may occur. This may be due to the tube 'clogging' or through patient position, with the catheter tip sitting against a vessel wall. The line may be flushed with saline, although this must be done with strict asepsis. Discontinuing the feed, e.g. for procedures, should be avoided. If this is required, the line should be flushed and locked according to organizational policy. It may be appropriate to discard any remaining solution and commence the next 24 hours' feed at the arranged time. However, this will reduce the patient's nutritional and fluid intake, and appropriate observations should be made, including those for rebound hypoglycaemia. Long delays in the delivery of PN should be avoided. Any catheter fracture should be reported immediately and the patient should be observed for signs of air embolus/ haemorrhage.

Phlebitis

Phlebitis is an acute inflammation of a vein directly linked to the presence of any vascular access device (Jackson 1998). The risk of phlebitis in central access is lower than with peripheral devices and PICC lines because of the fast dilution of fluid by the blood; however, all vascular access sites should be routinely assessed for signs and symptoms of phlebitis (RCN 2005). Phlebitis scoring tools should be incorporated into this practice (Jackson 1998).

Indications for assistance

Ideally a multidisciplinary team should oversee the nutritional management of the parenterally fed patient. This team will include dieticians, medical staff, ward/ community-based nurses, specialist nurses, pharmacists, and members of other professions allied to medicine.

Observations and monitoring

Because of the high infection and metabolic risks associated with PN, a rigid framework of observations should be followed (see **Box 10.13**).

Special considerations

Patients on PN therapy at home will require:

- Access to education, training, and information about managing their therapy.
- Access to appropriate resources.
- Support in managing their therapy.

NICE (2006) states that 'all people in the community having parenteral nutrition should be supported by a coordinated multidisciplinary team which includes input from specialist nutrition nurses, dieticians, GPs, pharmacists and district nurses.'

Procedure

Preparation

Prepare yourself

Wash your hands, put on a clean plastic apron. Ensure you are familiar with the electronic infusion device.

Box 10.13 Observations to undertake during parenteral feeding

- **General observations:** mental state, skin colour/tone.
- **Temperature:** should be recorded 4-hourly in initial stages; this frequency may be reduced in long-term, established community patients. An increased temperature would alert the practitioner to infection.
- **Pulse/blood pressure:** 4-hourly unless long-term, established patient. An increased pulse may indicate inflammatory response. The blood pressure may well be normal in compensation or may become lower than normal in late stages of systemic infection/sepsis.
- **Fluid balance** (continual).
- **Blood glucose:** near patient testing to detect hypo/hyperglycaemia (see Section 10.2). Four-hourly from initiation of therapy until stable. In the sick/diabetic patient this monitoring should continue until therapy is well established. The patient

should also be monitored for any obvious signs of hypo/hyperglycaemia.
- **Weight:** daily, as an indicator of fluid balance and to assess nutritional status.
- **Blood chemistry:** to include urea, creatinine, standard electrolyte screen, liver enzymes, phosphate, magnesium, and trace elements. Bloods will be required daily in early treatment; trace elements need only be measured weekly. The frequency of observation will decrease as the patient becomes more established on therapy. Regular monitoring will highlight biochemical derangement early.
- **Blood count:** to include white cell count, haemoglobin, and platelet count. White cell count may be an early indicator of infection.

Other aspects of care should also be assessed to prevent deterioration, for example regular oral assessments.

Prepare the patient

See Discussing the procedure box.

Prepare the equipment

- Ensure that the PN fluid is correct against the prescription, within valid expiry date, and noted for use on correct date. In some organizations this process will involve qualified nurses.
- Ascertain that the bag's patient registration number corresponds with prescription/patient.
- Ensure that the bag of feed has been stored according to the manufacturer's recommendations and local policy.
- Check that the PN fluid is not contaminated/separated/precipitated.
- Ensure that the electronic infusion device is plugged into the mains supply.

Discussing the procedure with the patient and family

- Explain why the patient is receiving PN.
- Discuss the procedure of connection to PN.
- Explore any anxieties or fears about therapy, encourage questions.
- Explain observations and subsequent ongoing care/therapy as a result of PN administration.
- Discuss potential effects that may arise from the administration of PN fluid.
- Educate the patient to be vigilant and report signs of infection.
- Explain any sounds/displays emitted from the electronic infusion device.
- Educate the patient to report any alarm sound from the pump.

Step-by-step guide to administering parenteral nutrition

Step		Rationale
1	Introduce yourself, confirm the patient's identity, explain the procedure, and obtain consent.	To identify the patient correctly and gain informed consent.
2	Combine the component admixtures of the PN fluid if required.	To prepare the solution for administration.
3	Open sterile dressing pack.	To create sterile field.
4	Place sterile administration set, gloves, and any connectors/filters on sterile dressing pack with any other equipment required.	To prepare sterile equipment for use.
5	Hang PN fluid container on drip stand. Spray the connecting port on the bag with alcohol spray/swab according to organizational policy. Allow to dry.	To allow gravity priming of administration set. To prevent contamination at PN reservoir.
6	Donning a pair of sterile gloves, assemble the administration set and filter (if used). Connect the administration set to the port on the bag without touching the set spike or inner aspect of the infusion port. Keep the distal end of the administration set on the sterile field.	To maintain asepsis/prevent contamination.
7	Prime the administration set/filter (if used). Ensure clamp is 'on'.	To purge the set of air and prevent air embolus.
8	Clean the access site/port with alcohol spray/swab according to organizational policy. Allow to dry. Place a sterile dressing towel underneath the access port. Discard sterile gloves.	To maintain asepsis/prevent contamination.
9	Apply a fresh pair of sterile gloves. Ensure that the access line is clamped. Remove the line bung.	To prevent air embolus. To access line.
10	Using a 10 ml syringe, aspirate the line, withdrawing at least 5 ml of fluid. Longer tunnelled lines may require a greater volume to be aspirated.	To remove any previous flush/Heparin solution from line. To assess line patency.
11	Flush the line using at least 5 ml of sterile 0.9% sodium chloride solution.	To assess line patency.

12	Connect the primed administration set to the access port.	To deliver PN solution.
13	Load administration set into electronic infusion device.	To administer feed correctly.
14	Programme the total volume to be infused and the hourly rate of infusion into the electronic infusion device as appropriate. Press 'run' or appropriate button on device.	To administer feed at correct rate/volume (this will be governed by PN prescription). To commence therapy.

Following the procedure

- Observe the patient for an acute allergic reaction as this may occur with the administration of any intravenous injection/fluid.
- Commence ongoing observations as outlined in Box 10.13.
- Reinforce patient education.
- Sign the appropriate documentation to record administration.

Reflection and evaluation

When you have administered PN to a patient, think about the following questions:

1 Were you able to answer the patient's questions?
2 How will you monitor the effectiveness of the therapy?
3 Is a goal of meeting nutritional needs via another route a realistic possibility? If yes, in what time span? And what factors will influence this?
4 Did the patient experience any alteration in their own body image?

Further learning opportunities

At the next available opportunity, discuss with the nutritional team the patient's PN prescription and how this was calculated/formulated.

Reminders

Don't forget to:

- Document the procedure.
- Educate the patient to report signs and symptoms of infection.

Patient scenarios

Consider what you should do in the following situations, then turn to the end of this skill to check your answers.

1 A patient presents himself to the surgical ward on a Sunday afternoon. He is normally on a home PN regime supported by a community multidisciplinary team. He complains of feeling feverish and has localized redness around his tunnelled line. What would your course of action be?
2 A patient in the critical care unit has been commenced on a PN regime following an extensive small bowel resection. The electronic infusion device starts to alarm occlusion. What would your course of action be?

Website

http://www.oxfordtextbooks.co.uk/orc/ endacott

You may find it helpful to work through our short online quiz and additional scenarios intended to help you to develop and apply the skills in this chapter.

References

Beghetto MG, Victorino J, Teixeira L, and Azevedo MJ (2005). Parenteral nutrition as a risk factor for central venous catheter-related infection. *Journal of Parenteral and Enteral Nutrition,* **29**, 367–73.

Brown J (1989). Peripherally inserted central catheter use in home care. *Journal of Intravenous Therapy,* **12**(3), 144–50.

Colagiovanni L (1997). Parenteral nutrition. *Nursing Standard,* **12**(9), 39–43.

Dougherty L and Lister S (2008). *The Royal Marsden Hospital manual of clinical nursing procedures*, 7th edition. Blackwell Publishing, Oxford.

EPIC (2001). Guidelines for preventing infections associated with insertion and maintenance of central venous catheters. *Journal of Hospital Infection*, **47**, 47–67.

Hearing SD (2004). Refeeding syndrome is under diagnosed and under treated, but treatable. *British Medical Journal*, **328**, 908–9.

Jackson A (1998). Infection control: a battle in vein; infusion phlebitis. *Nursing Times*, **94**(4), 68–71.

Leather A, Bushell L, and Gillespie L (2003). The provision of nutritional support for people with cancer. *Nursing Times*, **99**(46), 53–5.

McGee DC and Gould MK (2003). Preventing complications of central venous catheterization. *New England Journal of Medicine*, **348**, 1123–33.

McWhirter JP and Pennington CR (1994). Incidence and recognition of malnutrition in hospital. *British Medical Journal*, **308**, 945–8.

Mercadante S (1998). Parenteral versus enteral nutrition in cancer patients: indications and practice. *Cancer Care*, **6**, 85–93.

Merrer J, De Jonghe B, Golliot F *et al.* (2001). Complications of femoral and subclavian venous catheterization in critically ill patients: a randomized controlled trial. *Journal of the American Medical Association*, **286**, 700–7.

National Institute for Health and Clinical Excellence (2006). *Nutrition support in adults: oral nutrition support, enteral tube feeding and parenteral nutrition, Clinical Guideline 32*. DH, London.

Pittet D, Tarara D, and Wenzel RP (1994). Nosocomial bloodstream infection in critically ill patients: excess length of stay, extra costs and attributable mortality. *Journal of the American Medical Association*, **272**, 1589–601.

Royal College of Nursing (2005). *Standards for infusion therapy*. RCN, London.

Stehle P (2007). Development of liver dysfunction under artificial nutrition: a reason to modify nutrition therapy in the intensive care unit? [online] **http://www.ccforum.com/content/11/1/112** accessed 09/09/08.

Todd J and Hammond P (2004). Choice and use of peripherally inserted central catheters by nurses. *Professional Nurse*, **19**(9), 493–7.

Useful further reading and websites

Ingram P and Lavery I (2005). Peripheral intravenous therapy: key risks and implications for practice. *Nursing Standard*, **19**(46), 55–64.

Oie S and Kamiya A (2005). Particulate and microbial contamination in in-use admixed parenteral nutrition solutions. *Biological and Pharmaceutical Bulletin*, **28**(12), 2268–70.

Zurcher M, Tramèr MR, and Walder B (2004). Colonization and bloodstream infection with single-versus multi-lumen central venous catheters: a quantitative systematic review. *Anaesthesia and Analgesia*, **99**, 177–82.

Tutorial on refeeding syndrome: **http://www. ccmtutorials.com/misc/phosphate/page_07.htm**

 Answers to patient scenarios

1   The immediate concern with this patient is catheter-related sepsis. Patient assessment should include a set of baseline observations including temperature. A comprehensive history taken from the patient will identify any other possible causes of infection. Microbiological samples will be required including 'fresh stab' blood cultures and a swab of the line site; blood cultures should also be taken from the PN line. Blood should also be taken for standard biochemical and haematological tests. A medical review should be requested at the earliest opportunity. The results of this review may include stopping the feed and possibly removing the line. If this does occur, rebound hypoglycaemia may ensue and glucose should be monitored. The patient should have contact numbers of his multidisciplinary support team. This team should be contacted at the earliest opportunity for advice/ support. Ideally the patient's management will consist of observing for systemic inflammatory response/decompensation, and anti-bacterial/antifungal therapy. The patient should be kept under close observation.

2   Initially the electronic infusion device and the administration set and access device should be checked for signs of malfunction or kinking. The patient's position should also be checked. If no cause for occlusion is found, the infusion device should be stopped and the access device should be aspirated

and flushed using an aseptic technique. If the access device is blocked and this is not remedied by changing patient position, expert advice should be sought. If the PN fluid is off for a period of time, observation should be made for rebound hypoglycaemia.

10.8 **Abdominal palpation**

This is an advanced skill. You *must* check whether you can assist with or undertake this skill, in line with local policy.

Definition

Abdominal palpation is examination of the patient's abdomen by touching. This section will focus mainly on the general principles of abdominal palpation in the context of clinical practice, and each technique will be described in detail.

Abdominal palpation is a crucial part of the abdominal examination as it often reveals the most information. Successful palpation requires appropriate examination technique, relaxed abdominal muscles, and patient cooperation. A complete abdominal palpation includes general palpation (light and deep), and palpation for liver, spleen, kidneys, abdominal aneurysm, gall bladder, and urinary bladder. Palpation of gravid uterus in pregnancy will not be covered in this section.

It is important to remember that:

- This skill is part of the complete abdominal examination. In addition to palpation, a complete assessment of the abdomen consists of inspection, **percussion**, and auscultation.
- Even though not all nursing staff are expected to perform all the skills described in this section, some nurses (e.g. community-based nurses) may find the information helpful and relevant to their roles.
- To get the most of out this skill, the patient should be appropriately positioned and exposed, with the presence of a chaperone if necessary.

Prior knowledge

Before carrying out abdominal palpation, make sure you are familiar with the surface anatomy of the abdomen and the various structures found inside the abdominal cavity.

Background

Basic anatomy of the abdomen

The abdomen is the part of the body situated between the chest and pelvis. The abdominal cavity is enclosed by the abdominal wall (front, sides, and back), which is formed by abdominal muscles, the vertebral column, and iliac bones. The abdominal cavity contains the organs of the digestive system such as the stomach, small intestine, colon, and appendix. In addition, organs such as the liver, gall bladder, and pancreas can be found in association with the digestive tract. Other important abdominal organs include the spleen, kidneys, and adrenal glands. Major vessels such as the abdominal aorta and inferior vena cava are situated within the abdominal cavity. The **peritoneum** is a membrane that forms the lining of the abdominal cavity. Most of the abdominal organs are covered by peritoneum. It provides support to the abdominal organs and contains blood vessels, lymphatic vessels, and nerves.

Surface anatomy

Traditionally, the abdomen is divided into nine regions (see **Figure 10.25**) for descriptive purposes by two horizontal lines and two vertical lines (Douglas *et al.* 2005). The upper horizontal line lies at the level of the first lumbar vertebra; it is also known as the transpyloric plane as it crosses the pylorus of the stomach. This plane is situated halfway between the suprasternal notch and the top of the symphysis pubis. The lower horizontal line (transtubercular plane) passes through the upper borders of the iliac crests at the level of the fifth lumbar vertebra. The two vertical lines pass vertically from the midinguinal points (point midway between the anterior superior spine and the pubic symphysis on each side) towards the midclavicular points.

A simpler way to divide the abdomen is into four quadrants at the level of the umbilicus.

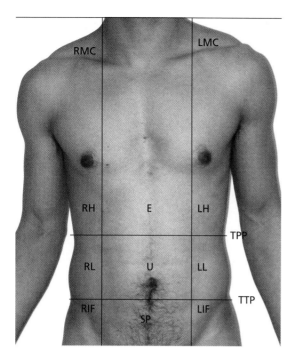

Figure 10.25 The nine regions of the abdomen. LMC – left midclavicular line; RMC – right midclavicular line; TPP – transpyloric plane; TTP – transtubercular plane. RH – right hypochondrium; LH – left hypochondrium; E – epigastrium; RL – right lumbar region; LL – left lumbar region; U – umbilical region; RIF – right iliac fossa; LIF – left iliac fossa; SP – suprapubic region (hypogastric region).

Abnormal findings on general palpation

Tenderness

A sign of discomfort during palpation. Tenderness is usually a useful indication of underlying pathology but it can be due to patient anxiety in the absence of other symptoms.

Rebound tenderness

This is a sensitive sign suggesting underlying peritoneal irritation or peritonitis. The sign is elicited when the abdominal wall is gently and slowly compressed, and is released rapidly, at which point the patient feels a sudden stab of pain. The alternative method to demonstrate the sign is to percuss gently over the area of tenderness on the abdominal wall.

Guarding

Voluntary guarding happens when the patient voluntarily contracts the abdominal muscles as a result of tenderness or anxiety. In the absence of other features of acute abdomen, voluntary guarding is unlikely to be abnormal. Involuntary guarding is seen in peritonitis as a result of a reflex contraction of the overlying abdominal muscles.

Rigidity

This is constant involuntary contraction of the abdominal muscles. Board-like rigidity is a term used to describe contraction of the muscles of the entire abdominal wall as a result of generalized peritonitis.

Mass

Generally masses are not palpable, but there are exceptions in thin patients (Douglas *et al.* 2005):

- The lower edge of the liver may be palpated just below the right costal margin. Sometimes Riedel's lobe, which is an anatomical variant of the right lobe of the liver, may be mistaken for a pathological finding.
- The aorta may be palpable as a pulsatile swelling (transmitted pulsation) above the umbilicus.
- The lower pole of the right kidney may be felt in the right flank.
- The sigmoid colon (when loaded with faeces) may be felt in the left iliac fossa.

Abnormal findings of various organs on palpation

Hepatomegaly

Hepatomegaly, or hepatic enlargement, can be a result of any longstanding liver disease. As the liver enlarges, it can extend inferiorly. It is not possible to palpate the superior edge of the liver. The aim of liver palpation is to feel if the lower border of the liver is palpable (Cox and Roper 2006).

Splenomegaly

The spleen lies under the left costal margins along the ninth, tenth, and eleventh ribs. The spleen has to increase in size threefold before it becomes palpable. As the spleen enlarges, it extends from the left costal margins inferiorly and medially towards the right iliac fossa. A 'notch' may be palpable in a massive splenomegaly. The aim of splenic palpation is to detect the spleen as it moves down against your fingers (Talley and O'Connor 2006). Characteristics of spleen: dull to percussion, moves down with inspiration, cannot get above it, and cannot ballot.

Enlarged kidneys

A grossly enlarged kidney is readily detected on palpation. Kidney enlargement of lesser extent can be detected using a bimanual technique (Douglas *et al.* 2005).

Abdominal aortic aneurysm

This is dilatation of the aorta and is found at the midline of the abdomen, above the umbilicus. The characteristic of an aneurysm is expansile pulsation, which should be differentiated from transmitted pulsation.

Abnormal gall bladder

The commonest pathology that affects the gall bladder is gall stones. This usually leads to a thickened and fibrotic gall bladder that is not palpable. A palpable gall bladder in the presence of jaundice can be a result of carcinoma of the pancreatic head, carcinoma of the ampulla of Vater, or common bile duct obstruction secondary to gall stones (Verghese and Berk 1986). Gall bladder enlargement without jaundice is seen in mucocoele (gall bladder fills with mucus), empyema (infected mucocoele), or acute cholecystitis.

Distended urinary bladder

An empty urinary bladder is impalpable. Urinary retention is commonly seen in elderly men with prostatic enlargement that obstructs the urinary flow. An enlarged urinary bladder due to acute urinary retention has to be drained by insertion of a urinary catheter; this is usually followed by great relief for the patient and disappearance of the palpable swelling.

If a palpable mass appears superficial, it may be arising from within the anterior abdominal wall instead of the abdominal cavity. This can be confirmed by asking the patient to tense the abdominal muscles by lifting the head; an abdominal wall mass will still be felt, whereas a deep mass will not.

Box 10.14 Describing an abdominal mass

- *Site:* which region(s)?
- *Size:* use a tape measure to quantify.
- *Attachment:* is it arising from the abdominal wall or abdominal cavity?
- *Mobility:* is it mobile or fixed?
- *Surface:* smooth or irregular? Overlying skin changes?
- *Edge:* well delineated or ill-defined? Regular or irregular? Sharp or rounded?
- *Consistency:* soft, rubbery, or hard?
- *Tenderness:* this suggests inflammation or distended capsule.
- Movement with respiration?
- *Pulsatility:* this suggests a vascular cause.
- Overlying temperature?
- *Percussion note:* resonant or dull?
- *Bruit:* this suggests a vascular cause.

Context

 ### When to use abdominal palpation

The aim is to check if there is any area of tenderness on the abdomen and to assess if there is any abnormal abdominal mass and/or enlarged abdominal organs.

 ### When not to use abdominal palpation

If the patient refuses to be examined, you should respect their wishes.

Alternative interventions

There are times in clinical practice when general palpation does not yield much information to help make a definite clinical diagnosis. For instance, a patient's clinical examination findings may not match with their history. One may need further investigation such as blood tests and imaging tests to assess the matter further.

Indications for assistance

If the patient shows signs of peritonitis or findings are controversial, help from a doctor should be sought immediately. Patients who have an obese abdominal wall or are on long-term steroid therapy may not have the

Box 10.15 Palpable intra-abdominal mass at different regions

Right iliac fossa mass

■ Caecum: carcinoma, Crohn's disease, tuberculosis.
■ Appendix: abscess.
■ Ovary: cyst, carcinoma.
■ External iliac artery: aneurysm.
■ Pelvic kidney.
■ Psoas muscle: abscess.

Left iliac fossa mass

■ Sigmoid colon: diverticular disease, carcinoma.
■ Ovary: cyst, carcinoma.
■ External iliac artery: aneurysm.
■ Pelvic kidney.
■ Psoas muscle: abscess.
■ Faeces.

Hypogastric/suprapubic mass

■ Sigmoid colon: carcinoma.
■ Ovary: cyst, carcinoma.
■ Uterus: fibroid, pregnancy.
■ Urinary bladder: urinary retention, carcinoma.

Epigastric mass

■ Stomach: carcinoma, pyloric stenosis in babies.
■ Liver: enlarged left lobe (e.g. carcinoma).
■ Gall bladder: mucocoele or empyema.
■ Pancreas: carcinoma, cysts, pseudocyst.
■ Aorta: aneurysm.

classical findings when presenting with acute abdomen; a second opinion should be obtained from doctors if in doubt.

Procedure

Preparation

Prepare yourself

● Wash and dry hands
● Ensure your hands are warm
● Always examine from the patient's right side

Prepare the patient

● Ensure privacy of patient and consider using a chaperone if necessary.
● Obtain consent.
● Explain the procedure to the patient, including the purpose of the examination.

Prepare the equipment/environment

● Ensure there is adequate lighting and warm surroundings.

Step-by-step guide to general palpation

Step		Rationale
1	Introduce yourself, confirm the patient's identity, explain the procedure, and obtain consent.	To identify the patient correctly and gain informed consent.
2	Ensure patient is lying flat on one pillow with arms alongside body; ensure patient is comfortable in this position. Kyphotic patients and those with dyspnoea may need more than one pillow.	Ensures complete relaxation of abdominal wall muscles.
3	Expose patient from nipples to pubic symphysis (**Figure 10.26**).	Ensures adequate exposure.
4	Ask if there is any area of discomfort/pain before the examination and ask patient to report any tenderness during the examination.	This helps to detect underlying pathology.
5	Use the flat of your right hand. Start with light palpation in each region. Palpate gently and systematically, covering the whole abdomen, avoiding sudden or jerky movements. Avoid examining areas of discomfort or tenderness first. Watch patient's face for signs of pain. All movements of the hand should take place at the metacarpophalangeal joints (the knuckles).	To detect areas of tenderness and superficial masses. Examining tender areas first may make subsequent assessment difficult.
6	Perform deep palpation by pressing down on the abdomen more firmly. Warn the patient before doing so.	To detect intra-abdominal masses. The patient may find deep palpation very uncomfortable, especially in the presence of localized and/or generalized peritonitis.

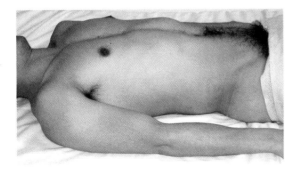

Figure 10.26 Position of patient and exposure of abdomen.

Step-by-step guide to checking for hepatomegaly

Step	Rationale
1 Remain kneeling down and start palpating from the right iliac fossa.	Liver enlarges and extends inferiorly. If palpation for liver started at the hypochondrium, the lower border of a massively enlarged liver would be missed.
2 Use the finger pads (or radial border of your right hand) and keep your hand flat on the abdomen.	This is the sensitive part of the hand.
3 Ask patient to take deep breath in (and out) following your instruction. As the patient breathes in slowly, apply some gentle pressure on the abdomen and advance your hand progressively up the right-hand side of the abdomen. Advance a couple of centimetres at a time, repeating the request to breathe in, until an edge is detected or you reach the right costal margin.	The liver descends during inspiration. You are feeling for an 'edge' that should descend to meet your fingers.
4 If the lower edge of the liver is felt, assess the surface of the liver and its consistency. Measure the size from the costal margin to the liver edge.	This will give you some clues about the underlying pathology of liver enlargement.
5 Percuss for both upper and lower border of liver span. The upper border of the liver is level with the sixth rib in the midclavicular line and the lower border at the level of the costal margin. The normal liver span is less than 13 cm.	Normal liver can be pushed down (and its lower edge become palpable) as a result of hyperinflation of the lungs such as in emphysema.

Step-by-step guide to checking for splenomegaly

Step		Rationale
1	Start palpating from the right iliac fossa.	The spleen extends inferiorly and medially as it enlarges.
2	Use the finger pads and keep your hand flat on the abdomen.	This is the sensitive part of the hand.
3	Ask patient to take deep breath in (and out) following your instruction. As the patient breathes in slowly, apply some gentle pressure on the abdomen and advance your hand diagonally up the left hypochondrium. Advance a couple of centimetres at a time, repeating the request to breathe in, until an edge is detected or you reach the left costal margin.	The spleen descends during inspiration. You are feeling for an 'edge' that should descend to meet your fingers.
4	If the edge of the spleen is not (or is only just) palpable, roll the patient onto their right side (towards you) and repeat the steps above. Palpate with right hand while left hand presses forward on the patient's left lower ribs from behind ('tipping the spleen').	With the help of gravity and 'tipping' of the spleen, a mildly enlarged spleen may become palpable using these manoeuvres.
5	Percuss from the right iliac fossa to left hypochondrium.	This helps to confirm a splenomegaly.

Step-by-step guide to checking for enlarged kidneys

Step		Rationale
1	Stand at the patient's right side and place your left hand behind their back below the lower ribs (renal angle). Place your right hand flat on the abdomen on the flank, lateral to the rectus muscle.	This is an attempt to capture the kidney between your hands.
2	Press down with your right hand while flexing upwards with the fingers of your left (balloting).	An enlarged kidney can be felt to float upwards and hit the anterior (right) hand.
3	Repeat this on the other side.	To check the other kidney.

Step-by-step guide to checking for abdominal aortic aneurysm

Step		Rationale
1	Stand at the patient's right-hand side and place one hand on the midline of the patient's abdomen, above the umbilicus.	The abdominal aorta bifurcates at the level of the umbilicus.
2	If pulsation of the aorta is prominent, place your fingers on either side of the borders (**Figure 10.27**). Your fingers will be pushed up and outwards if it is an aneurysm (also known as expansile pulsation). A transmitted pulsation (e.g. a mass over aorta) will lift your fingers up but not outwards.	To determine whether an aneurysm is present.

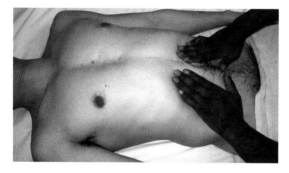

Figure 10.27 Fingers across abdominal aorta for detection of expansile pulsation.

Step-by-step guide to checking for abnormal gall bladder

Step		Rationale
1	Gently palpate the patient's right upper quadrant. A palpable gall bladder is bulbous, rounded, and focal. It moves inferiorly on inspiration below the right costal margin.	To check for abnormal gall bladder.
2	If cholecystitis is suspected, look out for Murphy's sign by asking the patient to breathe in as you examine the right hypochondrium. The sign is present if the patient catches their breath when your hand presses on the inflamed gallbladder.	To confirm cholecystitis.

Step-by-step guide to checking for distended urinary bladder

Step	Rationale
1 Gently palpate the patient's abdomen, starting from the umbilical region and moving towards the suprapubic region. An enlarged urinary bladder is typically smooth, firm, and oval-shaped. It is impossible to feel its lower edge. It is felt in the hypogastric region and can extend to the umbilicus. The patient may feel the urge to urinate as you press over the enlarged urinary bladder.	To check for an enlarged bladder.
2 If you suspect a palpable urinary bladder due to retention, percuss over it.	In the presence of urinary retention, the urinary bladder is dull to percussion.

Following the procedure

Thank the patient, help them to dress, and document findings in the notes. Do not forget to wash your hands once you finish your examination.

Recognizing patient deterioration

Contact the doctor immediately when features such as worsening of abdominal pain and/or progressive deterioration of bedside observations (heart rate, temperature, respiratory rate, and blood pressure) are found in patients presenting with acute abdomen.

Reflection and evaluation

When you have completed abdominal palpation on a patient, think about the following questions:

1 Were you able to palpate the abdomen systematically?
2 Were you able to answer the patient's questions?
3 Were you able to interpret the physical examination findings in light of the patient's medical condition?

Further learning opportunities

At the next available opportunity, try examining patients of different sizes.

- Do all their abdomens feel the same?
- Do you have to apply pressure on the abdomen differently for different patients?

Reminders

Do not forget to:

- Position patient appropriately and examine patient from the right.
- Enquire if the abdomen is tender before proceeding and examine area(s) of discomfort last.
- Perform light then deep palpation systematically throughout the nine regions. Use the flat of your hand and avoid sudden/jerky movements.
- Watch patient's face constantly for signs of tenderness.

Patient scenarios

Consider what you should do in the following situations, then turn to the end of this skill to check your answers.

1 A 65-year-old lady has severe kyphosis. She has been having abdominal pain for the past 3 days. How should she be positioned prior to the abdominal examination?

2 An 18-year-old man was admitted with an acute abdomen and refused to be examined because of the intensity and severity of his abdominal pain. What is the most appropriate way to manage this problem?

3 A 48-year-old man has been diagnosed with chronic myeloid leukaemia. You are about to palpate his spleen. Where in his abdomen would you start?

Website

 http://www.oxfordtextbooks.co.uk/orc/ endacott

You may find it helpful to work through our short online quiz and additional scenarios intended to help you to develop and apply the skills in this chapter.

References

Cox NLT and Roper TA (2006). *Clinical skills*. Oxford University Press, Oxford.

Douglas G, Nicol F, and Robertson C (2005). *MacLeod's clinical examination*, 11th edition. Elsevier Churchill Livingstone, London.

Talley NJ and O'Connor S (2006). *Clinical examination: a systematic guide to physical diagnosis*, 5th edition. Elsevier Churchill Livingstone, Marrickville.

Verghese A and Berk SL (1986). Courvoiser's law. *Lancet*, **1**(8492), 99.

Useful further reading and websites

Goldberg C and Thompson J (2004). *A practical guide to clinical medicine*. University of California, San Diego [online] **http://medicine.ucsd.edu/clinicalmed/ introduction.htm** accessed 08/07/07.

Mangione S (2000). *Physical diagnosis secrets*. Hanley and Belfus, Philadelphia.

 Answers to patient scenarios

1 Patient comfort is the priority. The patient should be lying supine and may need more than one pillow in this case.

2 Reassurance with adequate analgesia (opiate) prior to abdominal examination.

3 The patient may have a massive splenomegaly, in which case you need to start palpating from the right iliac fossa.

10.9 Abdominal paracentesis Ⓐ

This is an advanced skill. You *must* check whether you can assist with or undertake this skill, in line with local policy.

Definition

Abdominal paracentesis (abdominal tap) is an invasive procedure that involves removing peritoneal fluid that has accumulated in the abdominal (peritoneal) cavity, a condition known as ascites. It is performed via insertion of a fenestrated catheter through the abdominal muscles into the peritoneal cavity (Dougherty and Lister 2008).

There are two types of abdominal paracentesis:

1 *Diagnostic* – a small amount of peritoneal fluid is removed for diagnostic purposes.

2 *Therapeutic* – a large amount (can be up to several litres) of peritoneal fluid is removed for symptomatic relief of ascites.

It is important to remember that:

This skill is normally performed by clinicians and assisted by nurses. However, nurses should have a good understanding of the skill prior to assisting.

Prior knowledge

Before assisting with abdominal paracentesis, make sure you are familiar with:

- Anatomy of the peritoneum
- Pathophysiology of ascites
- Causes of ascites
- Clinical features of patients with ascites

Background

Peritoneum

The peritoneum is a serous membrane that consists of an outer layer (parietal peritoneum) and an inner layer (visceral peritoneum). The parietal peritoneum is attached

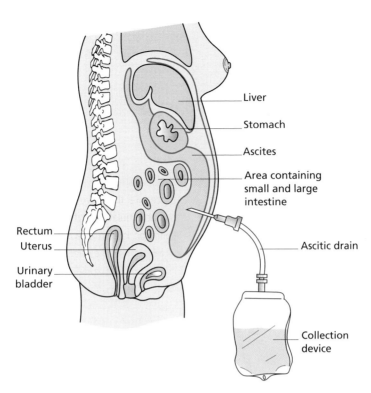

Figure 10.28 Lateral view of female peritoneum with ascites.

to the abdominal wall and the visceral peritoneum is wrapped around the internal organs that are located inside the abdominal cavity. The peritoneal cavity is a space between these two layers, which consists of a small amount of serous fluid (about 50 ml) that allows the two layers to glide freely over each other.

The omentum is a sheet of fat that is covered by the peritoneum. The greater omentum is attached to the bottom edge (greater curvature) of the stomach, and hangs down in front of the intestines. Its other edge is attached to the transverse colon. The lesser omentum is attached to the top edge (lesser curvature) of the stomach, and extends to the undersurface of the liver.

The mesentery is made up of a double layer of visceral peritoneum that contains blood vessels, nerves, and other structures between these layers (Faiz and Moffat 2006).

Common pathology of the peritoneum

Pneumoperitoneum is the presence of gas within the peritoneal cavity. This condition may occur when a hollow viscus (e.g. stomach, intestines) perforates, and can also be created iatrogenically when a laparoscopic procedure is performed (e.g. laparoscopic cholecystectomy).

Peritonitis is a condition characterized by inflammation of the peritoneal lining, which may occur either by perforation of intra-abdominal organs or by spread of infection through the walls of abdominal organs.

Ascites is an accumulation of excess fluid within the peritoneal cavity (see **Figure 10.28**).

Pathophysiology of ascites

The pathophysiology of ascites is multifactorial and is still poorly understood (Becker *et al.* 2006, Moore and Aithal 2006). In the presence of malignancy, ascites may result from blockage of lymphatic drainage by tumour cells, which prevent absorption of intraperitoneal fluid and protein. In the presence of high protein concentration in many patients with malignant ascites, alteration in vascular permeability results in the development of ascites. Hormonal mechanisms are involved when the subsequent reduction in circulating blood volume as a result of decreased lymphatic absorption causes activation of the renin–angiotensin–aldosterone system, leading to sodium retention.

Portal hypertension (which favours transudation of fluid into the peritoneal cavity) and sodium and water retention (seen in patients with cirrhosis) are implicated in the pathogenesis of non-malignant ascites.

Causes of ascites

Traditionally, ascites is divided into 'exudates' and 'transudates' based on the concentration of protein in the ascitic fluid. Ascitic protein concentration of more than 25 g/litre is 'exudates' and less than 25 g/litre is 'transudates'. The reason for this subdivision is to help classify the cause of ascites. However, there are misconceptions in clinical practice. For instance, up to 30% of patients with uncomplicated cirrhosis have an ascitic protein concentration of more than 25 g/litre (Becker *et al.* 2006, Moore and Aithal 2006).

The serum ascites–albumin gradient (SA–AG) is far superior in categorizing ascites, with 97% accuracy. It can be calculated via the following formula:

SA–AG = serum albumin concentration – ascitic fluid albumin concentration

Based on the SA–AG, the causes of ascites where SA–AG is more than 11 g/litre are cardiac failure, nephrotic syndrome, and cirrhosis. Where SA–AG is less than 11 g/litre, the causes are pancreatitis, tuberculosis, and malignancy.

Cirrhosis of the liver is the commonest cause of ascites (75%), the remainder being malignancy (10%), cardiac failure (3%), tuberculosis (2%), pancreatitis (1%), and other rare causes.

Clinical features of ascites

The symptoms related to ascites may vary from patient to patient and depend on the quantity of ascitic fluid. The patient may be asymptomatic if there is a small amount of ascitic fluid. On the other hand, the patient may complain of abdominal fullness/distension, abdominal pain, early satiety, or dyspnoea.

The accuracy of detecting ascites clinically depends largely on the amount of ascitic fluid present and the body habitus of the patient. It may be technically more difficult and challenging to detect ascites in obese patients. Typically, findings of ascites include generalized abdominal distension with flank fullness, shifting dullness, and a positive fluid thrill (only in massive ascites). Imaging modalities such as abdominal ultrasound scan and CT scan can be used to confirm the presence of ascites if physical examination is equivocal.

Context

 When to use abdominal paracentesis

Abdominal paracentesis is performed for the following reasons:

- To evaluate the underlying cause of ascites (diagnostic study).
- To provide symptomatic relief in patients with large-volume ascites.

 When not to use abdominal paracentesis

There are no contraindications as such for this skill, but one has to be aware of the conditions that may increase the risk of complication when the skill is performed (McGibbon *et al.* 2007):

- Blood coagulation disorder (e.g. low platelet count, prolonged prothrombin time).
- Infection of the abdominal wall.
- Intestinal obstruction.
- Pregnancy.
- Poor patient cooperation.
- Previous multiple abdominal surgeries.

In difficult cases, an ultrasound-guided approach should be considered to minimize potential complication.

Alternative interventions

In addition to abdominal paracentesis, depending on the underlying cause, the following treatments have been suggested for ascites (Becker *et al.* 2006):

Dietary salt
No added salt diet of 5.2 g salt/day (i.e. restrict salt intake to 90 mmol salt/day).

Diuretics

In cirrhotic ascites, spironolactone is currently the first line treatment. If this fails, furosemide should be added with careful monitoring of biochemical (blood urea and electrolytes levels) and clinical profiles.

Transjugular intrahepatic portosystemic shunt (TIPS)

A transjugular intrahepatic portosystemic shunt (TIPS) is a percutaneously created connection within the liver between the portal and systemic circulations. A TIPS is placed to reduce portal pressure in patients with complications related to portal hypertension. This procedure has emerged as a less invasive alternative to surgery in patients with end stage liver disease.

The goal of TIPS placement is to divert portal blood flow into the hepatic vein, to reduce the pressure gradient between the portal and systemic circulations. Shunt patency is maintained by placing an expandable metal stent across the intrahepatic tract. TIPS could be used for the treatment of refractory ascites requiring repeated therapeutic abdominal paracentesis.

Liver transplantation

Liver transplantation should be considered in patients with cirrhotic ascites.

Indications for assistance

More than one nurse may be appropriate when extra help is needed, e.g. in mobilizing and positioning of patient and reassuring patient in difficult situations. In addition, if the vital signs are abnormal following the procedure, further medical assessment may be needed.

Procedure

Abdominal paracentesis is performed using the aseptic technique by a trained doctor, who is assisted by a nurse throughout. The following steps are recommended, but skills and resources may vary locally (Dougherty and Lister 2008).

Preparation

Prepare yourself
Wash and dry hands.

Prepare the patient

- Ensure privacy of patient and consider using a chaperone if necessary.
- Obtain consent.
- Explain the procedure to the patient, including the purpose of the examination.

Prepare the equipment/environment
Ensure there is adequate lighting and warm surroundings. Equipment needed includes:

- Sterile abdominal paracentesis set (containing trocar and cannula, connector to attach to the cannula, disposable scalpel, suturing equipment, swabs, and towels).
- Sterile gloves.
- Sterile dressing pack.
- Sterile receiver.
- Sterile specimen pots.
- Needles and syringes.
- Antiseptic solutions.
- Local anaesthetics.
- Sterile drainage bag or container.
- Clamp.
- Tape measure.
- Weighing scales.

Step-by-step guide to abdominal paracentesis

Step		Rationale
1	Introduce yourself, confirm the patient's identity, explain the procedure, and obtain consent.	To identify the patient correctly and gain informed consent.
2	Check if patient is allergic to antiseptic solution, dressing, or local anaesthetics.	Minimizes possibility of allergic reaction.
3	Ensure patient empties urinary bladder.	Minimizes risk of bladder injury.
4	Measure abdominal girth using tape measure at the umbilical level (before and after procedure).	Provides an indication of fluid shift and shows if procedure has been beneficial.
5	Lie the patient supine in bed with the head raised at a 45° angle with a back rest.	With the aid of gravity, this allows fluid to accumulate at the lower abdomen and makes drainage easier.
6	Wash hands using antibacterial solution and apply sterile gloves using aseptic technique.	Minimizes the risk of local and/or systemic infection.
7	Expose the abdomen, then prepare the abdomen aseptically and drape it with sterile towels.	Minimizes the risk of local and/or systemic infection.
8	Administer local anaesthetics at the point of entry. NB entry point may be just beneath the umbilicus, lateral to the rectal sheath, or a point marked via ultrasound scan prior to the procedure.	Reduces pain associated with the procedure and facilitates patient cooperation throughout it.
9	Gently introduce trocar and cannula once the local anaesthetics have taken effect.	To allow drainage of ascitic fluid.
10	Remove the trocar.	This allows the fluid to drain.
11	Collect the ascitic fluid drained from the cannula and send samples for cytological, microbiological, and biochemical analysis.	To investigate the cause of ascites if not already known.
12	Connect cannula to a drainage bag via connector if it is to remain *in situ* and secure drain with sutures. Apply sterile dressing.	Ensures cannula remains *in situ* and reduces risk of local and/or systemic infection.

Following the procedure

- Clear and tidy up the area, ensuring sharps are properly disposed of to minimize risk of injury to staff and patient.
- Document the procedure appropriately.
- Monitor the patient's blood pressure, pulse, respiratory rate, temperature, and nature and rate of drainage. Observe for evidence of shock or infection and ensure satisfactory drainage.
- Monitor fluid and electrolyte balance. Paracentesis of less than 5 litres of uncomplicated ascites should be followed by plasma expansion with a plasma expander (e.g. Gelofusine® or Haemaccel®), and volume expansion with albumin is unnecessary (Moore and Aithal 2006).
- Following removal of a large amount of ascitic fluid, fluid moves from the intravascular space and reaccumulates in the abdominal cavity. Problems of electrolyte imbalance and hypovolaemia may be present.

Complications related to abdominal paracentesis

The following are known complications related to abdominal paracentesis (McGibbon *et al.* 2007):

- Bleeding when abdominal wall vessels are injured (abdominal wall haematoma).
- Hypovolaemia or hypotension if large amount of fluid is drained without replacement.
- Injury to bowel and/or urinary bladder, especially when the patient is uncooperative or technique is poor.

Recognizing patient deterioration

- If continuous bleeding occurs at site of cannula, apply firm pressure with sterile dressing and contact doctor for urgent review.

- If patient develops fever and the ascitic fluid appears cloudy, this may suggest spontaneous bacterial peritonitis. Send ascitic fluid for microbiological analysis and contact doctor for review.

Reflection and evaluation

When you have assisted with abdominal paracentesis, think about the following questions:

1. Was the patient well informed before the procedure?
2. Were you able to answer the patient's questions?
3. Was the procedure well tolerated by the patient?

Further learning opportunities

At the next available opportunity, try to assist different medical staff in performing abdominal paracentesis.

- Does it make any difference to the comfort of the patient when different techniques are used?

Reminders

Don't forget to:

- Obtain informed consent before procedure.
- Use aseptic technique.
- Ensure patient is comfortable throughout.
- Document clearly following procedure.
- Clear area following procedure.
- Monitor vital signs and fluid and electrolyte balances if excessive fluid drained.
- Measure abdominal girth before and after procedure.
- Weigh patient.

Ⓠ Patient scenarios

Consider what you should do in the following situations, then turn to the end of this skill to check your answers.

1. A 58-year-old alcoholic male presented with confusion, jaundice, and gradual abdominal distension. What is the most likely cause of his abdominal distension?
2. A 74-year-old female is about to have a diagnostic abdominal paracentesis. What would you tell her?
3. A 66-year-old man has had multiple abdominal surgeries in the past and is about to undergo abdominal paracentesis. What would be the safest option?

Website

 http://www.oxfordtextbooks.co.uk/orc/ endacott

You may find it helpful to work through our short online quiz and additional scenarios intended to help you to develop and apply the skills in this chapter.

References

Becker G, Galandi D, and Blum HE (2006). Malignant ascites: systematic review and guideline on treatment. *European Journal of Cancer*, **42**, 589–97.

Dougherty L and Lister S (2008). *The Royal Marsden Hospital manual of clinical nursing procedures*, 7th edition. Blackwell Publishing, Oxford.

Faiz O and Moffat D (2006). *Anatomy at a glance*, 2nd edition. Blackwell Publishing, Oxford.

McGibbon A, Chen GI, Peltekian KM, and Van Zanten SV (2007). An evidence-based manual for abdominal paracentesis. *Digestive Diseases and Sciences* [online abstract from SpringerLink database] **http://www.springerlink.com/content/ 0770265064948w50/** accessed 03/07/07.

Moore KP and Aithal GP (2006). Guidelines on the management of ascites in cirrhosis. *Gut*, **55**, 1–12.

Useful further reading and websites

Goldberg C and Thompson J (2004). *A practical guide to clinical medicine*. University of California, San Diego [online] **http://medicine.ucsd.edu/clinicalmed/ introduction.htm** accessed 08/07/07.

Gompertz RHK, Rhodes M, Poston G, Decadt B, and Armitage J (2000). *Churchill's house surgeon's survival guide*, 2nd edition. Churchill Livingstone, London.

Smith EM and Jayson GC (2003). The current and future management of malignant ascites. *Clinical Oncology*, **15**, 59–72.

 Answers to patient scenarios

1 This patient has ascites secondary to cirrhosis.

2 It is important to explain to the patient in simple terms what the procedure entails before obtaining informed consent. Ensure she is comfortable throughout.

3 In this case, the patient may have developed adhesions from his previous operations. To minimize injury to his internal organs and related complications, an ultrasound-guided procedure will be safest.

11 Musculoskeletal system

Skills

11.1 Moving and handling patients

Definition

As a result of illness or disability, many patients will require assistance with moving and repositioning themselves. Patients' dependence on the assistance of carers may range from slight to total, and this dependence may be temporary or permanent.

The health care worker has a responsibility to reduce, as far as possible, the risk of handling-related injuries to themselves, their colleagues, and their patients. This can only be achieved by taking a cautious and thoughtful approach to patient movement and handling.

Decisions on moving and handling patients will range from how to provide the most appropriate coaching and equipment to facilitate patients in being as independent as possible, to choosing between manual and mechanized approaches to moving more dependent patients.

It is important to remember that:

The manual handling of loads in the workplace is comprehensively regulated by health and safety legislation, principally the *Manual Handling Operations Regulations (MHOR) 1992* (amended: Health and Safety Executive (HSE) 2004a) and the *Health and Safety at Work Act 1974*:

- You must have a reasonable knowledge of local health and safety policies.

- You must have received the structured basic training in movement and handling deemed mandatory for your organization.
- You should never attempt to operate patient-linked equipment without adequate training in its use. 'Adequate' in this context means that you have received structured, appropriate training in the use of specified equipment, are personally confident of your knowledge and competence, and a qualified nurse has verified and confirmed your competence.
- The use of equipment does not reduce the need for personnel. One nurse should focus on operating the equipment while another is carefully observing the patient for any signs of discomfort or the development of any hazards.
- Equipment must be maintained according to a regular schedule and more frequently if showing any signs of wear. Most hoists have a 'return for inspection' date on them – these dates should be conscientiously observed.

The MHOR (1992) guidelines (HSE 2004a: 4) define an employer's duty as follows:

> *Each employer shall, so far as is reasonably practicable, avoid the need for his employees to undertake any manual handling operations at work which involve a risk of their being injured. Where that is not reasonably practicable they must make a suitable and sufficient assessment and take appropriate steps to reduce the risk of injury to those employees arising out of their undertaking any such manual handling operations to the lowest level reasonably practicable.*

While employers have duties as described, it must not be forgotten that every individual worker has obligations under the *Health and Safety at Work Act 1974* and the MHOR (1992/2004a) guidelines to:

- Follow appropriate systems of work laid down for their safety.
- Make proper use of equipment provided for their safety.
- Cooperate with their employer on health and safety matters.
- Inform the employer if they identify hazardous handling activities.

- Take care to ensure that their activities do not put others at risk.

(HSE 2007b: 1)

A qualified nurse will often find themselves to be representing both their employer as the shift supervisor, and themselves and their colleagues as employees. Thus they must have a good grasp of how this legislation applies to their own area. They will be responsible for ensuring that safe systems of work are practicable and observed.

Regardless of status, any employee, including a learner, has clear obligations to cause no harm to others in the workplace. The workplace will include a patient's home for those working in the community.

Remember too that patients have the right to influence significantly and make decisions about their own health care plans. Their needs, wishes, and safety need to be balanced against those of the health care workers providing their care.

Prior knowledge

Before undertaking any patient handling activities, make sure you are familiar with:

1 The main principles within the *Manual Handling Operations Regulations* (1992). These are summarized on and linked to the Health and Safety Executive's website (see Useful further reading).

2 The *Guide to the Handling of Patients* (Smith 2005) is an excellent and detailed resource for all involved in patient handling. In particular you should understand which patient handling manoeuvres are hazardous or should be avoided – these are clearly outlined in the chapter on controversial techniques by Ruszala (2005).

3 The Royal College of Nursing (RCN) *Code of Practice for Patient Handling* (2002) highlights major hazards to carers and suggests how these might be managed at an organizational level.

4 The main elements of performing a manual handling risk assessment and examples of generic manual handling assessment charts can also be accessed from the Health and Safety Executive website (see Useful further reading). These elements are discussed briefly in the next section.

5 The core elements of the *Disability Discrimination Act 1995*, which broadly reinforces that one person may not be treated less favourably than another merely because of a disability.

6 As a nurse you must always uphold the basic principles of the Nursing and Midwifery Council (NMC) *Code of Professional Conduct* (2004). In the context of patient handling, particular consideration should be given to treating the patient as an individual, obtaining informed consent to treatment, and involving patients in care decisions.

7 The local Trust policy on moving and handling patients.

Background

The movement and handling of patients carries significant risk of injury to both the patient and the patient handler. For all UK employees, the most common kind of over 3-day injury was sustained while handling, lifting, or carrying, accounting for 41% of all such injuries in 2006/07. The reported total of these injuries that year was 46–152 (HSE 2007a).

Statistics for injuries to patients caused by poor handling are not collated as systematically, but one of the most common types of patient injury linked to poor handling is damage around the armpit and shoulder (Lindgren *et al.* 2007). The brachial plexus (nerve junction) is located beneath the axilla; excessive pressure here can cause damage to nerves supplying areas of the arm, hands, shoulder, and neck.

More significantly, pulling a patient by the arm can result in subluxation (dislocation) of their shoulder (Owen 2003). Apart from the pain and discomfort caused to the patient, there may be major long-term implications for their potential recovery from, for example, a stroke if their ability to participate fully in early rehabilitation activities is impaired by such an injury.

To understand fully the risks and hazards posed by the handling of patients, you should review the following:

- Anatomy and physiology of the musculoskeletal system.
- Biomechanics of human movement.
- Ergonomics applied to the handling environment.
- Risk assessment of patient handling activities.
- Balanced decision-making.

Anatomy and physiology of the musculoskeletal system

Pay particular attention to reviewing the structure of the spine, major joints, and the muscles of the torso. Review different types of muscle tissue, muscle function, and tissue adaptation. Recognize common musculoskeletal disorders (MSDs) and consider their causes.

Biomechanics of human movement

Biomechanics relate to how the body is subjected to and responds to forces and stresses exerted by and upon it. Efficient human movement should allow the achievement of physical goals with as little effort and risk of injury as possible. Thoughtful planning of handling manoeuvres should reduce the impact of these forces and stresses as much as possible.

Gravity is perhaps the most significant force acting on our bodies. The loads we move are governed by it but, more importantly, nearly all human movement is set against gravitational pull. Simply standing still or sitting requires a great deal of organization on the part of our postural management systems to maintain balance and a comfortable position.

Certain postures are less stressful than others, mainly because they involve balanced positions – for example the body is said to be in balance if the line of gravity falls within the person's base of support (Brown and McLennan 2007).

When standing, a person's centre of gravity lies within the pelvis, level with the second sacral vertebra. The line of gravity is described as a perpendicular line that travels down through the centre of gravity to the ground, as shown in **Figure 11.1** (Foss and Farine 2007).

When we adopt different positions our centre of gravity shifts. When it shifts enough that the line of gravity no longer lies within our base, then we are out of balance and need to move or else use a great deal of muscular stiffening and tension to prevent ourselves from overbalancing.

A good example of this is a stooped position. Projecting the spine forwards, with the heavy cranium on its distal end, effectively displaces a large amount of our weight, and therefore our centre of gravity, forwards. As shown in **Figure 11.2**, when we draw a line from above down through the new centre of gravity and onto the

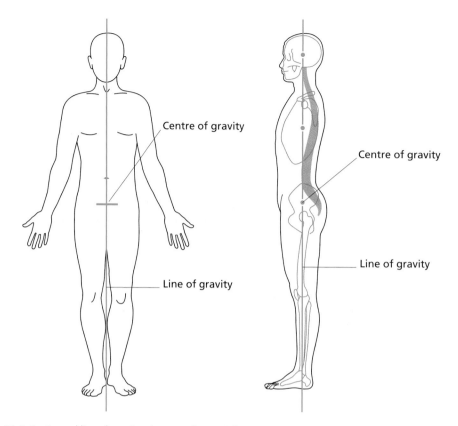

Figure 11.1 Centre and line of gravity when standing upright.

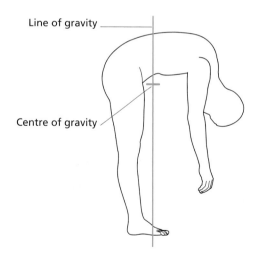

Figure 11.2 Unstable centre of gravity when bent over.

ground, we find that the line of gravity has moved to the very front of the base created by our feet. Thus we are unstable, under stress, and prone to injury.

In a similar way, holding a load away from the body moves our centre and line of gravity out from our base.

Therefore, in practice it is always good to keep any load as close to your centre of gravity as possible, with the risk of injury increasing significantly the further away the load is held from the body (HSE 2004a).

Simple advice on good biomechanical handling principles includes:

- Plan each part of the sequence.
- Position yourself to be stable and comfortable.
- Be close to your load.
- Don't move out of balance or twist.

Consideration of good biomechanical principles may make you less prone to injuries; however, people frequently and unexpectedly injure themselves when moving very trivial loads (Dolan and Adams 2005), so biomechanics as a sole predictor of the likelihood of injury has limitations.

Biomechanical considerations are complex and so patterns of safe and efficient human movement are extremely difficult consciously to remember and apply in varied practical situations. A 2 year study of 163 female health care workers in Denmark (Jensen *et al.* 2006) found that despite significant training input, there was no significant reduction in the incidence of lower back pain. The Health and Safety Executive (HSE 2007c) also concede that training focused on handling techniques is often not applied in the workplace – they suggest that improvements are most likely to result from training that raises awareness of ergonomic factors and changes the workplace culture to one that is more risk aware through improved risk assessment and reporting.

Ergonomics applied to the handling environment

Ergonomics in the handling context is largely concerned with assessing and optimizing the working environment and designing safe methods of working within it (systems of work). Environments that compel workers to bend, reach, twist, stoop, lift, and even remain static have been identified as posing risks for the development of musculoskeletal disorders (Hignett 2005).

The main ergonomic issues in the work environment are space constraints, heights and widths of working surfaces, distances of travel, load characteristics, and available equipment. The types and frequencies of routine tasks can also be added to this list.

Space to move is vital for safety and the use of equipment, yet many health care environments were poorly designed at the time of building. Since the 1980s, health service architects have increasingly designed health care environments with a view to ergonomic factors. Much health care now, however, is provided in old buildings and in the patient's own home.

Adjustable height trolleys and beds allow the nurse to adopt more stress-neutral positions that suit their individual requirements and thus reduce stooping and lower back stress (Griffiths 2006). However, even though a bed may be height adjustable, the carer must not lose sight of the fact that its width defeats one of the key biomechanical principles for safe handling – it distances you from your load. Beds are an inescapable factor in health care and almost always compromise the handler's optimum positioning by separating them from their patient.

Other available equipment may include heavy duty lifting equipment, but there is definite ergonomic value in minor pieces of equipment such as transfer boards and handrails that promote a patient's self-caring capacity or allow them to assist in manoeuvres.

Lloyd (2003) considers that shear forces in the anterior–posterior and lateral planes are a major contributor to back injuries among nursing professionals. He explains that nursing tasks, unlike most manufacturing tasks, involve mainly horizontal load transfers. He describes the spine as analogous to a column of blocks, which can withstand substantial forces acting from above along its length, but which easily collapses when subjected to fairly minor forces from the side.

Ergonomic analysis of the tasks that are routinely carried out should be made and those tasks that potentially involve twisting or the exertion of sideways forces identified as posing increased risk of injury. In addition to these generic risk assessments, additional individual risk assessments should be made for each patient.

Risk assessment of patient handling activities

The basic elements that should constitute a risk assessment are outlined in **Table 11.1**. They can be seen to form the acronym ELITE, standing for Environment, Load, Individual, Task, and Equipment.

These recommendations are generic and need to be adapted to local requirements. At the earliest opportunity you should familiarize yourself with the existing protocols for risk assessment within the areas where you will be working. Legislation states these must be systematically carried out, documented, and kept current (HSE 2004a).

Charney (2003) states that a proper safe handling policy cannot be fully implemented until:

- Sufficient and suitable handling equipment and furniture is in place.
- The environment is made suitable, for instance by enlarging cubicles or installing extra handrails.
- Staff are provided with appropriate training – in particular on risk assessment and how to use equipment.

Balanced decision-making

When deciding what will be the most appropriate method or system of work for moving and handling a patient,

Table 11.1 ELITE assessment

Problems to look for	Reducing risk
In the environment, are there: ■ Constraints on posture? ■ Awkward heights and depths of work surfaces? ■ Poor lighting? ■ Uneven or slippery floor surfaces? ■ Excesses of heat, cold, or humidity?	Can you: ■ Create more space? ■ Adjust heights and depths? ■ Improve lighting? ■ Improve flooring? ■ Control temperatures?
Are the loads/patients: ■ Heavy, bulky, or unwieldy? ■ Too large to see around? ■ Sharp, hot, or soiled? ■ Angry or aggressive? ■ Uncooperative or confused?	Can you make the load/patient: ■ Smaller? ■ Safer to hold? ■ Less angry? ■ More cooperative? If not, use equipment and additional personnel.
For the individual (the handler) – does the job: ■ Need unusual strength or skill? ■ Demand special training? ■ Endanger those with health problems or disabilities, or varied heights and builds? ■ Endanger pregnant workers?	Can you: ■ Mechanize all or part of the task? ■ Provide special training? ■ Support workers with special considerations?
Do the tasks involve: ■ Twisting, stooping, or reaching? ■ Holding loads away from the body? ■ Repetitive handling? ■ Supporting a load for prolonged periods? ■ Strenuous pushing or pulling?	Can you: ■ Mechanize the process? ■ Improve workplace layout? ■ Alter the process? ■ Provide support for loads? ■ Reduce load or friction, or mechanize?
Is equipment: ■ Easily available? ■ The right type for that task and environment? ■ Well maintained? ■ Easily manoeuvrable?	Can you: ■ Obtain what is needed? ■ Carry out planned maintenance? ■ Service wheels, adapt floor surfaces, create space?

Adapted from HSE 2004b

more has to be taken into account than simply employee safety. A number of additional factors must be considered, for example:

- A patient may refuse to be moved by a mechanical device.
- Moving a patient mechanically on every occasion may increase their level of dependence by denying them opportunities to participate in self-care and thereby develop and recover strength and capability.

- A system that reduces carer risk by reducing how much personal care is given – for example by leaving a patient to become soiled and attending to them less frequently – will impact significantly on that patient's dignity and comfort.
- Modifications to a patient's home to facilitate safe handling for carers may be unacceptable to the patient and other householders.
- Moving a dependent patient from the floor represents a very high risk to handlers – does this mean the

patient should a) be left where they fall, or b) have their mobility restricted to reduce the risk of falling?

Both patients and carers have rights to safety, dignity, and choice. Many of these rights are enshrined in legislation such as the *Human Rights Act 1998* and within various standards for care, patient choice, and disability rights. The management of situations like these will often depend on exercising some degree of compromise. Rigidity should be avoided and thoughtful risk assessments must be carried out that take appropriate account of patient choice and individual circumstances.

As in all professional decisions, choices must be justifiable against good evidence and take account of all parties involved. In patient care planning this is commonly referred to as 'balanced decision-making', and in the patient handling context is discussed in some depth with many more practical examples by Michael Mandelstam (2005) in the strongly recommended *Guide to the handling of people* (Smith 2005).

Context

 ## When to assess a patient's capacity to weight bear and stand

Assess and regularly reassess every patient who needs assistance with movement. Their capacity to weight bear and cooperate may vary from day to day and even throughout the day. This assessment might form part of the 'Load' section of a full manual handling assessment. This skill is also fundamental to any patient handling task involving a standing patient.

 ## When not to assess a patient's capacity to weight bear and stand

A number of patients will be clearly incapable of reliable weight bearing. Patients who are obviously fully lucid can usually discuss their own capability. An aggressive and uncooperative patient will require additional staff and often equipment if their movement cannot be delayed until they are more amenable. Considerable communication skills (see Chapter 2) may need to be employed.

Alternative interventions

There is no substitute for thorough individual patient assessment.

Potential problems

During assessment: look for any sign of discomfort such as grimacing, guarding (protecting painful areas), or favouring certain areas of the body. Also any muscle spasm or any complaints of lightheadedness. Patients with neurological impairments such as stroke or multiple sclerosis often have more complex handling needs.

Indications for assistance

A second carer may sometimes be needed for assistance and safety – particularly if the patient's cooperativeness is in question, or they appear in any way unpredictable. Some patients may benefit from a more specialized assessment, for example by a physiotherapist or a movement and handling advisor.

Interpreting readings

The main factors to assess will be balance, stability, comfort, confidence, strength, and stamina.

Special considerations

Particular difficulties may be experienced by patients who:

- Have had a period of prolonged immobility.
- Have been sedated.
- Are obese.
- Have a neurological impairment such as multiple sclerosis or a previous stroke.
- Have experienced recent fractures – especially of the femur.
- Have missing or non-functional limbs.
- Have had recent surgical operations – standing for the first time after an operation may cause unexpected discomfort when tensing muscles not used while lying or sitting.
- Have any history of postural hypotension (a drop in blood pressure when upright).

These patients should have primary assessments carried out by an experienced nurse or an appropriate specialist.

Procedure

Preparation

Prepare yourself

- Read through any available documentation for the patient, paying particular attention to their diagnosis, medical history, and presence of any of the factors mentioned in the special considerations.
- Consider the documented results of any previous mobility assessments.
- The assessment must be done from scratch where you do not know the patient and they seem confused.
- Decide if you will need assistance or special equipment like a standing hoist or walking frame.
- Where appropriate, discuss the patient's mobility with their relative or primary carer.

Prepare the patient

- Explain the process and purpose of the assessment and obtain their consent.
- Ensure they are wearing non-slip shoes or slippers.
- Be sure they are dressed appropriately and won't be unnecessarily exposed.
- This is a good time to evaluate their general lucidity and cooperativeness.
- Allow any previous sedation to wear off. Some patients may need ongoing sedation, but this does not mean that they should necessarily be confined to a bed or chair for long periods without some exercise. The level of sedation must be assessed as allowing safe standing with supervision and minimal assistance.

Prepare the equipment/environment

- Start with the patient in a good chair, ideally with arm rests. The patient should be assessed from a sitting position in a chair that allows them to place their feet fully on the floor and, where possible, to assist themselves by using the arm rests. The chair should be neither too low nor too deep. Patients being cared for in the community may need to have more suitable furniture such as profiling beds or suitable chairs installed in their home – these are sometimes given on a lease or loan basis or can be fully provided by the caring organization, which may be the NHS or local authority. A walking frame may be useful for the patient to bear some weight through their arms when standing and also to increase the size of their base if balance is suspected to be poor.
- For an unknown and unpredictable patient, consider first assessing their ability to tolerate taking their weight through the legs and being upright by using a standing hoist for a brief period.
- Clear enough surrounding space for the nurse(s) to position themselves comfortably near the patient.
- Consider having a stool nearby for your comfort when assessing the patient's lower limbs.

Discussing the procedure with the patient and family

- Explain the procedure to the patient and advise them about what they will need to do.

- Explain why it is important to undertake the procedure safely.

Box 11.1 Consultation

It may be best for an experienced physiotherapist to assess patients with significantly impaired mobility and to advise on mobilization plans.

An occupational therapist will be able to provide advice on suitable mobility equipment and aids, while also conducting assessments of the patient's mobilizing capacity.

If the patient is recently post-operative or has had recent fracture repair, the surgeon should have declared the patient suitable for mobilization.

Step-by-step guide to assessing capacity to weight bear and stand

Step	Rationale
1 Introduce yourself, confirm the patient's identity, explain the procedure and obtain consent.	To identify the patient correctly and gain informed consent.
2 Visually assess the patient while sitting, paying particular attention to their posture and sitting balance. Are they erect or slumped?	If the patient cannot comfortably maintain sitting balance, it is unlikely they will manage standing balance without difficulty. A stooped or off-balance posture will displace their expected centre of gravity.
3 Ensure the patient can place both feet flat on the floor, slightly apart and offset.	Feet must be fully in contact with the ground for stability and sensory feedback to nerves and muscles. A comfortable stance with feet slightly offset improves standing stability.
4 For standing, the heel of one foot should ideally be positioned about 10 cm behind that knee joint (Carr and Shepherd 2003). This should be the strongest leg if there is a difference between them. The other foot can be slightly forwards of the first (see **Figure 11.3**).	At least one foot should be under the centre of gravity, which, when sitting, is above the mid-thigh area. Motion from sitting is in a forward direction as well as up – a posteriorly positioned (set behind) foot helps to move the body in a forward direction. This foot will be the main weight-bearing one; the other will act to control forward motion if placed slightly ahead.
5 Next evaluate the muscle strength of the patient's upper limbs – ask them to squeeze your hands with theirs and to flex and extend their arms against moderate resistance provided by you. Assess for general strength and any inequality between sides.	The patient will need some arm strength and coordination to push on the arms of the chair.
6 Then assess the lower limbs: ■ Press down on their knees and ask them to raise each foot from the floor in turn. ■ Press on each shin and ask them to straighten the leg against moderate resistance provided by you. ■ With each foot separately raised slightly off the floor, and with your hand behind the heel, ask them to draw the leg back towards themselves against moderate resistance.	The patient will need reasonable leg strength and coordination to stand. Assessing them while sitting is better than discovering too late that they have a significant weakness not noted on visual assessment.
7 Take the lower leg passively from flexed to straight, closely observing the patient for any signs of discomfort (see Section 11.2).	Patients who have neurological impairment or have been immobile for long periods may not be able to execute movements through their full range of motion due to contraction (shortening) of the muscles and tendons.

continued overleaf

8	By gently manipulating foot and ankle with leg partially extended (see **Figure 11.4**), assess the ability of the foot to dorsiflex (rise upwards towards the shin from the ankle).	A fixed ankle means the lower leg will be kept perpendicular to the floor and prevent positioning for dynamic movement forwards and up.
9	Also assess the ability of the patient's arms to move through a normal range of flexion and extension with some rotation at the shoulder by asking them to perform the movements or by taking the forearm and gently moving it while supporting the shoulder.	Arm range of motion may also be reduced and therefore compromise the patient's ability to use their arms to assist and steady the manoeuvre.
10	While gently performing all of the above, closely observe for signs of pain, discomfort, and also muscle cramps.	If any of these signs are significantly present it may be best to pursue a passive exercise regime with the patient before placing full weight-bearing and mobilizing demands on them.
11	Ask the patient to use the arms of the chair and move or shuffle themselves towards the front of the seat. Closely observe their agility, balance, and posture during this phase.	It is much easier to stand from the front of a seat than deep in the back. If the patient struggles with merely moving to the front of the chair, this is a strong indication that a second handler will be required for the safety of both patient and nurses.
12	With the patient at the front of the seat, ask them to place both hands on the chair arms and reassess feet for optimum positioning.	The patient can assist and steady themselves with their arms and be well positioned for optimum use of the body's natural levers in standing.
13	Discuss the next phase of standing with the patient.	Ensures they are ready and understand what is expected of them.
14	Ask them initially to relax down and then to stand by first looking ahead and then taking the torso over the thighs by moving their shoulders forwards.	Relaxing down is a precursor to moving up – it undoes the postural stiffening that occurs when the trunk has been static and so facilitates a more dynamic start to the manoeuvre. Looking ahead helps to align the spine in a more upright shape. With the head looking forward lumbar curvature is present – it is easier to move the spine and surrounding structures when it is fully erect rather than when slumped. Moving the shoulders over the thighs takes the torso forwards in the horizontal part of standing and arranges the weight more over the legs and centre of gravity.
15	Almost simultaneously they should then push with arms and legs to move to a standing position, following the top of the head forward and up.	The legs, helped by the arms, will drive the final upward part of the movement out of the chair – the head should still be gazing forwards and lead the rest of the body upwards.

16	If the patient is particularly frail or lacks confidence, they may take this manoeuvre to a point where they just clear the seat and then sit down again. For some, however, it will be easier to stand fully than to stand partially – this staging is often more about confidence than lack of strength.	The patient may increase their strength, coordination, and confidence by practising manoeuvres in small stages with the 'safety net' of the chair below them.
17	Once they are upright, observe and assess the patient's capacity to balance and effectively weight bear in the standing position. Instability or poor balance will generally be obvious. Some postural sway is not necessarily a sign of instability. Allow a few minutes standing to evaluate strength and stamina and ask if they have any sense of dizziness. Do not expect too much from patients who have not stood for some time.	To assess balance and ability to stand. Being able to sway and cope with a rapidly changing position without falling is a sign of postural competence.
18	It may be of benefit for some to have a walking frame positioned conveniently ahead of them.	A walking frame can be held for added stability or, for some, to practise straightening up when they have not been upright for some time.
19	If the patient cannot stand, investigate the reasons for this and, if not contraindicated, try again later. If you can see no clear reason for them being unable to stand and the patient cannot explain, ask for a specialist opinion, e.g. a physiotherapist.	Moving from sitting to standing involves a very complex series of connected movements and capabilities, more so than stair climbing and even walking. For some patients there will need to be a period of exercise and rehabilitation before competence can be regained.
20	Once you have assessed the patient's standing, carefully supervise them while sitting back down. Take time to position yourself, the patient, and the chair carefully before commencing. Ensure that the chair is well positioned and stable, and ask the patient to use the arms of the chair to help lower themselves.	Sitting involves a backward descent that requires a lot of muscular control to be achieved smoothly. If the chair is well positioned, the patient will ultimately finish in a seated position through simple gravity.
21	Be wary of the potential for the patient to lose muscular control as the angle at the knee becomes more acute. However, don't try to arrest this sudden descent.	The majority of people who have had a period of immobility are likely to lose this control abruptly before regaining the surface of the chair. You may injure yourself.

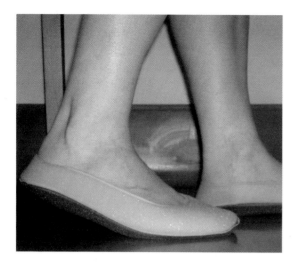

Figure 11.3 Angle of foot dorsiflexion for standing.

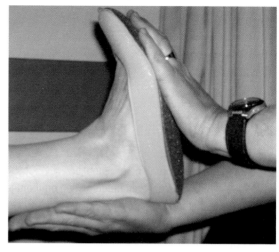

Figure 11.4 Assessing the patient's capacity to dorsiflex.

Following the procedure

- Discuss with the patient how they feel the manoeuvre went and address any expressed concerns or preferences where possible – what made it easier or harder for them?
- Observe the patient for:
  - signs of any potential problems – dizziness, fatigue, pain, cramp
  - level of patient fatigue
  - persisting pain or discomfort.
- A patient with contracted muscles, particularly behind the knee, will not be able to stand fully erect – this may resolve over time with a regimen of stretching exercises, but you need to be aware of it through thorough assessment as described.
- Patients who complain of dizziness should be evaluated for postural hypotension by comparing lying and standing blood pressure measurements.
- As soon as possible after this assessment, document your findings in the patient's notes. Discuss with colleagues how the result will affect the planning and execution of that patient's care.
- Ensure that the patient's individual manual handling risk assessment documents are updated, including recommendations on how and with how many personnel the tasks to be undertaken with and by that patient should be approached. Include the need for any items of equipment or handling aids and any comments on the environment.

Reflection and evaluation

When you have assessed capacity to weight bear and stand, think about the following questions:

1. Did anything you did cause the patient unnecessary discomfort?
2. Did you feel that the assessment involved any risk to you, the patient, or any assistant?
3. Could you have communicated your instructions more effectively?
4. Were you surprised by any effect or event during the assessment?
5. Did your colleagues disagree with any of your conclusions?

If you answered yes to any of the above, consider how you might modify or improve your approach in future.

Further learning opportunities

Spend more time closely observing human movement and try mentally to break common manoeuvres down into their component parts. Particularly note the influence on moving of different positions of the limbs, trunk, and head. For example, try to stand from sitting without using your arms and with your head looking down. Compare this to standing by following your erected head from the seat – the latter should be significantly easier. Apply this to patient movement – ask patients to raise their gaze and follow their heads up when moving in any direction except down.

Try to stand with both feet set out in front of you. This is asking too much of the body's levering system – at least one foot needs to be moved back to drive you forwards and up.

If you can appreciate the biomechanical impact of these simple things, you will be much better at assisting and advising patients. This will also increase your ability to recognize abnormalities and to help patients who are struggling to regain their mobility.

Your skills in risk assessment probably need to be developed and much improved before taking on the role of the nurse in charge of a clinical area or a patient caseload. Scrutinize as many workplace assessments as you can.

Consider ways of adapting patient mobilization and handling tasks between the hospital and the home. Discussions with the occupational therapist will be particularly beneficial here.

Reminders

- Listen carefully to the patient – they know themselves better than anyone.
- Some patients may need to work through a whole movement in small stages – little and often is better than setting unrealistic goals.
- The only person who can take full responsibility for their own safety during handling tasks is you – assess and plan carefully.
- Patient handling has formed the focus of this section but you will also find yourself handling a wide variety of inanimate objects that will represent significant injury risks to you.
- It is your duty to observe any prescribed safe systems of work, i.e. the method, staff, and equipment recommended to perform certain tasks.

 Patient scenarios

Consider what you should do in the following situations, then turn to the end of this skill to check your answers.

1 Mr Brown is unable to weight bear and it is recommended that he be moved using a hoist. However, he refuses to be lifted mechanically. How could you manage this potentially hazardous situation?

2 You are awaiting a new admission to your ward and a very obese patient subsequently arrives on a trolley.

You see from the documentation that arrives with her that her last recorded weight was 30 stones or 191 kg. What are your immediate priorities?

3 A patient is discharged home from hospital into your care. Her mobility is significantly reduced following a stroke. Hospital staff were unsure of her capacity to manage on her own but the patient insisted on returning home. When you first visit her it is quickly apparent that she has only very limited capacity to care for herself. What will you do?

Website

 http://www.oxfordtextbooks.co.uk/orc/ endacott

You may find it helpful to work through our short online quiz and additional scenarios intended to help you to develop and apply the skills in this chapter.

References

Brown A and McLennan A (2007). Moving and handling. In EM Jamieson, LA Whyte, and JM McCall, eds. *Clinical nursing practices*, 5th edition, pp. 213–8. Churchill Livingstone, Edinburgh.

Carr J and Shepherd R (2003). *Stroke rehabilitation: guidelines for exercise and training to optimize motor skill*. Elsevier Science Limited, Philadelphia.

Charney W (2003). Introducing a safer patient handling policy. In W Charney and A Nelson, eds. *Back injury among health care workers: causes, solutions and impacts*, pp. 73–80. CRC Press, Taylor and Francis Group, London.

Dolan P and Adams MA (2005). Biomechanics of low back pain. In J Smith, ed. *The guide to the handling of people*. 5th edn. pp 45–55. Back Care, Teddington.

Foss M and Farine T (2007). *Science in nursing and health care*, 2nd edition. Pearson Education, London.

Griffiths H (2006). Manual handling risk management: critical care beds and support systems. *Nursing Standard*, **20**(32), 45–53.

Health and Safety Executive (2004a). *Manual handling. Manual Handling Operations Regulations 1992 (amended). Guidance on Regulations L23*, 3rd edition. HSE Books, Sudbury.

Health and Safety Executive (2004b). *Getting to grips with manual handling: a short guide* [online] **http://www.hse.gov.uk/pubns/indg143.pdf** accessed 05/01/08.

Health and Safety Executive (2007a). *Kinds of accident – fatal, major and over-3-day injuries* [online] **http://www.hse.gov.uk/statistics/causinj/index.htm** accessed 02/01/08.

Health and Safety Executive (2007b). *The regulations – advice for workers and employers* [online] **http://www.hse.gov.uk/msd/pushpull/regulations.htm** accessed 02/01/08.

Health and Safety Executive (2007c). *The Manual Handling Operations Regulations 1992 (amended) (MHOR) OC 313/5* [online] **http://www.hse.gov.uk/foi/internalops/fod/oc/300-399/313_5.pdf** accessed 04/01/08.

Hignett S (2005). Ergonomics in health and social care. In J Smith, ed. *The guide to the handling of people*, 5th edition, pp. 37–44. BackCare, Teddington.

Jensen LD, Gonge H, Jors E *et al.* (2006). Prevention of low back pain in female eldercare workers: Randomized controlled work site trial. *Spine*, **31** (16), 1761–9.

Lindgren I, Jonsson A-C, Norrving B, and Lindgren A (2007). Shoulder pain after stroke: a prospective population based study. *Stroke*, **38**, 343–8.

Lloyd J (2003). Biodynamics of back injury: manual lifting and loads. In W Charney and A Nelson, eds. *Back injury among health care workers: causes, solutions and impacts*, pp. 27–35. CRC Press, Taylor and Francis Group, London.

Mandelstam M (2005). Manual handling in social care: law, practice and balanced decision making. In J Smith, ed. *The guide to the handling of people*, 5th edition, pp. 15–30. BackCare, Teddington.

Nursing and Midwifery Council (2004). *The NMC code of professional conduct: standards for conduct, performance and ethics*. NMC, London [online] **http://www.nmc-uk.org/aDisplayDocument.aspx?DocumentID=201** accessed 10/09/08.

Owen B (2003) Magnitude of the problem. In W Charney and A Nelson, eds. *Back injury among health care workers: causes, solutions and impacts*, pp. 5–14. CRC Press, Taylor and Francis Group, London.

Royal College of Nursing (2002). *Code of practice for patient handling*. RCN, London.

Ruszala S (2005). Controversial techniques. In J Smith, ed. *The guide to the handling of people*, 5th edition, pp. 273–290. BackCare, Teddington. 273–290.

Smith J, ed (2005). *The guide to the handling of people*, 5th edition. BackCare, Teddington.

Useful further reading and websites

Nelson A (2006). *Safe patient handling and movement: a practical guide for nurses and other health care professionals*. Springer Publishing Company, New York.

Disability Discrimination Act (1995): **http://www.opsi.gov.uk/acts/acts1995/ukpga_19950050_en_4#pt3–pb1-l1g21**

Health and Safety Executive: **http://www.hse.gov.uk/**

 Answers to patient scenarios

1 Moving a non-weight bearing patient without a hoist would put staff and patient at unacceptable risk. Solutions mainly involve use of communication skills:

- Try to discuss the patient's reasons for refusing the hoist – some may be irrational or based on erroneous beliefs; others may reflect a single bad experience.
- Point out that the hoist is a much safer option for him as well as the nurses.
- Some patients find the slings uncomfortable – ensure they are applied correctly but, more importantly, ensure the patient is only suspended for the seconds it takes to move them.
- Use the correct size and style of sling for that patient.
- If you seem unsure, the patient will detect this, so being fully confident in your ability to operate the hoist safely is important. Practise with colleagues until you have this level of confidence and easy competence.
- Using the hoist routinely for any patient who cannot adequately assist lets all patients see that this is the normal procedure and they have not been singled out for personal reasons.
- If the patient is not persuaded, involve an external arbiter such as the local movement and handling advisor. They will have experience of similar situations and can often be a more acceptable source of guidance to the patient.
- If the patient remains adamant, then you will have to involve the movement and handling advisor and the local health and safety representative in designing an acceptable safe system of work for that individual.

2 Firstly, this patient should not have arrived with her weight unannounced like this. Bariatric (very obese) patients should have been previously assessed and the results and recommendations communicated effectively.

- You will need a special bed. Most beds and hoists will only have safe working limits of 25–30 stones or 159–191 kg.
- It is important to arrange transfer onto a suitable bed quickly as the trolley may be unsafe and you will be unable to adjust her position should her condition deteriorate.
- Keep the patient informed about what is happening and try to reassure her that she can be well managed.
- Most NHS Trusts now own one or two beds, chairs, and hoists for patients up to 40 stones or 254 kg, but these may already be in use. Additional equipment is usually obtained on short-term lease from local suppliers, but this may take some time to arrange. This underlines the need to give clear advance notice to anywhere the patient is to be transferred or admitted to.
- Involve a movement and handling advisor at the earliest possible stage. All of this patient's care will be complicated by her weight, and various systems will need to be devised for safe handling. These must be effectively communicated to all staff involved in her care.
- Specially designed or adapted equipment – theatre tables, X-ray tables, transfer trolleys, and ambulances – will need to be arranged.

3 This patient should have had a full and comprehensive assessment of her ability to manage at home before discharge – this should include:

- A physiotherapy assessment to describe and quantify her mobility.
- An occupational therapy assessment to examine her disabilities and evaluate what equipment and adjustments to her home might help her to self-care.
- A social work assessment to consider her eligibility for support, both financial and in carer terms.
- If the local authority is expected to fund her care, they must agree to accept her as a client and may prefer that she be managed in a care home setting.
- While the patient has every right to demand to return to her own home, she must accept that she does not have the right to demand all the care that return entails, particularly when other options more acceptable to the above parties exist.

- This is an example where balanced decision-making is needed as well as good communication with the patient and between services. The cost of providing round-the-clock personal care to individuals is too high for many authorities and patients are often only deemed suitable for home care when it can be provided more cost-effectively than by other means.

11.2 **Passive movements**

Definition

Passive movements are where the health care worker repeatedly moves a joint through the available range of movement without any active participation or resistance from the patient. Stretches include 'any therapeutic manoeuvre designed to lengthen (elongate) pathologically shortened soft tissue structures and thereby to increase range of motion' (Kisner and Colby 2007).

It is important to remember that:

- The purpose of passive movements is to ensure sufficient length of **connective tissues**, thus allowing the available joint range of movement to be achieved.
- They can be used both as a treatment for an active condition and as a preventative measure.
- While it is essential to maintain the range of movement at any joint, there are circumstances whereby potentially serious adverse effects could be observed, e.g. soft-tissue contractures.

Prior knowledge

Before attempting passive movements, make sure you are familiar with:

1 Anatomy of the musculoskeletal system.
2 Microbiology of muscle fibres.
3 Physiology of muscle function.
4 Pathophysiology of common conditions requiring passive movements, e.g. strokes, cerebral palsy, critical care patients.
5 Pharmacology of drugs that have direct effects on neuromuscular activity.

Background

What happens during a stretch?

When a muscle is placed into a stretched position, some of its fibres will stretch while others will remain relaxed. The degree of stretch achieved depends on the amount of fibres allowed to stretch.

Proprioceptors are present throughout the body to detect position and movement. The two main proprioceptors involved in stretching are found in the muscle fibres and the muscle tendons. The stretch receptors are found within the muscles, and the Golgi tendon organ is located in the tendon near the end of the muscle fibres.

A muscle stretch also causes the stretch receptors to lengthen. They are sensitive to both the length of the stretch and the speed at which the stretch is carried out. When a muscle stretch is completed, a sensory message is then relayed that elicits the stretch reflex (see **Figure 11.5**). The role of this reflex is to combat the change in muscle length by initiating muscle contraction. The more rapid the stretch, the greater the counteractive muscle contraction will be.

When the muscles contract there is a resultant tension generated where the Golgi tendon organ is situated. When a muscle contraction exceeds a certain limit, the Golgi tendon organ elicits a lengthening reaction, which in turn causes muscle relaxation. As it is both the muscles and tendons that undergo stretching, this may be more appropriately termed 'connective tissue stretching' (Taylor *et al.* 1997).

How long should a stretch be held?

A stretch needs to be held for a period of time between 10 and 30 seconds (Jones and Barker 1996, Bandy *et al.* 1997). One of the main reasons for this is that it allows the stretch receptors to become accustomed to the new position, desensitizing them. This in turn decreases the strength of the counteractive muscle contraction so a greater stretch can be achieved. Another important point to consider is that a stretch that is held for a longer period of time is more likely to trigger the lengthening reaction from the Golgi tendon organ, causing further relaxation of the stretched muscle. **Figure 11.6** shows the correct technique for stretching the Achilles tendon.

What happens as a result of immobility?

It has long been recognized that prolonged periods of immobility (i.e. bed rest) following disease or trauma are detrimental. Bird (1997) stated that joint mobility is often found to be lacking due to underuse, secondary to a joint not being taken through its full range of movement. Bloomfield (1997) stated that within a matter of days of bed rest beginning, adaptations could be observed within muscle and bone. These findings were supported by LeBlanc *et al.* (1997). From their experimental work into the unloading of limbs during space flight (i.e. non-weight bearing), they concluded that bed rest produced significant muscle atrophy, the extent and rate of which were muscle specific.

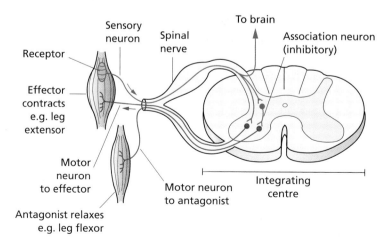

Figure 11.5 The stretch reflex.

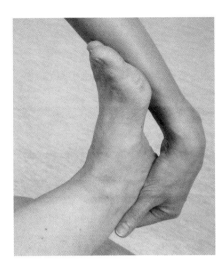

Figure 11.6 The correct technique for stretching the Achilles tendon.

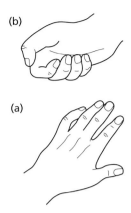

Figure 11.7 Extensor shortening. (a) This hand position contributes to extensor shortening, reducing the ability to grasp objects. (b) This hand position helps prevent extensor shortening.

Earlier work by St.-Pierre and Gardiner (1987) looked in depth at the morphological changes of muscle tissue following immobilization. They found that the extent to which a muscle atrophies is dependent on the type of muscle fibres (fast- and slow-twitch), the length of time immobilized, and the positions in which associated joints were fixed. It was stated that the postural muscles (i.e. slow-twitch) tended to atrophy at a quicker rate than fast-contracting muscles. They also found that the rate of atrophy was rapid in the first few weeks of immobility and then slowed down in its progression. Lastly, and possibly most importantly, the muscles that were allowed to be fixed in a shortened range atrophied to a greater degree. The shortened muscles lose their extensibility, resulting in a loss of joint range. Muscles positioned in an elongated position atrophied at a slower rate.

While this is an important point, it must be remembered that while one group of muscles is in a lengthened position, the opposite groups of muscles are shortened. For example, it is common practice to position patients' hands flat on the bed. However, this leads to shortening of the wrist and finger extensors, resulting in an inability to grasp objects (which is far more functional). One way of combating this is to ensure the hands spend an equal amount of time in both extended and flexed positions (seek guidance from the physiotherapy service in the event of any neurological insult) – see **Figure 11.7**.

Normal joint ranges of movement

Normal ranges of movement are the measured degrees of a movement in the person without any pathology present. There are set ranges for all of the main articulations of the body. The major articulations are shown in **Table 11.2**.

Different types of end feel

The term 'end feel' is reserved to describe how a joint feels when it has reached the end of the available range of movement. It is typically used to aid the practitioner in assessing whether or not any pathology is present. The different types of end feel are shown in **Table 11.3**.

Hand placement during passive movements

The correct placement of hands and the provision of adequate support during passive movements are essential for an effective assessment/treatment. The patient should be supported to enable them to relax and be comfortable. In addition to this, the hands should be placed as close as possible on either side of the joint. This is not possible when mobilizing proximal joints (i.e. hips and shoulders). In this case the hands and forearms should support as much of the limb as possible to reduce any distraction trauma to the joint. Finally, it should be

Table 11.2 Main ranges of movement

Upper limb		
Shoulder	Forward flexion	160–180°
	Extension	50–60°
	Abduction	170–180°
	Lateral rotation	70–90°
	Medial rotation	80–90°
Elbow	Flexion	140–150°
	Extension	0°
Wrist	Flexion	80–90°
	Extension	70–90°
Fingers (MCP)	Flexion	85–90°
	Extension	0°
Thumb	Flexion	50–55°
	Extension	0°
	Abduction	60–70°
	Opposition	tip to tip
Lower limb		
Hip	Flexion	110–120°
	Extension	10–30°
	Abduction	30–50°
	Adduction	30°
	Lateral rotation	40–60°
	Medial rotation	40–60°
Knee	Flexion	135°
	Extension	0°
Foot and ankle	Plantarflexion	50°
	Dorsiflexion	20°
	Inversion	45–60°
	Eversion	15–30°

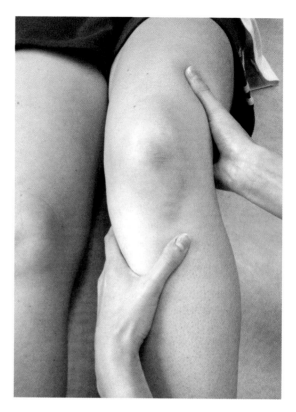

Figure 11.8 The correct hand position for knee flexion and extension.

movement of the nurse's upper torso or body weight that results in the joint movement, and not the gripping or pulling movements of the hands. This could result in potential pain for the patient and an inadequate technique. **Figure 11.8** shows the correct hand position for knee flexion and extension.

Context

 When to use passive movements

Passive movements are used when a patient is unable to move their joints actively through the full range of movement either due to a disease process or following long-term inactivity. They are also used to decrease the risk of complications during inactivity by:

- Minimizing the development of contractures.
- Maintaining muscle elasticity.
- Aiding circulation.
- Decreasing pain.

Another indication for completing passive movements is when advised to do so by the physiotherapist.

Despite the benefits of passive movements, they do have several limitations, and cannot compensate for the loss of active movement. This is the case regardless of how frequently they are done. The limitations of passive movements are that they:

- Do not prevent muscle atrophy.
- Do not maintain or improve muscle strength.
- Do not aid circulation as much as active muscle contractions do.

Table 11.3 Different types of end feel

End feel	Description	Example
Normal		
Bone-to-bone	Hard end feel that is painless.	Knee extension.
Soft tissue resistance	Soft feeling to end of range as soft tissues become compressed.	Knee flexion (restricted by calf muscles on hamstrings).
Tissue stretch	Springy end feel.	Wrist flexion.
Abnormal		
Spasm – early	Likely to resist movement early on in the range, more protective in nature.	Resisting due to acute inflammation.
Spasm – late	Likely to guard against further movement in the case of instability and also irritability of the movement.	Taking a joint into a position whereby the stabilizing structures are deficient.
Bone-to-bone	As for normal bone-to-bone but occurring much sooner than expected.	Loss of range due to bony osteophytes from an inflammatory arthropathy.
Empty	Movement is only limited by the presence of severe pain. There is no physical block felt to the movement.	Fractures, tumours, bursitis.

 ## When to use passive stretches

Passive stretches are used when a reduction of normal joint range of movement is observed during passive movements. The indications for their use include:

- When a range of movement is lacking due to contractures or adhesions.
- When a limited range of movement may lead to joint deformities.
- When a the reduced range of movement may interfere with the functioning of opposite muscle groups (e.g. contractures of the hamstrings inhibiting quadriceps contraction).
- To aid circulation to the extent that active muscle contractions do.

 ## When not to use passive movements

Passive movements should be avoided (or completed with caution following guidance) in the following circumstances:

- Where there are any concerns over the procedure.
- Where there is soft tissue damage (i.e. ligament, tendon, or muscle).
- Where there is active joint pathology present that could be exaggerated.
- When there is active joint pathology present and passive movements could cause pain (ensure adequate analgesia prior to commencing).
- Specific operation notes that stipulate restrictions (e.g. following orthopaedic or vascular surgery).
- Cardiovascular or neurological instability.

 ## When not to use passive stretches

Passive stretches should be avoided in the following circumstances:

- Following a recent fracture.
- When signs of acute tissue trauma are observed (e.g. increased temperature, swelling, redness, pain, or loss of function).
- When contractures are intended and provide the patient with increased functional abilities (e.g. those with spinal injuries).

Alternative interventions

Other considerations for the patient requiring passive movements include referral to the physiotherapy service, use of **continuous passive movement** equipment, and regular changes in the patient's position.

Potential problems

As these are manual treatment techniques they carry with them certain potential problems, including:

- Eliciting pain.
- Overstretching of connective tissue.
- Damage to recent surgery.
- Eliciting cardiovascular or neurological instability.

Indications for assistance

It is essential to understand normal joint ranges and when not to complete passive movements. Always seek guidance from the physiotherapy service and discuss any restrictions with the medical team responsible for the patient.

Interpreting readings

- Eliciting pain: any abnormal movements or joint positions and excessive stretching are likely to result in a pain response.
- Overstretching of connective tissue: any overstretching of connective tissue (see Table 11.2 for normal ranges) is again likely to result in a pain response.

Specific observations

During the procedure it is imperative that any signs of discomfort or pain are observed for, as well as any abnormal neuro-musculoskeletal responses. These can include:

- Patient demonstrating facial features of grimacing.
- Observing for the physiological signs of pain, including increases in heart rate, blood pressure, and respiratory rate.
- Protective spasm of the muscle groups being stretched (automatic response to inhibit any further stretching, thus limiting pain).

Special considerations

- Age of the patient: with elderly patients, remember that their normal joint range may be significantly less than that stated under the normal ranges in Table 11.2. Also, their tissues may have lost some elasticity so any stretches would need to be completed more slowly than usual.

- Location: if undertaking this skill in the patient's home, remember to make sure that the working environment is safe and that there is enough space available for you to complete the procedure appropriately.

- Chronic arthropathies: remember that with arthritis, any movements during an acute flare-up could result in increased pain, protective muscle spasm, and a further reduction in range.

Procedure

Preparation

Prepare yourself

- Ensure you understand the reasons why you are undertaking passive movements and/or stretches, what to observe, what ranges of movement are expected, and what the possible detrimental effects are.
- Wash your hands.

Prepare the patient

- Ensure that the procedure is fully explained to the patient. Allow them to ask any questions they may have and answer them as fully and honestly as possible (within your professional boundaries).
- Gain verbal consent from the patient. If unable to gain consent, ensure you are familiar with the *Mental Capacity Act (2005)*.

Prepare the environment

- Ensure when mobilizing the patient's limbs that their dignity is maintained at all times.
- Ensure, wherever possible, that the environment is warm so as to allow as much relaxation of connective tissue as possible.
- Wear gloves to minimize the risk of any cross-infection.

Discussing the procedure with the patient and family

- Explain why passive movements and/or stretches need to be done.
- Explain that the procedure may feel uncomfortable as structures are being stretched, but that it shouldn't be painful.
- Make the patient aware that if the discomfort increases or the procedure becomes painful, they should inform you so that the treatment can be altered or the session stopped.
- If the movements and/or stretches only need to be done on one limb or the limbs on one side of the body, then demonstrate initially on the patient's unaffected limb(s).

Step-by-step guide to passive movements

Step		Rationale
1	Introduce yourself, confirm the patient's identity, explain the procedure, and obtain consent.	To identify the patient correctly and gain informed consent.
2	Ensure that you and the area are prepared for the intervention.	To allow for patient dignity and comfort to be maintained at all times.
3	Ensure that the patient is in a comfortable position.	To allow the patient to relax, minimizing counterproductive muscle spasm.
4	Position yourself appropriately and move as necessary to complete the movements.	To prevent any unnecessary strain on your back and ensure the movements are completed in a smooth and rhythmical manner.
5	Position your hands on either side of the joint being moved, as close as possible.	To allow for the movement to be controlled, therefore decreasing the occurrence of sudden movements.
6	Move the joint through the available pain-free range.	To minimize any secondary complications of immobility.
7	Ensure that the movements are performed in a rhythmical manner with an even tempo.	To allow the patient to relax fully and not need to guard the movement (i.e. prevent further movement).
8	At the end of available joint range, if necessary, apply a passive stretch.	To counter any loss of range secondary to connective tissue shortening.

continued overleaf

9	Slowly return the limb to the resting position. Reposition the patient as necessary to attempt to keep the increased range.	To allow for any gained range to be maintained.
10	Explain to the patient that the procedure is now complete.	To keep the patient informed of any treatment process.
11	Ensure that the environment is left as clear and clutter-free as possible.	To maintain a safe environment for both staff and patient.
12	Remove any protective clothing and wash your hands.	To maintain hand hygiene and infection control measures.
13	Document treatment session including any observations and outcomes.	As a communication tool and as a legal document.

Following the procedure

Following the intervention it is necessary to document which joint movements have been completed and the ranges of movement achieved. From this it is possible to create a treatment plan, monitor progress, and refer on to any other staff as appropriate (i.e. medical team and physiotherapists).

Recognizing patient deterioration

- Is the range of movement decreasing from the initial assessment?
- Is there an increase in the amount of discomfort/pain demonstrated by the patient?
- Are there any systemic changes to the limbs (e.g. changes in temperature, swelling, discoloration)?

Reflection and evaluation

When you have undertaken passive movements and/or stretches with a patient, consider the following questions:

1 Did the patient demonstrate any form of discomfort or pain during the procedure?
2 Did the passive movements and/or stretches demonstrate any problems with the patient's range of movement, given what the normal ranges are?
3 Did their ranges of movement match with what was expected given the patient's medical condition?

4 Are the ranges of movement being maintained to their optimum or are the stretches improving the given range over time?

Further learning opportunities

At the next available opportunity, try out some passive movements on different groups of people. Consider the following:

- Does the age of the person make a difference to the available range of pain-free movement?
- Do people of a similar age have similar ranges of movement?
- Does the position of the person make a difference to the range of movement?

Have someone try out passive movements on you. Consider the following:

- Is there a period of time at which the procedure becomes uncomfortable?
- Does the positioning of their hands make a difference to the comfort of the procedure?

Reminders

- Always consider the environment and the comfort and dignity of the patient.
- Be guided by medical restrictions and the advice of the physiotherapists.

- Record which joints are moved and their ranges of movement if necessary.
- Inform the appropriate staff of any abnormalities observed.

Patient scenarios

Consider what you should do in the following situations, then turn to the end of this skill to check your answers.

1 While attempting passive movements you identify that your patient is grimacing. What would your course of action be?
2 Your patient has recently had surgery to their lower limb and there is no plan documented in the medical notes. You are verbally instructed following a ward round to 'move the leg'. How would you proceed?
3 There is a new patient admitted to your ward with generalized weakness and lack of movement. There is no obvious medical cause for their immobility, but the patient is sleepy and doing very little. What would your next steps be?

Website

http://www.oxfordtextbooks.co.uk/orc/ endacott

You may find it helpful to work through our short online quiz and additional scenarios intended to help you to develop and apply the skills in this chapter.

References

Bandy WD, Irion JM, and Briggler M (1997). The effect of time and frequency of static stretching on flexibility of the hamstring muscles. *Physical Therapy*, **77**(10), 1090–6.

Bird SR (1997). *Exercise physiology for health professionals*. Nelson Thornes Ltd, Gloucestershire.

Bloomfield SA (1997). Changes in musculoskeletal structure and function with prolonged bed rest. *Medicine and Science in Sports and Exercise*, **29**(2), 197–206.

Jones K and Barker K (1996). *Human movement explained*. Butterworth-Heinemann Ltd, Oxford.

Kisner C and Colby LA (2007). *Therapeutic exercise – foundations and techniques*, 5th edition. FA Davis Company, Philadelphia.

LeBlanc A, Rowe R, Evans H, West S, Shackelford L, and Schneider V (1997). Muscle atrophy during long duration bed rest. *International Journal of Sports Medicine*, **18**, S283–5.

St.-Pierre D and Gardiner PA (1987). The effect of immobilisation and exercise on muscle function: a review. *Physiotherapy Canada*, **39**(1), 24–32.

Taylor DC, Brooks DE, and Ryan JB (1997). Viscoelastic characteristics of muscle: passive stretching versus muscular contractions. *Medicine and Science in Sports and Exercise*, **29**(12), 1619–24.

Useful further reading and websites

Clarkson HM (2005). *Joint motion and function assessment: a research-based practical guide*. Lippincott Williams and Wilkins, Philadelphia.

Lieber RL (2002). *Skeletal Muscle Structure, Function and Plasticity: The Physiological Basis of Rehabilitation*. Lippincott Williams and Wilkins, Philadelphia.

Norkin CC, White DJ, and White J (1995). *Measurement of joint motion*. FA Davis, Philadelphia.

http://www.askoxford.com/concise_oed/passive

http://www.askoxford.com/concise_oed/movement

http://www.cmcrossroads.com/bradapp/docs/rec/ stretching/stretching.pdf

http://www.csp.org.uk

Answers to patient scenarios

1 It is important to identify the cause of the pain – generalized movements, or is there a specific joint and movement responsible? The procedure should be abandoned at this point. In either case it would be appropriate to notify the medical team and request a review of the prescribed analgesia.
2 It would be reasonable to request that the medical team document in the medical notes a post-operative plan, indicating if there are any restrictions. Even if there are no restrictions, the medical instructions should still be documented (to aid communication and as evidence of their request).
3 It would be necessary to complete a series of passive movements as an assessment tool. Obtain baseline joint ranges and refer on to the appropriate physiotherapy staff.

11.3 **Application of a cervical collar**

Definition

A cervical collar is a method of providing support to or immobilization of the cervical spine. Cervical collars are either rigid or soft. Rigid collars are used in possible cervical spine injuries following trauma. Soft collars are not commonly used and are for support in severe whiplash, after spinal surgery, and in degenerative spinal diseases such as arthritis.

It is important to remember that:

- There are different sizes and makes of both rigid and soft collars available.
- It is important to measure for a collar accurately. An ill-fitting collar can do as much harm as going without.
- A collar alone does not immobilize the cervical spine; blocks and straps are also required for complete immobilization (JRCALC 2006).
- All patients are individuals and, although they may have similar injuries, their injury will still be individual to them. The impact a possible injury may have upon the patient may cause them to react in different ways, e.g. some patients are distressed and others may be quite aggressive.

Prior knowledge

Before undertaking application of a cervical collar, make sure you are familiar with:

1 The anatomy of the cervical spine and neck muscles.
2 The manufacturer's recommendations for use of the cervical collar.
3 The history of the accident/injury, i.e. how the trauma was sustained. By understanding the circumstances leading up to a trauma event, the event itself and the possible injury patterns can be predicted.

Background

Anatomy of the cervical spine

The vertebral column provides protection for the spinal cord. The vertebrae are held together by a series of ligaments and intervertebral discs. There are seven cervical vertebrae, which are the smallest and most flexible of the vertebrae. C1, also called the atlas, supports the head and articulates with the occipital condyles of the skull. This vertebra is different to the rest of the vertebrae as it does not have a spinous process or vertebral body. C2, also called the axis, has a vertical projection called the odontoid peg that articulates with the atlas (C1).

Common trauma mechanisms involved

To appreciate the importance of a correctly fitting rigid collar, it is useful to consider the mechanisms of injury involved in trauma and how the cervical spine can be damaged:

- Spinal injuries commonly affect the younger population and are more common in males than females at a ratio of 3:1. The initial carers of this group of patients must provide optimal care and treatment to minimize injury wherever possible (Greaves *et al.* 2008).
- Forty per cent of spinal injuries occur in the cervical region, so protection of the cervical spine is essential in all patients who are at risk of having such an injury (see next section). The rigid cervical collar has been a great addition to the successful management of cervical spine injuries. There are a variety of manufacturers and styles available, and each includes detailed instructions of how to use, measure for, and apply them.

Examples of injuries that may require rigid cervical collar placement

- Road traffic collisions (RTCs) resulting in sudden onset of neck or back pain.
- Serious assault resulting in loss of consciousness or serious injury above the clavicular region, e.g. blunt trauma to the head, attempted strangulation.

- Head injury with loss of consciousness.
- Fall greater than one and half times the person's height resulting in head injury, neck or back pain, or loss of consciousness.
- Sport injuries – rugby and diving most common.

As some patients self-present to Emergency Departments with a history that falls into one of these categories, nurses need to understand the importance of taking a history from a patient to ascertain what first line treatment is required.

Importance of history taking

Taking a thorough history of the events leading up to the trauma and also the trauma itself can help to predict the possible injuries the patient may have:

- If the patient had a front collision in a car and there was a 'bull's eye' mark in the windscreen, this can be indicative of both a head injury from the impact of hitting the windscreen and a possible spinal injury due to hyper-flexion of the neck prior to impact.
- If the patient dived into a shallow pool and hit their chin on the bottom, this can be indicative of a compression injury to the cervical spine.
- If the patient was involved in an RTC and was either ejected from a vehicle or off a motorbike, this may result in a hyper-extension injury to the cervical spine.

(Although these examples show what could possibly happen to the cervical spine, it should be noted that there could be other injuries that also need consideration.)

To understand the use of soft collars, it would also be useful to understand degenerative diseases such as arthritis and how the cervical spine can be affected. Pre-existing diseases such as arthritis and spondylosis reduce the force required to injure the spine.

Context

 ### When to use a rigid cervical collar

A cervical collar is used to support the cervical spine and to prevent movement of the head, which can cause further injury. It is used when injury to the cervical spine is suspected or confirmed.

 ### When not to use a rigid cervical collar

If the patient has a curvature of the cervical spine due to a degenerative disease, the application of a rigid collar can cause additional problems such as damage to the spinal cord and paralysis (Webber *et al.* 2002).

 ### When to use a soft cervical collar

A soft cervical collar can be used if there is degenerative disease of the cervical spine or after cervical spine surgery.

 ### When not to use a soft cervical collar

There are no contraindications to the use of a soft collar.

Alternative interventions

Hard blocks can be placed on either side of the head along with straps across the forehead and chin that are extended onto the bed. These additional forms of support are always used in conjunction with rigid collars but can be used alone if there are contraindications to rigid collars. Any form of support is better than no support at all (Kwan *et al.* 2001).

Potential problems

- Increase in level of pain, tingling/pins and needles/numbness in limbs that was not present before (also beware of spinal injuries). Bear in mind that rigid collars are not completely comfortable and can cause discomfort to some patients.
- Difficulty in swallowing and/or breathing can occur if the collar is too tight or ill-fitting (Kreisler *et al.* 2000).

Specific observations

Remember that it is necessary to take into account any other injuries and use the level of observation required for them.

One of the main observations required is to observe the patient's level of consciousness, especially if a head injury is also evident. The patient's sensation in their limbs also has to be assessed at least hourly for the presence of tingling, pins and needles, and numbness, all of which can be either due to a spinal injury or to an adverse reaction to the rigid collar.

Once the cervical collar is *in situ* the patient is unable to move, so they should not be left unattended due to the risk of vomiting and aspiration.

If a spinal injury above the level of the sixth thoracic vertebra is suspected, the sympathetic nervous system may be compromised, resulting in bradycardia (pulse below 60 bpm) and hypotension (systolic below 120 mmHg) (JRCALC 2006).

Special considerations

- Young children and the elderly do not tolerate rigid collars very well.

- Patients with claustrophobia also tend to be more susceptible to panic attacks while wearing a collar.

Procedure

Preparation

Prepare yourself

- Ensure you fully understand the complete procedure.

- Ensure universal precautions are undertaken where necessary.
- Request help from a colleague: it is a two person technique as one person needs to support the neck throughout (Bache *et al.* 2003).
- Ensure you are familiar with the manufacturer's instructions on how to use the collar.
- Undertake a full set of neurological observations before and after the procedure, including sensory and motor examination of all four limbs.

Prepare the patient

- Give full explanations regarding the whole procedure to the patient, ensure they understand what to expect, and gain their verbal consent.
- Reinforce the need for them to keep still.
- Remove any neck jewellery and earrings, as these will show up on X-ray and could lie in front of a possible bony injury and hide it.

Prepare the equipment

- Correctly sized rigid collar.
- Suction in case the patient vomits during the procedure.
- Blocks and straps.

Step-by-step guide to applying a cervical collar

Step		Rationale
1	Introduce yourself, confirm the patient's identity, explain the procedure, and obtain consent.	To identify the patient correctly and gain informed consent.
2	Measure patient's neck using your fingers. Measure how many finger widths there are from the top of the shoulder to immediately below the chin. Patient should be in a supine position with someone standing at the head of the bed, immobilizing the head and neck by placing the palms of their hands on either side of the head with their index finger stabilizing the mandible.	To ensure correct fit.

3	Select the correct collar using your fingers. Measure the depth of the hard part of the collar as per manufacturer's instructions and choose the most appropriate size.	To ensure correct fit.
4	Apply the collar: slide the flat back part of the collar behind the patient's neck, underneath clothing, and place the front of the collar underneath their chin. Secure the collar using the Velcro strap. Ensure the patient's neck, the front of the collar, and the bottom of the collar conform to one line with the patient's nose and navel in line (see **Figure 11.9**).	To ensure correct fit and placement.
5	Reassure the patient: talk to them and ensure they still understand what is happening and what is going to happen to them. Reinforce the need for them to keep still.	To reassure the patient, gauge level of consciousness, and encourage cooperation with the procedure.
6	Document the size of collar used and the time it was applied.	Good practice; document all activities.
7	Observe patient: take into consideration any other injuries, level of consciousness, any increase in pain, tingling, pins and needles, numbness in limbs, anxiety levels. Repeat full set of neurological observations.	To assess for any deterioration in condition.

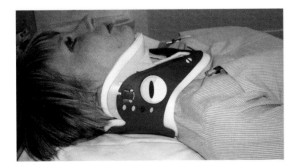

Figure 11.9 Ensure the patient's neck, the front of the collar, and the bottom of the collar conform to one line with the patient's nose and navel in line.

Following the procedure

Step 7 of the procedure needs to be repeated at regular intervals until an injury is either confirmed or ruled out and the collar is removed, to ensure no exacerbation of the possible injury has taken place.

Reflection and evaluation

When you have applied a cervical collar, think about the following questions:

1   Reflect upon the specific incident. What was wrong with the patient and why did they require a rigid collar?
2   Look at the whole patient and their scenario. How did you feel throughout the episode?
3   Were you adequately guided and supervised throughout? If not, why? Was there a specific reason?
4   How did the patient feel after the application of the collar?
5   Have you experienced wearing a rigid collar? If not, try it!

Further learning opportunities

Practise applying a rigid collar. It will be useful at this stage for you to practise this skill on your colleagues.

Reminders

Don't forget:

- Use the correct landmarks when measuring for the collar.
- Explain fully to the patient what the procedure is and what they can expect.
- Document all events accurately.
- Ensure the collar is fitted correctly.
- Do not leave a patient in a cervical collar unattended due to their inability to move.

 Patient scenarios

Consider what you should do in the following situations, then turn to the end of this skill to check your answers.

1   Patient A has had a hard collar in place for 10 minutes and now states that it feels very uncomfortable

and he wants it removed. However, the doctor says it needs to stay in place until he has been X-rayed. What would you do?
2   Patient B needs a hard collar fitting but states he has arthritis of his cervical spine. What would you do?
3   Patient C has a hard collar *in situ*. She develops an increase in pain and becomes disorientated, and starts pulling at the collar. What other information would you like and what would you do?

Website

 http://www.oxfordtextbooks.co.uk/orc/ endacott

You may find it helpful to work through our short online quiz and additional scenarios intended to help you to develop and apply the skills in this chapter.

References

Bache J, Armitt C, and Gadd C (2003). *Handbook of emergency department procedures*, 2nd edition. Mosby, Oxford.

Greaves I, Porter K, and Ryan J (2008). *Trauma care manual*, 3rd edition. Arnold, London.

Joint Royal College Ambulance Liaison Committee (JRCALC) (2006). *Clinical practice guidelines* [online] **http://jrcalc.org.uk**

Kreisler N, Durieux M, and Spiekermann B (2000). Airway obstruction due to a rigid collar. *Journal of Neurosurgical Anaesthiology*, **12**, 118–9.

Kwan I, Bunn F, and Roberts I (2001). Spinal immobilisation for trauma patients, Cochrane Review. *Cochrane Database Systematic Reviews*, **2**, CD002803.

Useful further reading and websites

Davies G, Deakin C, and Wilson A (1996). The effect of a rigid collar on intracranial pressure. *Injury*, **27**, 647–9.

Gwinnutt C and Driscoll P (2003). *Trauma resuscitation: the team approach*, 2nd edition. Bios Scientific Publishers Ltd, London.

Houghton L and Driscoll P (1999). Cervical immobilisation – are we achieving it? *Pre-Hospital Immediate Care*, **3**, 17–21.

http://www.instantanatomy.net
http://www.trauma.org

Answers to patient scenarios

1 This patient requires reassurance, but in addition you need to find out why the patient finds it so uncomfortable. Is he in pain or does he just not like it? Reiterate why the collar needs to be on and the risks of removing it before X-rays have been taken. Check his observations.

2 What type of arthritis does he have – has he got a deformity of his cervical spine? Check his observations including motor and sensory function in all four limbs. Is he in pain, and has the pain changed or increased? Any discrepancies – inform the doctor or nurse practitioner who is looking after him.

3 Check this patient's observations – has she become hypoxic? Is she confused? Was she confused before? Is she in pain? Has she got any other injuries that could be causing further problems? Reassure her as much as possible and get her reassessed.

11.4 **Application of slings**

Definition

A sling, also called a triangular bandage, is used as a method of support for an injured upper limb. There are two different methods of application depending on the reason it is required:

1 A **broad arm sling** is the standard method of application of a sling and is generally used for fractures to the forearm and upper arm.

2 A **high arm sling** is a modified version of the broad arm sling, which is generally used when a higher elevation is required, e.g. if there is gross swelling to the hand.

It is important to remember that:

- The sling must be applied correctly to avoid complications.
- The patient may require analgesia prior to the application.
- The patient should be advised to observe for swelling after the application (depending on reason for application).

Prior knowledge

Before undertaking application of a sling, make sure you are familiar with:

1 The basic anatomy of the upper limb.
2 The patient's injury.

Background

The broad arm sling has been used for many years for elevating the upper limb. The elevation provides support and subsequent pain relief for an injury to the upper limb. The high arm sling is a modification of the broad arm sling and provides a higher amount of elevation. A high arm sling is also sometimes known as an elevation sling.

The broad arm sling has many uses but its main function is support for the upper limb. It is used to provide immobilization, resulting in pain relief for fractures of the upper limb, e.g. clavicle, wrist, and hand (Cooke 2007). The high arm sling is used when higher elevation is required for the upper limb, e.g. swelling to the hand in cellulitis (Jevon and Cooper 2008).

Fractures

There are six main groups of fractures:

1 Open – where there is a break in skin integrity over or close to the break.
2 Closed – where the skin remains intact.
3 Comminuted – where there are more than two segments of bone.
4 Greenstick – where the bone is 'buckled', i.e. broken on one side but still intact on the other.
5 Impacted – where both ends of the fracture site have been driven into each other.
6 Displaced – where one or both ends of the fracture are out of alignment.

History taking

As with all patients who have an injury, it is important to find out how the injury occurred in order to ascertain if there are any other injuries. For example, if the patient is complaining of wrist pain after falling onto their outstretched hand, it is possible that they may have an injury higher up the arm (e.g. clavicle) from the impact of the fall onto the hand and the transmission of energy up the arm.

The pain in most types of fractures is caused by the bone ends moving. The application of a sling to immobilize the arm reduces the movement, thus reducing the pain. In addition, for the fracture to heal, the fracture site needs to be immobilized to allow the formation of new bone in between the bone ends.

Context

 When to use a broad arm sling

The types of injury this sling is used for are fractures or soft tissue injuries to the:

- Hand
- Wrist
- Forearm
- Elbow
- Upper arm
- Shoulder
- Scapula
- Clavicle

The broad arm sling holds the arm in a neutral 90° angle at the elbow. This position provides the required support while also providing elevation to reduce any existing swelling and prevent any further swelling.

The broad arm sling is mainly used for patients with fractures or soft tissue injuries to the wrist, forearm, elbow, humerus, scapula, and clavicle, and also after the reduction of a dislocated shoulder. The sling can be applied at the time of injury to provide pain relief and support and also after any relevant treatment. In addition the broad arm sling can be used to provide elevation for patients with cellulitis or infections, e.g. olecranon bursitis of the upper limb.

 When not to use a broad arm sling

There are very few contraindications to using a broad arm sling, but if the patient has the following it should not be used:

- An allergy to a material in the sling.
- Neck problems, e.g. severe arthritis, which make it uncomfortable or painful to use one.

- An increase in pain in the affected area following the application, e.g. with a fractured radius/ulna prior to application of the plaster. Application of a sling can cause more pain and so the affected arm should be supported on a pillow until plaster can be applied.

 When to use a high arm sling

The high arm sling is mainly used for fractures, soft tissue injuries, or cellulitis of the hand. In addition this sling can be used to elevate an injured arm or hand to stop haemorrhage, along with a pressure dressing.

 When not to use a high arm sling

Again, the contraindications to using a high arm sling are minimal, but remove the sling if the patient has any of the following:

- An allergy to a material in the sling.
- An increase in pain following application.

Alternative interventions

There is only one alternative to broad arm and high arm slings and that is the 'collar and cuff'. This is a piece of foam covered in fine netting. It is applied in a figure of eight around the neck and the affected wrist. However, it does not provide any support to the elbow or forearm so its uses are not as wide as those of slings.

Procedure

Preparation

Prepare yourself

Ensure that you fully understand how to apply the sling you require. Also, is the sling to be applied under or over the patient's clothing?

Prepare the patient

Ensure the patient fully understands the procedure. Remove all jewellery from the patient's neck and affected arm.

Prepare the equipment

Triangular bandage, scissors, and tape.

Step-by-step guide to application of a broad arm sling

Step		Rationale
1	Introduce yourself, confirm the patient's identity, explain the procedure, and obtain consent.	To identify the patient correctly and gain informed consent.
2	Place sling against body with the long edge parallel to the sternum, the opposite point toward the patient's elbow on the affected side, and the upper end on the patient's opposite shoulder.	To ensure correct application.
3	Elevate the patient's affected arm to 90° over the top of the sling (see **Figure 11.10**).	To ensure correct positioning of the patient's arm.
4	Position sling by extending the lower end over the arm and shoulder of the affected side.	To ensure correct support.
5	Secure the sling by tying the ends behind the patient's neck. Secure the elbow with tape (see **Figure 11.11**).	To secure the sling in place.

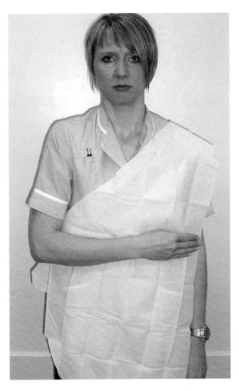

Figure 11.10 Elevate the patient's affected arm to 90° over the top of the sling.

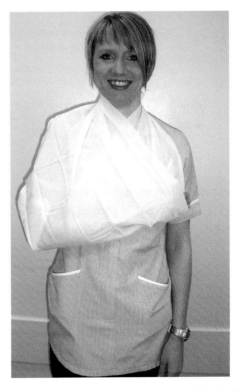

Figure 11.11 Secure the sling by tying the ends behind the patient's neck and secure the elbow with tape.

Step-by-step guide to application of a high arm sling

Step		Rationale
1	Introduce yourself, confirm the patient's identity, explain the procedure, and obtain consent.	To identify the patient correctly and gain informed consent.
2	Position the patient: put their affected hand on their opposite shoulder.	To ensure correct position.
3	Place the sling over the top of the patient's affected arm with the short corner at the elbow (see **Figure 11.12**). Bring the lower end of the sling underneath the affected arm and around the patient's back.	To ensure correct position.
4	As the ends of the sling meet between the patient's shoulder blades, tie them there. Secure the elbow with tape.	To secure sling in place.

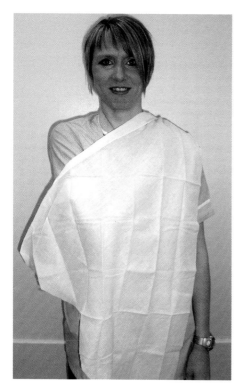

Figure 11.12 Place the sling over the top of the patient's affected arm with the short corner at the elbow.

Following the procedure

- If required, check the patient's radial pulse prior to plastering, e.g. in cases of a suspected fracture to the forearm or elbow.
- Provide the patient with follow-up advice regarding what exercises they need to do, e.g. if they have a fracture to the forearm and it is in plaster they need to exercise their fingers, elbow, and shoulder to prevent stiffening of the muscles.

Reflection and evaluation

When you have applied a sling, think about the following questions:

1 How did you feel?
2 Were you supervised and supported during the procedure?
3 Were you able to apply the sling without any problems? If not, what problems did you have?
4 Have you rectified these problems? If not, what action plan have you constructed to assist you?

Further learning opportunities

Practise the skills of applying a broad arm and high arm sling. It is a good idea to practise on your colleagues while supervised.

Reminders

- Do not forget to remove the patient's jewellery before application of a sling.
- Explain to the patient what you are going to do.
- Provide the patient with the correct advice following the application of the sling.

Patient scenarios

Consider what you should do in the following situations, then turn to the end of this skill to check your answers.

1 Patient A has a suspected fracture to the elbow, which is not in plaster. You have applied a sling but they complain of an increase in pain. What do you do?

2 Patient B requires a broad arm sling but is allergic to the material. What do you do?

3 Patient C requires a high arm sling but refuses to take their necklace off. What do you do?

Website

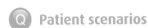 **http://www.oxfordtextbooks.co.uk/orc/ endacott**

You may find it helpful to work through our short online quiz and additional scenarios intended to help you to develop and apply the skills in this chapter.

References

Cooke M (2007). *Pre-hospital care.* Churchill Livingstone, Edinburgh.

Jevon P and Cooper L (2008). First aid – Part 6 – application of slings. *Nursing Times,* **104**(4), 26–7.

Useful further reading and websites

Greaves I and Porter K (2007). *Oxford handbook of pre-hospital care.* Oxford University Press, Oxford.

McRae R and Esser M (2008). *Practical fracture treatment,* 5th edition. Churchill Livingstone, Edinburgh.

St Johns Ambulance (2006). *First aid manual,* 8th edition. Dorling Kindersley, London.

Answers to patient scenarios

1 Remove the sling and support their arm on a pillow until they have been X-rayed. Also ensure they have been given some pain relief. Check their radial pulse to ensure there has not been a change in their perfusion. Document your findings.

2 Do not apply a sling – use a collar and cuff.

3 Explain to the patient that the necklace may rub on their neck as the sling will lie over the top of it and it will become very sore. If they still refuse to remove it, ensure they understand the possible complications, document your discussion, and get the patient to sign it.

Glossary

Active (closed) wound drainage Drain attached to a vacuum container and drainage is encouraged by a gentle negative pressure.

Acute abdomen Condition characterized by sudden, severe pain in the abdomen often requiring urgent diagnosis. Treatment can involve surgery.

Acute haemolytic reaction An immunological response due to incompatible blood groups.

Acute wound A recent injury in which the surface of the skin is torn, pierced, cut, or broken.

Adipose tissue Fat under the skin and surrounding major organs, providing stored energy, insulation, and protection.

Adjuvant drugs Drugs used to treat conditions that in turn provoke pain.

Adrenergic response (or 'fight or flight' syndrome) When threatened the sympathetic nervous system reacts with a general discharge priming the individual for fighting or fleeing. This response is recognized as the first stage of a general adaptation syndrome in response to stress, pain, and cardiovascular failure.

Aerosolize Turn into a form of fine droplets that has the appearance of steam.

Afterload Pressure in the aorta and pulmonary artery that has to be overcome by ventricular contraction.

Agglutinogens Antigens found on red blood cells responsible for determining the ABO blood group classification.

Agonal respirations Slow (3–4 per minute), shallow, irregular respirations caused by cerebral ischaemia.

Air embolism Presence of air in a vein. May happen during placement, manipulation, or removal of a catheter. Symptoms include dyspnoea, chest pain, reduced consciousness, visual disturbances.

Alzheimer's disease A progressive form of dementia characterized by loss of memory, loss of concentration, abnormal perception, and eventually personality change.

Ambulatory cardiac monitoring A method of recording an ECG over a 24-hour period, often referred to as a 24-hour tape.

Amyloidosis A wide range of rare conditions that result in pathological aggregation of extracellular amyloid deposition. Can be inherited or acquired; systemic or organ-specific.

Anaemia A shortage of red blood cells associated with pallor, weakness, breathlessness, and reduced energy.

Anaesthesia The absence of normal sensation, especially sensitivity to pain, as induced by an anaesthetic substance, hypnosis, or as occurs with traumatic or pathophysiological damage to nerve tissue.

Anal fissure A small tear in the anal mucosa.

Anal pruritus Intense anal itching.

Anaphylaxis Extreme sensitivity to a substance such as a protein or drug.

Anastomosis Surgical joining of two ends of bowel; may be stapled or hand-sewn.

Angioedema Rapid swelling of the skin, mucosa, and submucosal tissues.

Angiogenesis Production of new blood vessels. In a healing wound new vessels grow into a loop, and when seen in the lighter pink connective tissue of the wound bed, they have the appearance of deep-red granules (called granulation tissue).

Angiotensin-converting enzyme (ACE) inhibitors Drugs that relax the muscles of blood vessels. ACE inhibitors prevent an enzyme in the body from producing angiotensin II, a substance that affects the cardiovascular system, including narrowing blood vessels which can cause high blood pressure and force the heart to work harder.

Antacid A drug, usually a base formula, which reduces gastric acid concentration.

Anthropometric Physical measurements of the human body.

Antibodies Molecules produced by B cells in response to stimulation by an allergen.

Anticoagulant A drug that interrupts the normal clotting (coagulation) of blood by preventing new clots from forming or an existing clot from enlarging.

Antimicrobial A substance that kills or inhibits the growth of microbes, such as bacteria, fungi, viruses, or parasites.

Aortocaval Relating to the aorta and vena cava.

Apex beat or apical pulse The furthermost point outwards (laterally) and downwards (inferiorly) from the sternum at which the cardiac impulse can be felt.

Apex–radial pulse deficit Difference in the number of apical beats compared with the radial pulse.

Apnoea The absence of observed breathing, e.g. sleep apnoea is apnoea seen when sleeping.

Appendicitis Inflammation of the appendix. One of the most common causes of acute abdomen worldwide. Mild cases settle without treatment, whereas the severe cases require appendicectomy (via an open surgery or laparoscopically).

Appliance (stoma) The bag or pouch worn over a stoma.

Apyrexia Absence of fever (high temperature).

Arrhythmia Abnormal heart rhythm.

Arteriovenous fistula A vein directly joined to an artery that can be needled to provide access to the circulation for haemodialysis treatments.

Arthritis Inflammation of the joints, caused by hardening and calcification of cartilage (osteoarthritis) or inflammation of tendon sheaths and membranes (rheumatoid arthritis).

Ascites A collection of excess fluid in the peritoneal cavity, traditionally classified into 'exudate' or 'transudate'. However, the serum ascites–albumin gradient (SA–AG) is far superior in categorizing ascites.

Asepsis Without the presence of pathological microorganisms.

Aseptic procedure A non-touch method used to keep equipment and people free from disease-causing microorganisms.

Aspartate aminotransferase (AST) An enzyme that is normally present in liver and heart cells.

Aspiration The accidental inhalation of food or fluids into the lungs.

Asthma A chronic condition characterized by inflammation of the airways.

Asymptomatic Shows no symptoms.

Atelectasis Lung collapse due to blocking of the airways (e.g. by a plug of sputum) and absorption of gas distal to the blockage, or to compression of the lung (e.g. by pulmonary tumours or pleural effusions).

Atherosclerosis Hardening of the artery walls by plaque made from cholesterol, platelets, and fibrin. The plaque may become so thick that the artery becomes blocked, or the plaque may become dislodged and block a narrower artery further along the circulation.

Atonic bowel Poor muscle tone within the colon.

Atraumatic Designed to avoid injury.

Atria The top chamber(s) of the heart.

Atrial fibrillation The individual contraction of heart muscle fibres that leads to a 'quiver' rather than a coordinated contraction. The stimuli from the atria will reach the atrioventricular node in an erratic fashion, leading to an irregularly irregular heartbeat.

Atrioventricular node Located between the atrium and the ventricle conducting the impulse to the ventricle.

Atrioventricular valves Valves lying between the atria and ventricles of the heart.

Attenuation Filtering of breath sounds generated from within the larger airways.

Audit trail Record of activity (e.g. record of all occasions when an individual patient record is accessed).

Auscultation Act of listening to sounds produced by the heart and lungs to aid diagnosis, usually with the aid of a stethoscope.

Auscultatory gap The absence of sound in phase 2 of the Korotkoff sounds.

Autonomic dysreflexia A syndrome that affects those with a spinal cord lesion above the mid thoracic level.

AVPU Simple neurological assessment. Is the patient **A**lert or do they respond only to **V**oice, or **P**ain, or are they **U**nresponsive?

Bacteraemia The presence of viable bacteria circulating in the bloodstream.

Bacteriostatic The property of reducing the harmful effects of bacteria.

Bariatrics The branch of health care that deals with the causes, prevention, and treatment of obesity.

Barrier cream Ointment, lotion, or similar preparation applied to exposed area of the skin to protect skin from exposure to various allergens or irritants.

Baseline (observations or data) An initial set of observations or data used for comparison or a control.

Basophil Type of white blood cell.

Bigeminy Cardiac arrhythmia where a regular normal beat is closely followed by an ectopic beat, creating a regularly irregular rhythm.

Biomechanics The science concerned with the internal and external forces acting on the human body and the effects produced by these forces.

Biomedical model Model that focuses on the physical processes, such as the pathology, the biochemistry, and the physiology of a disease.

BiPAP Bi-level, or biphasic, positive pressure ventilation (BiPAP Respironics, Inc.) provides a higher pressure during inspiration than during expiration, and can provide a back-up with a fixed inspiratory and expiratory ratio, i.e. it can support the patient's breathing if their respiratory drive is not well preserved.

Bleb Blister-like lesion/protrusion on pleura.

Blood type The two most important classifications of human blood type are ABO and the Rhesus factor (Rh factor).

Body mass index (BMI) A measure of body fat based on height and weight.

Bowel sounds Sounds caused by the propulsion of the intestinal contents through the lower alimentary tract.

Brachial Pertaining to the arm, typically denoting the area between neck and elbow, especially the axillary region.

Bradycardia Heart rate of 60 beats per minute or below.

Bradypnoea Respiratory rate of under eight breaths per minute.

Brainstem Comprises the medulla oblongata, pons, and midbrain. Connects the spinal cord to the remainder of the brain – the cerebral hemispheres and cerebellum. Responsible for essential functions such as breathing and cardiovascular function, and lesions here often result in death or serious impairment.

Bronchial breath sounds Loud, high-pitched sounds heard in inspiration and expiration, generated from within the trachea and large airways. Abnormal when heard over any other lung field.

Bronchoconstriction The closure of the airway in the lungs due to the tightening of smooth muscle tissue as a result of allergy, asthma, or exercise.

Bullae Over-distended, thin-walled sacs formed from damaged alveoli.

Bundle of His/Bundle branch A bundle of modified heart muscle fibres. It conducts the impulse from the AV node to the apex of the fascicular branches. It branches off into three bundle branches.

Cachexia State of severe muscle wasting and weakness occurring in the late stages of illnesses such as cancer.

Caldicott guardian The 1997 Caldicott Report recommended the establishment of Caldicott Guardians in the NHS to oversee access to patient-identifiable information.

Capillary refill time (CRT) A non-invasive test used to gain a rapid 'snapshot' assessment of tissue perfusion.

Carcinoma A malignant epithelial neoplasm that tends to invade surrounding tissue and to metastasize to distant regions of the body.

Cardiac arrhythmia A disturbance of the heart rhythm: the heart beats too fast, too slow, or irregularly.

Cardiac cycle The complete cycle of events in the heart from the beginning of one heartbeat to the beginning of the next.

Cardiac output The amount of blood ejected from the heart, measured in litres/minute. This is the product of stroke volume × heart rate. Stroke volume is determined by preload, contractility, and afterload.

Cardiac shunt A diversion of blood between sides of the heart or the great vessels.

Cardiomegaly Hypertrophy (enlargement) of the heart.

Cardiopulmonary resuscitation (CPR) An emergency procedure including artificial ventilation and cardiac compression.

Cardioversion A synchronized shock delivered by a defibrillator to restore normal sinus rhythm.

Carotene A fat-soluble pigment found in green and yellow leafy vegetables and yellow fruits.

Cataract A cataract is a clouding of the lens in the eye that may reduce vision.

Catheter A tubular, flexible surgical instrument that is inserted into a cavity of the body to withdraw, introduce, or allow drainage of fluid.

Cation A positively charged ion.

Cellulitis Infection and inflammation of the tissues beneath the skin.

Central cyanosis Central cyanosis is usually due to a respiratory problem that leads to poorer oxygenation in the lungs.

Central venous catheter A single or multiple lumen catheter inserted into a large central vein. Enables more accurate cardiovascular monitoring, fluid balance control, and administration of certain medications.

Central venous pressure The pressure within a central vein. It reflects venous tone, circulating volume, intra-thoracic pressure, and right-sided cardiac function.

Cerebellum The cerebellum sits between the cerebral cortex and the spinal cord.

Cerebral cortex (cerebral hemispheres, forebrain, cerebrum) The left and right cerebral hemispheres constitute the largest and most well-developed part of the brain. Each hemisphere is responsible for sensation and movement on one side of the body. The cerebrum also contains the limbic system (emotion), hippocampus (memory), the dominant language centres, and basal ganglia.

Cerebrovascular accident Interruption of blood flow to the brain resulting in compromise of neurological function in the affected area. This may be due to bleeding or thrombosis.

Charcoal filters These allow flatus to escape slowly through an activated charcoal filter designed to absorb odour.

Charriere A system of gauge measurement; 1 Charriere unit (expressed as Ch or Fr) is equal to one-third of a millimetre.

Chronic kidney disease (CKD) Long-term renal condition, often progressive and categorized in stages 1–5.

Chronic obstructive pulmonary disease (COPD) A disease characterized by progressive deterioration in lung function. As the condition deteriorates, sufferers will find it increasingly difficult to breathe and their ability to carry out exercise will decrease.

Chronic wound A wound that does not heal within a 12 week period is generally considered chronic.

Circadian rhythm The cycle of physiological activity over a day.

Cirrhosis A result of chronic liver disorder where liver tissue is replaced by scar tissue with regenerative nodules, leading to progressive loss of liver function. Commonly caused by alcoholism and hepatitis C.

Clot retention Retention of urine due to blood clots getting stuck in the drainage eyelets of a catheter.

Coagulopathy A disorder of normal clotting mechanisms, affecting the formation of clots. Can result in excessive bleeding and delayed wound healing.

Collagen A protein. The term collagen is frequently used to mean collagen fibres, but actually relates to a family of glycoproteins found in a range of sources including collagen fibres, reticulum fibres, and basement membranes. May be detected in wounds within the first 10 hours post-injury.

Colostomy Surgical opening into the colon through the abdominal wall with formation of an artificial opening (stoma) to allow the discharge of faeces into a lightweight bag attached to the skin. May be temporary or permanent.

Commensals Microorganisms commonly found in an area that do not cause infection at that site.

Compliance The extent to which a patient's behaviour matches the prescriber's recommendations.

Compliance aids Devices that can help a patient to take or use their medication including devices to help patients use their inhalers, administer eye drops, or monitor dosage systems.

Concordance Involvement of the patient in decision-making about their treatment in order to improve their compliance.

Contaminated A wound that contains microorganisms that do not necessarily impede wound healing.

Continuous renal replacement therapies A selection of treatment options similar to haemodialysis that are mostly used in the intensive care setting for patients who are too unstable to receive a more routine renal replacement therapy.

Contractility The strength of contraction of the heart muscle.

Contraction In the musculoskeletal context, the shortening of muscles and sometimes tendons when they are not stretched for prolonged periods due to immobility.

Contraindications Substance, usually another medication or alcohol, which is deemed inadvisable while taking a particular medication because of a likely adverse reaction.

Corneal abrasion A scratch on the surface of the cornea. Normally very painful.

Corneal arcus A creamy ring around the cornea indicating hyperlipidaemia.

Coronary arteries Blood vessels supplying the myocardium.

Cor pulmonale Enlargement of the right ventricle of the heart (and occasionally the left) due to disease of the lungs or pulmonary blood vessels.

CPAP A continuous level of positive airway pressure throughout the respiratory cycle, to keep the airways open. No ventilation is provided, and so the patient must be able to breathe spontaneously to use CPAP.

Crackles Discontinuous, explosive popping sounds originating from within the airways.

C-reactive protein A protein that appears in large quantities in the blood in the course of infections to assist in the destruction and removal of microorganisms.

Creatine kinase (CK) An enzyme that appears in multiple forms, found in high concentrations in heart and skeletal muscles, and (in smaller amounts) in brain tissue.

Creatinine A product of normal muscle and tissue breakdown.

Critical colonization A wound that contains microorganisms that may start to impede wound healing.

Crohn's disease A chronic inflammatory disease of the digestive tract.

CTPA Computed tomography pulmonary angiography.

Cushing's response A physiological response to raised intracranial pressure. In order to preserve blood supply to the brain, blood pressure rises, with a wide pulse pressure, and heart rate drops. It is a sign that pressure on the brain needs to be relieved urgently and often requires neurosurgical intervention.

Cyanosis A bluish colour of the skin and the mucous membranes due to insufficient oxygen in the blood.

Data Protection Act (1998) Legal framework governing the processing of information that identifies a living individual's personal data.

Debridement The removal of devitalized tissue and foreign matter from a wound.

Decalcification Removal of calcium from tooth enamel or bone.

Defecation The act of eliminating faeces.

Dehisce/dehiscence Parting of wound edges, often referred to by the term wound breakdown.

Dehydration Excessive loss of water from body tissues accompanied by a disturbance in the balance of essential electrolytes, particularly sodium, potassium, and chloride. May follow prolonged fever, diarrhoea, vomiting, acidosis, and other conditions in which there is a rapid depletion of body fluids.

Delirium (acute confusion) An acute failure of cognitive function seen in 20% of acutely ill hospital inpatients. Impairment of attention, memory, and abnormal perception such as visual hallucinations are seen. The condition classically fluctuates over time. There is often periodic drowsiness.

Dental caries Tooth decay producing holes in the teeth.

Dental plaque Layer of bacteria and debris that coats the teeth.

Deoxygenated haemoglobin Haemoglobin that has given up its oxygen to cells.

Dermis Thick, sensitive layer of skin or connective tissue beneath the epidermis that contains blood, lymph, vessels, sweat glands, and nerve endings.

Detached retina If the retina is weakened by a hole or tear fluid can seep underneath so that the retina becomes detached. When detached vision becomes blurred and dim.

Dextrocardia An unusual condition in which the heart is positioned on the right side of the chest – it is normally on the left (mirror-image).

Diabetes mellitus An endocrine disorder whereby the body is unable to utilize glucose effectively due to a deficiency of insulin production or action.

Diabetic ketoacidosis (DKA) A life-threatening condition occurring as a result of the body's inefficiency in utilizing glucose, thereby causing a build-up of ketones. This makes the pH of the blood acidic and causes a state of severe dehydration.

Diabetic retinopathy A potentially blinding complication of diabetes that damages the eye's retina.

Diaphoresis/Diaphoretic Perspiring profusely, or something which can cause increased perspiration.

Diastole The relaxation phase of the cardiac cycle.

Diastolic blood pressure The pressure exerted by the blood flow on the blood vessels when the ventricles are relaxed.

Distal phalanx End bone of a finger or toe.

Diuretic A drug that increases the output of urine by promoting the excretion of salts and water from the kidney.

Diverticular disease Formation of pockets in the wall of the large bowel that may become inflamed and infected with stagnant faeces.

Doppler Ultrasound device using reflected sound waves to evaluate blood flow through a blood vessel.

Dorsiflexion The turning upward of the foot or hand so as to reduce the angle between the top of the foot and the shin or the back of the hand and the forearm.

Dry eyes Also known as keratoconjunctivitis sicca. Occurs when the eyes don't make enough tears to keep them moist.

Dumping syndrome A collection of symptoms caused by rapid emptying of partially digested food into the duodenum. Symptoms can include dizziness, fullness, weakness, and diaphoresis. Hypoglycaemia may also be present. It may occur immediately after a meal (early dumping syndrome), or a few hours later (late dumping syndrome).

Duodenostomy Surgical opening into the duodenum through the abdominal wall.

Duodenum The first part of the small intestine, originating from the stomach and joining the jejunum. It is predominantly responsible for the breakdown of food.

Duty of confidence This arises when one person discloses information to another (e.g. patient to clinician) in circumstances where it is reasonable to expect that the information will be held in confidence.

Dyspareunia Abnormal pain during sexual intercourse.

Dysphagia A compromised or dysfunctional swallowing mechanism.

Dyspnoea Difficult or laboured breathing, shortness of breath.

Early Warning Score (EWS) A scoring system developed to enable early identification of patient deterioration. An EWS is calculated using five physiological parameters: mental response rate; pulse rate; systolic blood pressure; respiratory rate; and temperature. A sixth parameter, urine output, can also be added for acute patients.

Echocardiogram A test in which ultrasound is used to examine the heart.

Eczema A skin condition that can result in dry, red, and flaky skin which may feel hot and very itchy. Scratching can lead to damage and infection.

Elastin A protein in connective tissue that is elastic and allows many tissues in the body to resume their shape after stretching or contracting.

Electrocardiogram (ECG) A graphic recording of electrical waveforms produced by the electrical activity of the heart.

Electrolyte imbalance Incorrect balance between the different elements in the body tissues and fluids.

Electrolyte screen A set of blood investigations to check levels of basic blood electrolytes, e.g. sodium, potassium, calcium. Urea and creatinine may also be checked.

Emollient Emollients reduce water loss from the epidermis, by covering it with a protective film.

Encrustation Formation of a crust on the end of a tube (e.g. on to urological catheters), formation of a hard crust at the end of the catheter over time.

Endocarditis Inflammation of endocardium and heart valves.

Endoscopic tube A flexible scope used to view the interior surfaces of an organ.

End stage renal disease Irreversible failure of kidney function.

Enterocutaneous fistula A connection from a hollow viscus directly to the body surface.

Enzymes Proteins produced by living cells that catalyse chemical reactions in organic matter.

Epidermis The thin, outer layer of skin that is made up of several layers.

Epiglottitis Inflammation of the epiglottis (the flap of cartilage attached to the back of the tongue that protects the trachea during swallowing).

Epistaxis Nose bleed.

Erythema/Erythematous An abnormal redness of the skin caused by capillary congestion. It is one of the cardinal signs of inflammation.

Exsanguination The fatal process of total blood loss.

Extracellular matrix (ECM) The main component of the connective tissue of the dermis. Consists of water, glycosaminaglycans (e.g. hyaluronic acid), proteins such as collagen and elastin, fibronectin, vitronectin, and lamina.

Extravasation Infiltration of vesicant (irritant) medications or fluids into surrounding tissues, potentially causing tissue damage and necrosis.

Exudate Fluid that collects in a wound due to increased capillary permeability.

Familial adenomatous polyposis A condition in which multiple polyps are found throughout the gastrointestinal tract. This is inherited as an autosomal dominant trait.

Fibronectin A glycoprotein that helps prevent colonization of the mouth by bacteria.

Frank–Starling's Law of the Heart The force of recoil is proportional to the length the heart muscle is stretched.

Gastric stasis A delay in the emptying of the stomach contents into the small intestine. Gastric emptying is influenced by neuronal control, the amount and type of food in the stomach, as well as patency of the pyloric sphincter muscle. Other influencing factors include anxiety and electrolyte balance.

Gastrointestinal tract The system of body organs responsible for the acquisition of nutrients and expelling the waste products, also known as the alimentary tract.

Gastrostomy Surgical opening into the stomach through the abdominal wall, performed to feed a patient who has cancer of the oesophagus, tracheoesophageal fistula, or is expected to be unconscious for a prolonged period.

Glucagon A polypeptide hormone produced in the pancreas. It acts to increase blood glucose levels by mobilizing glucose stored in the liver as glycogen back into free glucose.

Glucometer An electronic device for analysing blood glucose levels.

Gluten intolerance A reaction to gluten (found in wheat and barley). Some people with gluten intolerance have coeliac disease, an autoimmune response to gluten.

Glycaemia Presence of glucose in the blood.

Glycogen The principal storage form of glucose within the body.

Glycolipids Lipids attached to carbohydrate; they provide energy and serve as markers for cellular recognition.

Glycoprotein Proteins that contain a carbohydrate component.

Granulation Soft, pink, fleshy projections that form during the healing process in a wound not healing by first intention.

Gravid Pregnant.

Growth factors Polypeptides produced by cells that stimulate them to proliferate.

Gyri Ridges on the cerebral cortex that represent areas of the brain with specific functions. They are generally surrounded by one or more sulci.

Haematoma A collection of blood; it can occur anywhere that bleeding occurs.

Haematuria The discharge of blood in the urine. The urine may be slightly blood-tinged (pink), grossly bloodstained, or a brown colour (indicating old blood).

Haemoconcentration Decrease in the volume of plasma in relation to the number of red blood cells; increase in the concentration of red blood cells in the circulating blood.

Haemodialysis A mechanical method for removing waste products and excess water from the blood.

Haemodynamic The movement of blood flow.

Haemoglobin A protein–iron compound in the blood, predominantly responsible for oxygen transport, which gives the blood its characteristic red colour.

Haemolysis The destruction of red blood cells and release of haemoglobin.

Haemorrhage Abnormal loss of blood from an artery, vein, or capillary.

Haemorrhoids Enlarged blood vessels in or around the lower rectum and anus.

Halitosis Bad-smelling breath.

Head injury A broad term encompassing any blunt or sharp injury to the head, which can result in skull fracture, intracranial haemorrhage, or diffuse brain injury (swelling).

Hepatitis Inflammation of the liver.

Hepatomegaly Enlarged liver. Can be detected using abdominal palpation and confirmed by ultrasound scan and CT scan of abdomen.

Hepatosplenomegaly Simultaneous enlargement of both the liver (hepatomegaly) and the spleen (splenomegaly). The causes include malaria, amyloidosis, sarcoidosis, lymphomas, leukaemias, and others.

Herniation A weakness in the muscle through which the underlying structures (e.g. bowel or stoma) can bulge.

Hip to waist ratio A measurement that may be used to detect obesity. It is determined by dividing waist circumference by hip circumference.

Hirschsprung's disease Characterized by the absence of ganglion cells in the distal bowel.

Histamine H2 receptor agonists A group of drugs that reduce gastric acid production by histamine H2 blockade.

Hydrocolloid paste Paste used to fill cracks, crevices, and gullies to level peristomal skin and achieve a leak-proof adherence to the skin.

Hypercapnia High carbon dioxide concentration, outside of normal limits, in arterial blood.

Hypercatabolic Excessive metabolic breakdown of substances or body tissue.

Hyperemesis Severe, persistent vomiting that can be associated with pregnancy.

Hyperglycaemia High blood glucose level (above 7 mmol/litre between meals, or above 8 mmol/litre within 90 minutes of eating).

Hyperkalaemia High serum potassium level.

Hyperlipidaemia High serum concentration of fats.

Hypernatraemia High serum sodium level (greater than 145 mmol/litre).

Hyperosmolar High osmotic concentration solution.

Hyperosmolar non-ketotic (HONK) coma A diabetic medical emergency occurring in type 2 diabetics. Characterized by hyperglycaemia and dehydration due to an increased osmotic effect of glucose.

Hypersensitivity Severe reaction to a drug, allergen, or other agent.

Hypertension Blood pressure greater than 140 mmHg systolic and/or 90 mmHg diastolic.

Hypervolaemia An overload of circulating blood volume.

Hypodermoclysis Subcutaneous infusion of fluids.

Hypoglycaemia Low blood glucose level (below 4 mmol/litre).

Hyponatraemic Low serum sodium level (less than 135 mmol/litre).

Hypoperfusion Inadequate perfusion of the tissues, which can lead to dysfunction, damage, and death.

Hypotension Low blood pressure (systolic pressure below 90 mmHg).

Hypothalamus Sitting just above the brainstem, the hypothalamus links the central nervous system to the hormonal endocrine system (pituitary). It secretes hormones that regulate temperature, hunger, thirst, and control of emotion and sexual drive.

Hypovolaemia Low blood volume.

Hypoxaemia Deficiency in the concentration of oxygen in arterial blood. It can be a result of poor passage of atmospheric oxygen to the blood as a result of lung disease, or inadequate or inappropriate flow of blood through the lungs.

Hypoxia Deficiency of oxygen in the tissues.

Iatrogenic A condition that has resulted from treatment.

Ileostomy Surgical opening into the ileum through the abdominal wall, with a bag to collect liquid contents from the small bowel. Allows faeces to bypass the colon (large bowel); constructed when the colon and/or anorectum are diseased.

Ileum The last part of the small bowel from 4.5 m (15 feet) to 9.5 m (31 feet) long.

Immunocompromised An immune system that has been impaired by disease or treatment.

Immunoglobulin Glycoprotein expressed from B lymphocytes and plasma cells.

Immunosuppression Suppression of the immune system, often caused by radiation or medication, for example chemotherapy or anti-rejection therapy following organ transplant.

Incontinence Uncontrolled leakage of urine or faeces.

Induration Hardening of an area of the body (e.g. a vein) as a reaction to inflammation.

Inert dilutent A substance without chemical properties that is used to dilute drugs, making them fit for aerosolization.

In extremis Latin phrase meaning 'at the point of death'.

Infiltration Fluids that are not irritant (vesicant) are accidentally infused into surrounding tissue.

Inflamed Body tissue that becomes red and swollen, in response to injury or infection.

Inflammation/Inflammatory response The complex biological response to harmful stimuli. This may be the result of exposure to an external pathogen/substance or an internal cause. Inflammation may be specific to a small area (localized response) or have effects on other body organs (systemic response).

Inoculation injury An injury sustained following contact with a 'sharp' or splashing of blood or body fluid onto mucous membranes or non-intact skin.

Insulin A hormone responsible for the uptake of glucose by cells, thereby lowering blood glucose.

International normalized ratio (INR) The time it takes blood to clot in comparison with the average clotting time. In a healthy person, the INR is 1.0; patients taking anticoagulant medication would typically have an INR in the range 2.0–3.0. An INR above 4.0 may indicate the blood is clotting too slowly, creating a risk of uncontrolled bleeding.

Inter-rater reliability Inter-rater reliability is the degree to which an assessment yields similar results for the same situation for more than one rater.

Interstitial A small space between parts of the body or in a tissue.

Intracellular space The space within the cell membrane.

Intracranial Within the skull.

Intravenous Within a vein. Commonly used to describe the therapeutic administration of drugs/fluids into a vein.

Intravesical Within the bladder.

Iritis Inflammation of the iris, and at times the ciliary body, located behind the iris.

Ischaemia Restriction in blood supply.

Ischaemic Restriction in blood supply with resultant damage of tissue.

Jaundice A yellow discoloration of the skin and whites of the eyes due to abnormally high levels of bilirubin (bile pigmentation) in the bloodstream.

Jejunostomy Surgical opening into the jejunum through the abdominal wall.

Jejunum The portion of the small intestine in between the duodenum and the ileum. It is predominantly responsible for absorption of nutrients.

Keloid A large firm mass of scar tissue that extends beyond the actual site of repair and tends to be darker than the surrounding skin. A keloid results from an abnormal over-healing response to injury.

Ketosis High concentration of ketones within the body, caused by an imbalance in fat metabolism.

Korotkoff sounds The sounds heard via a stethoscope during return of blood flow to an artery occluded by a sphygmomanometer cuff.

Kyphosis/kyphotic Abnormal curvature of the spine in the chest area causing the back to appear even more rounded than usual. From the Greek word 'kyphos' meaning 'hump'.

LA Refers to 'left arm' on ECG connectors and cables. However, placement is normally on the left shoulder or below the left clavicle.

Laceration A wound consisting of torn, cut, or punctured skin resulting in damage to the soft tissue underneath.

Lactate dehydrogenase (LDH) An enzyme present in a wide variety of organisms, including plants and animals.

Left lateral decubitus position Lying on the left side.

Left ventricular failure The failure of the left side of the heart to pump adequately, leading to pulmonary oedema. This is a complication of myocardial infarction and/or age.

Lipohypertrophy A complication of subcutaneous insulin injection; it is a build-up of fat below the surface of the skin, causing minor lumps up to the size of an orange. It is caused by repeated insulin injections at the same site or at sites nearby.

Liver enzymes Substances released from the liver that catalyse chemical reactions, for example aspartate aminotransferase (AST) and alanine aminotransferase (ALT). If the liver is injured, enzymes may be released into the blood.

LL Refers to 'left leg' on ECG connectors and cables. However, placement is normally the left lower thorax/hip.

Local action Medication affecting a specific part of the body.

Loculated fluid Fluid contained within a fibrous membrane.

Lysozyme Bacteriocidal protein found in saliva and tears.

Maceration Excessive moisture on the skin that may cause tissue damage.

Macrophages These play a role in protecting wounds against bacterial invasion and are phagocytic destroying. They also produce chemical mediators that are encouraged to the injured site in the first 24 hours, destroying clots and bacteria and allowing fluid-filled cavities to form, into which fibroblasts and endothelial cells can grow.

Magnesium A predominant intracellular anion used in energy metabolism and protein synthesis. Also involved in muscular activity and energy production.

Mandatory Constituting a demand (often legal).

Mast cell Type of white blood cell.

Mastectomy Surgical removal of one or both breasts, partially or completely.

MCL1 Refers to modified chest lead 1 (i.e. V1).

Medic alert bracelet An identification tag worn as a bracelet, neck chain, or on the clothing bearing a message that the wearer has an important medical condition that might require immediate attention. Some people prefer to carry it as a wallet card.

Medicines management A system of processes and behaviours that determines how medicines are used by the NHS and patients, enabling the best possible use of medicines.

Medulla The medulla lies in the lower part of the brainstem, above the spinal cord, below the pons, and anterior to the cerebellum. It is responsible for autonomic bodily functions: breathing, blood pressure, heart rate, and vomiting.

Meningitis Infection of the meninges, the membranes that cover the brain and spinal cord. It can be caused by bacteria or viruses.

Metabolic instability An acute dysfunction of metabolic processes. This may be related to acid–base imbalance or an imbalance between catabolism and anabolism as seen in patients with ongoing physiological stress.

Microorganism A living organism that is too small to be seen by the human eye, e.g. bacteria.

Micturition Passing urine.

Midbrain The upper part of the brainstem involved in relaying motor and sensory information to the cerebral cortex. Has a special function in filtering unwanted motor information. Lesions here can cause Parkinsonism.

Mid upper arm circumference The circumference of the left upper arm, measured at the midpoint between the tip of the shoulder and the tip of the elbow.

Monitored dosage system (MDS) Medication packed into blister packs or compliance aids such as 'dosette' boxes. Medication is placed into separate compartments for different times of day and days of the week. The MDS allows patients and carers to know what medication should be taken and when, and whether it has been taken.

Monocyte A leukocyte that is responsible for phagocytosis (ingestion) of foreign substances in the body.

Monophonic wheeze Single pitch and tonal quality heard over an isolated area.

Mucocutaneous Of, or pertaining to, the mucous membrane and the skin.

Mucus A white, slimy lubricant produced by the large bowel.

Multi-infarct dementia A common cause of dementia. Individuals with cerebrovascular atherosclerosis (stroke disease) are susceptible to numerous and repetitive small strokes that lead to atrophy and damage to the cortex.

Myocardium Heart muscle.

Nasopharyngeal airway A curved, rigid tubing that is passed via the nose into the patient's upper airway for the purposes of ventilation and suctioning.

Necrosis/Necrotic The local death of tissue. This tissue is often black/brown in colour and leathery in texture.

Nephrotic syndrome Disorder characterized by proteinuria (>3.5 g/day), hypoalbuminaemia, and oedema, occurring when the kidneys have been damaged, resulting in leakage of protein into the urine. Do not confuse with nephritic syndrome.

Neuropathic pain Results from a malfunction of the peripheral or central nervous system. It is often called nerve pain.

Neutrophils Remove and destroy bacteria and cellular debris by the actions of phagocytosis and proteolysis.

Nociceptive pain Caused by the activation of nerve receptors by a noxious stimulus. This may be caused by excessive heat, cold, stretching, or chemical irritation. This form of pain is sometimes termed inflammatory pain.

Nocturnal micturition Passing of urine during the night.

Normal flora Microorganisms that live in or on the body without causing disease.

Nosocomial infection Health care-acquired infection.

Nutrition The process of taking in and assimilating nutrients.

Nutritional support Any method of giving nutrients that encourages an optimal nutritional status.

Obturator A dead-end luer lock cap used to protect against bleeding out of or contamination entry into a line.

Oedema/Oedematous An abnormal and excessive accumulation of fluid within body tissues or body cavities, causing generalized or local swelling. An abnormal swelling in a plant caused by an accumulation of water in the tissues.

Oesophageal reflux The retrograde entry of stomach contents into the oesophagus. This is usually related to a failure of the gastro-oesophageal valve or as a result of delayed gastric emptying. Burning and inflammation can occur, with severe indigestion symptoms.

Open-angle glaucoma (Also called chronic glaucoma) is the most common type of glaucoma. This develops slowly so that any damage to the nerve and loss of sight is gradual.

Orogastric tube A tube inserted through the mouth into the stomach via the oesophagus. This may be inserted to aid drainage of gastric contents or to facilitate early enteral nutrition in specific patients.

Oropharyngeal (Guedel) airway A curved, rigid tube that is inserted into the patient's mouth to depress the tongue and allow passage of air into the patient's upper airway for the purposes of ventilation and suctioning.

Orthopnoea Shortness of breath on lying down.

Oscillometry The measure of a back and forth motion.

Oxygen saturation The measure of the amount of oxygen carried in the blood (SaO_2) on the haemoglobin molecules.

Oxyhaemoglobin Oxygen bound to haemoglobin.

Oxyhaemoglobin dissociation curve Oxygen saturation increases and decreases according to partial oxygen pressures in the blood, and this is described by an oxygen–haemoglobin dissociation curve. Oxygen will be nearly 100% at partial oxygen pressures of >10 kPa.

Palliative To soothe or relieve.

Pallor Pale skin colour.

Palpation/Palpating Examination by touch.

Palpebral conjunctiva Area around the eyelid.

Pancreatitis Acute or chronic inflammation of the pancreas.

Paralytic ileus A decrease in or absence of intestinal peristalsis.

Parenteral nutrition The provision of total or supplemental nutritional support directly into the bloodstream.

Paroxysmal nocturnal dyspnoea Sudden breathlessness that occurs at night when lying down.

Partial pressure of arterial oxygen The amount of oxygen carried by haemoglobin at any time relates to the partial pressure of oxygen to which the haemoglobin is exposed. In the lungs this is normally high and so oxygen binds easily to haemoglobin. However, this is not the case elsewhere in the body, and can change in disease states.

Passive (open) wound drainage The wound drain provides a sinus tract along which drainage escapes into a dressing or drainage bag.

Pathogenic Capacity to cause disease.

Pathological Relating to disease or arising from disease.

Pathophysiology Altered physiological processes associated with disease or injury.

Patient identifiable information Any information that may be used to identify a patient directly or indirectly. E.g. patient's name, post code, date of birth, video or audio data, NHS number, also rare diseases, drug treatments, or statistical analyses which have very small numbers within a small population.

Patient's own drugs (PODs) Any medication that a patient brings in to hospital with them. Can be prescribed, over-the-counter, alternative, or herbal medicines.

Percussion A physical examination technique in which various areas of the body (the chest, back, and abdomen) are tapped to determine by resonance the condition of internal organs.

Percutaneous Any medical technique that accesses underlying tissues by skin puncture rather than an 'open' approach.

Peri-arrest At the time of cardiac arrest.

Peridontal disease Chronic destruction of gums.

Peripheral Of or on the boundary of a surface or area (e.g., of an organ or the body).

Peripheral cyanosis Blue tint in fingers or extremities, due to inadequate circulation.

Peripheral vascular disease (PVD) Diseases of blood vessels outside the heart and brain. The most common cause is atherosclerosis or in some cases blood clots that lodge in the arteries and restrict blood flow.

Peripheral vasoconstriction Narrowing of blood vessels in the extremities of the body.

Peristalsis Wave-like muscular contractions of the alimentary tract.

Peristomal Pertaining to the area of skin surrounding a stoma.

Peritoneal dialysis Form of dialysis that uses the peritoneal membrane and specifically manufactured fluid to dialyse the patient.

Peritoneum A serous membrane that consists of an outer layer (parietal peritoneum) and an inner layer (visceral peritoneum). The parietal peritoneum is attached to the abdominal wall and the visceral peritoneum is wrapped around the internal organs that are located inside the abdominal cavity. The peritoneal cavity is a space between these two layers.

Peritonitis Inflammation of the peritoneum, which can be localized or generalized. This can be due to an infective or non-infective process and usually represents a surgical emergency. Symptoms are acute onset abdominal pain, tenderness, and guarding.

Petechiae Tiny flat, red, or purplish spots on skin or mucous membranes as result of bleeding capillaries.

pH The acidity or alkalinity of a solution; the hydrogen ion concentration reflected in a negative logarithmic scale.

Phagocyte White blood cells that can degrade infectious organisms by phagocytosis.

Pharmacokinetics The body's reaction to drugs, including their absorption, metabolism, and elimination.

Phlebitis Inflammation of the wall of a vein.

Phlebostatic axis The external reference point for the right atrium when the patient is supine. It is located in the fourth intercostal space on an intersection with the midaxillary line.

Phlegmasia cerulea dolens An uncommon severe form of deep venous thrombosis that results from extensive thrombotic occlusion of the major and collateral veins of an extremity.

Phosphate A salt of phosphorus. A component of nucleic acids and adenosine triphosphate. Predominantly found in the extracellular capacity.

Plasma volume expanders (PVEs) Any liquid used to replace blood plasma, usually a saline solution, often with serum albumins, dextrans, or other preparations. These substances do not enhance the oxygen-carrying capacity of blood, but merely replace the volume.

Platelets Platelets are fragments of megakaryocyte cells. They are active agents of inflammation and blood clot formation when blood vessel trauma occurs.

Pleural effusion An abnormal collection of fluid between the thin layers of tissue (pleura) lining the lung and the wall of the chest cavity.

Pleural rub Sound similar to creaking leather or walking on fresh snow, caused primarily by inflammation of pleural membranes.

Pleura/Pleural space Two membranes surrounding the lungs. The outer membrane is attached to the wall of the chest (the parietal pleura); the inner membrane is attached to the lung and other visceral tissues (the visceral pleura). Between the two membranes there is a small gap called the pleural cavity or pleural space.

Plexus A junction of a network of vessels or nerves.

Pneumothorax Air leakage into the space between the chest wall and the outer tissues of the lungs resulting in a collapse of the lung on the affected side. It can occur as a result of disease or injury, or spontaneously. Also known as a collapsed lung.

Polycythaemia Abnormal increase in the number of red blood cells due to excess production.

Polypharmacy Multiple drug therapies, more than four medicines.

Polyphonic wheeze Multiple pitches and tones heard over a variable area of lung, indicative of widespread bronchospasm.

Pons (pontine) An area of the brainstem responsible for relaying sensory information to the cerebellum and cerebrum. It may also have a role in dreaming. Lesions here can be catastrophic and are associated with bilateral constricted pupils.

Post-mortem Literally 'following death' – usually means the medical examination of the body in order to establish cause of death.

Postprandial After eating a meal

Postural hypotension (Usually rapid) fall in blood pressure when in an upright or standing position.

Precordial Relating to the area over the heart and lower chest.

Preload The degree of tension placed on the resting myocardial fibres at end-diastole just before the onset of systole (contraction). The main factor influencing preload is the venous return to the heart; end-diastolic blood volume.

Preprandial Before eating a meal.

Presbyopia A natural part of the ageing process of the eye. The elasticity of the lens is reduced, causing light to be focused behind the retina. This can lead to blurring and an inability to focus on objects close to the eye.

Primary intention (healing by) Wound edges are brought together and then held in place by mechanical means, e.g. sutures, clips, etc.

Prolapse The falling, sinking, or sliding of an organ from its normal position or location in the body, such as a prolapsed uterus.

Propellant An inert substance used to transport a drug out of a device at high pressure ready for inhalation.

Prophylaxis Preventative.

Proptosis Forward projection or displacement of the eyeball.

Protease Enzyme that breaks down protein.

Protective wipes Applied to clean, dry peristomal skin to provide a film on the skin to act as a barrier to any leakage from a stoma.

Proteolytic Breaking down proteins.

Pruritis Itching.

Psoriasis A common, chronic skin disorder characterized by circumscribed red patches covered by thick, dry, silvery, adherent scales that are the result of excessive development of epithelial cells.

Public interest Exceptional circumstances that justify overruling the right of an individual to confidentiality in order to serve a broader societal interest. Decisions about the public interest are complex and must take account of both the potential harm that disclosure may cause and the interest of society in the continued provision of confidential health services.

Pulmonary artery Blood vessel that leads from the right ventricle to the arteries of the pulmonary circulation.

Pulmonary aspiration Accidental inhalation of secretions, fluid, or foreign substances into the trachea, bronchus, or lungs.

Pulmonary embolism This occurs when a blood clot forms in the lungs (having moved from a site of formation elsewhere) and blocks the lungs' arterial blood supply. It can cause severe collapse, even death, and can be treated with anticoagulants.

Pulmonary oedema The accumulation of fluid in the lungs leading to impaired gas exchange, potentially causing respiratory failure.

Pulse The expansion and recoil of the artery as a result of contractions of the left ventricle.

Pulse deficit The difference between the apical rate and the pulse rate is the 'pulse deficit'; this deficit is greater when the ventricular rate is high.

Pulse pressure The pressure difference between the systolic and diastolic blood pressure (SBP − DBP = PP).

Purkinje fibres Part of the electrical system in the heart; the terminal fibres that innervate the ventricles.

Purulent Relating to, containing, or consisting of pus.

Purulent wound exudate Thick, yellowish or green wound drainage; contains microorganisms.

QRS Part of the P-QRS-T configuration of the cardiac electrical cycle.

RA Refers to 'right arm' on ECG connectors and cables. However, placement is normally on the right shoulder or below the right clavicle.

Radio-opacity From radio-opaque, not transparent to X-ray.

Raised intracranial pressure (ICP) Increasing pressure in the skull due to brain swelling or brain haemorrhage. Pressure leads to poor blood supply and increased risk of ischaemic stroke. At its most severe, the brain starts to herniate out of the skull through its foramina towards the spinal canal leading to death

Raynaud's phenomenon A disorder that affects the blood vessels in the fingers, toes, ears, and nose. Characterized by episodic spasms, called vasospastic attacks, which cause the small blood vessels to constrict and change colour, leading to cold and painful extremities.

Rectal prolapse Partial protrusion of the rectum through the anus.

Rectus abdominus sheath One of a pair of anterolateral muscles of the abdomen, extending the whole length of the ventral aspect of the abdomen.

Red eye A non-specific term to describe an eye that appears red due to illness or injury.

Regurgitation (gastric) Passive backward flow of stomach contents into the oesophagus and mouth.

Renal replacement therapy A term used to encompass haemodialysis and haemofiltration, treatments that take over the function of the kidneys in renal failure.

Renal transplantation Transplant of a donor kidney into a patient with chronic kidney disease.

Reticular formation A poorly defined area of the brainstem that appears to control physical behaviours such as sleep and alertness. It contains the ascending reticular activating system (ARAS), an area important in maintaining conscious level.

Retraction Pulling back.

Reversibility (of asthma) The extent to which symptoms of asthma can be reduced by the use of bronchodilator medications (which work to open up the airways) and by steroid medications (which work to reduce the airways' inflammation).

Rigor A shaking that occurs during a high fever.

Rigor mortis Latin phrase meaning muscle stiffening following death.

RL Refers to 'right leg' on ECG connectors and cables. However, placement is normally the right lower thorax/hip.

Rod A plastic rod/bridge used in the formation of a loop colostomy that keeps the loop of bowel in place and prevents it from retracting into the abdomen. The rod can be removed 7–10 days after surgery.

Sanguinous wound exudate Blood-stained wound drainage.

Sarcoidosis A disease affecting the immune system characterised by non-caseating granulomas. Lymph nodes and any organs can be affected but pulmonary involvement is the most common presentation.

Sclerosed Hardened, or indurated, by sclerosis.

Secondary intention (healing by) The wound is left open and heals by the process of granulation and epithelialization.

Sedatives Drugs that depress the central nervous system resulting in drowsiness, amnesia, and reduced anxiety. Examples are opiates and benzodiazepines.

Self-administration of medication While in hospital, patients administer their own medication under the supervision of nursing staff. Also known as **self-medication**.

Semi-lunar valves Heart valves shaped like a half-moon located between the aorta and the left ventricle (aortic valve) and between the pulmonary artery and the right ventricle (pulmonary valve).

Senile macular degeneration When the central area of the retina starts to break up or disintegrate, often with some bleeding at the back of the eyes. The central visual field is disturbed but peripheral vision remains unaffected.

Sepsis A systemic inflammatory response caused by infection in the circulation.

Serosanguinous wound exudate Thin/watery and pink/red wound drainage. Contains plasma and a few red blood cells.

Serous wound exudate Clear or slightly yellow wound drainage; contains plasma and water.

Shock Failure of the circulatory system to maintain adequate perfusion of the vital organs and tissues. Causes are many and varied; it is commonly categorized as hypovolaemic, septic, cardiogenic, or distributive.

Shunting The process of red blood cells passing through the pulmonary circulation and not being reoxygenated, resulting in hypoxia.

Side effect Undesirable secondary effect of a drug.

Sinoatrial node Group of modified cardiac cells located in the right atrium generating an electrical impulse (pacemaker) for the cardiac cycle.

Sinus rhythm Cardiac conduction generated from the sinoatrial node.

Skin abrasion An injury where the skin is scraped off against a rough surface usually only taking off the surface layer of skin, leaving a raw, tender area underneath.

Skin fold thickness A measurement using subcutaneous fat to estimate an individual's body fat.

Skin protective wafers Sheet or ring applied around a stoma to improve the seal if leakage problems occur.

Skin turgor Ability of the skin to change shape and return to normal (elasticity).

Slough Dead tissue (verb: to shed).

Sphygmomanometer Equipment used to measure blood pressure.

Spirometry Detects and measures airway obstruction by measuring forced expiratory volume in 1 second and forced vital capacity.

Splenomegaly Enlargement of spleen caused by infection, lymphoma, and leukaemia.

Stomatitis Inflammation of the mouth.

Stridor Harsh, high-pitched sound heard during inspiration; indicates laryngeal/tracheal obstruction.

Stroke volume (SV) The volume of blood ejected by each contraction of the ventricle. It is regulated by preload, contractility, and afterload. The normal SV for an adult is 70 millilitres (ml) per beat.

Subacute endocarditis Inflammation of the inner lining of the heart and valves caused by infection.

Subconjunctival haemorrhage One cause of a red eye: caused by a small bleed behind the conjunctiva. It can look alarming, but it usually causes no symptoms and is harmless.

Subcutaneous Beneath the skin.

Subluxation The dislocation of a joint. Usually the unseating of a bone from its position in the joint, frequently seen in the shoulder.

Subungual Under a nail.

Sulci (Latin: 'furrows') Depressions or fissures in the surface of the brain.

Supine Laying flat on the back.

Supraorbital ridge The bony area above the eye where the eyebrow lies. Pressure here results in pressure on the supraorbital nerve, which is intensely painful.

Synchronized cardioversion Synchronized defibrillation of the heart to restore a normal rhythm with output.

Syncope Transient loss of consciousness.

Systemic action Medication affecting a system of the body, distinct from having a local effect.

Systemic vascular resistance (SVR) Resistance to blood flow in the systemic circulation, which depends on the viscosity of blood, length of vessels, and radius of vessels.

Systole The phase of the cardiac cycle when the heart muscles of either the atria or ventricles are contracted.

Systolic blood pressure (SBP) The pressure exerted by the blood flow on the blood vessels when the ventricles contract.

Tachycardia Heart rate of 100 beats per minute or above.

Tachypnoea Fast respiratory rate (above 30 breaths per minute).

Telemetric/Telemetry Method for remote monitoring of patients, for example ECG.

Thomboembolism Blockage of a blood vessel by a clot.

Thrombophlebitis Inflammation of a vein associated with/as a result of clot formation.

Thrombosed Affected with or obstructed by a clot of coagulated blood.

Trace elements Elements present in very small amounts in the body including iron, chromium, cobalt, copper, iodine, manganese, selenium, zinc.

Tracheal stenosis Damage to the trachea caused by trauma or intubation, which can cause the trachea to be narrowed.

Traction Literally means steady pulling. It is used to align fractures that are too difficult to align with a plaster cast.

Transcutaneous electrical nerve electrical nerve stimulation (TENS) A self-contained portable system that involves the passage of an electrical current between two self-adhesive electrodes placed on the skin either side of a painful area or sensory nerve supplying the area of pain.

Transduced Conversion of pressure readings into a waveform.

Transurethral resection of the prostate (TURP) Surgery carried out via the urethra to remove prostatic tissue that may be obstructing the urinary tract.

Tunnelled line An intravenous line that has been tunnelled under the subcutaneous layer prior to vein entry.

Type IV contact dermatitis Inflammation and itching of the skin. A type IV (or delayed) reaction involves T cells and tends to be an allergy to minute quantities of a substance.

Ultrasound An ultrasound produces a 3D (three dimensional) image by echo analysis, which provides the practitioner with a view of the vein under the skin.

Universal donor A person whose type O Rh– negative blood may be safely transfused into people with other blood types.

Universal recipient A person who has blood type AB positive and is therefore able to receive blood from any other group in the ABO system.

Urea The product of protein metabolism, formed in the liver and excreted by the kidneys.

Ureterostomy Surgical creation of an opening from a ureter to the surface of the body or into another outlet, such as the rectum.

Urethral stricture Narrowing within the urethra causing difficulty passing urine; a form of bladder outflow obstruction.

Urostomy Surgical creation of an external opening into the ureter, which usually involves bringing the ureter to the skin surface so that urine can drain into an appliance.

Urticaria Raised red skin welts.

Validity In statistics a valid measure is one that is measuring what it is supposed to measure. Validity implies reliability (accuracy).

Vasoconstriction A narrowing of the lumen of blood vessels.

Vasovagal (syncope) Stimulation of the vagus nerve often following pain, trauma, or fright; ultimately causing cerebral ischemia and loss of consciousness. Also known as vasodepressor syncope.

Veins Carry de-oxygenated blood at low pressures from the body back to the heart. Superficial veins lie near to the body's surface. Deep veins, which are used for central venous catheters, lie close to arteries.

Venospasm Spasm (contraction) of a vein.

Ventricular Pertaining to the lower chambers of the heart.

Verification of death Can be provided by a registered medical practitioner or a Registered Nurse who has undergone specialist training.

Vesicant A substance that causes blisters.

Vocal cord paralysis Weakness of one or both of the vocal cords. It may decrease the effectiveness of coughing, swallowing, and sneezing.

Vocal resonance Sound of speech transmitted through the chest wall to a stethoscope.

VQ scan A nuclear scan to look at both airflow (ventilation) and blood flow (perfusion) in the lungs.

Wheeze High or low-pitched continuous musical tone produced by airflow vibrating compressed or narrowed airways.

White cell count The number of white blood cells (leucocytes) in the blood, essential for immune response.

White-coat hypertension High blood pressure as a result of the anxiety experienced by patients when consulting a health care worker.

Work of breathing The amount of energy expenditure used to achieve adequate gaseous exchange between atmospheric air and the blood.

Wound closure The bringing together of wound edges using fixation appropriate to the location and type of wound.

Wound drainage Steps taken to prevent fluid accumulating in the wound bed.

Xanthomata Yellowish deposits of lipids around eyes.

Xerostomia Dryness of the mouth.

Xiphoid process An extension to the lower part of the sternum.

Z-track injection A method of injecting medication into a large muscle. It seals the medication deeply within the muscle and allows no exit path back into the subcutaneous tissue and skin.

Index